Progress in
Cancer Research and Therapy
Volume 5

CANCER INVASION AND METASTASIS: BIOLOGIC MECHANISMS AND THERAPY

Progress in
Cancer Research and Therapy

Progress in
Cancer Research and Therapy
Volume 5

Cancer Invasion and Metastasis: Biologic Mechanisms and Therapy

Edited by

Stacey B. Day, M.D.,
Ph.D., D.Sc.
Member and Professor
Sloan-Kettering Institute for
Cancer Research and Therapy
New York, New York

W. P. Laird Myers, M.D.
Chairman, Department of Medicine
Memorial Sloan-Kettering Cancer
Center
New York, New York

Philip Stansly, Ph.D.
National Cancer Institute
National Institutes of Health
Bethesda, Maryland

Silvio Garattini, M.D.
Director
Istituto di Ricerche Farmacolo-
giche "Mario Negri"
Milan, Italy

Martin G. Lewis, M.D., M.R.C.(Path.)
Director, Cancer Unit
McGill University
Montreal, Quebec, Canada

Raven Press ■ New York

Raven Press, 1140 Avenue of the Americas, New York, New York 10036

Main entry under title:

Cancer invasion and metastasis.

   (Progress in cancer research and therapy; v. 5)
   Includes bibliographical references and index.
   1. Metastasis. 2. Cancer. I. Day, Stacey B.
II. Series. [DNLM: 1. Neoplasm metastasis.
2. Neoplasm metastasis--Therapy. W1 PR667M
v. 5 / QZ200 C21525]
RC269.C35   616.9'94'07   77-83695
ISBN 0-89004-184-9

Foreword
Cancer Metastases: The Scientific Assault
on a Fearsome Process

Man loathes that which he fears. We all fear and hate cancer more than any other disease. Indeed, when asked what they fear the most, 65% of Americans say cancer. They do not say death, war, atomic destruction, economic catastrophy, vascular disease, old age, or even environmental abuse. They now say cancer. The reason for this fear is that cancer not only kills but kills in such a destructive and often demeaning way. It is such a frequent disease that no one can escape the threat of its ravages. Otherwise rewarding lives are often robbed of meaning by an illness that can destroy the brain and mind, produce intolerable pain (e.g., by invading the bones), invade and destroy the liver or lungs, and suppress the bone marrow, thus interfering with a vital defense against infection and the ability to coagulate the blood. The protean manifestations of cancer that stem from damage to almost every organ or tissue derive from the fact that cancer is invasive and can spread to distant organs by metastasis.

Cancer would not be such an awful disease were it possible to prevent or control its metastatic spread. Consequently, the understanding of metastases and development of means to treat, control, and prevent these distant extensions lie at the very heart of our efforts to conquer cancer. Were it possible to treat or prevent metastases, surgery, radiation, and chemotherapy might be more effective.

A hope deriving from studies of osteogenic sarcoma and breast cancer, that adjuvant chemotherapy can effectively treat very early metastases, currently generates much excitement in the clinical field. This hope also lies behind intensive efforts to apply immunotherapy even before the scientific basis for this pursuit has been developed for human cancer. Yet, ability to prevent metastases or even to treat early metastases after they have occurred could make conventional modalities of cancer therapy much more telling.

Although propensity to metastasize often reflects the size of the primary tumor, too often metastases are not predictable. In some forms of cancer, they notoriously occur early, even before the primary cancer can be detected. Examples of such treacherous cancers are oat cell carcinoma of the lung and opthalmic malignant melanoma. These forms of cancer and many others can represent disseminated disease when first encountered clinically. In almost all forms of human cancer, however, present difficulty in predicting when disease is localized or disseminated makes approaches to the application of adjuvant chemotherapy statistical and consequently halting and uncertain.

A recent surge of inquiry represented by the chapters in the present volume reveals promise that the biological revolution is beginning to address the fascinating challenge of metastatic neoplastic disease. Progress made in a very short time seems promising. As is to be expected, much of the new information from these analyses contains surprises and there is much to encourage hot pursuit.

Among the important observations on the nature of metastases are the following: (1) cancer cells that adhere to one another firmly are more likely to be successful as metastases than those not so adherent; (2) immunological processes directed against tumor can favor the metastatic event; (3) the propensity for cancer cells to metastasize is not stochastic but clearly reflects the operation of epigenetic control; (4) successful metastases of cancers seem to be dependent on relations of the surface chemistry of the cancer cells to one another, and to vessel walls. The biochemical characteristics of the cancer cells thus far elucidated show features reminiscent of embryonic cells which must move about the embryo and often invade, but which do so in this phase of development under precise control. Indeed, the very chemistry of the surface glycolipids and glycoproteins involved as determinants or at least intimate concomitants of the metastatic process seems to share features involved in surface recognition that are fundamental to many biological phenomena. These include such diverse processes as feeding of amoeba, sexual interactions of bacteria or paramecia, aggregation of unicellular organisms, aggregations of embryonic cells in certain stages of development, ecotaxis of lymphoid cells, and even the fertilization of the egg.

It is clear from the present volume that fundamental chemical characteristics of metastatic cells, growth requirements of the metastatic cells, the act of metastasis and pharmacological influences on this biological process can now be systematically studied. Further, these studies are being carried out in a framework that will sooner or later be translatable into effective prophylaxis or therapy.

Indeed, splendid model systems for studying metastases of a wide variety of tumors have been introduced and the influences of pharmacological agents on the metastatic process are rapidly being catalogued. Ingenious new approaches are being developed and tested in these model systems, and numerous influences that facilitate or retard metastases have already been defined.

It would seem that the first toddling steps in developing a biochemistry, molecular biology, and pharmacology that will yield an understanding to prediction and control of metastases have already been taken. These first steps will contribute much needed understanding, and many new approaches to this most feared characteristic of cancer will be the consequence.

One can be certain that if the focus of study is maintained on fundamental explorations of the metastatic cells and the metastatic process, these toddling steps will strengthen into a firm walk and ultimately break into a run. These fundamental investigations, of course, must include constant comparison of the metastatic cancer cells with normal, fully differentiated cells, embryonic cells, normal lymphoid cells, as well as the primary cancer cells.

Analysis, in chemical terms, of the nature of the epigenetic controls in certain cancer cells that establish the characteristics essential to metastasize, must also be incisively studied. Vigorous development of this new biology and development of a concomitant pharmacology of metastases by investigations that include efforts to understand cell–cell interaction of normal cells in the basic terms, the travels of lymphocytes, movements and invasions of embryonic cells, and even invasion by placental membranes, will, I believe, yield most rapidly the needed ability to talk to the cells through their surfaces or through their surface-to-nuclear signals that can contribute much toward the inhibition of metastases of cancer.

Robert A. Good, M.D., Ph.D.
President and Director
Sloan-Kettering Institute for Cancer Research
New York

Preface

Notwithstanding the extraordinary increase in experimental resources, and in the wealth of information that is daily becoming available from research on the biology of the cancer cell, the major cause of death from cancer remains the disseminated and uncontrolled growth of tumor cells. Irrespective of conceptual views of the causation of the disease or the therapy recommended for a given patient, death is all too commonly associated with metastases in various organs and at various sites of the human body. Given enough time, almost every malignant neoplasm will spread from its primary site; yet it is precisely the mechanism of this spread associated with the phenomenon of growth in distant locations that is so relatively poorly understood in the biology of cancer diseases. It is precisely in our inability to master the inductive process, to comprehend or define the absolute mechanism(s) of spread, and to limit or alterably eradicate distant new growth spread of cancer that we fail.

In recent years, there has been a move toward an understanding of many regulatory and control mechanisms that occur in presumably physiologically normal as well as in aberrant or cancer cells. Investigative research in molecular and enzyme metabolism, cell regulation, biomembrane control and gene expression, endocrine concepts and transport physiology have opened new vistas for the experimental cell physiologist. The immunologist too has expressed his interest, and in studies on the cell surface there is a growing confidence in the belief that tumor-specific antigens, aided and abetted by genetic control mechanisms, will ultimately surrender to cellular engineering, immunologic manipulation, and immunotherapeutic control. Yet nonetheless patients die. Even though the *cause* of cancer is important, in the clinical case it is the *spread* — the phenomenon of metastasis — that is of much more immediate concern in the human situation.

I believe it was with this sensitivity, fortified by a perspective that developmental hypotheses and experimental data are of little consequence without a structured understanding, that so distinguished a group of physicians and scientists met in New York in December 1976. Many investigators present had spent long years devoted to research of biological problems in metastasis control. All were drawn from intellectually multidisciplinary directions, and together, in an interdisciplinary forum, these discussants sought to bridge the gap between scientific knowledge and the patient's needs. One might more easily have negotiated the rapids between scylla and charybdis! Approaches to study and elucidation of the control of metastases in cancer are difficult. The dimensions of the problem are wide,

ix

and the expression of the "variables" as formulated in the minds of different investigators, often from different parts of the world, is rarely constant. Difficulties exist in developing a "universal" model that is reproducible and can reasonably be said to simulate the human disease. Variations and subtleties in biologic interpretation, and the arduous, slow nature of the experimental work, seldom accompanied by éclat or brouhaha, test both patience and probity in the investigators.

With so many apparent hazards, the carefully developed contributions to this text become most important, not only because they represent the work of the first major international gathering of scientific minds on this problem in over 4 years, but also because by force of this interdisciplinary interaction among multidisciplinary talents, it is evident, to this observer at least, that the research on metastasis is no longer a matter of cinderella biology knocking on the door of grant-supporting agencies who allocate funds for cancer research; it has (as it always *should* have merited) now reached wide professional notice. It is reasonably assured that future investigative studies will be more fully and favorably supported, for, in terms of patient needs, few programs are more relevant to the public in terms of direct-assisted research programs, than are enquiries into the biology of metastasis control.

I am confident that the very important contributions in this text will be well received and widely sought. They will, I believe, attest beyond affirmation that the patient's needs in the spread of cancer are problems foremost in some of the most able and critically perceptive minds in the fields of cancer biology today.

Stacey B. Day

Acknowledgments

This volume evolved from an International Interdisciplinary Workshop that met under the sponsorship of Memorial Sloan-Kettering Cancer Center, New York; The Division of Cancer Research Resources and Centers, National Cancer Institute, Bethesda; the Mario Negri Institute for Pharmacological Research, Milan, Italy; and the Mario Negri Foundation, New York.

At a time when financial support is critical and most difficult to enlist, the editors feel it important to acknowledge help from the private sector which made this meeting possible. Full and unstinted acknowledgment is made to the following corporations who gave valued assistance: Adria Laboratories Inc., Burroughs Wellcome Co., Ciba-Geigy Corporation, Hoechst-Roussel Pharmaceuticals Inc., Hoffmann-La Roche Inc., ICI United States Inc., Ives Laboratories Inc., Janssen R & D, Inc., Johnson & Johnson, Eli Lilly and Co., Ortho Pharmaceutical Canada Ltd., Pennwalt Corporation, Riker Laboratories, Inc., Sandoz Pharmaceuticals, E. R. Squibb & Sons.

Contents

Contributors

Peter Alexander
Division of Tumor Immunology
Chester Beatty Research Institute
Belmont, Sutton, Surrey, England

H. A. Atherton
Chemotherapy Department
Imperial Cancer Research Fund
Lincoln's Inn Fields
London, England

Richard S. Bockman
Laboratory of Calcium Metabolism
Memorial Sloan-Kettering Cancer
  Center
New York, New York 10021

Oscar Bodansky
Memorial Sloan-Kettering Cancer
  Center
New York, New York 10021

Tibor Borsos
Laboratory of Immunobiology
National Cancer Institute
National Institutes of Health
Bethesda, Maryland 20014

J. M. Brown
Department of Radiology
Stanford University Medical Center
Stanford, California 94305

Michael Brown
Department of Pathology
Tufts University School of Medicine
Boston, Massachusetts 02111

Gary R. Burleson
Lobund Laboratory
University of Notre Dame
Notre Dame, Indiana 46556

Monica Cairo
Department of Cancer Chemotherapy
  and Immunology
Istituto di Ricerche Farmacologiche
  "Mario Negri"
Milan, Italy

Walter P. Carney
Department of Microbiology
Jefferson Medical College
Thomas Jefferson University
Philadelphia, Pennsylvania 19107

W. J. Chauvin
Department of Pathology
University of Western Ontario
London, Ontario, Canada

J. Norris Childs
Chester Beatty Research Institute
Royal Cancer Hospital
Belmont, Sutton, Surrey, England

Amiel Cooper
Department of Pathology
Tufts University School of Medicine
Boston, Massachusetts 02111

Antonio L. Cubilla
Department of Pathology
Memorial Sloan-Kettering Cancer
  Center
New York, New York 10021

J. N. P. Davies
Albany Medical College
Albany, New York 12208

Stacey B. Day
Sloan-Kettering Institute for Cancer
  Research
New York, New York 10021

Charles DeLisi
Laboratory of Theoretical Biology
National Cancer Institute
National Institutes of Health
Bethesda, Maryland 20014

Maria Benedetta Donati
Laboratory for Hemostasis and
  Thrombosis Research
Istituto di Ricerche Farmacologiche
  "Mario Negri"
Milan, Italy

Pelham Douglas
Ludwig Institute for Cancer Research
Lausanne Branch
and
Department of Radiotherapy
Cantonal University Hospital
Lausanne, Switzerland

M. Dowsett
Department of Medicine
Marsden Hospital
Surrey, England

D. M. Easty
Department of Medicine
Marsden Hospital
Surrey, England

G. C. Easty
Department of Medicine
Marsden Hospital
Surrey, England

Isaiah J. Fidler
Basic Research Program
NCI Frederick Cancer Research
  Center
Frederick, Maryland 21701

Patrick J. Fitzgerald
Department of Pathology
Memorial Sloan-Kettering Cancer
  Center
New York, New York 10021

Judah Folkman
Children's Hospital Medical Center
Harvard Medical School
Boston, Massachusetts 02115

Giovanni de Gaetano
Laboratory for Hemostasis and
  Thrombosis Research
Istituto di Ricerche Farmacologiche
  "Mario Negri"
Milan, Italy

Silvio Garattini
Laboratory for Hemostasis and
  Thrombosis Research
Istituto di Ricerche Farmacologiche
  "Mario Negri"
Milan, Italy

Douglas M. Gersten
Basic Research Program
NCI Frederick Cancer Research
  Center
Frederick, Maryland 21701

Dorothy Glaves
Department of Experimental
  Pathology
Roswell Park Memorial Institute
Buffalo, New York 14263

Lester T. Goldstein
Department of Microbiology
Jefferson Medical College
Thomas Jefferson University
Philadelphia, Pennsylvania 19107

K. Hellman
Chemotherapy Department
Imperial Cancer Research Fund
Lincoln's Inn Fields
London, England

Yuhji Higuchi
Third Department of Internal
  Medicine
Tokushima University School of
  Medicine
Tokushima, Japan

J. P. Holmquist
Southern Research Institute
Birmingham, Alabama 35205

James T. Hunter
Laboratory of Immunobiology
National Cancer Institute
National Institutes of Health
Bethesda, Maryland 20014

Harry L. Ioachim
Department of Pathology
Lenox Hill Hospital
New York, New York 10021
and
Department of Pathology
College of Physicians and Surgeons
Columbia University
New York, New York 10032

S. E. James
Chemotherapy Department
Imperial Cancer Research Fund
Lincoln's Inn Fields
London, England

L. M. Jerry
McGill University Cancer Research
Unit
Montreal, Quebec, Canada

Steven E. Keller
Department of Pathology
Lenox Hill Hospital
New York, New York 10021
and
Department of Pathology
College of Physicians and Surgeons
Columbia University
New York, New York 10032

Alfred S. Ketcham
Division of Oncology
Department of Surgery
University of Miami School of
Medicine
Miami, Florida 33152

Jerome Kleinerman
Department of Pathology Research
St. Luke's Hospital
Cleveland, Ohio 44104

Tomowo Kobayashi
Cancer Chemotherapy Center
Japanese Foundation for Cancer
Research
Tokyo, Japan

L. Kopelovich
Cornell University Graduate School
of Medical Sciences
Memorial Sloan-Kettering Cancer
Center
New York, New York 10021

Irwin H. Krakoff
Vermont Regional Cancer Center
University of Vermont
Burlington, Vermont 05401

W. P. Laird Myers
Memorial Sloan-Kettering Cancer
Center
New York, New York 10021

Philip Levine
Memorial Sloan-Kettering Cancer
Center
New York, New York 10021
and
Ortho Research Foundation
Raritan, New Jersey 08869

Martin G. Lewis
Cancer Unit
McGill University
Montreal, Quebec, Canada

Lance A. Liotta
National Cancer Institute
National Institutes of Health
Bethesda, Maryland 20014

Phyllis H. Luckert
Lobund Laboratory
University of Notre Dame
Notre Dame, Indiana 46556

Preston A. Marx
Department of Microbiology
Jefferson Medical College
Thomas Jefferson University
Philadelphia, Pennsylvania 19107

Kathryn Mason
Section of Experimental
Radiotherapy
The University of Texas System
Cancer Center
M. D. Anderson Hospital and Tumor
Institute
Houston, Texas 77030

Douglas Miller
Department of Pathology
Tufts University School of Medicine
Boston, Massachusetts 02111

Giovanni Mistrello
Department of Cancer Chemotherapy
and Immunology
Istituto di Ricerche Farmacologiche
"Mario Negri"
Milan, Italy

Maria Luisa Moras
Department of Cancer Chemotherapy
and Immunology
Istituto di Ricerche Farmacologiche
"Mario Negri"
Milan, Italy

Susan Morgello
Department of Pathology
Tufts University School of Medicine
Boston, Massachusetts 02111

Luciana Mussoni
Laboratory for Hemostasis and
Thrombosis Research
Istituto di Ricerche Farmacologiche
"Mario Negri"
Milan, Italy

A. M. Neville
Department of Medicine
Royal Marsden Hospital
Surrey, England

Garth L. Nicolson
Department of Developmental and
Cell Biology
University of California
Irvine, California 92717

Sarkis H. Ohanian
Laboratory of Immunobiology
National Cancer Institute
National Insitutes of Health
Bethesda, Maryland 20014

Takao Okuda
Laboratory of Immunobiology
National Cancer Institute
National Insitutes of Health
Bethesda, Maryland 20014

Antonia Pearse
Department of Pathology
Lenox Hill Hospital
New York, New York 10021
and
Department of Pathology
College of Physicians and Surgeons
Columbia University
New York, New York 10032

Lester J. Peters
Section of Experimental Radiotherapy
The University of Texas System
Cancer Center
M. D. Anderson Hospital and Tumor
Institute
Houston, Texas 77030

J. Philips
Department of Pathology
University of Western Ontario
London, Ontario, Canada

T. M. Phillips
McGill University Cancer Research
Unit
Montreal, Quebec, Canada

Andreina Poggi
Laboratory for Hemostasis and
Thrombosis Research
Istituto di Ricerche Farmacologiche
"Mario Negri"
Milan, Italy

Morris Pollard
Lobund Laboratory
University of Notre Dame
Notre Dame, Indiana 46556

G. Poste
*Department of Experimental
  Pathology
Roswell Park Memorial Institute
Buffalo, New York 14263*

Trevor J. Powles
*Department of Medicine
Royal Marsden Hospital
Surrey, England*

J. W. Proctor
*Division of Radiation Oncology
Clinical Radiation Therapy Research
  Center
Allegheny General Hospital
Pittsburgh, Pennsylvania 15212*

Herbert J. Rapp
*Laboratory of Immunobiology
National Cancer Institute
National Institutes of Health
Bethesda, Maryland 20014*

Charles W. Riggs
*Information Systems Department
NCI Frederick Cancer Research Cen-
  ter
Frederick, Maryland 21701*

G. Rowden
*McGill University Cancer Research
  Unit
Montreal, Quebec, Canada*

Gerald Saidel
*Department of Biomedical Engineer-
  ing
Case Western Reserve University
Cleveland, Ohio 44106*

A. J. Salsbury
*Cardio-Thoracic Institute
Brompton Hospital
London, England*

A. H. Sanford
*Southern Research Institute
Birmingham, Alabama 35205*

Haruo Sato
*Department of Oncology
Research Institute for Tuberculosis,
  Leprosy, and Cancer
Tohoku University
Sendai, Japan*

Frank M. Schabel, Jr.
*Southern Research Institute
Birmingham, Alabama 35205*

Seymour I. Schlager
*Laboratory of Immunobiology
National Cancer Institute
National Institutes of Health
Bethesda, Maryland 20014*

L. Simpson-Herren
*Southern Research Institute
Birmingham, Alabama 35205*

Federico Spreafico
*Department of Cancer Chemotherapy
  and Immunology
Istituto di Ricerche Farmacologiche
  "Mario Negri"
Milan, Italy*

T. A. Springer
*Southern Research Institute
Birmingham, Alabama 35205*

Jan Stjernswärd
*Ludwig Institute for Cancer Research
Lausanne Branch
and
Department of Radiotherapy
Cantonal University Hospital
Lausanne, Switzerland*

Everett V. Sugarbaker
*Division of Oncology
Department of Surgery
University of Miami School of Medi-
  cine
Miami, Florida 33152*

Maroh Suzuki
*Department of Oncology
Research Institute for Tuberculosis,
  Leprosy, and Cancer*

Tohoku University
Sendai, Japan

Jerry Thornthwaite
Division of Oncology
Department of Surgery
University of Miami School of Medicine
Miami, Florida 33152

Eiro Tsubura
Third Department of Internal Medicine
School of Medicine
Tokushima University
Tokushima, Japan

Shigeru Tsukagoshi
Cancer Chemotherapy Center
Japanese Foundation for Cancer Research
Tokyo, Japan

Kenneth Tyler
Children's Hospital Medical Center
Harvard Medical School
Boston, Massachusetts 02115

Jan Vaage
Department of Cancer Therapy Development
Pondville Hospital
Walpole, Massachusetts 02081

B. A. Warren
Department of Pathology
University of Western Ontario
London, Ontario, Canada

Kent J. Weinhold
Department of Microbiology

Jefferson Medical College
Thomas Jefferson University
Philadelphia, Pennsylvania 19107

I. Bernard Weinstein
College of Physicians and Surgeons
Columbia University
New York, New York 10032

Leonard Weiss
Department of Experimental Pathology
Roswell Park Memorial Institute
Buffalo, New York 14263

E. Frederick Wheelock
Department of Microbiology
Jefferson Medical College
Thomas Jefferson University
Philadelphia, Pennsylvania 19107

Takashi Yamashita
Third Department of Internal Medicine
School of Medicine
Tokushima University
Tokushima, Japan

Eliyahu Yarkoni
Laboratory of Immunobiology
National Cancer Institute
National Institutes of Health
Bethesda, Maryland 20014

John M. Yuhas
Cancer Research and Treatment Center
and
Department of Radiology
University of New Mexico
Albuquerque, New Mexico 87131

Cancer Invasion and Metastasis: Biologic Mechanisms and Therapy, edited by S. B. Day et al. Raven Press, New York © 1977.

On the Nature of Metastasis

Stacey B. Day

Sloan-Kettering Institute for Cancer Research, New York, New York 10021

Peyton Rous said what men think determines what they do. And if it is true that science implies a responsible process of inquiry, then a gathering together of interested and informed investigators should provide opportunity for critical examination of the conditionings and conclusions on which the truth of their knowledge is based. Yet put to the test, few can really justify beliefs, attitudes, and doctrines postulated with respect to the nature of metastasis. And more so, would such beliefs presented be the ones most acceptable to "nonexperts"? And is there reasonably conclusive evidence for or against the opinions preferred or contested? Certainly these are difficult questions to propose. With this in mind, it seemed not unreasonable in developing a cooperative international interdisciplinary working group as met, to provoke them with some of these issues. Such matters as how do we know that a particular argument is valid? What shall we believe from among the multitude of data that we are presented? Why should we believe? These and so many other interpretive questions in a number of fields of thought impinge on critical scientific objectivity and color the background of the metastasis problem.

To these considerations quite obviously must be added others including the intellectual conceptualizations of the biology of cancer as seen by different scientists in different parts of the world. It was of interest to understand whether all participants at the cancer metastasis workshop on which this volume is based would share the same basic views on the nature of metastasis, and whether their views, as experts, could broadly be reconciled with present hypotheses and speculations on the nature of cancer.

To this end an exercise was posed to those members of the workshop who presented a paper at the conference. The form of the exercise requested the answer to three questions with a request that no one should exceed in his answer a discussion greater than three pages in length. The wording of the questions was chosen to reflect essentially variations on the same theme, the hope being to see through the answers in an effort to perceive in what precise way the respondent would handle the question, the better to obtain an idea as to how he was really likely to understand the nature of metastasis in respect of his views as to the nature of cancer. The following were the three questions posed:

1

1. Is a metastasis a cancer cell?
2. If it is a cancer cell, why is it so?
3. If a metastasis is not a cancer cell, why is it not?

No deviousness or invidious prospect was inherent in the exercise. Based on 21 responses, many of which, in general, broadly attempted to build answers around the questions, the response analysis can be tabulated below:

Is a metastasis a cancer cell (21 responses)?

Response	Number
Yes	12
No	5
Variable response (e.g., "A metastasis can be but is not necessarily a cancer cell.")	4

If this exercise resolved nothing else, it made it appear most unlikely that there was real uniform agreement as to what precisely is the nature of metastasis, at least as considered by the distinguished group of contributors assembled at this conference. And most if not all of them had devoted many scholastic years and much effort in research in this same field of study. Moreover, to the mind of this observer, this variation of opinion and disagreement of response is a most important vector. It pointed out, even before the meeting, the need for discussions on this subject, for it was evident in the considerable thought esablished in many of the replies that the manifold and conflicting aspects of the biological nature of metastasis are perplexing, even to those who have addressed the scientific problems involved over a long period of time.

For the patient with cancer, apprehensive of its spread and his own impending death, the problem of metastasis is in many ways *the problem* of cancer: metastasis is at the very heart of the biological problems posed by cancer research.

THE CLASSIC VIEWPOINT

I see no reason why the historical perspective (semantics, if you please) of the term *metastasis* is not a suitable starting point in a discussion on the nature of metastasis. I add here a grace note of qualification, that when I posed the question to my colleagues, I was hoping that some would move from a so-called *cellular* theory to more provocative and contemporary concepts that I would call *molecular* in nature. Included in such discussions would be those aspects surrounding virus pathophysiology of late years, as well as such theories based on molecular genetics (see later) and multistep biology. Of the assembled workshop only Dr. Sugarbaker, so it seemed to me, appeared to take into account possibilities for such "new" horizons, which he evaluated and then set aside in favor of the cellular theory.

The prefix *meta* is of course of Greek origin and designates *with, after, beyond,* often with the sense of "change" (metabolism, metastasis, metacarpal, metamorphosis, metaphysics). Elsewhere in this text Professor Davies has properly pointed out that neither invasion nor metastasis is peculiar to cancer. Both phenomena are biologically exemplified in many other ways including by the developing placenta from which fragments of chorionic tissue can on occasion spread to liver and lungs (J. N. P. Davies, *this volume*). Two or three medical generations ago *metastatic infections* were common, pneumococci in particular often entering the bloodstream from a diseased lung paving the way for pneumococcal inflammation in other tissues—endocarditis, pericarditis, arthritis, meningitis, otitis media, and peritonitis. Metastatic abscesses as complications of bronchopneumonia (metastatic cerebral abscess) and pyemia with lung abscess are familiar to any person who has so much as walked through a museum of pathology.

With respect to tumors and metastasis, in the view of the writer, the observations of Willis (1) are second to none:

> The development of separate secondary growths in parts of the body more or less remote from the primary growth is always clear proof that a tumor is malignant, no matter how slow its proliferation or how perfect its histological differentiation.
> Metastasis depends on the invasion of lymphatics, blood vessels, or serous or other cavities, and *the detachment and transfer of tumor particles*. [Italics added.] Not all kinds of malignant tumors produce metastasis: thus rodent carcinomas of the skin are invasive destructive growths of acknowledged malignancy, which however almost never metastasize; and while most gliomas of the brain are infiltrative and fatal tumors, apart from occasional dissemination in the cerebrospinal spaces, these tumors produce no secondary growths in other parts of the body. Moreover, in those classes of tumors which frequently do metastasize, e.g., carcinomas of the lung, stomach or breast, there occur members which fail to do so, even after a long period of active growth and the attainment of great size.

Reasonable study of the nature of metastasis (and of cancer) should leave room for evidence furnished by skeletal remains that disease, including cancer, is much older than man himself. A specimen of dinosaur (Apatosauros), whose age must be measured in millions of years, was discovered by Professor Roy Moodie in Wyoming with a bony tumor in the caudal vertebra. Tumors occur in all classes of vertebrates, and even in some invertebrates (the honey bee and the oyster). Thus although our knowledge of neoplasia has increased and become refined over the years, many basic features remain characteristic—e.g., the progressive growth of tumors uncoordinated with that of normal tissues and irrespective of the structure and functional requirements of the body, and persistence after cessation of the stimulus that presumably originally provoked the tumor.

Surgeons, who were among the first to face the challenge of metastasis, classically were taught this view (2):

> [A tumor] may be merely *locally malignant,* or more commonly become distributed all about the body following on the invasion of the blood and lymph vessels by the cells of the tumor, which are carried in the stream or rapidly grow along the lumina of the vessels, to distant parts; these scattered cells continue to grow, forming *metastases,* or secondary deposits of the original or primary growth.

Nor has the "metastasis of metastases" been a concept of recent date. Over 25 years ago a fundamental text of pathology (3) clearly stated:

> When the lymphatic glands have themselves become the seat of secondary growths, they in turn constitute new centers of infection, and may thus infect the more distant glands, the immediate adjacent tissues, or the blood stream.

And of metastasis:

> . . . breaking off of malignant cells into (lymph stream), by which they are swept into the regional glands (malignant embolism). Hence the cells develop into secondary tumors or metastases of the same nature as the parent growth.

Throughout these classic descriptions we see underlying comprehension of the spread of tumors, much as we recognize today. Then, as now, it appeared that tumor cells perform no useful function or service in the economy of the body. New growths, then, as now, seemed to be cell colonies in which, contrary to normal practice, the function of work had become subordinate to growth.

MORE CONTEMPORARY CONSIDERATIONS

If these descriptions are standard extant, why does one note an apparent difficulty in reaching agreement in answering or discussing a question posing the nature of metastasis? Part explanation may be an echo of what Peyton Rous (4,5) has called "the intermingling of the facts newly won . . . the 'hows' and the 'whys' as one might call them (and fortunately some are of both sorts)." Rous, too, predicated caution in his words "no one can tell what change or experiment may next reveal as concerns tumor causation."

Yet current studies, if anything, besides being evocative and challenging of intellectual thought, should find a place in the discussion of metastasis, not be hidden from sight. There are numerous experiments exciting in respect to metastases that might be mentioned, especially in the area of the disclosures provided by viruses, reciprocating partnerships between cells and viruses, as well as such matters as concern the exquisite host-within-a-host relationship of virus, cell, and organism. These and many other observations are provocative of thought in the domain of metastasis study. Thus studies such as the comparison of the distribution of tumors produced by intravenous injection of type 12-adenovirus and adeno-12 tumor cells (6) raise concepts for a role for presumably susceptible "target" cells (liver, kidneys, lungs, adrenals) and make appraisal of their relationship with "metastasis" intriguing.

Moreover, as was indicated earlier, broadly "molecular" aspects of the nature of metastasis merit attention. Farber (7) has summarized some of these approaches in the view that in cancer part of the whole perspective may be a combination of host response (immunologic) as well as some differences in the cells themselves. Writing on cancer as a *multistep* process, Farber says:

> Thus, malignant neoplasia is seen as a terminal phase of a process of cellular evolution in which the properties with which we identify cancer, namely the accumulation of cells showing uncontrolled or inadequately controlled *growth, invasion* beyond the normal confines of that cell population, ability to break off and grow at distant sites (*metastasis*) and often obvious *cytologic* abnormalities, especially of the nucleus, are relatively late manifestations. Biologically, these properties are not a tightly coupled package but rather are separate units of aberration.

Bross and Blumenson (8) among others have urged recognition that the overall process of metastasis in humans is a cascade or multistep process. With others, they argue that the start of the process is a clone of cells in a primary and the end is "generalized disease." In their view a given primary metastasizes to one or more "generalizing sites," and these in turn produce the generalized disease.

In new areas, too, would be such analyses as those of Bienengraber, Ernst, and Tessmann (9) who explored possibilities that genetic informational nucleic acid material from the cells of the primary tumor might elicit an analogous transformation of normal cells in addition to its localized process, and in so doing could be responsible for the production of metastases. Preliminary experiments with the injection of isolated DNA from Guerin rat tumors were not successful in promoting this sort of concept.

SOME OBSERVATIONS ON THE NATURE OF METASTASIS BY CONFERENCE RESPONDENTS

The following section presents some of the edited discussions reflecting views of various members of the conference on metastasis. Interpretation of differences is left as an intellectual exercise for the reader. I am grateful to those who have contributed their thoughts to this section, and whose views have added to the interest of the program, which had among its several goals the important one of trying to distinguish between speculations and established knowledge in the matter of the biology and the nature of metastasis. The following are some of the views suggested:

Theses that a Metastasis Is a Cancer Cell

Respondent: Yes, I think it is.

(a) From animal studies, it is apparent that some time after inoculation of tumor cells bioassay of various lymph nodes or organs proves the existence of tumor cells because of killing of host animals by systemic invasion.

(b) If a metastasis is not a cancer cell, therapeutic result after chemotherapy, radiotherapy, or surgery will be much more excellent than the current status.

(c) Suppose a metastasis is not a cancer cell, there must be some host control for the proliferation, but actually this is not so.

Respondent: Indeed, you are asking was Virchow correct when he queried "Metastatic diffusion takes place . . . by means of certain *fluids* and these possess the power of . . . reproduction of a mass of the same nature as the one which originally existed" (from *Cellular Pathology,* 1863).

It is my opinion that many compelling cases of circumstantial evidence refute any theory other than a cellular theory for metastasis. Cancer cells are found in the blood of patients who have grossly established metastases. Additionally, intravenous injection of tumor cells results in metastases in experimental tumor systems. Also, the spread of metastases follows consistent anatomical guidelines either to regional lymphatics or into usually the initial organ draining a given malignancy, further establishing circumstantial evidence. Lastly, the classic clinical pathologic studies in malignant melanoma and breast cancer by W. Sampson Handley show through the microscope the progression of cells into lymphatics and to the first set of regional lymph nodes.

Therefore, in my opinion, although transmission of oncogenic materials remains a theoretic possibility in cancer metastasis, overwhelming circumstantial evidence from experimental and clinical systems favors strongly a cellular nature of metastasis.

Respondent: Yes, a metastasis is definitely a cancer cell. It is in fact the cancer cell "par excellence" because by seeding another area it demonstrates its capacity for autonomous growth, one of the characteristic features of a cancer cell.

Respondent: Cancer metastasis is, simply I think, the cancer cell itself. However, the biological phenomena of cancer metastasis are complicated. Many kinds of factors in host as well as tumor cell influence the process of metastasis. We usually consider this process divided into four steps, as (a) release of tumor cells from the primary tumor, (b) their migratory transport in the blood vessel, (c) lodgment of tumor cell at the target organ, and (d) extravascular growth of these lodged cells. So far as our studies on hematogeneous metastasis are concerned, blood coagulation plays a major role in the initial stage of tumor cell lodgment on capillary endothelium. I am expecting to find an important host factor in the process of metastasis.

For the final purpose of preventing metastasis, we must pay attention to the point of tumor cell release from the primary tumor. Immunoprophylactic studies on this point seem to me very attractive.

Respondent: When we consider the process of metastasis formation, such as liberation of tumor cell(s) from the primary site where that cancer developed, invasion in the tissue, intravasation into blood vessels or lymphatics, transfer of tumor cells, arrival of tumor cells in distant tissues and organs, behavior of those tumor cells in the microcirculation (embolism, transcapillary passage, deformation, adhesion, and lodgment), extravasation of tumor cells, and proliferation of tumor cells to form a metastatic focus, there is no doubt that a metastasis is due to a cancer cell. Of course, it is also true that every cancer cell does not always form a metastatic focus. In other words, it seems reasonable to say that only a few cells could be the seeds which grow to be metastatic foci even when a number of tumor cells had departed from the primary site.

Respondent: A metastasis is a single cell or collection of cells which will grow relentlessly and kill the host if not treated.

Metastases are made up of cancer cells because they are derived from cancer cells shed from a primary tumor. I do not think the word *metastasis* is appropriate to describe malignant cells that have been shed from a primary tumor and remain dormant for long periods if not permanently. A metastasis must be an actively growing entity.

Respondent: I accept the old argument of pathologists that the unequivocal characteristic of malignancy is metastasis; therefore, by definition, I have to agree that a metastasis is a cancer cell or a group of cancer cells. Semantics, however, does little to improve our understanding of a problem, and my belief that a metastasis is a cancer cell relies on the argument that all metastases are cancer cells but not all cancer cells have the capacity to metastasize.

My own bias is that a cancer cell is not a negative thing but is rather a normal cell which performs one of its functions to excess, be this a prolonged life span or an abnormally rapid rate of production. The metastasis is in the same way a positive step beyond the malignant state. This newly acquired function may be related to the ability to see into the hematogenous or lymphatic pathways, the ability to escape immunologic destruction, or the ability to bind to and invade the vascular wall. Whatever the specific characteristic or series of them which allows a cell to develop into a metastasis, it represents an adaptation to selective pressure which might otherwise prevent its survival. In summary, I view the cancer cell as one which has learned to overcome one of the selective pressures in the body, and a metastasis as a cancer cell which has learned to overcome those selective pressures which remain effective against cancer cells.

To me this represents the major problem in addressing metastatic disease, whether one considers cancer cells relative to normal cells or metastatic cells relative to nonmetastatic cells. We are talking about loss of a normal control function. My belief, or perhaps more accurately stated, my hope, is that a cell which avoids normal control function must somehow have associated with it a compromise which can be exploited. Elucidation of these compromises would appear to offer a greater likelihood of developing a general means of treating metastasis than would attempts to reinstate the control mechanism artificially.

Respondent: I believe all the evidence I know of points to the conclusion that the cells that make up a metastasis are cancerous in their nature. To my mind, the essential proof of this is that one can transplant metastatic cells and obtain a tumor that has the same essential characteristics (progressive growth and loss of cell control) of the original metastasizing tumor. The question is rather: are cells disseminated from a primary and eventually growing into a metastasis a statistical cross section of the general tumor population, or are they inherently endowed with somewhat specialized properties favoring or essential to their metastasizing capacity? Obviously I do not know the answer to this question. Probably it is a complex answer. Probably we are not dealing with black or white kinds of problems but with different degrees of gray.

Respondent: A metastasis is a group of cancer cells present *in vivo* at a site different from the site of origin of the malignant tumor. Avenues of metastasis include hematogenous and lymphatic dissemination and seeding of tumor along surfaces lining natural cavities. Whether growth by direct extension is considered metastasis is somewhat semantic and is usually judged by criteria of the distance of extension from the primary site and whether anatomic borders have been crossed between one tissue and another.

A number of qualifying statements must be added.

Location. The typical metastasis consists of tumor cells intermingled with and destroying normal tissue cells. How should we consider malignant cells present in the lumen of an organ in continuity with the "outside world," for instance, bronchogenic carcinoma cells free in the tracheobronchial lumen, or adenocarcinoma cells from a primary carcinoma of the cecum found free in the lumen of the colon? Are these cells capable of reattachment to the wall and invasive growth? Should malignant cells that have separated from a primary site and are found in the bloodstream be considered "metastatic"? By the conventional definition, these cells must first lodge, reattach, invade, and grow to constitute a metastasis.

Viability. The finding of malignant cells at a site different from their origin does not *per se* indicate their biological or clinical significance. This is especially true for cells found in those special locations described above but also pertains to small groups of malignant cells composing a conventional metastasis. Numerous tumor and host factors could result in failure of tumor growth and regression.

Single versus multiple sites of origin. When multiple carcinomas are found at homologous locations, it is frequently difficult or impossible to know whether each arose independently or whether one original tumor metastasized to the homologous site(s). The most common source of this ambiguity is the frequent occurrence of bilateral breast carcinomas, but a similar problem can exist with bilateral renal carcinomas and with multiple colonic carcinomas. This same question of unique versus multicentric origin exists for many lymphoid neoplasms which can present with simultaneous involvement of multiple sites.

Why is a metastasis a cancer cell? Judging from the qualifying statements in answer to the first question, it is apparent that there are ambiguities involved in deciding whether a given group of cancer cells constitutes a metastasis. There seems to be little ambiguity as to whether the cells constituting a given "metastasis" are cancer cells. There is no reason to think that once cancer cells have metastasized they lose any of the characteristics of cancer cells. One special question might be, Once cancer cells metastasize to a given distant site, do these metastatic cancer cells have the same, greater, or lesser propensity to "re-metastasize"? Since metastatic cells are cancer cells, they should be capable of further metastasis. If a selection process were involved in the original metastasis, it would be anticipated that the metastatic cancer cells would have an even greater tendency to again metastasize.

Theses with "Qualified" Responses to the Questions Posed

Respondent: A metastasis can be, but is not necessarily, a cancer cell. Metastasis is a process in which a pathogenic agent or pathologic process is transferred from one part of the body to another by a process other than direct extension. The pathologic condition may be caused by cancer cells, infectious agents, antigens, foreign bodies, or products of the body such as emboli. Doubtless this list could be extended. According to this definition, within the area of cancer a metastasis can be either a cancer cell or an agent that can induce a cancer cell. As an example, the dissemination of oncogenic viruses from the primary site of infection to distal sites could be described as a metastasis although this spread is commonly referred to as a viremia.

Respondent: A metastasis originates when one or more cancer cells with proliferative potential (that is, malignant stem cells) leave a primary tumor and lodge in another environment suitable for their growth. At this stage in development, the term *micrometastasis* is appropriate. The metastasis becomes clinically significant when sufficient proliferation has occurred to yield a tumor mass large enough to be detected.

Respondent: Metastasis is both a process and a lesion. I perceive metastasis as a process to be a series of events encompassing the dissemination of a tumor from a (usually) primary site to a distant site, and its subsequent arrest and growth.

A metastasis is, of course, the singular of metastases. I look on this abnormality as a tumor rather than a cancer cell, i.e., a lesion derived from the above process and consisting of cancer cells together with stroma and adventitious tissue of varying complexities.

Conceivably, metastasis could result not only from a wandering tumor cell but from a subcellular agent, such as a virus, emanating from a tumor.

Theses that a Metastasis Is Not a Cancer Cell

Respondent: Apart from the semantic point that a cancer cell is not a metastasis, only a potential metastasis, a metastasis may, of course, also refer to disseminated nonneoplastic diseases. A disseminated cancer cell must be implanted and multiplying before the result can be called a micrometastasis or metastasis, consequently, a metastasis is likely to quickly become a mixture of neoplastic cells and stroma.

Respondent: As a pathologist, I regard a metastasis as an established secondary tumor, growing by division, expanding, invading, and existing in spatial separation and in temporal separation in many cases from the primary growth from which it originated. The essence, then, of metastasis in cancer to me is the successful establishment of a colony of cells with its existing stroma and its vascular supply.

There is a difference between "metastasis" as a phenomenon, and thus not peculiar to cancer, and "a metastasis," which is an established secondary tumor. In a number of other conditions, migration of cells, organisms, and even inanimate matter (coal dust or asbestos fibers) is an observed phenomenon and has been termed metastasis, but the lesion which results is not usually regarded or termed "a metastasis."

I therefore do not regard a metastasis as "a cancer cell." I could not recognize it objectively as such and have some hesitation in accepting that a single cell migration can of itself produce what I call "metastasis." I accept that cancer, e.g., leukemia, can be mechanically transmitted by a single cell, but I doubt if this is the same phenomenon.

Respondent: Without further qualification, the answer to the question must be "no." Clearly, a cancer cell in culture is not a metastasis, nor is a dead cancer cell. I interpret the question as asking whether a living cancer cell, disseminated from a primary site, can be considered a metastasis. The word *metastasis* means literally "placed after" and was adopted as a clinical term to describe secondary growth of a cancer at a site which is noncontiguous with the primary site (10). As such, a detectable lesion is required to constitute a metastasis whether this lesion be clinically overt or only microscopic, i.e., a micrometastasis. To the pragmatic clinician, then, metastasis means tumor growth (or at least growth potential if treatment intervenes) at a site other than that of the primary cancer.

A cancer biologist, on the other hand, tends to consider metastasis as a dynamic *process* encompassing all the events between separation of a malignant cell from a primary neoplasm and its establishment as a progressive secondary growth. From neither point of view, however, can a single disseminated cancer cell be considered a metastasis.

Firstly, not all tumor cells have clonogenic potential, i.e., the ability to undergo unlimited proliferation. In experimental animal tumor systems, there is a wide variation in the number of viable tumor cells required to transplant the tumor even when immunologic considerations are factored out (11). Studies of human tumor autotransplantation (12), as well as inferential conclusions drawn from experience in the radiotherapy of human cancers, suggest that the proportion of clonogenic cells in many solid human tumors is very small.

Secondly, there is by no means any certainty that clonogenic cells entering the bloodstream will successfully survive and grow at a new location. In animals the efficiency of lung colony formation following intravenous injection of tumor cells is invariably lower than the efficiency of subcutaneous transplantation. Fidler (13) showed that after intravenous injection, the great majority of tumor cells die rapidly, and we have produced evidence that passive cell death rather than an active host defense is mainly responsible. It has long been observed that there is poor correlation between the presence of circulating tumor cells in the blood of cancer patients and their subsequent development of overt metastases (see 14). Furthermore, even if a clonogenic tumor cell survives the period of acute vulnerability soon after intravascular dissemination, there are still many "host factors" which may modify its ability to grow progressively. This, in my view, is the cardinal attribute of a metastasis.

Just as the term *cure* in oncology has come to have an operational rather than an absolute meaning, so I tend to think of metastasis as a cure-limiting phenomenon, and unless a cancer cell undergoes *progressive* secondary growth, it does not meet this criterion.

Respondent: A metastasis is a visible aggregate of multiplying tumor cells in an organ distant from the original site. Detection of individual tumor cells in the circulation does not necessarily imply that it will reproduce in another organ. A metastasis is not a cancer cell. It is an established and expanded focus of cancer cells.

CONCLUDING REMARKS

It is clear from these many thoughtful observations discussing the "nature" of metastasis that the problem is not amenable to clear-cut expression. The chapters presented in this volume emphasize the broad and interdisciplinary perspectives that the biology of metastasis encompasses, and they point up still the difficulty in expressing in a scientific sense those aspects of the biology of cancer that we may tend to assume are "simple" to understand. As we learn more of the nature of metastasis it seems certain that the true nature of the phenomenon retreats into further questions to be answered. One is almost tempted to believe, with Herbert Spencer, that the absolute is unknowable.

REFERENCES

1. Willis, R. A. (1950): *The Principles of Pathology*, p. 393. Butterworth and Co., London.
2. Romanis, W. H. C. (1948): *The Science and Practice of Surgery, Vol. 1, Ed. 8*, p. 176. J. and A. Churchill, Ltd., London.
3. Vines, H. W. C. (Ed.) (1949): *Green's Manual of Pathology, Ed. 17*. Bailiere, Tindall and Cox, London.

4. Rous, P. (1965): Viruses and tumor causation. An appraisal of present knowledge. *Nature,* 207:457–463.
5. Rous, P. (1959): Surmise and fact on the nature of cancer. *Nature,* 183:1357–1361.
6. Yohn, D. S., Weiss, L., and Neiders, M. E. (1968): A comparison of the distribution of tumors produced by intravenous injection of type 12 adenovirus and adeno-12 tumor cells. *Cancer Res.,* 28:571–576.
7. Farber, E. (1975): Biochemical pathology of chemical carcinogenesis. In: *Molecular Pathology,* edited by R. A. Good, S. B. Day, and J. J. Yunis, pp. 262–273. Charles C. Thomas, Springfield, Ill.
8. Bross, I. D. J., and Blumenson, L. E. (1976): Metastatic sites that produce generalized cancer: Identification and kinetics of generalizing sites. In: *Fundamental Aspects of Metastasis,* edited by L. Weiss. North-Holland Publishing Co., Amsterdam.
9. Bienengraber, A., Ernst, B., and Tessmann, D. (1965): Theory of tumor metastasis. *Zentralbl. Allg. Pathol.,* 107:445–450.
10. Willis, R. A. (1973): *The Spread of Tumors in the Human Body.* Butterworths, London.
11. Hewitt, H. B., Blake, E. R., and Walder, A. S. (1976): A critique of the evidence for active host defense against cancer based on personal studies of 27 murine tumors of spontaneous origin. *Br. J. Cancer,* 33:241–259.
12. Southam, C. M., and Brunschwig, A. (1961): Quantitative studies of autotransplantation of human cancer. *Cancer,* 14:971–978.
13. Fidler, I. J. (1970): Metastasis: Quantitative analysis of distribution and fate of tumor emboli labelled with ^{125}I-5-iodo-2'-deoxyuridine. *J. Natl. Cancer Inst.,* 45:773–782.
14. Griffiths, J. D., McKinna, J. A., Rowbotham, H. D., Tsolakidis, P., and Salsbury, A. J. (1972): Carcinoma of the colon and rectum: Circulating malignant cells and five year survival. *Cancer,* 31:226–236.

Cancer Invasion and Metastasis: Biologic Mechanisms and Therapy, edited by S. B. Day et al. Raven Press, New York © 1977.

Overview of the Biology and Pathology of Metastasis

J. N. P. Davies

Albany Medical College, Albany, New York 12208

It is not my task to anticipate the findings and conclusions of contributors to this volume but rather to draw the general picture of tumor invasion, in particular, that specific type of invasion we call metastasis. All of us in our various capacities and capabilities are attempting to grapple with what is, for the majority of patients with cancer, the central problem in clinical management, namely, the distal spread of cancer from its initial focus. The phenomenon of metastasis is only too familiar to clinicians and pathologists who are concerned with such patients. As long as any cancer remains localized, so long as it is not located in some vital spot or in some surgically inaccessible location, it is potentially and in many cases actually curable by local surgical incision. But either with invasion beyond restricted local limits or with distant spread the problems multiply and the prognosis worsens considerably.

Metastasis is the development of secondary tumors that are not in direct contact with the initial primary growth. Neither invasion nor metastasis is peculiar to cancer; both phenomena are exemplified by the developing placenta and the spread to liver and lungs of fragments of chorionic tissue which may implant and grow but which, with the cessation of the pregnancy, die and disappear. What is peculiar to cancer is the ability of the disseminated cells to continue to divide and thus increase in bulk. Here in itself is a problem. Do the metastases that continue to grow constitute a minority or a majority of the implants that have developed?

For the most part, cancer starts as a localized proliferation of cells, perhaps arising from a single cell, most probably from a focus of altered cells. The factors that induce and ensure the persistence of this proliferation are not our main concern but are of course highly germane to our major problems. As cell multiplication at the original focus continues, there is in most cases an increase in the volume of the local proliferating cell mass and a consequent rise in the local tissue pressures. Microscopically, and often with pigmented tumors clinically, we observe that around this central mass of proliferating cells, extensions of such cells develop in the interstices, the cracks and crevices, of the surrounding tissue. They dissect along tissue planes, may erode into vascular or lymphatic channels, and may extend for considerable distances while maintaining continuity with the initial cell mass. Often, however, we are able to recognize such extensions only by the secondary effects the emigrating cells produce, such as the fibrosis that may develop (for example, the *peau d'orange* skin change of invading breast cancer). Unhappily, there is no uniformity in extension, the boundaries being quite irregular in both lateral and depth penetration with superficial cancers, and in size, shape, and extent in central growths.

All this makes it certain that the extensions at any given point in time will be more widespread than clinical examination can determine, and thus the clinician is faced with the problem of complete excision. The initial focus must be cut out together with the probable area of extension, with the zone of potentially invaded tissue. Microscopy may be used to determine if the lines of excision are clear of growth, but in the end the extent of excision has to be determined subjectively by the surgeon because there is no sure method of detecting the limits of invasion. To remove too much may be harmful and disfiguring, yet removal of too little may lead to the dreaded disaster of local recurrence, which may be so difficult to treat.

To some extent local invasion can be regarded as a purely mechanical process; it can be duplicated somewhat by the accidental injection into human tissues of some foreign material under high pressure, as seen in accidents involving injection of lubricating grease, which can dissect along tissue planes, infiltrate tissue spaces, and be directed along diverse paths by fibrous barriers. Indeed, by injecting jelly spherules into gels resembling the normal surrounding tissues, Young was able to duplicate many of the clinical and pathological features of metastasis including vascular invasion. But local invasion is not solely a mechanical process for it is witnessed in tumors where there is no local volume or pressure increase. Cancer cells are motile, have decreased mutual adhesiveness and reduced contact inhibition, and can elaborate, or induce tissues to elaborate, substances that may lyse materials which impede the movements of cells throughout tissues.

Cancer cells can thus migrate and lose any connection with the parent growth. They may enter the bloodstream at an early stage and circulate. For many years, the fact that cancer cells circulated, especially during surgery, was regarded with dismay as tending to promote metastasis. Much attention was directed toward the identification and enumeration of such cells and to study of the consequences of such dissemination. Now views may be changing and some consider that such circulating cells, which usually do not survive long unless they implant, may favorably affect the prognosis. Thus it may be valuable to keep such cells in circulation by the use of fibrinolysins to prevent their implantation.

Metastasis is only a specialized type of invasion. We can see this beautifully illustrated in renal adenocarcinomas developing from renal tubular epithelium in an area where there are vast numbers of thin-walled veins to which the cancer cells, singly or *en masse,* gain speedy access. Thus renal carcinomas are notorious for the frequency with which an early clinical manifestation, perhaps the initial evidence of the cancer, is the development of a blood-borne metastasis at some far distant and often unusual site. Any experienced pathologist has seen an aural, nasal, or gastrointestinal polyp that is a metastasis from a renal carcinoma. Equally classic are the "cannonball" metastases that so speedily and massively develop in the lungs, but also seen are cases in which a solid column of cancer cells grows from the kidney into the renal vein, and along it into the vena cava and then may extend into the heart. The latter is invasion by permeation, but if single cells or clumps of cells break off and establish themselves, there is metastasis.

When the problems of invasion are studied, we see all the problems that we must consider with metastasis; almost every feature save one is unpredictable and even that is far from absolute. Thus with a fair degree of certainty we can predict that in the metastases that do occur the morphologic and functional features of the primary growth will be closely duplicated in the great majority of cases, over 80%. This is of immense benefit to the histopathologist who can often predict from study of a removed secondary nodule where the primary is located and its histologic type, which narrows the field of search for a primary. If there is a difference in morphology, the metastases usually are less well differentiated than the primary, although sometimes they are more differentiated. Independent of morphologic differences, there may be functional differences, thus in a pigmented melanoma the metastases may contain no pigment.

Although we can with some degree of confidence predict the likely morphology and function of the metastases from knowledge of the primary growth, and vice versa, almost every other aspect defies prediction. Metastasis is not necessarily proportional to the size of the primary; a minute primary may produce metastases enormous in both size and number, a bulky primary may produce no metastases or may produce them only late in time and few in number. Site may or may not have any influence on metastasis; the same applies to cell type, rapidity of growth, cytogenesis, or any of the features of the primary growth that we can recognize. Nor does invasion necessarily imply metastasis. Some cancers, e.g., basal cell carcinomas and ameloblastomas, classically invade widely and yet rarely metastasize, whereas others, such as melanomas, may show little local invasiveness yet produce widespread metastasis.

Moreover, we cannot relate the growth rate of the primary growth to that of the metastasis. The metastasis may flourish and the primary disappear as happens with some melanomas. Not all the metastases grow at the same rate, even in the same tissue or organ, and apparent "spontaneous" regressions of metastases are not all that unusual. When it was my lot, in the late 1930s, to observe numerous terminal cancer cases under treatment with lead and selenium compounds, I was astonished to note how often histologically verified skin metastases developed and regressed without treatment. Is it a coincidence that "spontaneous" regression has been noted with some frequency in the very renal adenocarcinomas that metastasize so readily? Sometimes regression may follow interruption of blood supply, but occasionally a whole crop of secondary nodules disappears, a feature not uncommonly seen in Kaposi's sarcoma.

Other features of the behavior of metastases are of enormous interest. On occasion, following apparent quiescence of activity many metastatic nodules all growing rapidly may suddenly appear in numerous sites, a veritable blizzard of metastasis. The obverse of this is the quite extraordinary degree of dormancy exhibited by some metastases. Thus a primary may be completely removed only for a secondary mass clearly identifiable as such, perhaps in a lymph node, to develop years later, sometimes after 30 or 40 years. If we could induce dormancy on metastatic nodules we would be much better off, and perhaps study of the factors producing this state would be of great benefit.

Although we cannot predict much about the behavior of primary growths in relation to the development of metastasis, we have a good deal of information on the routes of metastatic spread and can appreciate some of the local factors of importance in the actual development of a metastatic deposit. The two major routes of dissemination are by the lymphatics and the veins, both tubular systems with thin walls and sluggish flow of fluid. Thus the walls are easily breachable, there are channels in which cells can grow in continuity, and there is a flow in which cancer cells, singly or in masses, can be swept along to death or to lodgment with implantation and perhaps survival. This process of dissemination can be regarded from several aspects. The wider and more distant the dissemination of the cancer, the greater the likelihood that this dissemination has been via vascular channels. Ultimately, lymphatic drainage becomes blood vascular drainage because the large lymphatic trunks drain into the great veins in the neck.

The drainage of the small lymphatic vessels is to the draining lymph nodes, although these are often bypassed, and so the usual early location of metastasis is in the draining lymph nodes, initially in the peripheral sinuses — provided the nodes have not previously been blocked or damaged by some disease process. If this is the case there will be centrifugal rather than centripetal development of metastasis by retrograde lymphatic flow. This is something surgeons do not like to see, just as they dislike seeing centrifugal dissemination because of venous blocking. The more plentiful the venous or lymphatic drainage, the greater the likelihood that metastasis will develop at an early stage; but this does not always follow, and for many years controversy has raged as to whether there are reactive lesions in lymph nodes antecedent to the development of metastases which may limit the spread of cancer.

The inevitable fate of clumps of cancer cells in the blood is to arrest in one of the filtering organs: for the systemic venous system, in the lungs; for the gastrointestinal tract, in the liver; and for those which enter the vertebral vein interconnections, in the bones of the spine, pelvis, or skull. The frequency of metastasis in a particular location depends to some considerable extent on the site and type pattern of cancer in a particular community. Thus Virchow suggested that organs commonly the sites of metastasis were not usually common sites of primary tumor formation. This is instanced because it shows how things are different in various communities and how patterns of site and type change with time. Today Virchow would not claim this were he to see the great frequency of primary pulmonary cancer, for he instanced the lung as a rare site of primary tumors as compared with its frequent involvement in secondary growths. Conversely, in many tropical countries the liver is a major site of primary cancers as opposed to the frequency with which it is a major site of metastatic cancers in this country. This points to the changes in the patterns of metastasis with time and with different modalities of treatment. Thus nowadays one sees widespread vascular metastatic dissemination in cancers, such as carcinoma of the cervix uterus, that used to kill by the effects of local spread.

Just to speak of vascular dissemination is to cover our ignorance in what is an extremely complicated process. First of all, the cancer cells must implant, a process involving protection behind a fibrin barrier. Behind this the cells may survive for a long period but are not able to proliferate. To do this they have to penetrate the vascular wall; having done this, they must develop the necessary fibrous framework and the vascular connections; having done this, the cells can proliferate to invade locally and even to develop metastases of their own. We must consider every aspect of these processes from initial lodgment to established growth; but there is more to it than this. As in all pathology we have to consider the seed and the soil. There is no question that some cancers can grow only, or grow much more readily, in certain sites where the soil is favorable. There must be some special affinities. Thus we have the familiar phenomenon of the early development of metastatic cancer of the breast in the ovaries, often clinically undetectable but nevertheless such a common feature that many consider bilateral removal of the ovaries a necessary component of ablative surgery of breast cancer. Commonly in bronchogenic cancer there is bilateral involvement of the adrenal glands, where the pulmonary cancer cells flourish luxuriantly, whether by lymphatic or vascular dissemination. This has been found with certain experimental tumors which when disseminated by intravascular injection of tumor cells develop only in certain selected organs. The factors governing this await elucidation.

This of course raises the perplexing and often discussed question as to how far the experimental models actually mimic metastasis in the cancer patient. This is certainly something we shall have to bear in mind in our discussions. It is easy to devise methods of inoculating cancer cells which disseminate in experimental animals but not easy to equate these with other than some specific patterns of human metastasis. In particular, we have to consider the dormancy of metastases in human cancer; whatever the factors responsible, the existence of dormancy implies that viable cancer cells can exist in an established focus capable of proliferation but somehow restrained into long-term equilibrium with the body. Then this state of equilibrium is broken and growth restarts. How do these cells survive? How do they persist? Why do they start to proliferate? We do not know, and few problems in cancer have been so little studied.

This is indeed a matter of concern. Although the literature is considerable and many studies have been made, it is remarkable how little we know or understand about metastasis even on the purely morphological side. Few have studied metastasis in human cancer with the detail and care displayed by Rupert Willis (1–3), but despite this few complete autopsies have been made on human cancer cases. Usually the morphology of only a few meta-static deposits in each patient is studied, and there have been relatively few clinical studies. Yet it is the major clinical problem of cancer. And the fact remains that we cannot predict, diagnose, control, or successfully eliminate metastasis with any measure of success, yet the human economy can undertake the last three of these functions on occasion with a consider-able measure of success. But how? That is what we have to discover.

REFERENCES

1. Willis, R. A. (1934): *The Spread of Tumours in the Human Body, Ed. 1*. J. and A: Church-ill, London.
2. Willis, R. A. (1952): *The Spread of Tumours in the Human Body, Ed. 2*. Butterworths, London.
3. Willis, R. A. (1973): *The Spread of Tumours in the Human Body, Ed. 3*. Butterworths, London.

Cancer Invasion and Metastasis: Biologic Mechanisms and Therapy, edited by S. B. Day et al. Raven Press, New York © 1977.

The Cell Surface and Metastasis

G. Poste

Department of Experimental Pathology, Roswell Park Memorial Institute, Buffalo, New York 14263

The essential features of tumor cells that distinguish them from their normal counterparts are their abilities to proliferate in an uncontrolled fashion, invade normal tissues, and metastasize to distant sites, although these behavioral alterations are not always coupled. The complex interrelationships between these properties are well illustrated by such tumors as giant fibroadenoma of the breast which often grows quickly but does not metastasize, scirrhous carcinoma of the breast which grows slowly but often metastasizes, basal cell carcinoma of the skin which may show extensive growth and local invasion but rarely metastasizes, whereas the slow-growing carcinomas of the thyroid, prostate, and kidney frequently metastasize. In addition, tumors may display differing properties during different periods of their progression, and tumors ostensibly of the same type may show differing behavior in different patients and also respond differently to therapy.

It is now recognized that changes in the surface properties of tumor cells are probably important in determining aspects of their abnormal growth and social behavior. Within the primary tumor, alterations in the surface properties of tumor cells contribute to their escape from many of the controls and social restraints to which normal cells are subject. The proliferation of tumor cells is no longer effectively regulated by cell-to-cell contact interactions, and they are increasingly unresponsive to growth regulation by serum factors, hormones, and other agents that exert their effects after binding to the cell surface. Tumor cells can therefore achieve varying degrees of autonomy from normal growth restraints, and this ability is reflected in uncontrolled proliferation and progressive enlargement of the primary tumor. Altered surface properties of tumor cells may also result in aberrant cell-to-cell recognition, allowing tumor cells to escape from the control mechanisms responsible for maintaining proper cell position. In malignant lesions these processes are augmented by metastasis, in which the surface properties of tumor cells are important not only in the invasion of surrounding normal tissue (or tissues) and initial separation of cells from the primary tumor, but also in determining the subsequent pattern (or patterns) of cell distribution and establishment of metastatic foci. Finally, the outcome of the interaction of tumor cells with elements of the host immune apparatus in both primary and secondary tumors is influenced in large part by the surface properties of the tumor-cell population.

ANALYSIS OF THE SURFACE PROPERTIES OF MALIGNANT CELLS: EXPERIMENTAL APPROACHES AND PROBLEMS

The primary reason for comparison of tumor cells with their normal counterparts is to attempt to define features unique to tumor cells, which could form the basis for cancer therapy, perhaps via control of metastases. Since many of the basic surface functions of normal cells are maintained by tumor cells, it is not unreasonable to consider that certain of the altered surface properties found in tumor cells could result from subtle variation and modification of normal cell surface organization rather than involve gross departure. Such differences could involve additions or deletions of normal surface components resulting from quantitative and qualitative changes of both genetic and epigenetic origin. In addition, other alternations could simply arise from topographic redistribution and rearrangement of normal surface components in the absence of extensive chemical changes. This concept of topographic rearrangement of cell surface architecture in tumor cells is fully consistent with current views of plasma membrane structure, which indicate that the plasma membrane is a dynamic structure in which various components are able to undergo movement and redistribution within the membrane (see The Dynamic Nature of Cell Surface Organization, p. 26). However, in view of the fact that some 273 types of human cancers alone are classified and that similar diversity exists among the animal tumor models currently used in research, it would be remarkable if the surface differences identified in different types of tumor cells proved to be identical and did not vary quantitatively and qualitatively over a wide range. Yet in spite of these difficulties, the literature abounds with generalizations on the surface properties of cancer cells based on limited studies of one or, at best, a few cell types.

The majority of our knowledge on the altered surface properties of tumor cells has been derived from *in vitro* studies on cultured cells, particularly cell populations that have been rendered tumorigenic by exposure *in vitro* to tumor viruses or chemical carcinogens. I do not intend to discuss the inevitable question of how far information obtained *in vitro* is relevant to the situation *in vivo*. The relative simplicity of *in vitro* cell culture systems, the opportunities for detailed biochemical and genetic analyses on large uniform cloned populations of cultured cells, and the ability to directly study the cellular changes accompanying viral or chemically induced malignant transformation *in vitro* are powerful experimental approaches that would be impossible or difficult to pursue *in vivo*. It is important to recognize, however, that the *in vitro* characterization of the surface properties of normal and tumor cells still presents substantial problems, not the least of which are certain problems inherent in the technology of cell culture itself.

Many features of cellular organization are significantly affected by cultivation of cells *in vitro*. Awareness of the phenotypic changes that can be imposed in cell populations by cultivation *in vitro* is therefore of paramount importance if such techniques are to provide a meaningful experimental approach to the study of malignancy.

Many aspects of current procedures used in the isolation of cells from solid tissues and their subsequent propagation *in vitro* can produce changes in cell surface properties. A major problem concerns the use of enzymes, notably proteases, to disrupt tissues and to detach cells from substrates during routine subcultivation *in vitro*. Overt damage to the cell surface with resulting loss or reduction in cell viability is easily recognized, but there is still a general lack of appreciation of the more subtle changes and long-term selective effects that may arise from frequent sublethal modification of the cell periphery by enzymes and many other facets of the *in vitro* environment (58,108).

Once initiated in culture, mammalian cells undergo a myriad of phenotypic alterations, and this variability may be further reinforced by changes in the chromosome complement that emerge with prolonged cultivation *in vitro*. The problems posed by "instability" of various cellular properties, the current approaches used to limit such variation, and the availability of techniques for maintaining highly differentiated functions in cultured cells, including specific neoplastic cell characteristics, have been discussed at length in a recent symposium (68).

In view of the recognized instability of many features of the cellular phenotype *in vitro* and the role of culture conditions in contributing to cellular variation, it is obvious that data from *in vitro* studies on malignancy will always be open to question if strictly comparable normal and tumor cell populations are not used and if sufficient care is not exercised to ensure that the conditions for the growth of both normal and tumor cell populations are as far as possible identical. The type of medium, its pH, its serum supplement, the frequency and method of subcultivation, the nature of the substratum to which cells are attached, cell population density, and cell passage level are but a few of the factors that can exert important effects on the surface properties of cells in culture.

Another poorly understood factor that may well influence the phenotype of cultured cells is the geometry of the cell population (39). For example, in cell populations growing as monolayers attached to solid substrates, growth is essentially in two dimensions over the surface of the dish, and growth in a third dimension leading to an increase in the thickness of the monolayer is limited. Under these conditions cells increase their number indefinitely provided sufficient open space is available (this requirement being met by means of subcultivation and transfer to a new dish) and nutrient requirements are fulfilled. However, when the same cells are grown in suspension in agarose or methylcellulose (Methocel®), population growth occurs in three dimensions to form a spheroid, but unlimited growth does not occur despite the availability of space and nutrients. Spheroids grow to a limiting size, at which stage a peripheral rim of cells continues to proliferate while others in the center are dying, presumably due to inadequate diffusion of nutrients into the deeper regions of the spheroid. Since population growth in three dimensions more closely resembles the situation *in vivo*, the surface properties of tumor cells growing in spheroids might more accurately reflect that exhibited by the same cells growing *in vivo*. No data are presently available, however, to indicate how far the surface properties of cells differ when grown as monolayers and as spheroids.

Another problem facing investigators using cell culture techniques concerns the identity of cells that survive *in vitro*. The terms *fibroblasts* and *epithelial cells* are often used in the literature to describe cells under study, although in many instances these terms are applied merely on the basis of descriptive morphology rather than accurate identification of the tissue of origin. Although information on the precise histotypic origin of cultured cells may not be viewed as critical in experiments where neoplastic cellular transformation is induced *in vitro* (since the untransformed parent cell is usually known), this information is of more crucial importance for studies in which cultured cells are isolated directly from neoplastic tissues. In this situation it is obviously desirable to know the relationship of the cultured cells to those present in the original tumor in order that the properties of the newly isolated tumor cells can be compared with an appropriate normal cell type. Even to the naked eye recognizable tumors present a heterogeneous appearance and such heterogeneity extends to the cellular level. Actively growing, nongrowing, dying, dead, neoplastic, and normal cells of varying histotypic origins are all present in most tumors, often in contiguous areas of the same lesion. This dictates not only that it is extremely difficult to isolate pure populations of tumor cells in culture but also that identification of the nature of the isolated cells is of considerable relevance (14,25, 103,113).

Perhaps the most important question regarding the relevance of *in vitro* models for oncogenesis is the adequacy of the criteria used to define neoplastic transformation. A related question concerns the suitability of the experimental material selected as representative of normal and neoplastic cell populations.

By popular usage, the term *transformed* describes cells that display certain stable heritable alterations that have arisen either spontaneously following prolonged *in vitro* cultivation or after exposure of cells to tumor viruses or chemical carcinogens. Among the cellular alterations of this kind that have been widely used as markers for the "transformed" phenotype are acquisition of the potential for infinite growth *in vitro;* alterations in cell morphology and accompanying changes in social behavior such as the ability to grow to very high densities or grow in suspension; alterations in surface antigenicity; changes in cellular responsiveness to plant lectins; loss or simplification of cell surface glycoproteins and glycolipids; and altered sensitivities to attack by macrophages and lymphocytes. Unfortunately, in many studies the existence of morphological alterations and changes in the pattern of cell growth behavior *in vitro* and/or other *in vitro* criteria of the type outlined above have been used as the *sole* basis for assuming that the cell population has undergone neoplastic conversion, and the detection of surface alterations in such "transformed" cells is taken as evidence that the alterations are causally related to tumorigenicity even though the capacity of the cells to produce tumors *in vivo* has never been examined. This problem is illustrated by examination of Table 1 in a recent review by Glick (47), which lists a number of "membrane events associated with virus transformation *and tumorigenesis*" [italics added], although to the best of the author's knowledge none of the listed changes has yet been reliably correlated with the capacity of cells to cause tumors *in vivo*. All that can be stated with certainty at present is that the types of surface changes listed by Glick (and also in Table 1 of this chapter) have been detected with some degree of consistency in cultured cell populations after exposure to oncogenic viruses or chemical carcinogens, and that their appearance is associated with alterations in cell growth behavior *in vitro* (although not necessarily causally related). Not until detailed studies correlating these *in vitro* characteristics with the behavior of the same cells *in vivo* are completed can we make firm conclusions as to which surface alterations contribute to tumorigenicity (see Unsolved Problems, p. 39).

It would thus perhaps be desirable if the term *transformed* were restricted to describing cell cultures that have also been shown to be able to grow as tumors *in vivo*, or, alternatively, the term were qualified with respect to the type of change observed *in vitro*, i.e., morphological, antigenic, neoplastic, and so on.

The potential confusion inherent in the use of *in vitro* growth properties to classify cells as "normal" or "transformed" is also reflected in the widespread use of heteroploid established cell lines such as the BHK-21 hamster cell line as "normal" control cells for comparison with cells of the same type after "transformation" by tumor viruses. In this system, cells showing alterations in their *in vitro* growth behavior as a result of tumor virus infection are referred to as "transformed," whereas uninfected BHK-21 cells are referred to as "normal" or "untransformed" even though they can cause tumors when transplanted *in vivo* (23,56). Similarly, BALB/c mouse 3T3 cells, which have probably been used more extensively than any other cell type for studies on neoplastic transformation *in vitro*, have been shown recently to be tumorigenic in histocompatible mice when implanted attached

TABLE 1. *Cell surface changes associated with neoplastic transformation of cells cultured in vitro*

Property	Selected reviews
1. Changes in cell behavior influenced by cell surface organization	Folkman and Greenspan (39)
	Goldman et al. (49)
a. Decreased sensitivity to contact inhibition of movement	Trinkaus (106)
b. Decreased sensitivity to density-dependent growth inhibition	
c. Loss of "anchorage dependence" and acquisition of capacity for growth in suspension	
2. Changes in cell-to-cell and cell-to-substrate adhesiveness	Weiss (112)
a. Status uncertain	
3. Reduced cell-to-cell communication due to changes in the formation and organization of gap junctions	Sheridan (92)
	Weinstein et al. (109)
a. Status uncertain	
4. Changes in the structural organization of the plasma membrane	Edelman (29)
	Nicolson (70)
a. Increased mobility of integral membrane proteins and glycoproteins	Nicolson and Poste (71)
	Nicolson et al. (72)
b. Reduction in membrane-associated mircofilaments and/or other cytoskeletal elements	
5. Changes in cell surface charge	Weiss (111)
a. No consistent correlation between zeta potential and malignancy	
6. Changes in plasma membrane transport activities	Holley (53)
a. Enhanced transport of sugars	Pardee (75)
b. Enhanced transport of amino acids	
7. Changes in membrane-associated enzymes	Pardee (75)
a. Reduced adenyl cyclase activity	
b. Enhanced Na^+-K^+-ATPase activity and loss of growth-dependent changes in enzyme activity	
8. Changes in plasma membrane lipid composition and alterations in membrane "fluidity"	Nicolson (70)
	Nicolson et al. (72)
a. Status uncertain	
9. Changes in plasma membrane glycolipids	Brady and Fishman (10)
a. Incomplete glycosylation of glycolipids	Hakomori (51)
b. Reduced activity of specific glycolipid glycosyltransferases	Critchley and Vicker (22)
c. Increased reactivity of membrane glycolipids to antiglycolipid antibodies	
10. Changes in plasma membrane glycoproteins	Roblin et al. (89)
a. Incomplete synthesis of certain glycoproteins, especially lack of terminal sialic acid resulting from reduced sialyltransferase activity	Hynes (55)
	Gahmberg (42)
b. Increased production of fucose-containing sialoglycopeptides	
c. Loss of a high molecular weight (ca. 200,000–250,000 daltons) membrane glycoprotein (LETS protein; Z protein; FSA protein; galactoprotein A; L1 protein)	
d. Changes in glycopeptidyl-transferases	
11. Changes in membrane mucopolysaccharides	Roblin et al. (89)
a. Increased synthesis of hyaluronic acid	
b. Increased production of sulfated mucopolysaccharides	

TABLE 1. (*Continued*)

Property	Selected reviews
12. Changes in susceptibility to agglutination by plant lectins	Nicolson (69) Rapin and Burger (86)

13. Antigenic changes
   a. Novel tumor-associated transplantation rejection antigens
   b. Novel tumor-associated antigens not necessarily capable of evoking transplantation antigens
   c. "Embryonic" or "oncofetal" antigens
   d. Altered expression (deletion, reduction, increase) of normal cell- or tissue-specific antigens
	Coggin and Anderson (20)
	Klein (59)
	Smith and Landy (97)
	Ting and Herberman (105)

to 3-mm glass beads. Cells derived from these tumors were capable of producing lethal tumors on subsequent transplantation in the absence of beads (8,9). Inoculation of cells or beads alone did not produce tumors. These observations suggest that although 3T3 cells are not completely transformed and are not tumorigenic, they can perhaps be viewed as in a "preneoplastic" state which may be related to their status as an established cell line having the capacity for infinite growth *in vitro*.

These findings emphasize the need for caution in viewing such cells, or perhaps any established cell line, as "normal," at least when compared with diploid, primary, or low-passage secondary "normal" cell strains having limited growth potential *in vitro*. A further shortcoming in the use of spontaneously transformed established cell lines as "controls" for comparison with virally or chemically transformed cell populations is the known aneuploidy of many such lines, particularly those of murine origin, since this increases the risk of genetic drift and alterations in cell properties with passage *in vitro*. Recognition of these difficulties has dictated that many investigators are now returning to use normal cell populations obtained directly from body tissues as primary diploid cultures and which are then transformed by tumor viruses, etc., after only limited passage *in vitro*.

Information on the ability of cultured cells to cause tumors when implanted *in vivo* is not only essential for rigorous definition of neoplastic transformation but is also important if we are to define functional relationships between expression of particular cell surface alterations in cells *in vitro* and the capacity of the same cells to induce tumors, to invade, and to metastasize *in vivo*. The availability of the congenitally athymic nude mutant mouse has introduced exciting new opportunities for analyzing tumor cell behavior *in vivo*. The defect in their cell-mediated immune response enables nude mice to accept heterotransplants of a wide variety of normal and neoplastic tissues. The lack of immune rejection response permits *in vivo* transplantation studies to be done routinely with human tumor cells and animal tumor cell populations derived from noninbred strains. Previously, transplantation of such cells could be accomplished only by immunosuppression of recipient animals or by inoculation of cells into immunologically privileged sites such as the hamster cheek pouch and the anterior chamber of the eye or artificial privileged site systems such as alymphatic skin islands (118) and Millipore diffusion chambers (1), all of which posed significant technical and/or interpretational problems. Further advantages of tumor transplantation in nude mice are that the acceptance percentage is reasonably high and serial transplantation of tumors is possible enabling observations to be made on changes in the surface properties of tumor cells during tumor progression using sequential passaging *in vitro* and *in vivo*. In addition, the isolation of tissue culture lines from human tumors growing in nude mice offers new opportunities for the establishment of tumor cell lines from material which may be extremely difficult to cultivate *in vitro* when isolation is attempted from surgical biopsy material (67).

Isozyme analyses, assays of hormone production, and karyotypic, histologic, and immunologic studies indicate that tumors transplanted into nude mice maintain their original properties during serial passage over long periods (83,98). However, of potential significance for studies on the invasive and metastatic potential of transplanted cells is the finding that most of the tumors transplanted into nude mice to date form localized and well-encapsulated lesions and do not appear to metastasize. However, Giovanella et al. (46) and Giovanella and Stehlin (45) have reported both invasive and metastatic behavior in human tumor xenografts growing in nude mice.

Most of the points discussed in this section would seem to be stating the obvious. Unfortunately, the reader need make only the most casual excursion into the literature to see that these considerations are often overlooked. In too many cases, painstaking research using sophisticated techniques has produced information of limited value because of selection of unsuitable experimental material and/or the use of inappropriate test conditions for the comparison of normal and neoplastic cells.

CELL SURFACE ALTERATIONS IN MALIGNANCY

The Dynamic Nature of Cell Surface Organization

A general consensus has been reached in the last few years that the structure of biological membranes conforms to a number of basic principles (11,70,80,95,96). In brief, these are that: (a) the majority of the membrane lipids are arranged as a bilayer; (b) the bulk of the phospholipids are "fluid" under physiological conditions creating a lipid matrix with a viscosity equivalent to that of light mineral oil, although some classes of lipids may be immobilized in lipoprotein complexes or "solid" lipid islands; (c) the lipid bilayer is asymmetric (at least in all membranes examined to date) with particular phospholipids being distributed preferentially in the inner or outer halves of the bilayer; (d) the bilayer is not continuous but is interrupted by numerous proteins which are inserted to varying degrees into the bilayer (integral proteins) while other membrane proteins interact with the polar surfaces of the bilayer (peripheral proteins); (e) at least certain integral membrane proteins are believed to exist as oligomeric complexes, and complexes between integral and peripheral membrane proteins are also possible; (f) certain integral proteins actually span the lipid bilayer and have regions that protrude on both sides of the bilayer; and (g) cell membrane components (lipids, glycolipids, proteins, and glycoproteins) are capable of lateral movement within the membrane.

The surface membrane of cells in its most basic form can thus be viewed as a two-dimensional solution of a mosaic of integral proteins in a fluid lipid bilayer matrix.

The asymmetric distribution of components across the membrane permits membrane functions to be localized at different surfaces on the membrane (72). For example, membrane glycoproteins and glycolipids exhibit striking asymmetry with their carbohydrate residues being exposed exclusively at the outer face of the plasma membrane where these residues act as specific receptors for antibodies, hormones, lectins, viruses, and other agents that have specific receptors on the cell surface (24,70). Maintenance of membrane asymmetry requires that components oriented to the outer face of the bilayer, no matter whether on the cytoplasmic face or to the external environment, should not be able to rotate from one membrane face to the other at any appreciable rate since this would eliminate asymmetry. Restrictions on such transmembrane rotations have already been demonstrated experimentally for phospholipids (66,72). Similarly, the very large free energy of activation required for transmembrane rotation of integral proteins suggests that such a process would also be unlikely for these components. Consequently, the fluid mosaic structure exists as a highly oriented solution of lipids and proteins which permits specific functional components to be oriented at different faces of the membrane. Such an arrangement is therefore well suited to the vectorial flow of information across the cell surface.

Evidence obtained in several laboratories has shown that, in contrast to the limited capacity of membrane components to undergo transmembrane rotation, membrane components are free to undergo rapid and reversible lateral translational diffusion within the plane of the membrane in response to a wide range of physiologic stimuli and experimental perturbations (28, 29,31,70,80).

Different membrane components appear to move laterally at quite different rates. Phospholipids diffuse rapidly, each molecule exchanging with its neighbor about 10^7 times a second, although this may be modified within specific regions or "domains" within the bilayer resulting from lateral separation of different lipids into distinct physical phases or sequestration of phospholipids around integral proteins (80). A number of integral membrane proteins and glycoproteins are also able to diffuse laterally within the membrane but at much slower rates than the lipids, whereas certain proteins appear to be relatively immobile or "anchored" within the membrane (71,80).

Identification of the mechanisms involved in controlling the different mobilities of these components, notably the integral proteins and glycoproteins, may be of considerable importance for understanding some of the altered surface properties displayed by tumor cells, since there is an increasing body of evidence to indicate that the intramembrane mobility of some integral proteins and glycoproteins may be increased in neoplastic cells (70,71).

With the recognition that the lipid phase of the plasma membrane was fluid, several investigators proposed that changes in the fluidity of membrane lipids might regulate the mobility of membrane components and that the greater mobility of certain components found in tumor cells might reflect an increase in the fluidity of membrane lipids in these cells. Although such a proposal is not theoretically unreasonable, supporting evidence is still lacking. Despite claims for such differences (47), convincing evidence for a significant difference in the fluidity of bulk membrane lipids in tumor cells and their normal counterparts has yet to be obtained (41,70).

More satisfactory evidence has been obtained to indicate that the translational mobility of certain classes of integral membrane proteins is controlled by cytoplasmic cytoskeletal elements composed of microtubules and microfilaments that appear to be "linked" in some way to integral membrane proteins (26,28,29,61,70,72). This concept has been termed transmembrane cytoskeletal control because any regulatory influence exerted by cytoskeletal elements on the mobility of integral membrane components will simultaneously affect components on the outer face of the membrane that are transmembrane linked to this cytoskeletal system.

Transmembrane control of the topographic distribution of cell surface components offers a potential mechanism whereby the cell can maintain highly ordered topographic displays or "patterns" of molecules on the cell surface. Such patterns might determine the specificity of surface organization in different cell types and even specific regions of the same cell. The existence of cell-specific patterns of surface components could thus constitute an important mechanism for determining cell contact and recognition phenomena and for transmission of cell positional information in tissues. In addition, topographic redistribution of surface components might occur in response to various environmental stimuli, offering a mechanism for rapid and reversible modulation of cell surface properties after interaction of such agents as mitogens, serum factors, hormones, lectins, and antibodies with the cell surface and also in response to contact interactions with other cells (28,29,61,70,80).

Although a high degree of speculation must currently surround the interpretation of information on this subject, sufficient experimental data are already available to support a functional relation between the topography and dynamics of surface macromolecules and the control of cell surface properties (80). This leads logically to the question of whether perturbation of the transmembrane control mechanisms regulating the mobility and distribution of surface components might be responsible for certain of the altered surface properties exhibited by tumor cells. This question will be discussed in more detail below.

Surface Properties of Tumor Cells

The many differences in surface properties that have been found between transformed cells and their normal counterparts are summarized in Table 1.

Most of the data in Table 1 have been obtained from studies on cultured rodent or avian cell populations transformed *in vitro* by oncogenic viruses or chemical carcinogens. Less information is available on the properties of human cells exposed to similar agents *in vitro* or human cells cultured directly from tumor biopsy material.

As mentioned earlier, the definition of the "transformed" phenotype used in different studies has been highly variable. Thus many of the data in Table 1 refer to changes detected in "transformed" cells showing loss of growth control *in vitro*. Although many of the cells in question have been shown to be capable of producing tumors *in vivo*, it should be borne in mind that in many instances the data on tumorigenicity and cell surface properties were not obtained at the same time. Evidence for the tumorigenicity of cultured cell populations used to study surface properties is often based on earlier work, in many cases done by different investigators, using cells presumed to be of the same type but which were almost certainly at a different passage level and which may also have been exposed to different selection pressures due to the use of slightly different culture techniques. The variability of cell culture populations and the risk of new variants emerging during continuous passage and/or under different culture conditions have been mentioned already and require no further emphasis.

An intriguing concept that is beginning to emerge from studies done in several laboratories is that certain of the surface alterations found in transformed cells might not necessarily require the acquisition of new "tumor-specific" surface components but might instead result from topographic rearrangement(s) of the existing surface components found in normal cells. For example, certain of the so-called transformed characteristics such as loss of LETS protein (large external transformation-sensitive protein), enhanced agglutination by plant lectins, changes in plasma membrane glycolipids, altered membrane permeability and transport, and certain antigenic alterations expressed by viral and chemically transformed cells can also be detected in normal cells during mitosis and/or in interphase normal cells after brief treatment with proteases or infection by nontumor viruses (64,78,81, 86), and yet other surface properties appear to be shared by transformed cells and fetal cells at specific stages in ontogeny (85).

A number of observations suggest that transmembrane control of the mobility and distribution of cell surface receptors is altered by neoplastic transformation (70,80). In addition, recent observations made in several laboratories (70) suggest that the number and/or organization of membrane-associated cytoskeletal elements implicated as the transmembrane control mechanism is altered following transformation. Although a causal relationship has yet to be defined between this alteration and changes in receptor mobility, it is noteworthy that the mobility of several classes of integral membrane proteins is higher in transformed cells (70). Also, experimental perturbation of cytoskeletal elements in normal cells leads to increased receptor mobility similar to that in transformed cells (79,82).

A potentially important observation has been made in two recent studies (4,30) showing that the organization of the network of membrane-associated microfilaments and microtubules in cells transformed by temperature-sensitive mutants of Rous sarcoma virus reverts from a disordered state at permissive temperatures to an ordered state at nonpermissive temperatures. Ash et al. (4) further showed that addition of protein synthesis inhibitors to cells growing at permissive temperatures causes the cells to change from a transformed morphology to normal. Interestingly, this reversion is also accompanied by decreased mobility of lectin receptors on the cell surface and reversion of the cytoskeletal elements from a disordered to an ordered state. These results suggest that the synthesis of an unstable product of the transforming gene of the temperature-sensitive virus is required to maintain at least some features of the transformed phenotype. The data also suggest that the product of the transforming gene directly or indirectly causes a perturbation and disaggregation of the cytoskeletal elements involved in transmembrane control of receptor mobility.

The fact that several of the altered surface properties displayed by transformed cells can be detected in normal cells within only a few minutes of exposure to proteases strongly suggests that the expression of these properties in transformed cells need not involve acquisition of novel cell surface determinants requiring new pathways of genetic expression. Rather, expression of these properties in transformed cells could arise simply from topographic redistribution of already existing surface components. The only involvement of new pathways of genetic expression in contributing to these alterations might be in altering the basic mechanism(s) underlying control of protease release and/or the release of proteolysis amplification factors such as plasminogen activator (see below).

In drawing attention to the existence of surface properties shared by both normal and tumor cells, it is not suggested that the presence of these properties in tumor cells is irrelevant to the neoplastic process. The continuous expression in tumor cells of "normal" surface properties that are ordinarily expressed in a very restricted fashion by nontumorigenic cells is clearly abnormal. In focusing attention on the similarities between the surface properties of normal and tumor cells, it is helpful to question whether a common mechanism might be involved in the expression of such properties in both cell types. If this were so, it would indicate that at least some aspects of the neoplastic cell phenotype can arise via alterations in mechanisms also operating in normal cells, although in a highly regulated, temporally restricted, and phase-specific fashion. An important corollary to such a possibility is that by identification of a common mechanism it might prove feasible to modify the malignant phenotype by imposition of the normal regulation mechanism.

The finding that surface alterations similar to those found in transformed cells can be induced in normal cells by brief treatment of their surfaces with proteases raises the obvious question of whether proteolytic modification of the cell periphery might be involved in the expression of these properties in tumor cells. Thus, in normal cells proteolysis might be restricted to limited parts of the cell cycle, whereas in tumor cells proteolysis of the cell surface might be occurring continuously as a result of release of proteases (or activators of serum-derived proteases) throughout the cell cycle and perhaps also by enhanced production and release of proteases.

There have been several reports (88,89) indicating that tumor cells release significantly greater amounts of proteases and glycosidases than their normal counterparts. Whether these enzymes play any role in altering the cell surface is unknown. It has been shown that factors released by tumor cells can modify the surface properties of normal cells in the direction of the transformed phenotype and can also stimulate the growth of normal cells and that these effects can be mimicked by treating normal cells with trypsin and other proteases (88,89). Although this suggests that any proteases released by tumor cells could well modify the cell surface, formal identification of the above cell factors as proteases is still awaited.

More substantial evidence for the involvement of proteases in producing some of the altered surface properties and abnormal growth characteristics displayed by transformed cells has been provided by the demonstration in several laboratories that transformed cells release a factor that activates serum plasminogen to generate the protease plasmin (18,87,89). This observation is of interest since it introduces an amplification step in which a serum component serves as a substrate for the production of a protease that could then bind to the cell surface and directly alter it. That plasmin generated by this route is able to bind to the cell surface and induce proteolysis of membrane components has already been demonstrated (89). Furthermore, treatment of normal cells with purified plasmin has been shown to induce loss of a high molecular weight glycoprotein that is characteristically absent from transformed cells and also to enhance cellular susceptibility to agglutination by plant lectins (48,89). Finally, other recent experiments in which the properties of transformed cells were compared after growth in medium with complete serum and in medium with plasminogen-depleted serum have shown that plasmin-mediated proteolysis is necessary for expression of a number of the altered morphological and growth properties displayed by transformed cells (88,89).

In addition to the possible contribution of plasmin-mediated proteolysis in producing surface alterations in tumor cells, experiments showing stimulation of cell growth by purified thrombin and the appearance of certain "transformed" cell surface characteristics in normal cells after treatment with thrombin (16) suggest that we must also consider the possibility that the thromboplastin activity displayed by cells could also contribute to proteolysis of the cell periphery. Furthermore, since thrombin is capable of activating serum plasminogen to plasmin, cells that generate thrombin would probably also stimulate plasmin formation.

If proteolytic modification of the cell periphery is responsible for certain of the altered surface properties found in tumor cells, it should be possible to modify the expression of these properties by inhibition of the proteolytic process. This possibility has been tested in numerous laboratories by cultivating cells in the presence of a wide range of protease inhibitors. Although certain technical problems are not always recognized in treatment of cells with protease inhibitors, not least their cytotoxicity (89), a large number of experiments have successfully shown that the abnormal growth properties and social behavior of transformed cells, plus several of the altered surface properties displayed by these cells, are lost or significantly reversed after cultivation in medium supplemented with protease inhibitors (89).

These experiments provide impressive circumstantial evidence to suggest that the surfaces of transformed cells, at least in the *in vitro* situation, are subject to modification by proteases and that proteolysis is responsible for certain altered surface properties and perhaps other phenotypic abnormalities exhibited by these cells. Further support for the view that proteolysis of the cell periphery might be responsible for at least some of the altered surface properties found in transformed cells is provided by the observation that expression of similar "transformed" cell properties in normal cells after infection with nononcogenic viruses is prevented if the infected cells are incubated with protease inhibitors (78).

In view of the striking similarities between transformed cells and normal cells after treatment with proteases or nononcogenic viruses, it is tempting to speculate that the restricted expression of similar "transformed" surface characteristics by normal cells during mitosis might also result from proteolysis of the cell periphery. Unfortunately, information on this subject is extremely scant, but it may be pertinent that Allison (2) has shown that extracellular release of lysosomal enzymes occurs immediately before cells enter mitosis. The contribution of proteolytic modification of the cell surface to the malignant phenotype *in vivo* is unknown. Several studies have shown that the specific activities of lysosomal enzymes are often increased in tumors compared with their tissue of origin (77). These findings have prompted proposals that release of lysosomal enzymes might facilitate the invasion of normal tissue by tumor cells and also favor detachment of cells from the primary tumor, thereby increasing the risk of metastases (see Cell Surface Alterations and Metastasis, p. 34).

In pursuing the theme that proteolytic modifications of the cell periphery, together with alterations in the regulation of this process, are important in determining aspects of the malignant cell phenotype, it remains necessary to indicate how proteolysis of the surface might produce the range of surface alterations observed in tumor cells. If, as proposed, normal cell surface organization is dependent on a highly specific topographic distribution of surface components, disruption of this pattern by loss or altered mobility and redistribution of even one class of component would affect the spatial relationships of many surface components. The spectrum of alterations in surface properties that might accompany such topographic redistribution would no doubt increase further if the mobility of a number of surface components were not subject to transmembrane control.

The disruption of preexisting topographic relationships of components on the cell surface by proteases could occur as a reversible phenomenon, whose duration would be restricted by the period of active proteolysis of the cell surface. Such a mechanism might explain the expression of "transformed" cell properties on normal cells during mitosis, whereas the continued expression of "mitotic" surface properties in tumor cells during interphase could be interpreted as indicating that proteolysis is occurring continuously. In either situation, proteolysis, by inducing topographic redistribution of surface components, could serve as a pleiotropic stimulus initiating a wide range of cell surface and metabolic alterations (55,75).

Many elements of the proposals presented above remain to be proven. Additional information is required to answer several important questions. If proteolysis of the cell periphery is responsible for some (or perhaps all) of the altered surface characteristics displayed both by cells and by normal cells during mitosis, then we might profitably investigate the cellular mechanisms involved in regulating the release of proteases, particularly in normal cells. However, as discussed later (p. 42), evidence is already available which suggests that plasminogen activator release by transformed cells may not be correlated with their tumorigenicity *in vivo*. It also remains to be shown precisely how proteolysis of components on the external face of the plasma membrane might alter the linkage of membrane components to regulatory elements on the inside of the membrane. Finally, more information is needed on the range of surface alterations that can result from dislocation of linkages between integral membrane components and membrane-associated cytoskeletal elements.

CELL SURFACE ALTERATIONS AND METASTASIS

Metastasis formation involves the sequential release of cells from the primary tumor, their dissemination to distant sites, and their arrest, survival, and proliferation in these new locations. The surface properties of cancer cells, as well as those of the host cells with which they interact, are thought to play an important role in determining each of these steps in the metastatic process.

Invasiveness is a fundamental attribute of malignant cells which confers on them the ability not only to infiltrate local tissue interstices but also to penetrate blood and lymphatic channels and the body cavities. Most experimental observations on the invasive behavior of tumor cells have focused on three aspects of cellular function: (a) motility, (b) adhesiveness, and (c) the production of lytic substances that may modify surrounding normal tissues to facilitate infiltration.

The simple enlargement of a tumor as a result of unchecked cell proliferation undoubtedly creates conditions at the tumor margin in which tumor cells are literally forced into the surrounding tissue. The development of edema at the edge of a tumor might also be expected to open up tissue spaces, thus facilitating the access of tumor cells to preformed tissue spaces. In addition, the well-known rounding up of mitotic cells and their decreased attachment to other cells (and substrates) might augment passive infiltration of this kind. It is clear, however, that rapid proliferation *per se* does not confer invasive potential. Regenerating adult tissues such as liver as well as embryonic tissues transplanted into adult hosts display mitotic rates which far exceed that of the most rapidly growing tumor, yet they do not invade. Conversely, certain tumors may characteristically show marked infiltration of normal tissues yet grow very slowly (114).

Active movement of tumor cells into surrounding tissues is generally acknowledged to be of major importance in invasion, but little information is available on the factors controlling cell locomotion *in vitro* yet alone *in vivo*. Even the well-publicized concept that the invasive behavior of tumor cells reflects the fact that they are no longer subject to contact inhibition of locomotion in the same way as normal cells can no longer be accepted as a valid generalization (106).

The trend in the literature has been to place considerable emphasis on the infiltration of tissues by single tumor cells. Examination of the literature suggests, however, that invasion of tissues by advancing multicellular tongues or cords of tumor cells may be equally or perhaps even more common (106). Progress of tumor tongues or whole tumor fronts is probably mediated by movement of cells at the edges of the cell sheet in a fashion analogous to the morphogenetic cell movements seen during epiboly in the early embryo (106). Locomotion of aggregates of tumor cells must also be considered (27,32).

The stimulus for tumor cell locomotion is unknown. Although cell proliferation and locomotion are normally under strict homeostatic regulation, the two processes need not be coupled. Experiments on cultured cells have shown that fibroblast locomotion can be stimulated in the absence of proliferation (43,60) and proliferation can be induced without accompanying locomotion (117). On the other hand, factors have been isolated from cultures of transformed cells that stimulate both proliferation and locomotion (13).

Whatever the stimulus for the initial invasion of surrounding tissues, further dissemination of tumor cells requires their separation from the primary tumor, either as single cells or as multicellular aggregates. Whether or not malignant cells will separate from the primary tumor depends on whether the forces promoting separation generated by such factors as cell and tissue movements, lytic enzymes, muscular contractions, or surgical handling exceed the cohesive-adhesive forces holding tumor cells together within the primary tumor.

Unfortunately, there has been an uncritical acceptance, notably in the clinical literature [for example, see p. 2 of the textbook by Willis (114)], of the concept that cancer cells are less adhesive than their normal counterparts and that this facilitates their separation and the eventual formation of metastases. This view originates from the work of Coman (21) who showed that cells could be detached more easily from certain carcinomas than from corresponding tissues. Coman interpreted this finding as indicating that the mutual adhesion of malignant cells was defective, hence their tendency to metastasize. Coman also suggested that defective cell adhesion was due in part to the paucity of hypothetical intercellular calcium "bridges" between the surfaces of adjacent cancer cells. However, Coman's experiments suffer from a number of limitations. The cells were pulled apart with small hooks in traumatic fashion, trauma was not rate controlled, too few different types of malignant cells were examined, and the validity and viability of at least some of his controls are doubtful. In addition, the basic hypothesis that cancer cells bind less calcium than normal cells is incorrect (110). Indeed, no meaningful information is yet available on the relative adhesiveness of normal and tumor cells. This situation reflects the technical problem that present methods for the measurement of cell adhesion, whether to other cells or to solid surfaces, do not measure the *strength* of adhesion(s) and measure only the *rate* at which stable adhesions are formed.

Of the possible factors responsible for cell separation, release from mechanical confinement will be considered first. Mutual attachment of cells within tissues is probably achieved both via specialized cell junctions and by submicroscopic physicochemical bonds between charged moieties on the surfaces of adjacent cells. Junctions in tumors can be markedly reduced compared to the corresponding normal tissue, but this is by no means a general finding (109). The suggested role of gap junctions as pathways for cell-to-cell communication and growth control (92) also introduces the additional possibility that defective junction formation might influence tumor cell behavior via more subtle pathways than mechanical restraint.

The use of various enzymes to disperse organized tissues into single cells for tissue culture prompts the question of whether the increased levels of various lytic enzymes found in many tumors (see below) might promote cell separation and detachment by weakening cell-to-cell adhesions and also facilitate invasion by breaking down the surrounding extracellular matrix. Several studies have shown that the intercellular regions of solid tumors contain a variety of enzymes capable of modifying cell surface properties and facilitating cell separation, although the amounts of enzymes vary markedly according to differences in local vascularity and the extent of necrosis (77,104,113). Prominent among the enzymes are the lysosomal hydrolases (77), release of which has been shown to promote cell detachment *in vitro* and to promote metastasis *in vivo* (113).

The possible role of proteases and collagenolytic enzymes released by tumor cells in modifying surrounding normal tissues so as to facilitate tumor cell invasion has also attracted attention (101). However, as with virtually all aspects of tumor cell behavior, generalization is difficult. Morphological observations of tumor cell invasion have revealed a broad pattern of behavior ranging from complete lack of lytic activity (15) to massive destruction of host tissues (114).

With the finding that many transformed cells display enhanced fibrinolytic activity due to an increased production of plasminogen activator, interest has been stimulated in the possibility that this property might facilitate tumor cell invasion and metastasis. However, as discussed later (p. 42), the correlation between plasminogen activator production and tumorigenicity is by no means certain. In addition, studies on plasminogen activator production by cloned B16 mouse melanoma variants selected for high and low invasive and metastatic potential have failed to reveal any correlation between these two properties (73).

Once metastasizing tumor cells have gained entry into the circulation, their surface properties will influence their interaction with other tumor cells, the various blood cells, the vascular endothelium, and factors in the circulation such as hormones and antibodies. These interactions assume varying importance in determining both the extent and location of metastatic foci.

Only a small fraction [< 1% in one study (33)] of circulating malignant cells survive to establish metastases. The mere presence of tumor cells in the circulation is not an indication that they will be able to implant and proliferate. Indeed, the frequency of circulating tumor cells in patients with malignancies does not show a reliable correlation with the development of metastases (35,90). In order to survive, circulating tumor cells must attach to the vascular endothelium and "escape" from the bloodstream. Two major factors act to impede contact and adhesion between the tumor cells and the vascular endothelium: the considerable mutual electrostatic repulsion generated by their net negative surface charges, and the boundary layer created at the endothelial surface by the moving stream of plasma (50,112). However, the fact that malignant cells do form hematogenous metastases indicates that they must succeed in adhering to the vascular endothelium, in spite of these viscous and electrostatic barriers.

Many observations of both human and animal tumors indicate that the arrest of tumor emboli in capillary beds is in some way associated with thrombogenesis. Arrested tumor emboli commonly are seen surrounded by fibrin and platelets (for references see review in 17). The possible role of microcoagulation around tumor cells as a major factor in arrest of tumor cell emboli is also supported by experimental data showing that a variety of anticoagulants have inhibitory effects on metastasis (see 37 and 90 for references). Boeryd (7) has cautioned that anticoagulants may merely alter the pattern of tumor cell arrest rather than reduce the total number of cells which become arrested (but see 36 and 52 for a conflicting view).

Although the formation of fibrin around tumor cells and the formation of adhesions with platelets and other tumor cells may promote the arrest of tumor cell emboli, the surface properties of the vascular endothelium appear to influence cell arrest. Warren (107) showed that adhesion of emboli composed of tumor cells and platelets to intact vascular endothelium was characterized by negligible production of fibrin and the emboli deteriorated rapidly. On the other hand, on areas of damaged or absent endothelium, the tumor cell–platelet emboli became firmly embedded in fibrin, and progressive passage of tumor cells through the fibrin layer and the vessel wall was observed. It is possible therefore that the fibrinolytic activity of intact endothelium (5) impedes the adhesion of tumor cells.

The possibility that tumor cells can modify the surface properties of vascular endothelium must also be considered. For example, retraction of endothelial or mesothelial cells can lead to exposure of the deeper layers of the vessel wall, and adhesion of tumor cells to such denuded areas has been seen in several studies (for references see 12 and 62). Although the exact causes of cellular retraction are unknown, endothelial contraction can be induced experimentally by histamine-type mediators and by thrombin (63, 93). Thus if tumor cells are able (directly or indirectly) to produce similar agents this may enable them to convert the relatively nonadhesive endothelial and mesothelial surfaces to a more suitable substrate for cell adhesion and arrest.

Detailed quantitative studies on the distribution and fate of radiolabeled tumor cells have shown that the site(s) of tumor cell arrest and implantation are nonrandom for many types of circulating cancer cells (35). There is also a large body of clinical observations which indicate that comparable tumors at similar sites in different patients exhibit a general tendency to metastasize to the same set of organs. These observations have given rise to the view that disseminating tumor cells may have special affinities for the organs in which they establish metastatic foci. The strongest evidence in support of this concept has come from the experiments of Fidler (35) who has success- fully selected a series of B16 mouse melanoma cell variants with enhanced metastatic capacity for particular organ systems. Nicolson et al. (73) have presented evidence that the enhanced metastatic behavior seen in these B16 mouse melanoma variants may reflect alterations in their cell surface characteristics. Comparison of high and low metastatic B16 variants re- vealed that high metastatic cell populations aggregated at faster rates both in homotypic cell mixtures and in heterotypic interactions with lymphocytes and platelets. The enhanced aggregation seen with these cells might well account for their higher metastatic potential since this property would favor the formation of multicellular emboli which are known to be more successful on a per cell basis in establishing metastases (34).

Once arrested, tumor emboli must penetrate the vessel wall in order to establish foci of viable cells in the surrounding tissues. The final phase of metastasis formation involves cell proliferation and the subsequent enlarge- ment of the metastatic focus. At this stage the vascularization and nutrition of metastatic foci (38) and their susceptibility to immunologic attack be- come important in determining the extent of growth.

The fact that cancer cells express novel tumor-associated antigens (Table 1) should result in their detection and destruction by the host immune ap- paratus. Theoretically, there are several mechanisms by which tumor cells might overcome the immune surveillance mechanisms of the host (54,59). Of obvious relevance to the present chapter are examples in which antigenic determinants are shed from the cell surface or are "masked" or redistributed in such a way as to reduce the ability of the host's immune systems to either detect or destroy the cell (or both).

Antigenic modulation is probably the best known example in which neo- plastic cells develop (or, more likely, preexisting cells possessing those characteristics are selected for survival in the face of an immune challenge, see 54) "immunoevasive" surface properties. Antigenic modulation occurs when certain tumor cells are exposed to antibodies against cell surface anti- gens; they then rapidly become insensitive to the cytotoxic effects of com- plement (74). Stackpole et al. (99) have examined the modulation of surface antigens on mouse lymphoma cells and found that antigens such as thymus- leukemia (TL) which undergo modulation are characterized by a relatively rapid mobility within the membrane and are easily redistributed by anti- bodies to form patches and caps. The ease with which TL antigens are re- distributed may well account for tumor cell escape from complement-mediated immunologic killing because a correct distribution and disposition of adjacent antibody molecules bound at the cell surface is necessary to initiate fixation of complement components (102). Capping or patching of antigens probably prevents complement binding by aggregating antigens and antibodies into large, immobilized complexes so that steric hindrance or antibody molecular distortions are deterred. Conversely, lack of antigen-antibody lateral mobility would inhibit close approach of surface-bound antibody molecules, again prohibiting complement attachment.

Another important means of tumor cell escape from immune destruction is by shedding of antigens or antigen-antibody complexes from the cell surface. These shed components or complexes make up a family of so-called blocking factors that interfere with host immunity against neoplasia, and their presence in the host above critical levels can result in effective neutralization of the cell-mediated arm of immunity against tumor cells (84).

Finally, the "masking" of new tumor antigens by other surface components has been proposed on several occasions as a possible mechanism permitting escape of tumor cells from immune surveillance. However, critical examination of the pertinent literature fails to provide any compelling evidence for this phenomenon [see review by Weiss (111)].

UNSOLVED PROBLEMS

Despite the large number of surface differences identified between normal and tumor cells over the past decade (Table 1), we still have little insight into how surface differences arise in tumor cells or how they are maintained. We are also ignorant of how individual alterations in surface properties contribute to the complex multicomponent phenotypic traits of tumorigenicity, invasiveness, and metastasis. For example, is the increased rate of plasma membrane transport found in many transformed cells (Table 1) fundamental to the ability of these cells to cause tumors? It may be that this alteration merely confers a useful growth advantage on tumor cells when competing with normal cells for nutrients and as such is unrelated to tumor formation *per se*. The same question could be asked of the many other surface changes identified in transformed cells *in vitro*.

These shortcomings in our understanding of the role of particular surface changes in determining the neoplastic phenotype stem largely from the widespread failure to supplement *in vitro* studies on cell surface properties with observations on the behavior of the same cells transplanted *in vivo*. Although the problems associated with transplantation of cells into immunocompetent hosts referred to earlier (p. 25) have probably contributed to this situation, the use of the nude mouse for assaying cellular tumorigenicity completely eliminates these earlier difficulties. Thus, with the availability of a simple and convenient system for routine testing of the tumorigenicity of both human and animal cells, it may be an appropriate time to reevaluate certain aspects of current research on cell surface changes in neoplasia. Rather than devote our entire research effort in this area to the search for yet more surface changes in transformed cells or to analyzing known surface alterations in more and more detailed molecular terms, it might be equally profitable to evaluate which of the many surface changes already identified in transformed cells are related to the ability of these cells to form tumors. Once this classification is completed, the next step would be to attempt to identify which surface changes are related to loss of growth control as opposed to invasiveness or metastatic capacity.

Although the assay of tumorigenicity is relatively straightforward, experimental characterization of the invasive properties of tumor cells in mammalian hosts is still difficult. Direct observation of local tissue invasion by tumor cells when injected into the capillary bed of transparent tissues such as the omentum or the rabbit ear chamber has been attempted. However, in most instances only the traffic of tumor cells within capillaries has been observed and little information has been obtained on the process(es) of cellular penetration through the vessel wall and subsequent infiltration of the perivascular tissues. Also, observations of cell behavior over several days are virtually impossible in this system. A number of ultrastructural studies of tumor cell arrest and penetration of blood vessels have also been reported (17). These have provided some insight into the structural nature of the initial adhesion of tumor cells to vascular endothelia and also on the route(s) of egress of tumor cells from capillaries. However, the static nature of all morphologic observations limits their value in revealing the cellular mechanisms underlying invasion.

The most useful assay for cellular invasiveness available at present is based on the infiltrative properties of cells when inoculated into the chorioallantoic membrane (CAM) of 8- to 10-day-old embryonated eggs (3,27,91). The ability of cells to invade the cell layers of the CAM also shows a good correlation with their tumorigenicity in nude mice (G. Poste, *unpublished observations*). Mareel et al. (65) have described a similar assay in which cells are grafted into the chick embryo blastoderm. Less complex *in vitro* assays involving the infiltration of tumor cells in organ cultures (117) or cell aggregates (44) have also been described, but the correlation between invasiveness in these situations and tumorigenicity *in vivo* has not been defined.

From this brief outline, it is clear that at least a minimum number of suitable assay systems are now available for correlating expression of particular cell surface properties *in vitro* with the ability to cause tumors, invade, and metastasize *in vivo*. Although such correlations can, of course, be made simply by mass screening of the *in vivo* growth properties of a large range of transformed cell populations with known surface characteristics, the same goal can perhaps be achieved more efficiently using transformed cell populations which have been deliberately selected for particular surface properties or combinations of properties. Similarly, *in vivo* selection for tumor cells showing particular behavioral patterns *in vivo* (see below) offers equally valuable material for *in vitro* studies.

Several systems of this kind are already available. Revertant transformed cells showing loss of some, but not all, of their transformed characteristics are particularly useful since cloned revertants displaying differing combinations of surface alterations can be isolated. By comparing the *in vivo* growth behavior and surface properties of revertants with the wild-type transformed parent cells and the original untransformed cell population, it should be possible to correlate the presence or absence of specific surface changes with tumor formation and/or metastasis *in vivo*.

The same strategy can be used with somatic cell hybrids produced by fusion of combinations of normal and transformed cells, transformed cells and revertant cells, and normal and revertant cells. Cloned hybrid cell lines produced from these cell combinations will express differing surface characteristics and exhibit differing tumorigenicity. Thus comparing the *in vivo* growth behavior of different hybrids it should again be possible to establish reliable correlations between expression of particular surface properties and the ability or inability of the cells to form tumors and to metastasize. The results of several studies using this type of experimental approach have been reported recently. These studies (40,57,94) indicate that the one *in vitro* property that consistently correlates with tumorigenicity *in vivo* is the ability of cells to form colonies in a semisolid growth medium such as methylcellulose (i.e., loss of anchorage dependence). Pollack et al. (76) have shown that loss of anchorage dependence in SV40-transformed rat cells also correlates with enhanced production of plasminogen activator, and they suggested that the latter property was probably also correlated with tumorigenicity. However, as discussed below, the correlation of plasminogen activator production with the neoplastic phenotype is by no means certain. Indeed, the correlation between loss of anchorage dependence and plasminogen activator production described by Pollack et al. for transformed rat cells does not appear to apply to all virally transformed cells. For example, Wolf and Goldberg (115) have described a series of cloned Rous sarcoma virus-transformed chick cells with low, intermediate, and high levels of plasminogen activator production which all grew equally well in methylcellulose.

Other parameters used to define loss of cell growth control *in vitro,* such as growth to high saturation density and ability to grow in low serum containing medium, do *not* show a close correlation with cellular tumorigenicity in nude mice (16,94,100).

Chen et al. (16) have claimed that the ability of a series of adenovirus-transformed cell lines to form tumors in nude mice is correlated with loss or marked reduction in the amount of LETS protein on the cell surface. However, observations on the relationship between expression of LETS protein and tumorigenicity in a series of chemically transformed mouse fibroblasts have failed to establish such a correlation (57).

Similar ambiguity surrounds the functional relationship between plasminogen activator production and tumorigenicity. Studies in several laboratories have detected enhanced production of plasminogen activator in cultures of human tumor cells and animal cells transformed *in vitro* by a variety of agents (89), prompting a variety of proposals that this enzyme may be important in malignancy. Some support for a functional relationship between production of plasminogen activator and tumorigenicity has been obtained by Christman et al. (18). These investigators found that suppression of tumorigenicity in B16 mouse melanoma cells by BrdU was accompanied by reduction in plasminogen activator production. It is clear, however, that enhanced production of plasminogen activator is not a general marker for tumorigenicity. Tumorigenic clones of human fibrosarcoma cells with low plasminogen activator activity have been described (57), whereas nontumorigenic (16) diploid lung and kidney cells produce high levels of plasminogen activator (5,6). Indeed, fibrinolytic activity is associated with a diverse range of normal cell types and may play a role in normal tissue repair processes (5).

Work on the *in vivo* selection of tumor cell variants displaying particular growth properties is just beginning. The feasibility of this approach has been demonstrated by the work of Fidler (35) mentioned earlier, in which a series of B16 mouse melanoma variants showing an increased capacity to form lung metastases in syngeneic C57B216 mice has been isolated. The application of similar *in vivo* selection methods to other metastasizing tumors, together with the isolation of variants that metastasize preferentially to specific target organs, is now emerging as a major area of research activity. It is thus anticipated that data obtained over the next few years from correlative *in vitro* and *in vivo* experiments using cell variants of this kind will substantially improve our understanding of the functional importance of cell surface changes in influencing the various stages of the metastatic process.

REFERENCES

1. Algire, G. H., Weaver, J. M., and Prehn, R. T. (1954): Growth of cells in in vivo diffusion chambers. 1. Survival of homografts in immunized mice. *J. Natl. Cancer Inst.,* 15:493–503.
2. Allison, A. C. (1969): Lysosomes and cancer. In: *Lysosomes in Biology and Pathology,* Vol. 2, edited by J. T. Dingle and H. B. Fell, pp. 178–204. North-Holland, Amsterdam.
3. Ambrose, E. J., and Easty, D. M. (1976): Cellular dynamics of human breast carcinoma. In: *Human Tumours in Short Term Culture,* edited by P. Dendy, pp. 45–54. Academic Press, London.
4. Ash, J. F., Vogt, P. K., and Singer, S. J. (1976): Reversion from transformed to normal phenotype by inhibition of protein synthesis in rat kidney cells infected with a tempera-

ture-sensitive mutant of Rous sarcoma virus. *Proc. Natl. Acad. Sci. U.S.A.*, 73:3603–3607.

5. Astrup, T. (1975): Cell-induced fibrinolysis: A fundamental process. In: *Proteases and Biological Control*, edited by E. Reich, D. B. Rifkin, and E. Shaw, pp. 343–356. Cold Spring Harbor Laboratory, New York.

6. Barlow, G. H., Reuter, A., and Tribby, I. (1975): Production of plasminogen activator by tissue culture techniques. In: *Proteases and Biological Control*, edited by E. Reich, D. B. Rifkin, and E. Shaw, pp. 325–332. Cold Spring Harbor Laboratory, New York.

7. Boeryd, B. (1965): Action of heparin and plasminogen inhibitor (EACA) on metastatic tumour spread in an isologous system. *Acta Pathol. Microbiol. Scand.*, 65:395–404.

8. Boone, C. W. (1975): Malignant hemangioendotheliomas produced by subcutaneous inoculation of BALB/3T3 cells attached to glass beads. *Science*, 188:68–70.

9. Boone, C. W., Takeichi, N., Paranjpe, M., and Gilden, R. (1976): Vasoformative sarcomas arising from BALB/3T3 cells attached to solid substrates. *Cancer Res.*, 36:1626–1633.

10. Brady, R. O., and Fishman, P. H. (1974): Biosynthesis of glycolipids in virus-transformed cells. *Biochim. Biophys. Acta*, 355:121–148.

11. Bretscher, M. S., and Raff, M. C. (1975): Mammalian plasma membranes. *Nature*, 258:43–49.

12. Buck, R. C. (1973): Walker 256 tumor transplantation in normal and injured peritoneum studied by electron microscopy, scanning EM and radioautography. *Cancer Res.*, 33:3181–3188.

13. Bürk, R. R. (1973): A factor from a transformed cell line that affects migration. *Proc. Natl. Acad. Sci. U.S.A.*, 70:369–371.

14. Cailleau, R. M. (1975): Old and new problems in human tumor cell cultivation. In: *Human Tumor Cells in Vitro*, edited by J. Fogh, pp. 79–114. Plenum Press, New York.

15. Carr, I., McGinty, F., and Norris, P. (1976): The fine structure of neoplastic invasion: Invasion of liver, skeletal muscle and lymphatic vessels by the Rd/3 tumor. *J. Pathol.*, 118:91–99.

16. Chen, L. B., Gallimore, P. H., and McDougall, J. K. (1976): Correlation between tumor induction and the large external transformation sensitive protein on the cell surface. *Proc. Natl. Acad. Sci. U.S.A.*, 73:3570–3574.

17. Chew, E. C., Josephson, R. L., and Wallace, A. C. (1976): Morphologic aspects of the arrest of circulating cancer cells. In: *Fundamental Aspects of Metastasis*, edited by L. Weiss, pp. 121–150. North-Holland, Amsterdam.

18. Christman, J. K., Acs, G., Silagi, S., and Silverstein, S. C. (1975): Plasminogen activator: Biochemical characterization and correlation with tumorigenicity. In: *Proteases and Biological Control*, edited by E. Reich, D. B. Rifkin, and E. Shaw, pp. 827–839. Cold Spring Harbor Laboratory, New York.

19. Clarkson, B., and Baserga, R. (Eds.) (1974): *Control of Proliferation in Animal Cells*. Cold Spring Harbor Laboratory, New York.

20. Coggin, J. H., Jr., and Anderson, N. G. (1974): Cancer, differentiation and embryonic antigens: Some central problems. *Adv. Cancer Res.*, 19:105–165.

21. Coman, D. R. (1944): Decreased mutual adhesiveness, a property of cells from squamous cell carcinomas. *Cancer Res.*, 4:625–629.

22. Critchley, D. R., and Vicker, M. G. (1977): Glycolipids as membrane receptors important in growth regulation and cell-cell interactions. In: *Dynamic Aspects of Cell Surface Organization*, edited by G. Poste and G. L. Nicolson, pp. 307–370. North-Holland, Amsterdam.

23. Defendi, V., Lehman, J., and Kraemer, P. (1963): "Morphologically" normal hamster cells with malignant properties. *Virology*, 19:592–598.

24. De Meyts, P. (1976): Cooperative properties of hormone receptors in cell membranes. *J. Supramol. Struct.*, 4:241–258.

25. Dendy, P. P. (Ed.) (1976): *Human Tumours in Short Term Culture*. Academic Press, London.

26. De Petris, S. (1977): Distribution and mobility of plasma membrane components on lymphocytes. In: *Dynamic Aspects of Cell Surface Organization*, edited by G. Poste and G. L. Nicolson. North-Holland, Amsterdam (*in press*).

27. Easty, D. M., and Easty, G. C. (1974): Measurement of the ability of cells to infiltrate normal tissues in vitro. *Br. J. Cancer,* 29:36–49.
28. Edelman, G. M. (1974): Origins and mechanisms of specificity in clonal selection. In: *Cellular Selection and Regulation in the Immune Response,* edited by G. M. Edelman, pp. 1–38. Raven Press, New York.
29. Edelman, G. M. (1976): Surface modulation in cell recognition and cell growth. *Science,* 192:218–226.
30. Edelman, G. M., and Yahara, I. (1976): Temperature-sensitive changes in surface modulating assemblies of fibroblasts transformed by mutants of Rous sarcoma virus. *Proc. Natl. Acad. Sci. U.S.A.,* 73:2047–2051.
31. Edidin, M. (1974): Rotational and translational diffusion in membranes. *Annu. Rev. Biophys. Bioeng.,* 3:179–201.
32. Enterline, H. T., and Coman, D. R. (1950): The ameboid motility of human and animal neoplastic cells. *Cancer,* 3:1033–1039.
33. Fidler, I. J. (1970): Metastasis: Quantitative analysis of distribution and fate of tumor emboli labeled with ^{125}1-5-iodo-2′-deoxyuridine. *J. Natl. Cancer Inst.,* 45:775–782.
34. Fidler, I. J. (1973): The relationship of embolic homogeneity, number, size and viability to the incidence of experimental metastasis. *Eur. J. Cancer* 9:223–227.
35. Fidler, I. J. (1976): Patterns of tumor cell arrest and development. In: *Fundamental Aspects of Metastasis,* edited by L. Weiss, pp. 275–289. North-Holland, Amsterdam.
36. Fisher, B., and Fisher, E. R. (1967): Anticoagulants and tumor cell lodgement. *Cancer Res.,* 27:421–425.
37. Fisher, B., and Fisher, E. R. (1976): Metastasis revisited. In: *Fundamental Aspects of Metastasis,* edited by L. Weiss, pp. 427–435. North-Holland, Amsterdam.
38. Folkman, J. (1974): Tumor angiogenesis. *Adv. Cancer Res.* 19:331–358.
39. Folkman, J., and Greenspan, H. P. (1975): Influence of geometry on control of cell growth. *Biochim. Biophys. Acta,* 417:211–236.
40. Freedman, V. H., and Shin, S. (1974): Cellular tumorigenicity in *nude* mice: correlation with cell growth in semi-solid medium. *Cell,* 3:355–359.
41. Gaffney, B. J., Branton, P. E., Wickus, G. G., and Hirschberg, C. B. (1974): Fluid lipid regions in normal and Rous sarcoma virus transformed chick embryo fibroblasts. In: *Viral Transformation and Endogenous Viruses,* edited by A. S. Kaplan, pp. 97–115. Academic Press, New York.
42. Gahmberg, C. G. (1977): Cell surface proteins: Changes during cell growth and malignant transformation. In: *Dynamic Aspects of Cell Surface Organization,* edited by G. Poste and G. L. Nicolson, pp. 371–421. North-Holland, Amsterdam.
43. Gail, M. H., and Boone, C. W. (1971): Density inhibition of motility in 3T3 fibroblasts and their SV40 transformants. *Exp. Cell Res.,* 64:156–162.
44. Gershman, H., and Drumm, J. (1975): Mobility of normal and virus-transformed cells in cellular aggregates. *J. Cell Biol.,* 67:419–435.
45. Giovanella, B. C., and Stehlin, J. S. (1974): Influence of the host's sex on the growth of human tumors heterotransplanted in "nude" thymusless mice. *Proc. Am. Assoc. Cancer Res.,* 15:23–25.
46. Giovanella, B. C., Stehlin, J. S., and Williams, L. J. (1974): Heterotransplantation of human malignant tumors in "nude" thymusless mice. II. Malignant tumors induced by injection of cell cultures derived from human solid tumors. *J. Natl. Cancer Inst.,* 52:921–927.
47. Glick, M. C. (1976): Cell surface changes associated with malignancy. In: *Fundamental Aspects of Metastasis,* edited by L. Weiss, pp. 9–23. North-Holland, Amsterdam.
48. Goldberg, A. R. (1974): Increased protease levels in transformed cells: A casein overlay assay for the detection of plasminogen activator production. *Cell,* 2:95–104.
49. Goldman, R., Pollard, T., and Rosenbaum, J. (Eds.) (1976): *Cell Motility. Cold Spring Harbor Conferences on Cell Proliferation,* Vol. 3. Cold Spring Harbor Laboratory, New York.
50. Goldsmith, H. L. (1976): Collisions of circulating cells with the vascular endothelium. In: *Fundamental Aspects of Metastasis,* edited by L. Weiss, pp. 99–120. North-Holland, Amsterdam.
51. Hakomori, S. I. (1973): Glycolipids of tumor cell membrane. *Adv. Cancer Res.,* 18:265–315.

52. Hilgard, P. (1973): The role of blood platelets in experimental metastases. *Br. J. Cancer*, 28:429–435.
53. Holley, R. W. (1975): Control of growth of mammalian cells in cell culture. *Nature*, 258:487–490.
54. Hyman, R. (1977): Somatic genetic analysis of the surface antigens of murine lymphoid tumors. In: *Dynamic Aspects of Cell Surface Organization*, edited by G. Poste and G. L. Nicolson, pp. 513–549. North-Holland, Amsterdam.
55. Hynes, R. O. (1976): Cell surface proteins and malignant transformation. *Biochim. Biophys. Acta*, 458:73–107.
56. Jarrett, O., and Macpherson, I. (1968): The basis of the tumorigenicity of BHK21 cells. *Int. J. Cancer*, 3:654–662.
57. Jones, P. A., Laug, W. E., Gardner, A., Nye, C. A., Fink, L. M., and Benedict, W. F. (1976): *In Vitro* correlates of transformation in C3H/10T½ clone 8 mouse cells. *Cancer Res.*, 36:2863–2867.
58. Kaighn, M. E. (1975): 'Birth of a culture'—source of postpartum anomalies. *J. Natl. Cancer Inst.*, 53:1437–1442.
59. Klein, G. (1975): Immunological surveillance against neoplasia. *Harvey Lect.*, 65:71–102.
60. Lipton, A., Klinger, I., Paul, D., and Holley, R. W. (1971): Migration of mouse 3T3 fibroblasts in response to a serum factor. *Proc. Natl. Acad. Sci. U.S.A.*, 68:2799–2801.
61. Loor, F., and Roelants, G. E. (Eds.) (1977): *B and T Cells in Immune Recognition*. John Wiley & Sons, Chichester, England (*in press*).
62. Lunscken, C., and Strauli, P. (1975): Penetration of an ascitic reticulum cell sarcoma of the golden hamster into the body wall and through the diaphragm. *Virchows Arch. [Pathol. Anat.]*, 17:247–259.
63. Majno, G., Sheg, S. M., and Leventhal, M. (1969): Endothelial contraction induced by histamine-type mediators; an electron microscopic study. *J. Cell Biol.*, 42:647–672.
64. Mannino, R. J., and Burger, M. M. (1975): Cell surface changes accompanying mitosis and transformation: Possible involvement in growth control. In: *Regulation of Growth and Differentiated Function in Eukaryote Cells*, edited by G. P. Talwar, pp. 27–39. Raven Press, New York.
65. Mareel, M., Vakaet, L. and DeRidder, L. (1976): Characterization of malignancy through transplantation into young chick blastoderms. In: *Biological Characterization of Human Tumors*, edited by W. Davis and C. Maltoni, pp. 367–369. Excerpta Medica, Amsterdam.
66. McConnell, H. M. (1975): Coupling between lateral and perpendicular motion in biological membranes. In: *Functional Linkage in Biomolecular Systems*, edited by F. O. Schmitt, D. M. Schneider, and D. M. Crothers, pp. 123–131. Raven Press, New York.
67. Merenda, C., Sordat, B., Mach, J. P., and Carrel, S. (1975): Human endometrial carcinomas serially transplanted in nude mice and established in continuous cell lines. *Int. J. Cancer*, 16:559–570.
68. New Horizons for Tissue Culture in Cancer Research. (1974): *J. Natl. Cancer Inst.*, 53:1429–1519.
69. Nicolson, G. L. (1974): The interactions of lectins with animal cell surfaces. *Int. Rev. Cytol.*, 39:89–190.
70. Nicolson, G. L. (1976): Trans-membrane control of the receptors on normal and tumor cells. II. Surface changes associated with transformation and malignancy. *Biochim. Biophys. Acta*, 458:1–71.
71. Nicolson, G. L., and Poste, G. (1976): Medical progress: The cancer cell: Dynamic aspects and modifications in cell surface organization. *New Engl. J. Med.*, 295:197–203 and 253–258.
72. Nicolson, G. L., Poste, G., and Ji, T. H. (1977): The dynamics of cell membrane organization. In: *Dynamic Aspects of Cell Surface Organization*, edited by G. Poste and G. L. Nicolson, pp. 1–73. North-Holland, Amsterdam.
73. Nicolson, G. L., Winkelhake, J. L., and Nussey, A. C. (1976): An approach to studying the cellular properties associated with metastasis: Some in vitro properties of tumor variants selected in vivo for enhanced metastasis. In: *Fundamental Aspects of Metastasis*, edited by L. Weiss, pp. 291–303. North-Holland, Amsterdam.
74. Old, L. J., Stockert, E., and Boyse, E. A. (1968): Antigenic modulation: Loss of TL antigen from cells exposed to TL antibody: Study of the phenomenon in vitro. *J. Exp. Med.*, 127:523–529.

75. Pardee, A. B. (1975): The cell surface and fibroblast proliferation: Some current research trends. *Biochim. Biophys. Acta*, 417:153–172.
76. Pollack, R., Risser, R., Conlon, S., and Rifkin, D. (1974): Plasminogen activator production accompanies loss of anchorage regulation in transformation of primary rat embryo cells by SV40 virus. *Proc. Natl. Acad. Sci. U.S.A.*, 71:4792–4796.
77. Poole, A. R. (1973): Tumor lysosomal enzymes and invasive growth. In: *Lysosomes in Biology and Pathology*, Vol. 3, edited by J. T. Dingle, pp. 303–337. North-Holland, Amsterdam.
78. Poste, G. (1975): Interaction of concanavalin A with the surface of virus-infected cells. In: *Concanavalin A*, edited by T. K. Chowdhury and A. K. Weiss, pp. 117–152. Plenum Press, New York.
79. Poste, G., and Nicolson, G. L. (1976): Calcium ionophores A23187 and X537A affect cell agglutination by lectins and capping of lymphocyte surface immunoglobulins. *Biochim. Biophys. Acta*, 426:148–155.
80. Poste, G., and Nicolson, G. L. (Eds.) (1977): *Dynamic Aspects of Cell Surface Organization*. North-Holland, Amsterdam.
81. Poste, G., and Weiss, L. (1976): Some considerations on cell surface alterations in malignancy. In: *Fundamental Aspects of Metastasis*, edited by L. Weiss, pp. 25–47. North-Holland, Amsterdam.
82. Poste, G., Papahadjopoulos, D., and Nicolson, G. L. (1975): Local anesthetics affect transmembrane cytoskeletal control of mobility and distribution of cell surface receptors. *Proc. Natl. Acad. Sci. U.S.A.*, 72:4430–4434.
83. Povlsen, C. O. (1976): A study of human tumors growing in nude mice. In: *Biological Characterization of Human Tumors*, edited by W. Davis and C. Maltoni, pp. 127–131. Excerpta Medica, Amsterdam.
84. Price, M. R., and Baldwin, R. W. (1977): Shedding of tumor cell surface antigens. In: *Dynamic Aspects of Cell Surface Organization*, edited by G. Poste and G. L. Nicolson, pp. 423–471. North-Holland, Amsterdam.
85. Proceedings of the Fourth Conference on Embryonic and Fetal Antigens in Cancer (1976): *Cancer Res.*, 36:3384–3546.
86. Rapin, A. M. C., and Burger, M. M. (1974): Tumor cell surfaces: General alterations detected by agglutinins. *Adv. Cancer Res.*, 20:1–91.
87. Reich, E. (1975): Plasminogen activator: Secretion by neoplastic cells and macrophages. In: *Proteases and Biological Control*, edited by E. Reich, D. B. Rifkin, and E. Shaw, pp. 333–341. Cold Spring Harbor Laboratory, New York.
88. Reich, E., Rifkin, D. B., and Shaw, E. (Eds.) (1975): *Proteases and Biological Control. Cold Spring Harbor Conferences on Cell Proliferation*, Vol. 2. Cold Spring Harbor Laboratory, New York.
89. Roblin, R., Chou, I.-N., and Black, P. H. (1975): Proteolytic enzymes and viral transformation. *Adv. Cancer Res.*, 22:203–260.
90. Salsbury, A. J. (1975): The significance of the circulating cancer cell. *Cancer Treatment Rev.*, 2:55–72.
91. Scher, C. D., Handenschild, C., and Klagsbrun, M. (1976): The chick chorioallantoic membrane as a model system for the study of tissue invasion by viral transformed cells. *Cell*, 8:373–382.
92. Sheridan, J. D. (1976): Cell coupling and cell communication during embryogenesis. In: *The Cell Surface in Animal Embryogenesis and Development*, edited by G. Poste and G. L. Nicolson, pp. 409–448. North-Holland, Amsterdam.
93. Shimamoto, T. (1974): A reaction with the vessel wall: Contraction of endothelial cells in thrombogenesis. *Thromb. Diath. Haemorrh.* [*Suppl.*], 60:5–15.
94. Shin, S., Freedman, V. H., Risser, R., and Pollack, R. (1975): Tumorigenicity of virus-transformed cells in *nude* mice is correlated specifically with anchorage independent growth in vitro. *Proc. Natl. Acad. Sci. U.S.A.*, 72:4434–4439.
95. Singer, S. J. (1974): Molecular biology of cellular membranes with applications to immunology. *Adv. Immunol.*, 19:1–66.
96. Singer, S. J., and Nicolson, G. L. (1972): The fluid mosaic model of the structure of cell membranes. *Science*, 175:720–731.
97. Smith, R. T., and Landy, M. (Eds.) (1975): *Immunobiology of the Tumor-Host Relationship*. Academic Press, New York.

98. Spang-Thomsen, M., and Visfeldt, J. (1976): Homozygous nu/nu mice with transplanted human malignant tumors. *Am. J. Pathol.,* 84:193–196.
99. Stackpole, C. W., Jacobson, J. B., and Lardis, M. P. (1974): Antigenic modulation in vitro. I. Fate of thymus-leukemia (TL) antigen–antibody complexes following modulation of TL antigenicity from the surfaces of mouse leukemia cells and thymocytes. *J. Exp. Med.,* 140:939–953.
100. Stiles, C. D., Desmond, W., Chuman, L. M., Sato, G., and Saier, M. H., Jr. (1976): Growth control of heterologous tissue culture cells in the congenitally athymic nude mouse. *Cancer Res.,* 36:1353–1360.
101. Strauch, L. (1972): The role of collagenases in tumor invasion. In: *Tissue Interactions in Carcinogenesis,* edited by D. Tarin, pp. 399–434. Academic Press, London.
102. Sundqvist, K.-G. (1977): Dynamics of antibody binding and complement interactions at the cell surface. In: *Dynamic Aspects of Cell Surface Organization,* edited by G. Poste and G. L. Nicolson. North-Holland, Amsterdam *(in press).*
103. Sykes, J. W. (1975): Separation of tumor cells from fibroblasts. In: *Human Tumor Cells In Vitro,* edited by J. Fogh, pp. 1–22. Plenum Press, New York.
104. Sylvén, B. (1973): Biochemical and enzymatic factors involved in cellular detachment. In: *Chemotherapy of Cancer Dissemination and Metastasis,* edited by S. Garattini and G. Franchi, pp. 129–138. Raven Press, New York.
105. Ting, C.-C., and Herberman, R. B. (1976): Humoral host defense mechanisms against tumors. *Int. Rev. Exp. Pathol.,* 15:93–152.
106. Trinkaus, J. P. (1976): On the mechanism of metazoan cell movements. In: *The Cell Surface in Animal Embryogenesis and Development,* edited by G. Poste and G. L. Nicolson, pp. 225–311. North-Holland, Amsterdam.
107. Warren, B. A. (1973): Environment of the blood-borne tumor embolus adherent to vessel wall. *J. Med.,* 4:150–177.
108. Waymouth, C. (1974): To disaggregate or not to disaggregate: Cell injury and cell disruption, transient or permanent. *In Vitro,* 10:97–111.
109. Weinstein, R. S., Merk, F. B., and Alroy, J. (1976): The structure and function of intercellular junctions in cancer. *Adv. Cancer Res.,* 23:23–89.
110. Weiss, L. (1969): The cell periphery. *Int. Rev. Cytol.,* 26:63–105.
111. Weiss, L. (1973): Neuraminidase, sialic acids and cell interactions. *J. Natl. Cancer Inst.,* 50:3–19.
112. Weiss, L. (1976): Biophysical aspects of the metastatic cascade. In: *Fundamental Aspects of Metastasis,* edited by L. Weiss, pp. 51–70. North-Holland, Amsterdam.
113. Weiss, L., and Poste, G. (1975): The tumor cell periphery. In: *Scientific Foundations of Oncology,* edited by T. Symington and R. L. Carter, pp. 25–35. Heinemann, London.
114. Willis, R. A. (1973): *The Spread of Tumours in the Human Body.* Ed. 3. Butterworths, London.
115. Wolf, B. A., and Goldberg, A. R. (1976): Rous sarcoma virus-transformed fibroblasts having low levels of plasminogenesis activator. *Proc. Natl. Acad. Sci. U.S.A.,* 73:3613–3617.
116. Wolff, Et., and Wolff, Em. (1975): Current research with organ cultures of human tumors. In: *Human Tumor Cells In Vitro,* edited by J. Fogh, pp. 207–240. Plenum Press, New York.
117. Yarnell, M. M., and Schnebli, H. P. (1974): Release from density-dependent inhibition of growth in the absence of cell locomotion. *J. Cell Sci.,* 16:181–188.
118. Ziegler, M. M., Miller, E. E., and Barker, C. F. (1973): Regional lympatics and the mechanism of action of neuraminidase. *Surgical Forum,* 24:290–292.

Cancer Invasion and Metastasis: Biologic Mechanisms and Therapy, edited by S. B. Day et al. Raven Press, New York © 1977.

Role of Surface Glycoproteins in Tumor Growth

Amiel Cooper, Susan Morgello, Douglas Miller, and Michael Brown

Department of Pathology, Tufts University Medical School, Boston, Massachusetts 02111

Our abhorrence of the human consequences of metastasis must in part be matched by a certain intellectual awe when considering the complicated and almost ritualistic pattern of events adapted by neoplastic cells in their quest for immortality akin, say, to our awe for the instinctual patterns of migration and reproduction of the salmon. But the very intricacy of the metastatic process confers multiple potential points of vulnerability to therapeutic intervention.

We are interested in the quantitation, isolation, biosynthesis, and shedding of surface membrane glycoproteins of neoplastic cells. Much of our work has employed the transplantable murine TA_3 adenocarcinoma system because of the positive correlation between a specific group of surface glycoproteins and allogeneic growth (1,2). We report our findings, using this system, of the relationship of surface glycoprotein to subcutaneous growth, and our preliminary attempts to select for TA_3 tumor cells capable of wide dissemination in syngeneic mice following tail vein injection.

METHODS

TA_3 Tumors

The TA_3-Ha and TA_3-St sublines (3–5) were maintained by weekly passage in syngeneic male or females 15- to 18-g A/HeJ mice in the ascites form. We injected 10^5 viable tumor cells intraperitoneally (i.p.), and approximately 10^8 cells were harvested after cervical dislocation 1 week later. Red cells and leukocytes were removed by low-speed centrifugation of the tumor cells. After they were washed three times with Hanks balanced salt solution (Hanks BSS), the tumor cells were enumerated with a hemocytometer and the viability (>95%) and purity (>95%) were established by trypan blue exclusion and by examination of cytocentrifuge preparations stained by the Giemsa method. The ability of the sublines to survive in allogeneic mice was tested by similar inoculation and harvesting, using CBA, DBA, or Balb/c mice (Jackson Labs).

Subcutaneous Growth

Groups of four to six syngeneic or allogeneic mice were inoculated with 10^6 viable tumor cells in a volume of 0.2 ml Hanks BSS under the skin of the back of the neck using a 1-ml syringe and number 23 needle. Tumor takes were assessed on days 10 to 14 by the presence of a firm nodule > 1 cm in diameter at the injection site. Histologic sections (H & E) were taken on occasion to verify tumor growth. The tumor cells were obtained in suspension form by mincing in cold Hanks BSS and gently pressing through a nylon tea strainer. The TA_3 tumors grown in solid form were readily dispersed without the need for harsher conditions such as calcium depletion or trypsin treatment. Any cell aggregates were removed by fine straining, and 1 g sedimentation for 10 min. The tumor cells were finally purified of any red cells, leukocytes, and dead cells by Ficoll-Hypaque gradient centrifugation (6). We layer 2 ml of the tumor cell suspension (10^7 to 10^8 cells) in phosphate-buffered saline, pH 7.2, over 3 ml of the standard Ficoll-Hypaque gradient and centrifuge at room temperature at 600 g for 12 min. The interphase white band containing the purified tumor cells is washed three times with cold Hanks BSS, and the cells are enumerated and assessed for purity (>90%) and viability (>80%).

Intravenous Inoculation

Employing a brass mouse restrainer to facilitate injection, we injected (number 23 needle) 10^5 to 10^6 viable single-cell suspensions of tumor cells in 0.2 ml of Hanks BSS in a lateral tail vein of groups of four to six syngeneic (A/HeJ) mice. The mice were sacrificed 14 to 18 days after injection and were autopsied to search for gross evidence of tumor growth. Tissues suspected of containing tumor nodules and occasional grossly uninvolved tissues were taken for histologic sections and microscopic evaluation. When tumor nodules of sufficient size or number were identified by gross examination, the tumor cells were obtained in suspension form and purified on Ficoll-Hypaque gradients as described above.

Measurement of Cell Surface GP-I Glycoprotein

We employed our automated hemagglutination-inhibition assay using the lectin of *Vicia graminea* to measure a specific family of glycoproteins, termed GP-I, on the surface of small numbers of viable tumor cells (2,5,7). Our previous studies demonstrated that this lectin, which binds to carbohydrate side chains with the sequence βGal-NAc Gal-O-serine(threonine) (8–10) and which agglutinates human blood type N red cells, is highly specific in the mouse for the GP-I glycoproteins found on the surface of the TA_3-Ha tumor cells but not appreciably on the TA_3-St subline or on normal mouse tissues (5). The GP-I glycoproteins, also termed epiglycanin (10), are an unusual group of the high molecular weight (up to 500,000 daltons) glycoproteins consisting of 75 to 80% carbohydrate in the form of numerous short and longer side chains attached to serine and threonine residues of the protein backbone by O-glycosidic linkages to the reducing terminal sugar α-NAc Gal (10,11). These glycoproteins, which are heavily sialylated, are present in very large amounts (approximately 4 mg/10^9 cells or about 5 million molecules per cell) on the surface of the TA_3-Ha subline (5,11) and can be readily removed by trypsin or papain cleavage yielding fragments with an average molecular weight of 200,000 daltons (11,12). The GP-I molecules are also shed from *in vivo* growing Ha, but not St, tumor cells (7). Using our automated hemagglutination-inhibition assay and using a sample of GP-I purified by gel filtration as a standard, we were able to quantitate the GP-I molecules on the surface of intact Ha tumor cells, and, because of the high sensitivity of the assay, we could measure the amount of released GP-I free in the ascites fluid and even in the serum of mice bearing TA_3-Ha cells in the ascites form (2,5,7). The GP-I molecules are believed to be responsible for the ability of the TA_3-Ha subline to grow in the ascites form in allogeneic mice (1,13,14) because of some masking or steric hindrance effect which renders the H-2 histocompatibility antigens relatively inaccessible (11,15,16). An alternative explanation (7) is that the GP-I molecules shed *in vivo* have a suppressive or blocking effect on alloantigen reactivity by the hosts.

In brief, our method of measurement of GP-I on the surface of viable TA_3 cells consists of pelleting by centrifugation serial numbers of each type of tumor cell in small plastic tubes (Beckman) and resuspending the cells in 100λ aliquots of a dilute extract of the *V. graminea* seeds containing the active lectin. After they are mixed at 4°C for 1 hr, the cells are pelleted and an aliquot of each supernatant is removed, further diluted, and subsequently used in the automated hemagglutination-inhibition system to determine what percentage of the lectin was adsorbed by each cell aliquot. This percent adsorption is determined by comparing the residual hemagglutinating lectin activity in each supernatant with the activity of a series of dilutions of the unadsorbed *V. graminea* lectin (2,5). This method is highly sensitive, allowing us to determine lectin binding by as few as 5×10^2 tumor cells having large amounts of the GP-I bearing the lectin receptors, and is very convenient for measuring the lectin binding by a number of different tumor samples, since the postadsorption supernatants can be frozen and measured subsequently. By plotting the percent lectin adsorption versus the log of the number of adsorbing cells, we obtain a sigmoid curve for each tumor sample and this allows facile comparison of the lectin binding potency, i.e., amount of GP-I, for different tumor lines or samples. We express the relative lectin binding ability of different tumor samples as the number of cells required to adsorb 50% of our standard dilute *V. graminea* lectin solution. A detailed description of the general methodology of auto-mated hemagglutination-inhibition is provided in a separate publication (17).

In vitro Glycoprotein Turnover Studies

Tumor cells grown *in vivo* in the ascites form were harvested, washed, and suspended at a concentration of 10^6 cells per milliliter in sterile minimal essential medium (MEM) (Microbiologic Associates) supplemented with 50 μg/ml gentamycin and 10% heat-inactivated fetal calf serum (Flow Labs). ^{3}H-glucosamine (10 Ci/mM, New England Nuclear) was added and the cells were cultured for 16 to 20 hr in a Bellco spinner flask. The cells were pelleted by centrifugation and a glycoprotein extract was prepared from each culture supernatant by adding perchloric acid to a final concentra-tion of 0.75M, which precipitated the proteins and left the glycoproteins in solution. After exhaustive dialysis to remove the perchloric acid and any remaining ^{3}H-glucosamine, the samples were lyophilized and redissolved in 10 ml of phosphate-buffered saline, pH 7.0, and applied to an upward flow column (90 × 2.5 cm) of Sepharose 4B equilibrated with the same buffer. Then 6.5-ml fractions were taken and the radioactivity determined by adding 0.5 ml of each fraction to 10 ml of Aquasol (New England Nuclear) and counting in a Packard Tri-Carb Liquid Scintillation Spectrometer. The GP-I levels were also measured on each fraction using the *V. graminea* lectin assay (7). A 50λ aliquot of each fraction was incubated with 50λ of our standard lectin solution, and after this was mixed for 1 hr at 4°C the percent inhibition of the lectin was determined using our automated assay. The unknown levels were expressed as micrograms of GP-I based on a standard inhibition curve using purified GP-I (7).

RESULTS

Ascites Growth of TA$_3$ Sublines

As has been extensively demonstrated, we showed that the TA$_3$-Ha sub-line when injected i.p. has the unusual property of growing in and killing allogeneic strains of mice as well as syngeneic mice. In contrast, the TA$_3$-St grows only in syngeneic strain A mice. Table 1 demonstrates that an i.p. injection of 10^4 viable Ha cells killed all syngeneic and most allogeneic recipients, whereas 10^4 viable St cells killed only the syngeneic mice. We have obtained similar results in more extensive studies using 10^5 cells for the challenge and using additional allogeneic strains as recipients. Post-mortem examinations showed large accumulations of hemorrhagic fluid containing numerous tumor cells in the peritoneal cavities. Aside from occasional small tumor nodules at the site of injection in the abdominal wall,

TABLE 1. *Lethality of TA₃ sublines for syngeneic and allogeneic mice[a]*

TA₃ subline	A/HeJ	CBA/J	DBA/J	Balb/cJ
Ha	4/4	3/4	4/4	4/4
St	4/4	0/4	0/4	0/4

[a] We injected 10^4 viable TA₃-Ha or TA₃-St i.p. into groups of 4 syngeneic (A/HeJ) or allogeneic mice, and the number of mice killed within 3 weeks was noted.

no other tumor was noted in the organs on gross examination, i.e., there did not appear to be metastasis out of the peritoneal cavity. However, further microscopic documentation is needed to establish this fact.

Frequent measurements of surface GP-I on ascites-grown TA₃ cells, using the *V. graminea* lectin assay, were in accord with published values (2,5), 50% adsorption achieved by 5×10^3 to 10^4 Ha cells harvested from either syngeneic or allogeneic mice and 50% adsorption by syngeneic-grown St cells requiring $> 10^6$ cells.

Ha Variant

In the course of allogeneic i.p. injections of TA₃-Ha cells, an occasional mouse is able to reject the tumor. One female CBA mouse, which appeared to have rejected the inoculation of 10^5 Ha cells, was found 8 weeks after injection to have two large subcutaneous (s.c.) tumors, one on the back and one on the thigh. This mouse was sacrificed and the abdominal site of injection and the peritoneal cavity were found to be free of tumor. Single-cell suspensions of viable cells were prepared from the s.c. thigh tumor, and these were injected i.p. and s.c. into A/HeJ and CBA/J mice. The tumors grew readily in the ascites form in all the i.p. injected mice and as solid nodules in all the s.c. injected mice. Because of the cytologic and histologic similarity of these tumor cells to the TA₃ cells, because the tumor readily grew in the ascites form on i.p. injection, because the tumor cells grew in both strains of mice, and because the cells were shown to have on their surface numerous receptors for the *V. graminea* lectin, our interpretation was that the two s.c. tumors in the original CBA mouse represented spontaneous metastases of a few Ha cells from the original peritoneal injection site and that these s.c. tumors were allowed time to grow to a large size because of the rejection of the rest of the i.p. inoculum by the mouse. These tumor cells have been maintained by continuous s.c. inoculation of A/HeJ mice and will be referred to as "Ha variant." We have not as yet examined the chromosomes of this line nor do we know if it is a stable variant. However, as described below, there is evidence that these cells differ in some respects from the parent Ha subline, and this indicates that the line might have arisen under selective pressure in the original CBA mouse.

Subcutaneous Growth of TA$_3$ Sublines

Because of the unusual origin of our Ha variant line, we were interested in testing the s.c. growth ability of the Ha and St sublines and the Ha variant in both syngeneic and allogeneic mice and also in comparing the surface GP-I levels on cells grown in the s.c. solid form as opposed to the ascites suspension grown cells.

We found that the three lines had a high "take" rate, close to 100%, when 5×10^5 to 10^6 viable cells were injected s.c. into syngeneic A/HeJ mice. Smaller numbers of cells failed to consistently give s.c. tumors, in contrast to the consistent transplantation of the Ha and St lines i.p. in syngeneic recipients with 10^3 to 10^4 viable cells. The differences between s.c. and i.p. growth were even more striking when using allogeneic (Balb/cJ and CBA/J) mice as recipients. As anticipated, the St subline failed to grow s.c. in allogeneic mice just as it has always shown strain specificity for ascites growth. The Ha variant, as might be anticipated from its metastatic origin to an s.c. site in a CBA mouse, had a high take rate s.c. and i.p. in allogeneic mice. However, the Ha subline, which consistently grows i.p. in allogeneic mice, gave a poor take rate s.c. in allogeneic mice. Injection of 10^6 viable ascites-grown Ha cells into CBA and Balb/c mice s.c. gave an overall take rate of $< 50\%$. Some mice failed to develop tumors at all, and some mice developed s.c. tumors but went on to reject these by 2 to 3 weeks. Other allogeneic mice were killed within 2 to 3 weeks by the s.c. Ha tumors, just as were all syngeneic mice killed by s.c. Ha tumors. In contrast, if 10^6 Ha cells were passaged sequentially in the s.c. form in syngeneic strain A and then passaged directly s.c. to Balb/c, the tumors grew much better, as if the prior s.c. passages in syngeneic mice had adapted them to s.c. allogeneic growth.

An explanation for these observations may lie in our results of measuring the *V. graminea* binding by the three tumor lines grown s.c. in A/HeJ mice (Table 2). St adsorbs the lectin very poorly when grown i.p. or s.c., in keeping with the absence of GP-I on this subline and in keeping with the inability to grow i.p. or s.c. in allogeneic mice. The lectin binding by Ha cells drops when it is first grown s.c. If a similar change is occurring in Ha cells placed s.c. in allogeneic mice, the implied low GP-I level could account for the poor growth since there is strong evidence that the GP-I is playing a role in permitting allogeneic growth. However, during sequential s.c. passages of Ha cells, there appears to be a selective or adaptive change with increased expression of GP-I approaching i.p. levels, and this could explain the better allogeneic s.c. growth after sequential s.c. passage. The Ha variant apparently has relatively high levels of GP-I because of an initial selection process during its incipiency or has developed high levels during sequential continuous s.c. passage.

TABLE 2. Vicia graminea *lectin binding by TA$_3$ tumor lines*[a]

TA$_3$ line	Mode of growth	V. graminea binding[b]
St	i.p.	1.8×10^6
St	1st passage s.c.	2.2×10^6
Ha	i.p.	8×10^3
Ha	1st passage s.c.	3×10^4
Ha	back to i.p.	10^4
Ha	8 consecutive s.c.	8×10^3
Ha variant	2 consecutive s.c.	10^4
Ha variant	8 consecutive s.c.	6×10^3

[a] All the TA$_3$ lines were grown, as indicated, in syngeneic A/HeJ mice.
[b] The value indicates the number of cells needed to adsorb 50% of a standard lectin solution.

Intravenous Injection of TA$_3$ Sublines

We were next interested in the relative abilities of the three TA$_3$ lines to form distant tumors following injection of viable cells into the lateral tail veins of syngeneic mice. Groups of A/HeJ mice received injections of 10^6 or 5×10^6 viable tumor cells into a tail vein and the animals were sacrificed and examined 2 to 3 weeks later. The distribution of tumors as noted grossly is shown in Table 3. Most mice had several tumor implants in the lungs regardless of the type of TA$_3$ cell injected (Fig. 1). However, the occurrence of tumors beyond the lungs was less frequent and varied with the cell type used for injection. No distant tumor implants occurred with St injections,

TABLE 3. *Tumor implants following tail vein injection of A/HeJ mice*[a]

Cell injected	No. of cells injected per mouse	No. of mice injected	No. of mice with lung implants	No. of mice with other implants
St (s.c.)[b]	10^6	4	3	0
St (i.p.)	10^6	10	8	0
St (i.p.)	5×10^6	3	3	0
Ha (s.c.)	10^6	13	12	4 (3 peritoneal, 1 s.c.)
Ha (i.p.)	10^6	4	3	2 (1 peritoneal, 1 s.c.)
Ha (i.p.)	5×10^6	4	4	2 (s.c.)
Ha variant (s.c.)	10^6	15	13	1 (s.c.)

[a] The mice were injected with tumor cells in a lateral tail vein. Animals were sacrificed 2 to 3 weeks later and examined grossly for tumor implants.
[b] The mode of growth of the cells used for injection is indicated in parentheses.

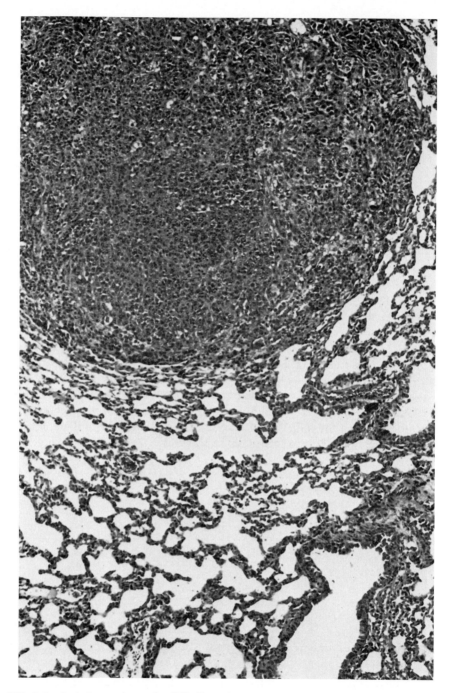

FIG. 1. Implantation and growth of TA$_3$-Ha cells in the lung following injection of 10^6 viable tumor cells into the tail vein of a strain A mouse 2 weeks previously.

whereas at least one mouse in the groups injected with the Ha or Ha variant cells developed a tumor implant remote from the site of injection and beyond the lungs.

Selection for TA$_3$ Cells Capable of Distant Implantation

We harvested and purified the tumor cells from the s.c. tumor nodule on the shoulder of the mouse injected with Ha variant cells. Each of six A/HeJ mice was injected with 10^6 of these cells in an attempt to enhance our chance of obtaining widespread tumor implantation. Of the six mice sacrificed 11 to 18 days later, one mouse had lung tumors only, one had peritoneal tumors only, three had lung and either liver, peritoneal, or s.c. implants, and one mouse had massive widespread tumor implantation in multiple organs including liver (Fig. 2), spleen, kidney (Fig. 3), lymph nodes, and peritoneum. There were only a few small lung implants in this animal. Thus, we had achieved a positive selection for widespread implantation and growth following tail vein injection of cells which had previously successfully implanted to a site beyond the lungs.

We then minced up the massively infiltrated liver of the latter mouse, obtained a single-cell suspension, and purified the viable cells, which were mainly tumor cells, on a Ficoll-Hypaque gradient. Next we injected 10^6 viable cells into the tail veins of four other A/HeJ mice and injected 5×10^5 tumor cells i.p. into a fifth mouse. Of the former group, which was sacrificed 2 weeks later, all had lung implants and three also had liver implants. This provided further strong evidence that we were achieving selection for distant spread. Tumor cells were harvested from the ascites fluid of the i.p. injected mouse. These ascites-grown cells derived from the massively infiltrated liver were propagated by weekly i.p. passage for several generations and were the source of the cells used for glycoprotein studies (see below).

Glycoprotein Studies on Cells Derived from Massive Liver Implantation

We measured the *V. graminea* lectin binding ability of the ascites-grown selected "metastatic" cells and of our standard Ha and St ascites lines (Fig. 4). The selected line gave 50% adsorption for 1.8×10^3 cells, whereas 4×10^3 Ha cells and 2×10^6 St cells were required to give similar adsorption of the lectin.

We then used the *in vitro* biosynthetic assay described under Methods to determine the quantitative profiles of *de novo* synthesized and shed glycoproteins for the ascites-grown selected cells and for ascites-grown Ha and St cells. The *in vitro* cultures for the selected line and for the Ha were done simultaneously and identically, whereas the St was done subsequently. For the selected "metastatic" cells and the Ha cells, 5×10^7 viable freshly harvested cells were cultured for 16 hr in 50 ml of culture medium containing

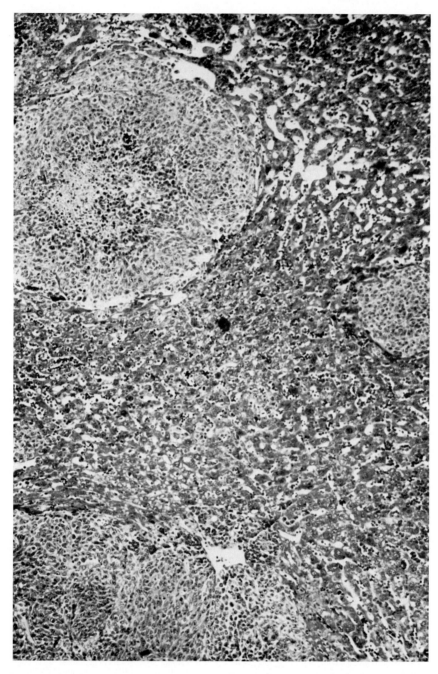

FIG. 2. Metastasis to the liver following tail vein injection of 10^6 viable tumor cells into a strain A mouse. The cells used for the injection had been in turn selected by previous implantation subcutaneously following tail vein injection of Ha variant cells.

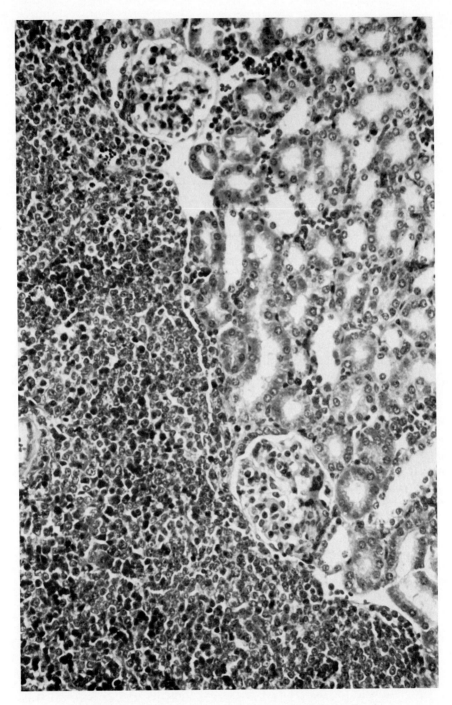

FIG. 3. Metastasis to kidney in same mouse described in Fig. 2.

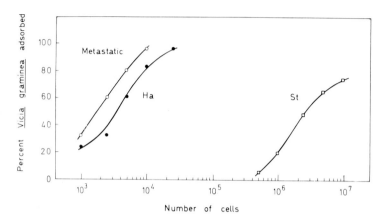

FIG. 4. Quantitative binding of the lectin of *V. graminea* by serial numbers of three TA$_3$ lines: Ha, St, and a line selected for high metastatic ability following tail vein injection in syngeneic A/HeJ mice. The metastatic line adsorbs the lectin approximately twice as well as the Ha on a per cell basis. The St binds very poorly.

20 μCi of ^{3}H-glucosamine. A Lowry protein determination on the two cell pellets was identical. The culture supernatants were handled as described, and 50% of the supernatant material for each cell type was applied sequentially to the same upward-flow Sepharose 4B column. Figure 5 shows the profiles of the radioactivity and the *V. graminea* lectin-inhibiting activity (GP-I) synthesized and released by the two cell types. In each instance there are three peaks of radioactive glycoproteins with an ascending shoulder on the third peak. For the "metastatic" selected cell, each peak is larger than the corresponding peak for the Ha, but the greatest difference is seen in the case of the second peak, which contains 2.7 times more radioactivity for the selected cell. The GP-I profiles show in each instance a very small peak, corresponding to the first radioactive peak, and larger peaks which trail the second radioactive peaks. This latter peak for the selected "metastatic" cells is approximately three times the corresponding Ha peak.

Figure 6 shows a similar experiment for the St cell. In this instance 3 × 10^8 cells were cultured in 300 ml of medium with 100 μCi of ^{3}H-glucosamine for 20 hr. Then 90% of the lyophilized glycoprotein extract of the supernatant was applied to the column. As would be anticipated (5,7), no higher molecular weight radioactive peaks are present, only the ascending shoulder and final peak. Likewise, no GP-I was present in any of the fractions (data not shown in figure).

DISCUSSION

Our rationale for undertaking these experiments was as follows: It has been extensively documented that the TA$_3$-Ha has the unusual ability to

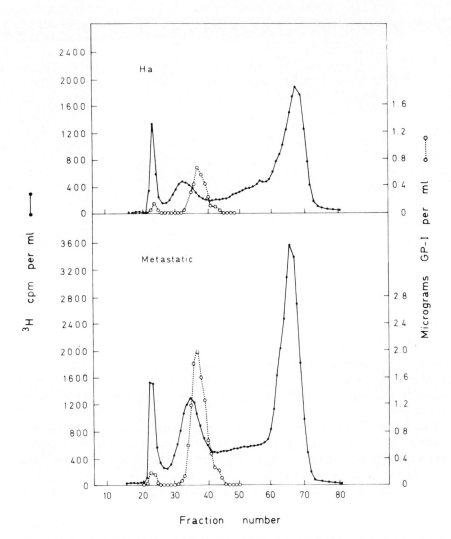

FIG. 5. Profiles of glycoproteins released *in vitro* by the Ha (*above*) and the "metastatic" (*below*) lines of the TA$_3$ tumor. First 5×10^7 viable cells were cultured for 16 hr with ^{3}H-glucosamine, then a perchloric acid extract of the culture supernatants was fractionated on an upward-flow column of Sepharose 4B. The solid lines represent the radioactivity in the *de novo* synthesized and released glycoproteins. The dotted lines represent the GP-I levels as determined by the *V. graminea* lectin inhibition assay.

grow in allogeneic mice, and this has been attributed to the large amount of high molecular weight glycoproteins, GP-I, on the surface (1). TA$_3$-St lacking this group of molecules is able to grow syngeneically but, like most transplantable tumors, will not take in allogeneic recipients. Further evidence for the role of GP-I surface glycoproteins in allogeneic growth in-

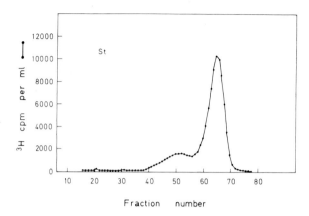

FIG. 6. Profile of glycoprotein release *in vitro* by TA₃-St cells. We cultured 3×10^8 cells for 20 hr with ³H-glucosamine, and the supernatant was fractionated as in Fig. 5. No GP-I was present as measured by the lectin assay. In addition, the higher molecular weight glycoproteins synthesized and released by the Ha and "metastatic" lines were absent from the St culture supernatant.

cluded our observations (2) that Ha cells cultured *in vitro* for several weeks lost surface GP-I and also lost the ability to grow in allogeneic, but not syngeneic, mice. Since many of the requirements for metastasis involve the tumor cell surface and since glycoproteins are believed to play an important role in cell-cell interaction, it seemed possible that TA₃ sublines differing dramatically in surface glycoprotein might have different syngeneic implantation and growth properties. This TA₃ model was also attractive because of the *V. graminea* lectin assay for the GP-I molecule. This assay enables us to measure GP-I levels on very few tumor cells, such as might be harvested from a metastatic site. We were further aided by the finding of the "Ha variant," which appears to have metastasized spontaneously from the i.p. injection site of the Ha tumor cells to the subcutaneous tissue of the back and the thigh.

The studies on s.c. injections of the TA₃ tumor lines demonstrated several facts. First, the GP-I levels on Ha cells grown for the first time at a s.c. site are much lower than when grown at an i.p. site. This probably accounts for the poor take rate of ascites-grown Ha tumors placed s.c. in allogeneic mice. However, another finding was that the low GP-I levels are reversible, as when the s.c. grown cells are put back i.p. or when the Ha is passaged sequentially in several recipients in the s.c. site. This latter finding explains the improved s.c. allotransplantability after several s.c. passages. We have no explanation for this reversible change in the level of GP-I expression but believe that this could have an important effect on the ability of a TA₃ line to implant or metastasize since a solid metastasis may be more akin to a solid s.c. growth than to the ascites form of growth.

Our selection experiments are patterned after those of Fidler (18,19). However, because all our lines gave lung implants upon tail vein injection whereas only those with known surface GP-I gave additional implantation to sites beyond the lung, we decided to use these latter implants as a source for further injection. It was of interest that of those implants which occurred outside of the lungs, many were to the s.c. tissue as had been true for the original spontaneous metastasis of the Ha variant. It is perhaps significant that our most promising results in attempting to select for distant tumor implantation following tail vein injection have come from "progeny" of the Ha variant line. The successful selection for high-rate spread to the liver followed the injection of cells from a distant s.c. implant site, which had in turn resulted from Ha variant injection. In another series of selective passages not reported here, we started with Ha variant cells and selected for very high rate implantation in the lungs.

Once we achieved a measure of selection in terms of implantation to the liver following i.v. injection, we wanted to test our hypothesis that the glycoprotein on the surface of the selected cells would be qualitatively or quantitatively altered. By passaging the "selected" cells in the ascites form for several generations we were able to show that they consistently had very large numbers of *V. graminea* lectin receptors, presumably because of large numbers of GP-I surface molecules. We were able to demonstrate, by using an *in vitro* synthesis technique, that the "selected" line was synthesizing and releasing into the medium nearly three times as much of the second peak material, which we believe comprises the bulk of GP-I, and twice as much of the first and third peaks, which we have not as yet characterized, compared with our standard Ha subline cultured under identical conditions. We were also able to show that the "selected" line released into the culture medium three times as much *V. graminea* lectin-inhibiting glycoprotein, which correlates well with the increase noted on the intact cell surface. We do not have evidence that these glycoprotein changes associated with the "selected" line are playing a causal role in permitting the enhanced spread of the tumor, but this is our current hypothesis. If true, the glycoproteins either could be functioning on the intact cell surface to modify in cell-cell interactions (20) or could be important after release *in vivo* from the cell.

ACKNOWLEDGMENTS

This work was supported by research grants CA-19987 from the U.S.P.H.S. and BC-201 from the American Cancer Society. One of us (A.G.C.) is a recipient of U.S.P.H.S. Career Development Award CA-70680. We thank Denise Willette for her excellent technical assistance and Steve Halpern for the photography.

REFERENCES

1. Codington, J. F., Sanford, B. H., and Jeanloz, R. W. (1973): Cell-surface glycoproteins of two sublines of the TA₃ tumor. *J. Natl. Cancer Inst.*, 51:585.

2. Miller, D. K., Cooper, A. G., Brown, M. C., and Jeanloz, R. W. (1975): Reversible loss in suspension culture of a major cell-surface glycoprotein of the TA₃-Ha mouse tumor. *J. Natl. Cancer Inst.,* 55:1249.

3. Klein, G. (1951): Development of a spectrum of ascites tumors. *Exp. Cell Res.,* 2:291.

4. Hauschka, T. S., Weiss, L., Holdridge, B. A., et al. (1971): Karyotypic and surface features of murine TA₃ carcinoma cells during immunoselection in mice and rats. *J. Natl. Cancer Inst.,* 47:343.

5. Codington, J. F., Cooper, A. G., Brown, M. C., et al. (1975): Evidence that the major cell surface glycoprotein of the TA₃-Ha carcinoma contains the *Vicia graminea* receptor sites. *Biochemistry,* 14:855.

6. Boyum, A. (1968): Separation of leucocytes from blood and bone marrow. *Scand. J. Clin. Lab. Invest. [Suppl. 97],* 21:77.

7. Cooper, A. G., Codington, J. F., Brown, M. C. (1974): *In vivo* release of glycoprotein I from the Ha subline of TA₃ murine tumor into ascites fluid and serum. *Proc. Natl. Acad. Sci. USA,* 71:1224.

8. Uhlenbruck, G., and Dahr, W. (1971): Studies on lectins with a broad agglutination spectrum, XII. N-acetyl-D-galactosamine specific lectins from the seeds of *Soja hispida, Bauhinia purpurea, Iberis amara, Moluccella laevis,* and *Vicia graminea. Vox Sang.,* 21:338.

9. Springer, G. F., Codington, J. F., and Jeanloz, R. W. (1972): Surface glycoprotein from a mouse tumor cell as specific inhibitor of antihuman blood-group N agglutinin. *J. Natl. Cancer Inst.,* 49:1469.

10. Codington, J. F., Linsley, K. B., Jeanloz, R. W., et al. (1975): Immunochemical and chemical investigations of the structure of glycoprotein fragments obtained from epiglycanin, a glycoprotein at the surface of the TA₃-Ha cancer cell. *Carbohydr. Res.,* 40:171.

11. Codington, J. F. (1975): Masking of cell-surface antigens on cancer cells. In: *Cellular Membranes and Tumor Cell Behavior,* 28th annual symposium, MD Anderson Hospital and Tumor Institute, p. 399. Williams & Wilkins, Baltimore.

12. Slayter, H. S., and Codington, J. F. (1973): Size and configuration of glycoprotein fragments cleaved from tumor cells by proteolysis. *J. Biol. Chem.,* 248:3405.

13. Lippman, M. M., Venditti, I. M., Kline, I., and Elam, D. L. (1973): Immunity to TA₃ tumor subline that grows in allogeneic hosts elicited by strain specific TA₃ tumor cells. *Cancer Res.,* 33:679.

14. Nowotny, A., Grohsman, J., Abdelnoor, A., Rote, N., Yang, C., and Waltersdorff, R. (1974): Escape of TA₃ tumors from allogeneic immune rejection: Theory and experiments. *Eur. J. Immunol.,* 4:73.

15. Sanford, B. H., Codington, J. F., Jeanloz, R. W., and Palmer, P. D. (1973): Transplantability and antigenicity of two sublines of the TA₃ tumor. *J. Immunol.,* 110:1233.

16. Friberg, S., and Lilliehook, B. (1973): Evidence for non-exposed H-2 antigens in immunoresistant murine tumour. *Nature [New Biol.],* 241:112.

17. Cooper, A. G., and Brown, M. C. (1977): Automated hemagglutination inhibition. In: *Automated Immunoanalysis,* edited by R. F. Ritchie. Marcel Dekker, New York.

18. Fidler, I. J. (1973): Selection of successive tumor lines for metastasis. *Nature [New Biol.],* 242:148.

19. Fidler, I. J., Caines, S., and Dolan, Z. (1976): Survival of hematogenously disseminated allogeneic tumor cells in athymic nude mice. *Transplantation,* 22:208.

20. Winkelhake, J. L., and Nicolson, G. L. (1976): Determination of adhesive properties of variant metastatic melanoma cells to BALB/3T3 cells and their virus-transformed derivatives by a monolayer attachment assay. *J. Natl. Cancer Inst.,* 56:285.

Cancer Invasion and Metastasis: Biologic Mechanisms and Therapy, edited by S. B. Day et al. Raven Press, New York © 1977.

Modulation of the Expression of the Cancer Cell Phenotype

I. Bernard Weinstein

Columbia University College of Physicians and Surgeons, New York, New York 10032

Much of the emphasis in our discussions has been concerned with host factors as determinants in the process of metastasis—factors such as vascular integrity, fibrin and the coagulation mechanism, the immune system, macrophages, nutrition, and even iatrogenic factors. I would like to refocus our attention on the "gangster" itself, the cancer cell, since we know that in certain experimental models the injection of a single (or a few) cancer cells into a normal intact host can induce metastatic disease, in some cases with striking organ specificity. The phenomena I will describe indicate how the properties of dormancy, growth, or regression of metastases may in part be explained by stepwise alterations in the phenotype of the cancer cell itself.

One must emphasize that the carcinogenic process is multistep in its evolution and multifactorial in its etiology. This is well illustrated in the so-called two-stage skin carcinogenesis system (1–3). In this system a class of carcinogens called "initiating agents" can induce a latent change in cells which is manifest only when a second class of agents termed "promoters" is applied. Repeated application of the promoting agent leads to hyperplasia, and this is followed by the occurrence of benign and eventually malignant neoplasms. At the present time, we do not know with certainty whether the initiating events are due to mutation or to a stable epigenetic event, which steps in this multistep process are reversible, and at what steps the synthesis of specific biosynthetic products (such as plasminogen activator, tumor angiogenesis factor, or other growth factors) is switched on in the cancer cell.

Our research has been concerned with three factors that modulate, in a reversible manner, the expression of properties of the tumor cell phenotype by normal or cancer cells. These three factors are the phorbol ester-promoting agents (5,8), glucocorticoids (7), and the effects of temperature shifts in appropriate temperature-sensitive mutants of transformed cells (9). We have found that the phorbol esters, a potent class of tumor promoters, induce the synthesis of plasminogen activator and alter the cell surface glycopeptides of cells in culture. They also induce other changes in normal cells that mimic the properties of cancer cells (5,8). The exposure of transformed cells to phorbol esters further potentiates the expression of the transformed phenotype (5,8). On the other hand, glucocorticoids induce phenotypic changes in certain transformed cells so that their growth properties more closely resemble those of normal cells (7). Studies with a temperature-sensitive mutant of a transformed rat liver epithelial cell line also demonstrate the ability of the same cell line to reversibly express either the transformed or normal cell phenotype (9).

Thus the expression by cells of specific properties associated with the cancer cell phenotype is subject to induction by phorbol esters in normal cells and repression in cancer cells by glucocorticoids. Studies with other compounds and with temperature-sensitive mutants provide additional examples of modulation of the transformed phenotype (4,6). Normal cells, therefore, contain most (if not all) of the information for being cancer cells, but they carefully regulate the expression of this information. Cancer cells, on the other hand, express this information in a less controlled manner, but with appropriate agents one can still modulate its expression. The latter findings have obvious implications in terms of developing more specific approaches to cancer therapy, including the therapy of metastases.

A final, more speculative point is that the low concentrations at which the phorbol esters act, and the strict structural requirements necessary for their action in diverse species, suggest that they act by usurping an endogenous receptor normally used by a yet to be identified growth regulatory substance (5). We are currently searching for this substance in biologic fluids. The activity of this putative endogenous phorbol-like growth regulator could play an important role in the natural process of carcinogenesis and the expression by cancer cells of functions required for invasion and metastasis.

REFERENCES

1. Berenblum, I. (1975): Sequential aspects of chemical carcinogenesis: Skin. In: *Cancer,* Vol. 1, edited by F. F. Becker, pp. 323–344. Plenum Publishing Corp., New York.
2. Boutwell, R. K. (1974): The functions and mechanisms of promoters of carcinogenesis. *CRC Crit. Rev. Toxicol.,* 2:419–443.
3. Hecker, E. (1975). Cocarcinogens and cocarcinogenesis. In: *Handbuch der Allgemeinen Pathologie,* Vol. IV/6, Geschwulste, Tumors, II, edited by E. Grundmann, p. 651. Springer-Verlag, Berlin-Heidelberg.
4. Weinstein, I. B. (1976): In: *Advances in Pathobiology #4, Cancer Biology II, Etiology and Therapy,* edited by C. M. Fenoglio and D. W. King, pp. 106–117. Stratton Intercontinental Medical Book Corp., New York.
5. Weinstein, I. B., Wigler, M., and Pietropaolo, C. (1977): The action of tumor promoting agents in cell culture. Presented at a symposium on *The Origins of Human Cancer,* Cold Spring Harbor Laboratory, New York. (*in press.*)
6. Weinstein, I. B., Yamaguchi, N., Gebert, R., and Kaighn, M. E. (1975): The use of epithelial cell cultures for studies on the mechanism of transformation by chemical carcinogens. *In Vitro,* 2(3):130–141.
7. Wigler, M., Ford, J. P., and Weinstein, I. B. (1975): Glucocorticoid inhibition of fibrinolytic

activity production by tumor cells. In: *Cold Spring Harbor Symposium on Proteases and Biological Control,* pp. 849–856, Cold Spring Harbor Laboratory, New York.

8. Wigler, M., and Weinstein, I. B. (1976): A tumor promoter induces plasminogen activator. *Nature,* 259:232–233.

9. Yamaguchi, N., and Weinstein, I. B. (1976): Temperature sensitive mutants of chemically transformed epithelial cells. *Proc. Natl. Acad. Sci. U.S.A.,* 72:214–218.

Cancer Invasion and Metastasis: Biologic Mechanisms and Therapy, edited by S. B. Day et al. Raven Press, New York © 1977.

Blood Group Antigens in Adenocarcinoma Foreign to the Host

Philip Levine

Memorial Sloan-Kettering Cancer Center, New York, New York 10021; and Ortho Research Foundation, Raritan, New Jersey 00869

On analyzing the differences in the pathogenesis of ABO and Rh hemolytic disease, it became essential to study the structure of the fluid lipid bilayer of the red cell membrane. The ABO antigens as derived from extracts of red cell stroma are glycosphingolipids emanating from the sphingosine and extending as a chain of oligosaccharides above the outer layer. The Rh antigen is a lipoprotein which constitutes a part of the structural outer and perhaps also the inner layer adjacent to the cytoplasm. These brief introductory remarks are essential for a full understanding of the serologic and hematologic differences of ABO and Rh hemolytic disease as recently described (1).

Of the several different kinds of red cell antigenic specificities, only the glycosphingolipids play a significant role in adenocarcinoma and these are the ABO and P blood group systems (1–3). The MN antigenic structures as arising from specific amino acids of the polypeptide chain are important in terms of their precursor substance – the T antigen, particularly in adenocarcinoma of the breast (3).

In 1951 a 66-year-old woman (Mrs. D.J.) with gastric carcinoma (4) was the first individual found to be of the very rare (1:150,000) genotype *pp* (Tj(a-)) or genotype Tj^bTj^b with anti-$P_1P_2P^k$ (anti-Tj^a) in her serum (4,5). Prior to subtotal resection, attempts to find a compatible donor having met with failure, a biologic test to determine if she would tolerate 25 ml of incompatible P_1 blood resulted in (a) a severe transfusion reaction with eventual recovery and (b) an increase of her titer from 1:4–1:8 to 1:512. Subtotal gastric resection was carried out and the patient recovered without benefit of transfusions.

Fortunately, the gastric tumor was lyophilized from the frozen state and so a fine white powder was available for absorption tests to determine which antibody, if any, would be specifically absorbed by the tumor cells. Tests showed that 20 mg of the powder absorbed 16 to 32 agglutinating units of the patient's own complex of antibodies, of which anti-P_1 is the most important. Thus the malignancy contained an antigenic determinant which was foreign to the host — or an illegitimate blood group antigen in the malignant tissue resulting perhaps from a mutation (4).

It is of interest that no reference to the origin of this illegitimate red cell antigen in the tumor cells appeared in the literature or any of the standard texts on blood groups, although frequent reference is made to Sanger's findings on the relationship of Tj^a to the P system (5). In 1955 I was invited by Dr. J. Furth to participate in one of the sections on malignancies at the Gordon Research Conferences held at New London College, New London, New Hampshire, but the subject aroused little if any discussion. And so this story lay dormant until October, 1974.

On the occasion of a visit with Marcus (6; D. Marcus, *personal communication*), suggested to me by Dr. R. Rosenfield, the former demonstrated the sequence of the oligosaccharides showing P_1 specificity derived from extracts of red blood cells. Then Marcus pulled out from his collection the 1951 paper by Levine et al. (4) on the presence of $P_1P_2P^k$ antigens in the malignant gastric tissue of the *pp* patient. Both Dr. Marcus and I had known about and were mystified by a 1967 report of Hakomori et al. (2) on the biochemical isolation of neo-A antigen in the gastric adenocarcinoma in a group O patient. They isolated a glycosphingolipid from a gastric adenocarcinoma of a group O patient, but their final product failed to exhibit biochemical properties characteristic of group O. When rabbits were injected with this preparation, the animals produced anti-A. This indicated the presence of an illegitimate or neo-A red cell determinant in the malignant tissue of a group O patient. Hakomori et al. (2) were not aware of the parallel serologic observation in the P (Tj^a) system reported in 1951 (4).

In October, 1974, Marcus (*personal communication*) demonstrated to this author his findings on the sequence of the sugars found in glycosphingolipid extracts of P_1 red cells and also the series of sugars (from 1 to 5) which form chains emanating from the sphingosine of the outer layer. These are listed below. The term *ceramide* (cer) refers to sphingosine.

ceramide monohexoside	Glc-Cer
ceramide dihexoside (lactosyl)	Gal($\beta,1\rightarrow4$)Glc-Cer
ceramide trihexoside (P^k antigen)	Gal($\alpha,1\rightarrow4$)Gal($\beta,1\rightarrow4$)Glc-Cer
globoside (P antigen)	-Gal($\alpha,1\rightarrow4$)Gal($\beta,1\rightarrow4$)Glc-Cer
	GalNAc($\beta,1\rightarrow3$)
paragloboside	-GlcNAc($\beta,1\rightarrow3$)Gal($\beta,1\rightarrow4$)Glc-Cer
	Gal($\beta,1\rightarrow4$)
P_1 antigen	-GlcNAc($\beta,1\rightarrow3$)Gal($\beta,1\rightarrow4$)Glc-Cer
	Gal($\alpha,1\rightarrow4$)Gal($\beta,1\rightarrow4$)

glc is glucose; gal is galactose; NAcGl is *N*-acetylglucosamine; and NAcGal is *N*-acetylgalactosamine

Immediately after the conference with Marcus, I contacted Dr. O. B.

Bobbitt of Charlottesville, Virginia, who referred the case to me in 1951, to update the subsequent history of Mrs. D.J., the *pp* propositus.

The following highly significant information was revealed:

1. Mrs. D.J.'s parents were double first cousins, thus raising the incidence of genotype *pp* from the random 1:150,000 to 1:4 in this family.
2. Mrs. D.J.'s younger sister had the same rare genotype *pp;* she died of carcinoma of the uterus in 1962.
3. Histologic examination revealed that the lesions in the uterus and the stomach were identical (J. Furth, *personal communication*).
4. Familial malignancy is a common event, but the 1951 study presents the first pedigree in which the familial malignancy of the patient and her sib is associated with another genetic property, i.e., the P system on chromosome 6 which carries also the HLA antigens (W. Bodmer, *personal communication*).
5. Mrs. D.J. survived for 22 years and died of old age in 1973 with no evidence of metastases. There was no autopsy and the family refused to permit exhumation. This aspect is discussed in the chapter on immunotherapy (P. Levine, *this volume*) where evidence is presented that a specific immunologic mechanism prevented formation of metastatic areas in this patient and allowed the patient to survive for 22 years (1,7).
6. In 1975, 24 years later, the lyophilized tumor, well preserved in refrigeration at −20°C, was found by my associate Mario Celano.

A sample was sent to Dr. S. Hakomori for biochemical study and the findings in his first preliminary experiment can be summarized as follows (S. Hakomori, *personal communication*): "0.5 gram of Tj^a tumor was extracted from chloroform-methanol (2:1) and the total neutral glycolipid fraction was obtained by DEAE-Sephadex A25 column, and was further purified by acetylation procedure. The migration rate of the major glycolipid present in this fraction on thin-layer chromatography was slower than the migration rate of a ceramide pentasaccharide of rabbit erythrocytes."

Thus Hakomori in 1975 confirmed biochemically the results of the serologic absorption tests made with the identical malignant tissue in 1951 as reported by Levine, Bobbitt, Waller, and Kuhmichel (4). Confirmation of Hakomori's findings was reported by Hakkinen (8) in 1970 when he demonstrated spots of anti-A immunofluorescence in six adenocarcinomatous stomachs, four of group O and two of group B patients.

It is to be expected that if the titer of anti-A is monitored in the seven cases of illegitimate neo-A antigens on malignant tissues once the diagnosis is established, the titer should drop during the period of early growth of the malignancy by virtue of specific *in vivo* absorption. However, the possibility of a therapeutic approach by increasing the titer of anti-A can now be readily subjected to testing. In increasing the titers of anti-A, the injection of minute quantities of incompatible group A red cells rather than the water-soluble A product seems preferable since the immunization would then be carried out with glycosphingolipids, which characterize blood group substances common to red blood cells, tissue cells, and the illegitimate neo-A antigen in adenocarcinomas (1).

In the proper setting very low titers of anti-A may add to the diagnostic criteria of suspected adenocarcinoma in patients of group O or B. The lesion need not be limited to the stomach as shown in the 1951 propositus D.J., whose sister B.D. died from adenocarcinoma of the uterus – granting that here a different blood group system is involved. In view of the accidentally successful outcome in the 1951 patient D.J. involving the p-P_1 mutation, the outlook for equally successful therapeutic results in O→A or B→A illegitimacy should be hopeful. Surely, this is an area of cancer therapy which has been grossly overlooked and long neglected, probably because the emphasis in the past has been on immune surveillance by the K variety of T lymphocytes and on chemotherapy and surgery.

As to the mechanism involved, one may speculate that this state of affairs may result from an error in transcription from DNA to RNA and/or in translation from RNA to protein synthesis (enzymes such as transferases). In the most frequent type, i.e., the unexpected appearance of neo-A determinant in a group O individual, all that is required is the addition via the transferase of N-acetylgalactosamine by the donor uridine diphosphate molecule to that galactose to which fucose is attached. Apparently this change is strictly limited to the malignant tissue. Can this be brought about by some failure in the function of the regulator gene mechanism controlling the structural gene?

It is hoped that experts in the multidisciplinary areas of DNA, RNA regulator, and structural genes and enzymes will ask key questions and thus find the essential experimental models to resolve this fundamental issue. In the case of the T precursor to M and N, perhaps the error preventing the expression of M and N in the malignancy results from the failure in production of sialidase transferase required for deposition of sialic acid.

In any event these unexpected developments, which were first revealed by serologic procedures in 1951, can now be subjected to more definitive biochemical approaches thanks to the notable contributions from the laboratories of Hakomori and Marcus. The highly surprising element derived from these serologic and biochemical observations supplies what appears to be a logical basis for an entirely new approach for immunotherapy with human blood group isoimmune antibodies specific for the antigenic determinant demonstrated in the malignant tissue. Whenever Nature on rare occasions is made to expose one of her numerous mysteries and secrets, it almost always reveals the mantle of utter simplicity. This by itself would seem to offer a bright outlook for successful therapy for a particular and rather frequent type of malignancy. And about this we should know more in the not too distant future.

If future studies confirm that mutations involving gene products of the ABO, MN, and P systems result in a specific histologic type of malignancy, i.e., adenocarcinomas, then the same principle may be assumed to apply to sarcomas. What is now urgently required is a programmed study of the biochemical nature of the several different antigenic varieties of sarcomas. When such information becomes available, the next step is to determine whether specific immunologic therapy is applicable, perhaps again by virtue of cytotoxicity.

REFERENCES

1. Levine, P. (1976): Biological and clinical significance of differences between RBC membrane (Rh) and non-membrane (ABH, MN, P) antigenic sites. *Rev. Fr. Transfus.,* 19:213.
2. Hakomori, S., Koscielak, J., Bloch, H., and Jeanloz, R. W. (1967): Immunologic relationship between blood group substances and fucose-containing glycolipid of human adenocarcinoma. *J. Immunol.,* 98:31.
3. Springer, G., Desai, R. R., and Scanlon, E. F. (1976): T precursor to M and N in breast cancer. *Cancer,* 37:169.
4. Levine, P., Bobbitt, O. B., Waller, R. K., and Kuhmichel, A. (1951): Isoimmunization by a new blood factor in tumor cells. *Proc. Soc. Exp. Biol. Med.,* 78:218.
5. Sanger, R. (1955): An association between the P and Jay systems of blood groups. *Nature,* 176:1163.
6. Naiki, M., and Marcus, D. (1975): An immunochemical study of the human blood group P_1, P and P^k glycosphingolipid antigens. *Biochemistry,* 14:4837.
7. Levine, P. (1977): Heredity in cancer. *Seminar in Oncology (in press).*
8. Hakkinen, I. (1970): A like blood group antigen in gastric cancer cells of patients in blood groups O and B. *J. Natl. Cancer Inst.,* 44:1183.

This work was supported in part by National Cancer Institute grant #1 RO1 CA-20660-01.

Cancer Invasion and Metastasis: Biologic Mechanisms and Therapy, edited by S. B. Day et al. Raven Press, New York © 1977.

Specific Immunotherapy for Adenocarcinoma with Anti-A and Anti-P₁ for Prevention of Metastasis

Philip Levine

Memorial Sloan-Kettering Cancer Center, New York, New York 10021; and Ortho Research Foundation, Raritan, New Jersey 00869

In the previous chapter, reference was directed to the 66-year-old patient, Mrs. D.J., who in 1951 following subtotal gastrectomy for removal of an adenocarcinoma survived 22 years until 1973 when she died of old age. At no point in the 22 years following her gastrectomy was there any evidence of metastases. The patient was in group O and her red cells contained an agglutinogen believed to be the first example of a newly discovered blood group system (1). Sanger (2) in 1955 showed this antigen, previously named the Tj^a anti-Tj^a system, to be a part of the P system discovered by Landsteiner and Levine in 1927. (The term Tj^a was derived from T for tumor and j for the initial of her family name, Jarrel.) Her red cells were identified as containing agglutinogen p (incidence 1:150,000), and her serum contained a complex of three antibodies identified as anti-$P_1P_2P^k$ which agglutinate and hemolyze all red cells except the rare p (titer 1:4 to 1:8).

Can this case be considered as a surgical cure or is this an example of a spontaneous cure resulting from a long-standing remission? Everson (3) in a review of more than 1,000 patients' histories states that certain types of malignancies "may undergo temporary or permanent spontaneous regression of partial or complete extent." He lists neuroblastoma, hypernephroma, choriocarcinoma, and malignant melanoma (28, 21, 13, and 13 patients, respectively). His series includes five patients each with carcinoma of the breast, uterus, colon, and rectum, and three patients with gastric carcinoma.

Soon after my visit with Marcus, and updating the events from 1951 to 1974, it became quite evident that the long survival may have been associated with the very high titer (1:512), which resulted from the intravenous injection of 25 ml incompatible blood as a biologic test for compatibility (1,4). Although the high-titered antibody must have diminished over the years, sufficient residual antibody remained to prevent any malignant cells from taking hold long enough to establish metastatic areas. This is highly likely if it could be shown that the cytotoxicity is attributable to IgG molecules, which are known to be characterized by very long duration in the absence of further antigenic stimulation. In analogy of p to group O, it is known that the antibodies found in the serum of all *pp* individuals tested are mixtures of IgG as well as IgM molecules (5,6).

Evidence that formation of metastatic areas was prevented by the continued action of IgG molecules on P_1 sites is derived from an unexpected source. This refers to the high incidence of spontaneous abortions among women of genotype *pp*. The initial observations were made in 1954 in a series of ten *pp* women (and three men) scattered over the five continents; seven women varying in age from 27 to 66 had only 11 living children and 18 abortions (7). It is of interest that the 11 children were born to Mrs. D.J., who had 4 children, and her compatible sib with 7 full-term children (Table 1).

It is now universally accepted that the high incidence of abortions in *pp* women is statistically significant. Race and Sanger list 10 *pp* women studied because of a history of abortions who had only two children and 53 abortions. Among 31 families with *pp* women studied because of transfusion requirement, pregnancies, or consanguinity, there were 57 live children and 49 abortions. These findings are summarized in Table 2.

In the analysis of the 10 *pp* women, it was assumed that their husbands were homozygous for P_1, i.e., genotype P_1P_1 so that the fetus in all pregnancies is heterozygous and could be only of genotype P_1p. As regards the

TABLE 1. *Incidence of abortions in 7 pp families*

						Obstetrical history	
Family	Location	Case	Sex	Age	Blood group	Full term	Abortions
I	Virginia, U.S.A.	1. DJ[a]	F	66	O	4, l & w[b]	0
		2. BD	F	45	O	7, l & w	0
II	South Africa	3. MC	F	37	O	None	4
III[c]	Australia	4. -[a]	F	23	O	None	1
		5. -	F	19	O		
IV	Poland	6. Za	F	30	A	None	4
V	Michigan, U.S.A.	7. EE[a]	F	30	O	None	3
		8. GG	M	36	A		
VI	Canada	9. E1	F	33	O	None	0
VII	Japan	10. Rit.Ho[a]	F	27	A	None	6
		11. Ris.Hag	F	22	A	None	0
		12. Yoi.Hag	M	17	O		
		13. Yas.Hag					

[a] In the four families with more than one example, the asterisk refers to the first sibling in whose serum the antibody was first found. This observation led to the study of the sera of the siblings.

[b] l & w indicates living and well.

[c] The red cells of the parents and four other siblings reacted with anti-Tj[a] and the red cells of the parents and one other sibling reacted with anti-Tj[a].

Modified after Levine and Koch (7) with permission.

TABLE 2. *All pp women with anti-$P_1P_2P^k$*

Families (No.)	Live children	Abortions	Reason for serum exam.
31	57	49	Sib of propositus Antenatal test Preop cross-match
10	2	53	Abortions

Modified after Race and Sanger (8) with permission.

two exceptions, one should exclude previous marriages, errors in typing for P_1, or illegitimacy.

In the 31 families with *pp* women listed in Table 2, 8 with only one pregnancy were excluded from Table 3 because they could not provide any information. Of the remaining 23 families, 8 were selected because they produced only live children and there were no abortions. It is assumed that their husbands were homozygous for P_2, i.e., genotype P_2P_2. Both living children and abortions in about equal numbers, 27 and 31, respectively, were recorded for 12 families. Such a distribution would be expected if the genotype of their husbands were P_1P_2 so that P_1p fetuses would abort and only P_2p fetuses would survive.

Among the 31 *pp* women, 3 were included as sibs of proposita listed among the 31, but not among the 10 who had 53 abortions (Table 2). In these three families there were 4, 3, and 7 pregnancies, respectively, each ending in abortion. Accordingly, these are added to the 10 to make 13 families with only 2 living children and 67 abortions.

These findings in a retrospective study clearly establish that the anti-P_1 of the anti-$P_1P_2P^k$ complex in the *pp* women and the high-titered antibody in the *pp* patient exerted a highly specific cytotoxic effect on P_1 sites whether they be P_1 sites on the tissues of the early P_1p fetus or the illegitimate P_1 sites in the malignant tissue.

TABLE 3. *All pp women with anti-$P_1P_2P^k$*

Families (no.)	Live children	Abortions	Presumed genotype of husband
8[a]	26	0	P_2P_2
12	27	31	P_1P_2
13[b]	2	67	P_1P_1
33	55	98	

[a] Eight families with 1–0 or 0–1 deleted.
[b] Three families of the 31 with 0–14 included.
Modified after Race and Sanger (8) with permission.

In the previous chapter the sequence of the sugars in the glycosphingo-lipid chain was given to form the following: antigen P^k globoside, paraglo-boside, and the final product P_1. Antigen p is a ganglioside with sialic acid (nana) added to the terminal galactose in paragloboside (9).

In addition to the role of O→A or B→A mutations as shown biochemi-cally by Hakomori et al. (10) and immunologically by Hakkinen (11), a third blood group system is involved in relation to adenocarcinoma of the breast and probably also of other organs. This refers to the ongoing studies of Springer, Desai, and Scanlon which indicate that the sialoglycopeptides M and N are demonstrable in all normal, benign, and malignant breast tis-sues. Their precursor substance—the T antigen—lacking sialic acid is present exclusively in malignant breast tissue. From this point on, the anal-ogy to illegitimate antigens neo-A in adenocarcinoma of the stomach, and probably also other organs, is remarkably parallel. Thus every normal serum has anti-T which tends to be diminished in titer by virtue of *in vivo* absorption. In uni- or bilateral mastectomies, Springer and co-workers have been attempting to increase the titer of anti-T by intradermal injection of a so-called vaccine consisting of antigen T extracted from (a) normal red cells and (b) the autologous adenocarcinomatous breast. To this a small quantity of BCG is added. Preliminary results in a limited number of pa-tients indicate that after several intradermal injections, the titer of anti-T is increased, hopefully to a level that will prove to be cytotoxic to the T anti-gen in the malignancy and hence to the malignancy itself, thus preventing metastasis (12).

Currently Springer, Desai, and Scanlon (12) have shown that in 21 out of 32 patients following mastectomy (not yet injected with their "vaccine"), the titer of anti-T is increased. Apparently anti-T is continually being ab-sorbed *in vivo* by the T antigen in the malignant breast tissue, and removing the absorbing breast tissue allows the titer to reach its physiologic level. It would seem that an identical state of affairs serves as a satisfactory ex-planation for the low titer of 1:4 to 1:8 in the 1951 patient of genotype *pp*.

The next logical step is to confirm these unexpected findings in selected patients with adenocarcinomas by increasing the titer of the antibody spe-cific for the illegitimate antigenic determinant in the malignant tissue. It is preferable to select patients with the frequent combinations of O→A or B→A presumed mutations (4). In this genetic system as well as in the P system (p→P_1) quantitative monitoring of the antibody acting specifically on the malignant tissue is expected to show that the initial titer will be low due to *in vivo* absorption. In the more frequent cases of groups O and B patients with neo-A determinants limited to the malignancy, attempts are underway to increase the titer of the incriminating anti-A by deliberate immunization of the patient preferably with very small quantities of incom-patible group A red cells.

REFERENCES

1. Levine, P., Bobbitt, O. B., Waller, R. K., and Kuhmichel, A. (1951): Isoimmunization by a new blood factor in tumor cells. *Proc. Soc. Exp. Biol. Med.,* 78:218.
2. Sanger, R. (1955): An association between the P and Jay systems of blood groups. *Nature,* 176:1163.
3. Everson, T. C. (1964): Spontaneous regression of cancer. *Ann. N.Y. Acad. Sci.,* 114:721.
4. Levine, P. (1976): Biological and clinical significance of differences between RBC membrane (Rh) and non-membrane (ABH, MN, P) antigenic sites. *Rev. Fr. Transfus.,* 19:213.
5. Wurzell, H. A., Gottlieb, A. J., and Abelson, N. M. (1971): Immunoglobulin characterization of anti-Tj^a antibodies. *Transfusion,* 11:103.
6. Pollack, M., Levine, P., and Cedergren, B. (1977): IgG as well as IgM molecules in sera of individuals of genotype *pp*. *In preparation*.
7. Levine, P., and Koch, E. A. (1954): The rare human isoglutinin anti-Tj^a and habitual abortions. *Science,* 120:239.
8. Race, R. R., and Sanger, R. (1975): *Blood groups in Man,* Ed. 6, p. 170, Blackwell Scientific Publications, London.
9. Marcus, D. M., Naiki, M., and Kundu, S. K. (1976): Abnormalities in the glycosphingolipid content of human P^k and p erythrocytes. *Proc. Natl. Acad. Sci. USA,* 73:3263.
10. Hakomori, S., Koscielak, J., Bloch, H., and Jeanloz, R. W. (1967): Immunologic relationship between blood group substances and fucose-containing glycolipid of human adenocarcinoma. *J. Immunol.,* 98:31.
11. Hakkinen, I. (1970): A like blood group antigen in gastric cancer cells of patients in blood groups O and B. *J. Natl. Cancer Inst.,* 44:1183.
12. Springer, G., Desai, P. R., and Scanlon, E. F. (1976): T precursor to M and N in breast cancer. *Cancer,* 37:169.

This work was supported in part by National Cancer Institute grant #1 RO1 CA-20660-01.

Cancer Invasion and Metastasis: Biologic Mechanisms and Therapy, edited by S. B. Day et al. Raven Press, New York © 1977.

Metastasis in Pancreatic Duct Adenocarcinoma

Antonio L. Cubilla and Patrick J. Fitzgerald

Department of Pathology, Memorial Sloan-Kettering Cancer Center, New York, New York 10021

Metastases of cancer are stereotyped and follow a reasonably predictable pattern, or, at the other extreme, are bizarre. All experienced oncologists are familiar with the latter type, which is often more spectacular than the former. Such examples as the initial clinical presentation of bilateral parotid swellings caused by metastases from an occult cancer of the breast and the appearance of a malignant cystosarcoma phylloides in the vaginal wall, also a metastasis from the breast, illustrate the folklore of oncology.

However, in the day-to-day study of large numbers of neoplasms at a cancer institute, it appears to us that most cancers have fairly characteristic routes of spread. Breast carcinomas, for the most part, take a lymph node pathway of spread. Decades of breast surgery have proven the statistical likelihood of a certain sequence of nodes being involved, and this is highly correlated with the probability of survival of the patient (1). A similar stereotyped pattern of spread is also true in many head and neck cancers with internal jugular lymph node involvement (2,3) and in the predictable retroperitoneal and parametrial pathways of spread of cancers of the cervix and body of the uterus (4). This does not mean that other avenues of spread are not used as well, but the former are more conspicuous.

Some tumors have a more variable pattern, and pancreas cancer may represent such a group.

Melanoma of extremities is indicative of a more variable group. It usually involves adjacent lymph nodes (5), but in a significant percentage of cases metastasizes widely. Generations of medical students have been inculcated with the diagnostic problem in a patient with liver metastasis of a melanoma from an unknown primary site; the problem is solved by the presence of a glass eye, indicating that a melanoma of the iris was probably the primary site.

The exotic are memorable. Cancers of the lung involve hilar or mediastinal nodes with distressingly frequent regularity, but rarely brain metastasis brings the patient to the psychiatrist or neurologist. The latter cases are long remembered after hundreds of other cases with the stereotyped metastases are forgotten. One of our favorites is fracture of the penis during love play occasioned by a penile metastasis from a cancer of the left nasal septum (6).

Some organs tend to invade adjacent structures, such as cancer of the cervix that frequently involves the ureter, or prostate cancer involving the bladder, and vice versa, and the gastrointestinal cancers that extend to contiguous loops of bowel, stomach, or colon. Choriocarcinoma is said to involve blood vessels primarily, and this is believed to explain its widespread metastasis. The presence of perineural sheath and vein involvement, as in prostate cancer, indicates that two or more portals of spread may be used by some cancers and suggests the complexity involved in any simple explanation of all clinical metastasis. Cancers have access to various routes of dissemination, and many use any and all on occasion. The lymph node spread of cancer is impressive, but the fact that most patients with breast cancer die of the disease in spite of radical excision of lymph nodes (1) may indicate that the routes of spread observed clinically may not necessarily be the only, or indeed the most significant, ones.

PANCREAS DUCT ADENOCARCINOMA

Pancreas cancer indicates the problem in trying to determine which potential routes of spread are responsible for the clinical appearance of metastases. In a study of about 800 patients listed as having cancer of the pancreas in the files of Memorial Hospital over a 24-year period, from 1949 to 1972, we found 508 cases with adequate clinical, surgical, and pathological material for study (7). We have broken these cases down into 10 morphologic types (8). The commonest one, pancreatic duct adenocarcinoma, comprising almost 400 cases, will be used to illustrate metastatic spread of the cancer.

It is assumed (but not necessarily correctly) that the presence of metastatic growth in adjacent lymph nodes indicates that lymphatic pathways have been invaded. But the presence of metastases in the lungs is more difficult to interpret since there is no direct evidence to indicate how the cancer arrived there, whether through lymphatic or blood vessel channels or a combination of both. The matter of selective growth of the metastasis may also be a factor—one organ may seem to favor the growth of metastases from another. For example, the adrenal is said to be a "fertile garden" for lung metastases. A complicating factor in assessing early routes of metastasis from pancreas cancer arose from the fact that about 85% of the patients were discovered to have the disease when the disease had already spread beyond the pancreas.

The most commonly involved organ in metastasis from cancer of the pancreas is the liver (Fig. 1, Table 1). Venous involvement is conspicuous (Fig. 2), and presumably this is the means by which the portal system is involved and becomes the conduit for liver metastasis from tumors of the gastrointestinal tract. However, the portal vein is also directly involved by

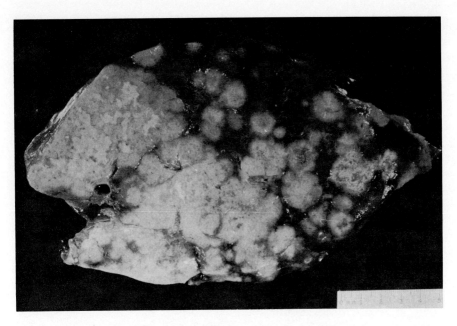

FIG. 1. Cut surface of liver showing diffuse and extensive metastases from pancreas duct adenocarcinoma.

TABLE 1. *Metastasis recorded at admission and/or exploratory laparotomy (262 patients)*

Site	No. patients	(%)
Liver	107	(41)
Peritoneum	65	(25)
Regional lymph nodes	52	(20)
Lung pleura	13	(4)
Lymph nodes, widespread	9	(3)
Skin	9	(3)
Cervix, vagina	8	(3)
Bone	8	(3)
Gallbladder	2	
Adrenal	2	
Brain	2	
Kidney	1	Each less than 1%
Thyroid	1	
Breast	1	
Ureter	1	

Metastases apparent to the surgeon at exploratory operation or to the internist on first examination.

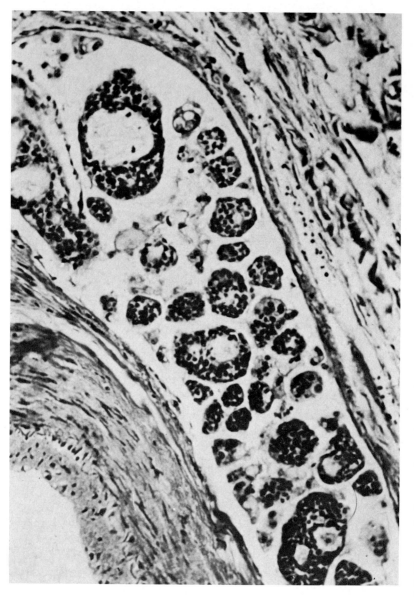

FIG. 2. Clumps of adenocarcinoma in a small vein of the pancreas. Artery negative. Pancreas duct adenocarcinoma (×182).

retroperitoneal spread, and invasion of the vessel wall can be found on occasion.

A common site of involvement is the peripancreatic lymph node system (Fig. 3) (9).

PRESENTATION OF CLINICAL METASTASIS

One of the problems in understanding clinical metastasis is who first sees metastasis and at what stage of the disease. As he opens the abdomen and sees a large pancreas cancer, the general surgeon is impressed with this cancer as being an intraabdominally spreading lesion, for at exploratory surgery the most commonly involved organs are liver (Fig. 1), peritoneal implants (Fig. 4), and regional nodes (Fig. 3, Table 1). The oncological surgeon fortunate enough to encounter an earlier case without liver or peritoneal involvement searches for peripancreatic node involvement (Fig. 3), retroperitoneal spread, or involvement of the celiac axis vessels or portal vein, factors affecting the possibility of resection and the probability of survival of the patient (Table 2). Occasionally, the gastroenterologist is surprised to find neck node metastasis as the presenting sign of what eventually is proven to be a pancreas cancer (Table 3), notwithstanding the absence of jaundice, back pain, or other signs or symptoms said to suggest a pancreas site of origin.

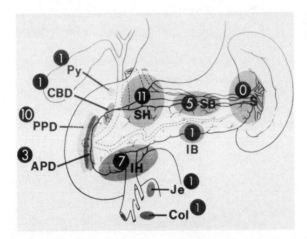

FIG. 3. Analysis of 25 pancreata resected for cancer of the head of the pancreas. The closer the cancer to the duodenum, the more the posterior (PPD) and anterior (APD) pancreaticoduodenal nodes are involved. The more distal to the ampulla of Vater, the more frequently the superior (SH) and inferior (IH) head of the pancreas lymph nodes are involved in cancer of the head of the pancreas. Je, jejunum; Col, colic; Py, pyloric; SB, superior body; IB, inferior body.

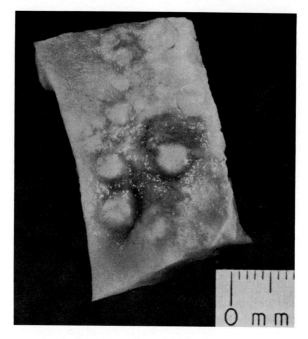

FIG. 4. Peritoneal implants from duct cell adenocarcinoma of the pancreas.

In most patients who have died of the disease, autopsy reveals widespread metastases but it should be noted that 4% of our patients died without metastases (Table 4).

LYMPH NODE INVASION

Lymph node invasion is important from the standpoint of the surgeon and his attempt at extirpation of the disease because the extent of lymph node involvement with cancer is related to survival (Table 2) (7). However, the

TABLE 2. *Stage of disease and survival (317 patients)*

Stage[a]	No. cases	Percent	Median survival (months)
I	47	13	11
II	65	19	5
III	205	68	3
Total	317	100	

[a] In stage I the cancer is confined to the pancreas, in stage II regional lymph nodes are involved, and in stage III the cancer had spread beyond the pancreas and adjacent lymph nodes (7).

TABLE 3. *Presenting site of metastasis, primary site unknown (50 patients)[a]*

Site	Total no. patients	Head	Body and tail	Site not specified
Lymph nodes	22	5	16	1
Left neck	11	1	10	0
Right neck	5	2	3	0
Inguinal	4[b]	0	3	1
Axillary	1	1	0	0
Multiple nodes	1	1	0	0
Skin	8	2	6	0
Bone	8	0	6	2
Lungs	4	3	1	0
Liver	3	2	1	0
Cervix, vagina	3	2	1	0
Brain	2	0	2	0
Total	50	14	33	3

[a] First clinical presentation from occult cancer in 50 of 380 patients. Note much higher frequency of patients with cancer of body and tail than with the more frequent cancer of the head of the pancreas.
[b] Metastasis in 1 patient found at operation for incarcerated hernia which contained metastasis.

TABLE 4. *Metastasis from pancreatic duct carcinoma at autopsy (118 patients)*

Site	Total	Head (61 patients)		Body-tail (57 patients)	
		No.	Percent	No.	Percent
Liver	90	43	70	47	82
Regional lymph nodes	84	43	70	41	72
Peritoneum	65	31	51	34	60
Lung and pleura	59	26	43	33	58
Adrenal	31	9	15	22	39
Bone	28	8	13	20	35
Systemic lymph nodes	28	17	28	11	19
Kidney	14	7	13	7	12
Skin	9	4	7	5	9
Thyroid	8	5	8	3	5
Heart	7	2	4	5	9
Ovary	7	4	7	3	6
Brain	6	3	5	3	6
Vagina	3	2	4	1	2
Gallbladder	3	0	0	3	6
Cervix	2	1	2	1	2
Rectum	2	0	0	2	2
Urinary bladder	1	1	2	0	0
Testis	1	1	2	0	0
Seminal vesicle	1	1	2	0	0
Corpus uteri	1	0	0	1	2
None	4	3	5	1	2

degree of lymph node involvement with cancer requires detailed examination of surgically resected specimens to determine if nodes are involved (9). In the Whipple operation specimen we found an average of 33 lymph nodes of which an average of 1 was positive; in total pancreatectomy specimens an average of 41 lymph nodes were examined and an average of 3 were positive; and with regional pancreatectomy (10) specimens an average of 70 nodes were found and an average of 5 showed cancer (9).

The distribution of lymph nodes with head of the pancreas cancers seems, in preliminary studies, to be fairly regular in 11 of 25 cases. The superior head group of nodes contained cancer; and the closer to the ampulla of Vater the tumor, the more posterior pancreaticoduodenal (PPD) nodes and also the anterior pancreaticoduodenal (APD) nodes were involved (Fig. 3) (9). The involved nodes seemed to be those closest to the tumor and the ones most likely to drain the tumor sites.

Survival was related to lymph node involvement. Patients with stage I lesions survived twice as long as those with stage II cancers, but there was less difference in mean survival between stages II and III (Table 2). Other factors such as site of origin and size of the original tumor are also related to survival (7).

NERVE SHEATH INVOLVEMENT

Nerve sheath involvement occurred in most cases of pancreas cancer (Fig. 5). This has been thought to explain the back pain that occurs in many cases, but there are far more pancreas cancer patients with nerve sheath involvement than those with back pain (11,12).

ISLET INVOLVEMENT

We found that in a small percentage of patients with pancreatic duct adenocarcinoma there was islet invasion (Fig. 6). The islet is well vascularized and this raises the question of whether this might be a route of metastasis in some cases. It also, incidentally, reopens the possibility that the relatively high incidence of diabetes and hyperglycemias in pancreas cancer patients may be related, in part, to involvement of islets.

DIRECT INVASION OF CONTIGUOUS ORGANS OR TISSUES

Posterior spread of pancreas cancer with involvement of the celiac axis vessels and the portal vein is an important extension of the disease that has defeated earlier surgical attempts at complete excision of the cancer. With the development of vascular surgery and replacement of vessels with grafts, the surgeon may attempt to resect this area, including portal vein and mesenteric vessels, and replace portions or all of these vessels by grafts, as

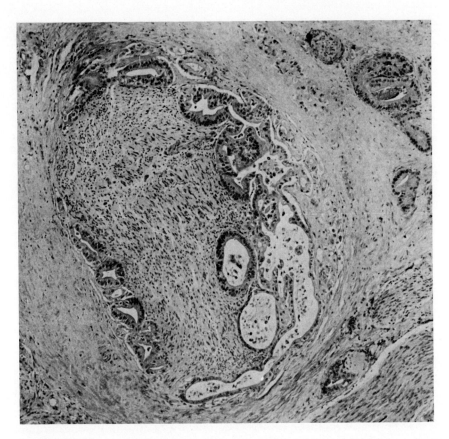

FIG. 5. Pancreas nerve involvement by duct cell adenocarcinoma of the pancreas — a very frequent occurrence (×200).

Fortner et al. (10) have done. Adjacent organs became involved in the course of the disease as with other sites of abdominal cancer (Table 5). The duodenum, in cases of cancer of the head of the pancreas, and stomach, from cancers of the body and tail, are most frequently involved. The peritoneum is involved in the majority of our cases that die of the disease (Fig. 4). The pancreas does not have a distinct capsule, and the absence of the customary organ barrier has been used to explain the extensive retroperitoneal and possibly peritoneal involvement.

WIDESPREAD METASTASES

The widespread metastases (Fig. 7) (Table 4) found at autopsy of the patient dying of cancer of the pancreas may not give a true picture of the sequence of spread of cancer because routes used early in the course of the

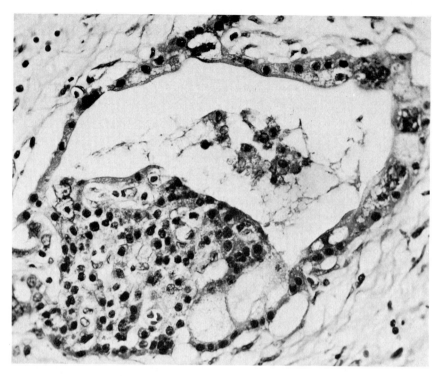

FIG. 6. Pancreatic duct cancer invading periphery of islet of Langerhans (×367).

disease may be overshadowed by the greater growth of tumors from other avenues used later.

Metastasis to the pancreas itself is uncommon (Fig. 8), in contrast to direct invasion from other cancers such as gastric, duodenal, or periampullary cancer.

TABLE 5. *Organ directly invaded (at autopsy) by pancreas duct cancer (75 patients)*

Anatomical site invaded	Total no. patients	Primary site		
		Head No. (%)	Body No. (%)	Tail No. (%)
Duodenum	30	24 (67)	6 (24)	0 (0)
Stomach	20	9 (25)	10 (40)	1 (7)
Spleen	8	0 (0)	3 (12)	5 (36)
Left adrenal	5	0 (0)	1 (4)	4 (29)
Transverse colon	6	1 (3)	3 (12)	2 (14)
Left kidney	2	0 (0)	1 (4)	1 (7)
Jejunum	3	1 (3)	1 (4)	1 (7)
Ureter (right)	1	1 (3)	0 (0)	0 (0)
Total (%)	75	36 (48)	25 (33)	14 (19)

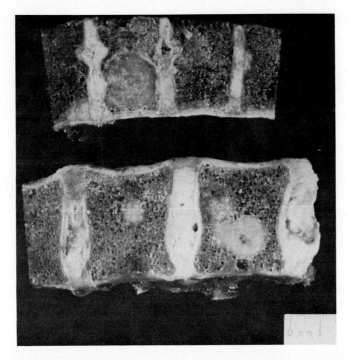

FIG. 7. Metastases to vertebral bodies from pancreas duct adenocarcinoma.

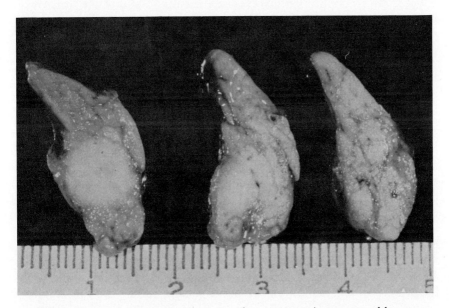

FIG. 8. Very rare metastases to pancreas from osteogenic sarcoma of femur.

The high correlation of lymph node involvement and survival may occur only because it indicates the overall extent of cancer metastases at that time, e.g., small foci of blood-borne metastasis, hidden to clinical examination, may explain why most patients with breast cancer eventually die of the disease in spite of radical resection of the cancer and the regional lymph nodes (2) and why resection of pancreas cancer even when lymph nodes are negative gives a median survival of only 11 months (Table 2).

HOST REACTION AND THE CANCER CELL

In view of current interest in the immunological response to cancer, although a desmoplastic reaction is common in pancreas cancer with abundant masses of dense collagen similar to that of infiltrating duct cancer of the breast, there is relatively little conspicuous lymphocytic or histiocytic response except in relation to duct obstruction and the degeneration, necrosis, and inflammation response associated with it. In only 5% of our 380 cases of pancreas duct adenocarcinoma were a significant number of lymphocytes present. Associated with the focal obstruction and necrosis was the usual acute inflammatory response, primarily of polymorphonuclear leukocytes with a few macrophages (8).

It should be pointed out that invasion of or metastasis to lymph nodes is not necessarily associated with widespread metastasis, as in pancreas cancer. With papillary cancer of the thyroid, e.g., lymph node spread is very frequent, yet metastases elsewhere are uncommon and only 5 to 10% of patients with lymph node involvement eventually die of the disease (13). Host reaction to the cancers, or the characteristics of the thyroid and pancreas cancer cells, must be greatly different in these two extremes of the cancer metastasis spectrum.

SUMMARY

Cancer of a visceral organ such as the pancreas appears to invade the organ early in the course of the disease, following fairly predictable routes to adjacent peripancreatic nodes, and also invades blood vessels (venous) and nerve sheaths. Later extension to adjacent organs and implantation on peritoneal surfaces appear to occur. As in all types of cancer, there are unusual sites of metastasis — 6% presented clinically as metastases to nonvisceral lymph nodes (Table 3).

It must be emphasized that our data were collected very late in the course of the disease — *in situ* carcinoma may have existed for years (14) and how long the invasive period was prior to the appearance of clinical signs and symptoms is not known. One cannot from the material assess the relative importance of lymphatic, venous, nerve sheath, or islet cell involvement in determining metastasis. Lodgment and growth in lymph nodes may reflect local circumstances as well as intrinsic aggressiveness of the cancer cell.

Animal models of pancreas cancer (14–17) wherein one can follow the stages from papillary hyperplasia through atypia and carcinoma *in situ* to invasive cancer may be of considerable aid in unraveling the complexities of the relative importance of routes of spread in this visceral cancer.

In attempting to understand the phenomenon of metastasis in human cancer, it appears that the ability of the cancer cell to breach basement membranes and to invade lymphatics and small blood vessels is one of its deadliest early characteristics. One might assume that this is because of the acquisition of a lytic enzymatic property, newly developed during the transformation process.

The explosive burst of metastases seen in this cancer may indicate that a clone, or a few clones, of malignant cells which had acquired the ability to penetrate basement membranes or other boundaries became increasingly predominant in the cancer cell population, possibly with the aid of some extra organ factor favoring their growth, and the preferential multiplication of the cells with these characteristics explains the rapid overwhelming of tissue and cellular barriers.

ACKNOWLEDGMENT

This work was aided by contracts NO1-CB-43232 and NO1-CP43975 from the National Cancer Institute.

REFERENCES

1. Adair, F., Berg, J., Joubert, L., and Robbins, G. F. (1974): Long-term followup of breast cancer patients: The 30-year report. *Cancer,* 33:1145–1150.
2. Cady, B., and Catlin, D. (1969): Epidermoid carcinoma of the gum. *Cancer,* 23:551–569.
3. Exelby, P. E., and Frazell, E. L. (1969): Carcinoma of the thyroid in children. *Surg. Clin. North Am.,* 49:249–259.
4. Fridell, G. H., and Parsons, L. (1961): The spread of cancer of the uterine cervix as seen in giant histological section. *Cancer,* 14:42–54.
5. Wanebo, H. J., Woodruff, J., and Fortner, J. G. (1975): Malignant melanoma of the extremities: A clinicopathologic study using levels of invasion (microstage). *Cancer,* 35: 666–676.
6. Pack, G. T., and Booher, R. J. (1949): Localization of metastatic cancer by trauma. *N.Y. State J. Med.,* 49:1839–1841.
7. Cubilla, A. L., and Fitzgerald, P. J. (1977): Pancreas cancer: I. Duct adenocarcinoma (*Submitted for publication*).
8. Cubilla, A. L., and Fitzgerald, P. J. (1975): Morphological patterns of primary nonendocrine human pancreas carcinoma. *Cancer Res.,* 35:2234–2246.
9. Cubilla, A. L., Fortner, J. G., and Fitzgerald, P. J. (1977): Lymph node involvement in pancreas cancer (*in preparation*).
10. Fortner, J. G., Kim, D. K., Cubilla, A. L., Turnbull, A. D., Pahnke, L. D., and Shils, M. E. (1977): Regional pancreatectomy (en bloc pancreatic, portal vein and lymph node resection). *Ann. Surg.* (*in press*).
11. Bowden, L., and Pack, G. T. (1969): Cancer of the head of the pancreas. A collective re-

view of the experiences of the Gastric Service of the Memorial Cancer Center 1926–1958. *G.E.N.,* 23:339–367.

12. Die Goyanes, A., Pack, G. T., and Bowden, L. (1971): Cancer of the body and tail of the pancreas. *Rev. Surg.,* 28:153–175.
13. Tollefsen, H. R., DeCosse, J. J., and Hutter, R. V. P. (1964): Papillary carcinoma of the thyroid: A clinical and pathological study of 70 fatal cases. *Cancer,* 17:1035–1044.
14. Cubilla, A. L., and Fitzgerald, P. J. (1976): Morphological lesions associated with human primary invasive nonendocrine pancreas cancer. *Cancer Res.,* 36:2690–2698.
15. Pour, P., Kruger, F. W., Althoff, J., et al. (1974): Cancer of the pancreas induced in the Syrian golden hamster. *Am. J. Pathol.,* 76:249–358.
16. Reddy, J. K., and Rao, M. S. (1975): Pancreatic adenocarcinoma in inbred guinea pigs induced by *N*-methyl-*N*-nitrosourea. *Cancer Res.,* 35:2269–2277.
17. Longnecker, D., and Crawford, B. (1974): Hyperplastic nodules and adenomas of the exocrine pancreas in azaserine-treated rats. *J. Natl. Cancer Inst.,* 53:573–577.

Cancer Invasion and Metastasis: Biologic Mechanisms and Therapy, edited by S. B. Day et al. Raven Press, New York © 1977.

Tumor Angiogenesis: Its Possible Role in Metastasis and Invasion

Judah Folkman and Kenneth Tyler

Department of Surgery, Children's Hospital Medical Center, Harvard Medical School, Boston, Massachusetts 02115

The vascularization of solid tumors has until recently occupied an insignificant niche of tumor biology. However, angiogenesis is assuming a more central position because the idea has been developed that the vessels interspersed in a solid tumor may be a control point in the growth of the tumor (10). Furthermore, tumor invasion and metastasis may be facilitated after the onset of vascularization has occurred.

PRESENT STATUS OF TUMOR ANGIOGENESIS

Tumors Induce Neovascularization

What do we know about tumor angiogenesis? First, we know that malignant tumors do not make their own vessels, but *induce* them from the host. This has been demonstrated in the hamster cheek pouch (15), the rat dorsal air sac, the anterior chamber of the rabbit eye (14), and in the chick embryo (8). However, the best evidence comes from the implantation of tumors in the rabbit cornea (13). The cornea is 12 mm in diameter and approximately 1 mm thick. It consists of layers of collagen, in which blood vessels and lymphatics are absent. The nearest blood vessels lie at the edge of the cornea in the limbus. Pieces of tumor, or normal tissue, 1 × 1.5 mm, can be implanted into small pockets made in the cornea. These pockets can be accurately placed so that they lie at any distance up to 6 mm from the limbal vessels. The distances can be measured with a stereoscopic slit lamp to ±0.1 mm. A variety of mouse, rat, rabbit, and human tumors placed in these pockets, or tumor cells from tissue culture, will induce new vessels to grow from the limbus and through the corneal stroma toward the tumor. Of interest is that the edge of a tumor implant must be within 2.5 to 3.0 mm of the limbus before vessel induction occurs. New vessels usually begin growing at an average rate of 0.2 mm per day, but as they approach the tumor, may increase their growth rate to 0.6 to 0.8 mm per day, and then penetrate the tumor implant.

Do normal tissues stimulate neovascularization? K. Tyler (*unpublished data*) in our laboratory showed that tissues such as heart, kidney, and thyroid from adult rabbits do not become vascularized in the cornea. These grafts do not stimulate neovascularization in the host. Even when they are brought into apposition with the limbus, they fail to anastomose with the host vessels. Embryonic tissues, however, will connect up with the limbal vessels, but only if the graft is placed in apposition to the limbal vessels (Fig. 1). By 36 to 48 hr, the white avascular graft suddenly becomes pink, as blood flows through its vessels. One can occasionally see the actual anastomosis of the graft vessels to the host. However, if such an embryonic graft (e.g., embryonic rabbit heart) is withdrawn from the corneal edge by only 0.1 mm, no vessels ever cross this short distance to the graft (Fig. 2). The graft is unable to stimulate neovascularization in the limbal vascular bed. Likewise, embryonic grafts that are implanted at 0.5, 1, and up to 2 mm from the limbal edge, cannot stimulate vessels. This simple system thus reveals a major operational difference between malignant and nonmalignant tissue. Small implants of neoplastic tissues can induce proliferation of vessels across distances of up to 3.0 mm in the cornea, whereas embryonic implants of the same size or larger cannot induce vessels across any measurable distance, but require instead direct apposition to host vessels before they will anastomose.

Ausprunk et al. (3) in our laboratory have also demonstrated this dif-

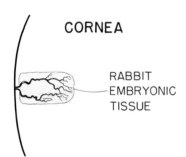

CORNEA

RABBIT
EMBRYONIC
TISSUE

FIG. 1. Vascularization of embryonic tissue implanted in the cornea compared to tumor implanted in the cornea when both grafts are placed in apposition to the limbal vessels. The intact vessels of the embryonic graft anastomose to the host vessels. By contrast, the original vessels within the tumor graft disintegrate, and new vessels are induced from the host.

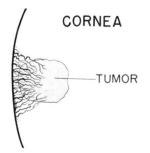

CORNEA

TUMOR

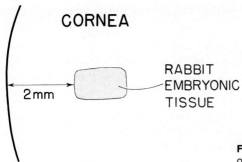

CORNEA

2mm

RABBIT
EMBRYONIC
TISSUE

FIG. 2. Comparison of corneal implants of embryonic tissue and tumor tissue when the grafts are placed at a distance from the limbal vessels. In this situation, the embryonic tissue is unable to attract new vessels, whereas the tumor graft does attract new vessels and becomes vascularized.

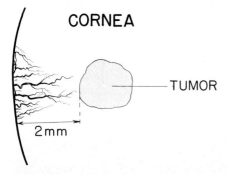

CORNEA

TUMOR

2mm

ference between tumor and normal tissues grafted in the chick embryo. They implanted tumor grafts and also grafts of normal adult and embryonic tissue into the chorioallantoic membrane, and studied their vascularization by looking at multiple histologic sections. Tumor grafts stimulated neovascularization, whereas normal tissues did not. Embryonic grafts could reestablish blood flow through their own vessels by anastomosis with host vessels, whereas adult tissues could not. However, neither of these "normal" tissues elicited neovascularization in the chorioallantoic membrane. Furthermore, the existing vessels within a tumor graft disintegrated shortly after transplantation so that the only vascularization possible for tumors was by stimulation of new capillary sprouts from the host. By contrast, the existing vessels of an embryonic graft remained intact and connected by anastomosis to the host vessels.

These corneal experiments and those in the chorioallantoic membrane provide further evidence that a diffusible substance, tumor-angiogenesis-factor (TAF) (9), travels from the tumor to stimulate host vessels. Although the ability to stimulate new vessel growth appears at the morphologic level to provide a qualitative difference between normal and malignant tissue, the difference may turn out to be only quantitative when the mechanism is more completely understood. It is conceivable that embryonic tissues also make

TAF, but at such low concentrations that this normal tissue must be in very close apposition to host vessels.

Vessel Proliferation Is Stimulated by a Diffusible Factor

A soluble material has been isolated from animal tumors and from tumor cells in culture and partially purified (12,16). It has not been found in primary cultures of normal cells, but is present in some long-established lines. This material, TAF, will stimulate neovascularization when placed on the chorioallantoic membrane of the chick embryo. More recently, we have incorporated it into slow-release polymer pellets which, when implanted into the rabbit cornea, also stimulate neovascularization (17). These controlled-release polymer pellets have enabled us to study in more detail the initial events of tumor-induced capillary proliferation.

Fenselau and Mello (6) have shown that extracts of Walker carcinoma will stimulate proliferation of bovine aortic endothelium in tissue culture. Suddith et al. (21) showed that tumor-conditioned medium would stimulate human umbilical vein endothelial cells in culture. Birdwell et al. (4) showed that conditioned medium from transformed cells stimulated DNA synthesis in bovine aortic endothelium. It remains to be seen whether these results are attributable to TAF or to other factors.

New Capillary Sprouts Originate from Endothelial Cells in Venules

Ausprunk and Folkman (1) implanted fragments of V-2 carcinoma into rabbit corneas. The preexisting limbal vessels and new capillary sprouts were examined daily. One day after tumor implantation, endothelial cells and preexisting blood vessels resembled regenerating endothelium. By 2 days, these endothelial cells penetrated the basal lamina and began to migrate toward the tumor stimulus. This generally occurred only in endothelial cells on the side of the venule facing the tumor or TAF implant. Pseudopods of endothelial membrane extruded between the fragmented basement membrane. There was active endothelial cell migration out into the cornea prior to any incorporation of ^{3}H-thymidine which began at 2 days and reached a peak of 8%-labeling index by day 3. New capillary sprouts were obvious by day 4, and were cannalized from the earliest stages. In the advancing capillary sprout, the migrating cells in the lead did not usually incorporate ^{3}H-thymidine but those cells just behind them did continue to proliferate and incorporate ^{3}H-thymidine. Continuous venous blood flow was established when two sprouts connected with each other to form a capillary loop. The loop itself then advanced and appeared like a bucket handle extending out from the venule. Usually the tip of a capillary loop with blood flowing in it would be the first vascular tissue to enter or penetrate the edge of the tumor or to arrive at the TAF pellet.

Rapid Tumor Growth Follows Vascularization

When a tumor is implanted into the cornea, or when a small tumor spheroid is implanted in the anterior chamber near the iris vessels, the exact onset of vascularization of the tumor can be observed. During the avascular stage, when new capillaries are still growing toward the tumor but have not yet *penetrated* it, the tumor remains small (1 to 3 mm in diameter), grows slowly, or often stops growing, but remains viable. Within 1 to 2 days after the tumor has been penetrated by new capillary sprouts, rapid tumor growth begins and the implant may reach 16,000 times the volume of the original avascular mass in less than 2 more weeks. One gains added insight by asking the question, "How large can a tumor become without blood vessels?" A general answer that would account for most solid tumors, except (perhaps) for chondrosarcoma, is that a tumor mass beyond a few millimeters in diameter, and a population density of more than 1 million cells, is not usually attainable without penetration of the mass by new blood vessels. This conclusion is drawn from the study of tumor spheroids of Brown–Pearce carcinoma floating in the anterior chamber of the rabbit eye (14), from observation of metastases of human retinoblastoma in the vitreous (9), and from measurements of mouse melanoma, V-79 hamster lung cells and L-5178Y mouse leukemia cells growing in soft agar as spheroids (11). All of these studies suggest that as tumor cells accumulate in a three-dimensional configuration (usually spheroidal), they reach a population size where simple diffusion of nutrients and wastes limits further expansion. While cells within the spheroid may continue to proliferate and die, an equilibrium is reached between new and dying cells so that the avascular mass itself appears to become dormant. This is a form of "population dormancy." The individual cells are not dormant.

These observations are, nevertheless, only indirect evidence. Stronger evidence for this supposition will come when tumor-induced angiogenesis can be blocked or inhibited in an experimental animal.

Newly Formed Capillaries Regress when the Tumor Stimulus Is Removed

Ausprunk and Falterman (2) have also studied the sequence of events in capillary regression. Vascularization was induced in rabbit corneas by silver nitrate burn or tumor implant (Brown–Pearce tumor that regresses spontaneously), or by an implant of slow-release polymer pellet containing sodium hydroxide or a tumor cell extract with angiogenesis activity. After the stimulus was discontinued (e.g., removing the polymer pellet), small secondary and tertiary vessel branches at the very tip of the capillaries disappeared in the first week. Larger vessels became thinner and blood flow stopped by 3 weeks. A few bloodless vessels persisted for 10 weeks. The earliest events occur at the very tip where there is endothelial cell damage after approximately 16 hr. Platelets stick to the damaged endothelial cells, and small clots form. The degenerating cells are then removed by macrophages and the vessel gradually shrinks back to its primary venule.

A POSSIBLE ROLE OF ANGIOGENESIS IN METASTASIS

The Primary Tumor: Relationship of Angiogenesis and Cell Shedding

Liotta and Kleinerman (18) showed that when the T-241 sarcoma was implanted in the thigh of the C57BL/6 mouse, no tumor vessels could be demonstrated in the implant prior to 4 days after transplantation. On day 4, small capillaries were found in the peripheral region of several tumors and on day 5 all tumors contained small vascular sprouts generally at the periphery of the tumor mass. No tumor cells were identified in the venous effluent before day 5, and this implies that few or no cells leave the tumor until *after* the new capillary sprouts have penetrated its periphery. These workers found a linear relationship between the density of perfused vessels of a diameter greater than 30 μm and the concentration of both total tumor cells and tumor cell clumps escaping from the tumor.

As the tumor grew (e.g., after day 12), the ratio of vessels greater than 30 μm to vessels less than 30 μm increased. This would permit tumor cell clumps of more than six to seven cells to leave the tumor.

Liotta et al. (19) have also shown that the number of metastatic foci increases roughly in proportion to the clump size. In addition, they demonstrated that up to 1.5×10^5 tumor cells may enter the circulation over a 24-hr period. Butler and Gullino (5) showed that 3.2×10^6 tumor cells per day enter the venous effluent from an embryonic carcinoma. These studies imply that vascularization of a tumor may be one of the steps necessary (although not sufficient) for cells to escape from a primary tumor into the circulation.

Indirect evidence to support this idea comes from the study of a variety of human carcinomas. During the *in-situ* phase of carcinoma of the cervix, breast, colon, bladder, or skin, the tumor is small (a few millimeters in diameter), rests above an intact basement membrane, and is *avascular*. Vessels have not penetrated from beneath the basement membrane through it and into the tumor. The *in-situ* stage may exist for years, and this prolonged period is also commonly free of metastases. Metastases usually appear *after* the primary tumor has become vascularized. If this were in fact not the common pattern, the clinical presentation of human cancer would be much different than we know it. The majority of patients would first present themselves with many established metastases, but the primary lesion would still be *in situ* or undetectable. In practice, such a presentation pattern is the exception.

Relationship of Angiogenesis to Growth of the New Metastasis

Once a few tumor cells or a clump of circulating cells have arrested in a capillary bed (i.e., the lung), little or no growth occurs here. Although there are exceptions, Wood (22) observed with time lapse movies of the rabbit ear chamber that circulating tumor cells stuck to the capillary endothelium, then moved through the basement membrane of the capillary and out into the extravascular space. There they stopped, began to proliferate, and then attracted new capillary sprouts that grew toward the new metastasis from nearby venules. G. Nicolson (*personal communication*) has observed in mice receiving melanoma cells intravenously that in hundreds of metastatic implant studies by histologic sections of lungs, there were only one or two examples of tumor growth within the blood vessels. All of the other tumor cells began to proliferate after they had escaped from the vascular lumen. Thus, a metastatic implant may need to recapitulate the induction of new vessels similar to the primary tumor in order that further growth can occur. However, dormant metastases may result from a variety of different mechanisms.

Relationship of Angiogenesis to Dormancy of a Metastasis

That metastases may lie dormant has been shown in a variety of experimental systems. Experiments by Fisher and Fisher (7) are perhaps the most compelling. Tumor cells were injected into the portal vein of rats. Liver metastases would appear after prolonged periods of time, but only after the animal had been exposed to blunt abdominal trauma. Presumably, the tumor cells lay dormant in the liver until somehow stimulated by the trauma.

By what conceptual framework can we account for this strange behavior? Before invoking obscure mechanisms such as steroid levels, or subtle immune changes, we must consider that angiogenesis may relate to the dormancy of metastases in at least one of three ways: (a) It is possible that tumor cells might become embedded between the endothelium and the basement membrane of a venule for long periods before migrating into the extravascular tissue. (b) It is possible that once outside the vascular lumen, a small population of tumor cells might remain in the avascular phase for some time and thus would be dormant because of the limitations of simple diffusion on further growth. (c) Finally, some metastatic tumors may temporarily stop growing even after vascularization. Although the onset of vascularization will permit the maximum growth for a given tumor, and although this growth is usually continuous, there are certain clinical cases in which vascularized metastases in the lung appear temporarily to stop growing for many months. There is no known explanation for the dormancy of a vascularized metastasis.

IS ANGIOGENESIS RELATED TO TUMOR INVASIVENESS?

Again, the evidence is sparse, and one can only speculate that the onset of neovascularization may in some way facilitate or activate the capacity of a tumor nodule to invade and destroy neighboring normal tissues. Proliferating capillaries themselves seem to be invasive. When new capillaries grow into the rabbit cornea, they are able to intrude between layers of tightly packed collagen. When new vessels grow into cartilage, there is associated chondrolysis (20). An avascular tumor implant in the rabbit cornea always remains as a thin plaque of cells (two to three cell layers thick) trapped between the collagen lamellae. The tumor never invades into adjoining lamellae. However, once the tumor has become vascularized, it is very destructive, and is capable of invading through layers of collagen to the outer aspect of the cornea. If the association of vascularization of a tumor with its increased invasive capacity continues to hold up, then it will be important to search for the mechanism of this synergism between a normal and malignant tissue.

SUMMARY

In summary, we have proposed a two-phase model for growth of solid tumors, in which the second phase begins after the tumor is penetrated by new vessels from the host. In this chapter, we have gathered the current evidence for the idea that this second phase (i.e., the vascularized tumor) facilitates metastasis and invasion. Furthermore, the avascular tumor (first phase) appears to shed metastases rarely, if at all, and it may not be invasive. In animals with experimental tumors, the *avascular* phase is so brief that it must be prolonged artificially to display its differences from the *vascular* phase. However, in human cancer, the *avascular* phase (*in-situ* carcinoma) is often years longer than the *vascular* phase, and the differences between them are more apparent.

ACKNOWLEDGMENT

This work was supported by grant #2RO1 CA14019 from the National Cancer Institute.

REFERENCES

1. Ausprunk, D., and Folkman, J. (1977): Migration and proliferation of endothelial cells in preformed and newly formed blood vessels during tumor angiogenesis. *Microvasc. Res.,* 14:53–65.
2. Ausprunk, D., and Falterman, K. (1976): Sequence of events in regression of capillaries. *J. Cell Biol.,* 70:209 (abstract).
3. Ausprunk, D., Knighton, D., and Folkman, J. (1975): Vascularization of normal and neoplastic tissues grafted to the chick chorioallantois. *Am. J. Pathol.,* 79:597–610.

4. Birdwell, C. R., Gospodarowicz, D., and Nicolson, G. L. (1977): Factors from transformed and untransformed 3T3 cells stimulate proliferation of cultured vascular endothelial cells. *Nature (in press)*.
5. Butler, T., and Gullino, P. (1975): Quantitation of cell shedding into efferent blood of mammary adenocarcinoma. *Cancer Res.*, 35:512.
6. Fenselau, A., and Mello, R. J. (1976): Growth stimulation of cultured endothelial cells by tumor cell homogenates. *Cancer Res.*, 36:3269.
7. Fisher, B., and Fisher, E. R. (1959): Experimental studies of factors influencing hepatic metastases. I. The effect of number of tumor cells injected and time of growth. *Cancer*, 12:926–928.
8. Folkman, J. (1974): Tumor angiogenesis. *Adv. Cancer Res.*, 19:331–358.
9. Folkman, J. (1974): Tumor angiogenesis factor. *Cancer Res.*, 34:2109–2113.
10. Folkman, J. (1975): Tumor angiogenesis: A possible control point in tumor growth. *Ann. Intern. Med.*, 82:96–100.
11. Folkman, J., and Hochberg, M. (1973): Self-regulation of growth in three dimensions. *J. Exp. Med.*, 138:745–753.
12. Folkman, J., Merler, E., Abernathy, C., and Williams, G. (1971): Isolation of a tumor factor responsible for angiogenesis. *J. Exp. Med.*, 133:275–288.
13. Gimbrone, M., Cotran, R., and Folkman, J. (1974): Tumor growth and neovascularization: An experimental model using rabbit cornea. *J. Natl. Cancer Inst.*, 52:413–427.
14. Gimbrone, M. A., Leapman, S., Cotran, R., and Folkman, J. (1973): Tumor angiogenesis: Iris neovascularization at a distance from experimental intraocular tumor. *J. Natl. Cancer Inst.*, 50:219–228.
15. Greenblatt, M., and Shubik, P. (1968): Tumor angiogenesis: Transfiltered diffusion studies in the hamster by the transparent chamber technique. *J. Natl. Cancer Inst.*, 41:111–124.
16. Klagsbrun, M., Knighton, D., and Folkman, J. (1976): Tumor angiogenesis activity in cells grown in tissue culture. *Cancer Res.*, 36:110–114.
17. Langer, R., and Folkman, J. (1976): Polymers for the sustained release of proteins and other macromolecules. *Nature*, 263:797–800.
18. Liotta, L. A., Kleinerman, J., and Saidel, G. M. (1974): Quantitative relationships of intravascular tumor cells, tumor vessels, and pulmonary metastases following tumor implantation. *Cancer Res.*, 34:997.
19. Liotta, L. A., Kleinerman, J., and Saidel, G. M. (1976): The significance of hematogenous tumor cell clumps in the metastatic process. *Cancer Res.*, 36:889.
20. Reddi, A. H., and Huggins, C. B. (1972): Biochemical sequences in the transformation of normal fibroblasts in adolescent rats. *Proc. Natl. Acad. Sci. USA*, 69:1601.
21. Suddith, R. L., Keely, P. J., Hutchinson, H. T., et al. (1975): In vitro demonstration of an endothelial proliferative factor produced by neural cell lines. *Science*, 190:682.
22. Wood, S. (1958): Pathogenesis of metastasis formation observed in the rabbit ear chamber. *Arch. Pathol.*, 66:550–568.

Cancer Invasion and Metastasis: Biologic Mechanisms and Therapy, edited by S. B. Day et al. Raven Press, New York © 1977.

The Tumor Dormant State

E. Frederick Wheelock, Lester T. Goldstein,
Kent J. Weinhold, Walter P. Carney, and Preston A. Marx

*Department of Microbiology, Jefferson Medical College,
Thomas Jefferson University, Philadelphia, Pennsylvania 19107*

The reappearance of overt tumor in patients months or years after successful treatment of a primary tumor by surgery, chemotherapy, or X-irradiation is not uncommon. The long delay prior to reappearance of clinically detectable tumor suggests that in such cases host regulatory mechanisms, immune or otherwise, have controlled tumor outgrowth following therapy. We shall refer to this clinically quiescent state as tumor "dormancy."

Evidence for the existence of tumor cells in a dormant state in clinically normal persons comes from a variety of histological studies. Beckwith and Perrin (1) found, in unselected autopsies of children up to the age of 3 months, small foci of cells resembling typical neuroblastomas in the adrenals at a frequency that was 40 to 50 times that expected from the actual incidence of clinical adrenal neuroblastoma. Similarly, Mortensen et al. (2) examined 821 unselected thyroids and found that 49.5% contained nodules, 17 of which were histologically malignant. Since the incidence of clinical thyroid cancer is about 6 per million, this finding of 2% incidence of histologically malignant lesions in unselected autopsies is much greater than would have been predicted. Similar findings were made in studies performed on carcinoma of the prostate by Ashley (3) and by Munsie and Foster (4). Following the introduction of smear cytology as a technique for early diagnosis of cervical carcinoma, vast numbers of "carcinoma *in situ*" cases were reported (5–7). Again, it is statistically evident that a large proportion of these "precarcinoma" lesions never develop into clinical disease. Clearly, some process, immunologic or otherwise, must act to restrain these "precancerous" cells from active growth to overt neoplasia.

To date few studies have been directed toward exploration of this tumor dormant state. Fisher and Fisher (8) described the first experimental model of tumor dormancy in 1959. They injected rats intraportally with 50 Walker-256 carcinosarcoma cells and then examined the rats 5 months later for hepatic tumor growth; none was evident. If, however, 3 months after injection of the cells the rats were subjected to repeated laparotomy and liver examination at 7-day intervals, 100% of the rats developed tumors within a few weeks. Eccles and Alexander (9) found that rats whose primary tumor transplants had been surgically removed were clinically normal for many months. However, these clinically normal rats, when subjected to whole-body X-irradiation, developed overt tumors from metastases that had apparently persisted in a dormant state following surgical removal of the primary implant.

On a theoretical basis, the following questions form a framework for further investigation.

1. How do tumor cells avoid outright destruction and establish a state of dormancy?
2. Are all tumor cells in the original tumor population equally capable of establishing a tumor dormant state or is there a selective process?
3. Is the tumor dormant state more characteristic of certain types of tumors than of others?
4. Does tumor dormancy involve an alteration in the rate of tumor cell division or is it simply a balance between tumor cell division and destruction?
5. What factors ultimately determine whether dormancy concludes in tumor cell outgrowth or tumor cell eradication?
6. What therapeutic regimen can be devised that will either promote eradication of dormant tumor or result in prolongation of the tumor dormant state?

At present, it is clear only that a delicate balance exists between tumor growth and tumor suppression in the animal host during tumor dormancy. We have attempted to understand this relationship and manipulate it in favor of the host. This chapter describes three experimental murine models of tumor dormancy currently under investigation in our laboratory. Each model system probably represents a different host response to the neoplastic process.

RESULTS

Friend Leukemia Virus

The first animal model employed to study tumor dormancy uses Friend leukemia virus (FLV), one of the several antigenically related murine oncornaviruses. Infection of adult DBA/2 mice with FLV produces, by day 21 post-infection, an erythroleukemia characterized by hepatosplenomegaly and large numbers of circulating erythroblasts. By 10 weeks, all mice have succumbed to the leukemia. FLV infects a variety of cell types, including lymphocytes, and infection leads to a rapid suppression of both humoral and cellular immunity. Reasoning that the immunodepression induced by FLV might be essential for its leukemogenicity, we sought ways to restore immune competence to FLV-infected mice and thereby permit the host to mount an immune response to the virus and to virus-transformed cells.

We found that 100% of infected DBA/2 mice were viremic and had large numbers of leukemic cells in their spleens by the third day after virus inoculation. An extensive search was made for a drug or biologic agent that could suppress FLV erythroleukemia when administered after systemic infection had been established. FLV leukemosuppressive activity was found in an extract of *Penicillium stoloniferum* cultures that had been infected with a double-stranded RNA containing mycophage (10,11). This extract, called statolon, could, when combined with chlorite oxidized oxyamylose (COAM), suppress erythroleukemia in 90% of FLV-infected mice (12). We have found that COAM-statolon treatment results in interferon production and suppression of FLV replication (13). Virus is rapidly cleared from the blood and most of the treated mice produce antibodies that neutralize the virus and lyse leukemic cells *in vitro* in the presence of guinea pig complement. Statolon-treated mice which suppress their FLV infection become clinically normal, and most display no gross pathologic, clinical, or hematologic manifestations of leukemia during their entire 2-year life span. However, late in life, some of these mice develop erythroleukemia from which FLV can be isolated (13). Attempts to isolate infectious FLV from the blood or spleens of these mice during remission have so far been unsuccessful. However, transfer of large numbers of spleen cells from mice in remission to normal mice does result in the production of FLV erythroleukemia in the recipients, indicating that the virus and/or leukemic cells were present in the clinically normal mice (13).

We have tested in a variety of assays lymphoid cells from clinically normal mice that harbor FLV and have been unable to demonstrate *in vitro* cell-mediated immune responses against FLV antigens even in the presence of virus-specific antibody. We have therefore focused our attention on the interferon production and humoral antibody responses. Interferon can be detected for 2 days after statolon inoculation, but it appears not to be the leukemosuppressive factor since COAM-statolon–treated mice that subsequently develop leukemia produce an interferon response that is indistinguishable from the response made in mice that suppress the virus to a dormant state. The major difference between the two groups of mice is the presence, in mice with dormant FLV infections, of antibodies that neutralize FLV and are cytolytic for virus-transformed cells.

In order to understand how such antibodies may be involved in leukemosuppression and FLV dormancy, we assayed the immunoglobulins in the sera of mice with dormant FLV infections by radioimmunoassay for specific binding to individual FLV antigens (14). As antigens in the assay, we used tissue culture grown ^{35}S-methionine-labeled FLV virions (15) disrupted with Triton X-100. Sera from mice with dormant FLV infections, mice with overt leukemia, and normal mice were assayed. Disrupted ^{35}S-labeled virions were mixed with the indicated serum, and an immune precipitate was formed by the addition of rabbit antimouse gammaglobulin. The resulting immune precipitate was analyzed for ^{35}S-labeled virion polypeptides by polyacrylamide gel electrophoresis. The results are shown in Table 1.

TABLE 1. *Comparison of relative levels of antibody to individual FLV-virion polypeptides in sera of DBA/2 mice with dormant versus overt FLV erythroleukemia*

Source of serum[b]	Presence of antibody[a] to virion polypeptide					
	gp69/71	gp43	p30	p15	p12	p10
COAM-statolon–treated dormant FLV-infected mice[c]	+	+	−	+	+	−
COAM-statolon–treated FLV leukemic mice	+	+	−	+	--	−
Untreated FLV leukemic mice	+	+	−	+	--	−
COAM-statolon–treated normal mice <22 weeks old	−	−	−	−	−	−
Normal mice <22 weeks old	−	−	−	−	−	−

[a] Detected by polyacrylamide gel electrophoresis of radioimmune precipitates. +, detected out to 1:320 dilution of serum; −, absent at 1:20 dilution of serum; --, absent at 1:10 dilution of serum.

[b] Serum was from one lot of DBA/2 mice all born within 1 week of each other.

[c] All infected mice received 2,000 LD_{50} of FLV administered i.p. COAM was given i.v. 2 days after infection (0.5 mg), and statolon was given i.v. 3 days after infection (5.0 mg).

Serum from dormant FLV-infected mice contained antibodies against the virion polypeptides gp69/71, gp43, p15, and p12. In contrast, serum from mice with overt leukemia contained antibodies against gp69/71, gp43, and p15 but did not contain antibody against p12. Antibody against virion p12 was readily detectable at a 1:320 dilution of serum from dormant FLV-infected mice but was not detected even at a 1:10 dilution of leukemic serum. Thus, there is at least a 32-fold difference in the levels of this antibody between mice with dormant FLV infections and mice with overt leukemia.

Since leukemic mice have depressed immune responses to a variety of nonleukemic antigens (16,17) and mice with dormant FLV infections are immunologically competent (18), the finding of FLV antibody in the sera of leukemic mice was unexpected. The absence of antibody to p12 in leukemic mice and its presence in FLV-dormant mice suggest that the humoral immune response to virion p12 may ultimately determine whether or not an FLV-infected mouse develops dormant or overt erythroleukemia.

L5178Y Tumor Cells — Syngeneic Mice

A second model for the study of tumor dormancy employs a methylcholanthrene-induced lymphoma, L5178Y, in its host strain of origin, the DBA/2 mouse. In this system, from 55 to 95% of specifically immunized mice establish a state of tumor dormancy following intraperitoneal challenge with live tumor cells. In the experiment to be described, a group of 27 female mice were immunized by intraperitoneal injection of 10×10^6 mitomycin C-treated tumor cells. Ten days later these mice and a group of five control mice were inoculated intraperitoneally with 5×10^4 live tumor cells. At various days thereafter, clinically normal mice randomly picked from the experimental group were sacrificed and their peritoneal and spleen cells placed into culture and observed for tumor cell outgrowth. Cultures were examined for the presence of increasing numbers of lymphoblastoid cells which, when transferred into culture vessels containing fresh medium, continued to proliferate. Some mice from the experimental group were reserved for long-term observation for tumor emergence. The results of this experiment are summarized in Table 2.

Table 2 shows that the five unimmunized mice succumbed to the tumor within 15 days of tumor cell inoculation. In contrast, all the mice in the immunized group remained clinically normal throughout the first 55 days. The first deaths in the immunized group occurred 60 days after challenge.

TABLE 2. *L5178Y tumor dormancy in DBA/2 mice*

| Cell inoculation[a] | Day relative to tumor cell challenge | Tumor outgrowth | | |
| | | Immunized | | Controls |
		In vitro	*In vivo*	*In vivo*
Mitomycin-L5178Y ⟶	−10			
Live-L5178Y ⟶	0			
	15		0	5
	30	3/5	0	
	49	2/2	0	
	55	4/7	0	
	60		2	
	80		6	
	110		1	
	150		1	
	170		1	
	205		1	
	Number positive/total	9/14	12/13[b]	5/5

[a] Immunization consisted of an i.p. inoculation of 1×10^7 mitomycin C-treated L5178Y cells.
Challenge consisted of an i.p. inoculation of 5×10^4 live L5178Y cells.
[b] One clinically normal mouse alive at day 270.

Additional deaths due to tumor were also observed during the subsequent 5-month period.

In the interval between days 30 and 55, when all mice were clinically normal, a total of 14 mice were sacrificed and examined for gross tumor. Spleen cells and peritoneal washout cells from those mice were placed into culture and tumor cells were isolated in cultures from 9 of these 14 mice. In no instance was the recovery of tumor cells from the peritoneal cavity associated with macroscopically detectable tumor nodules or an unusually high total peritoneal cell count at the time of harvest. In four of the nine mice from which tumor cells were recovered from the peritoneal cavity, tumor cells were also isolated from the respective spleen cell cultures.

L5178Y Tumor Cells — F_1 Hybrid Mice

The third tumor dormant model developed out of an investigation of the hybrid effect, a phenomenon in which small numbers of parental cells fail to proliferate or proliferate deficiently in F_1 hybrid mice. Snell (19) first described the hybrid effect with tumor cells in 1958, and in 1964 Cudkowicz and Stimpfling (20) reported that X-irradiated F_1 hybrids could reject parental hemopoietic bone marrow grafts. Cudkowicz and co-workers (21–25) subsequently reported that the mechanism was determined by non-codominately inherited Hh genes which map in the D region of the H-2 complex, and that the anti-Hh response is regulated by non-H-2 linked immune response genes. These Hh antigens have been shown to exist on both normal and neoplastic parental hemopoietic cells (26,27). Investigations carried out by Bennett (28) and by Kumar et al. (29) showed that the cell mediating the hybrid effect is a radioresistant bone marrow-derived cell which has been designated "M" cell (for marrow derived). Expression of the hybrid effect is impaired by treatment with [89]Sr (28,29) or antimacrophage agents (25), suggesting that the M cell may be a macrophage-like cell or at least require such a cell for expression of its activity.

In order to determine if the hybrid effect was operative on the DBA/2-derived L5178Y lymphoma cell in BDF$_1$ mice (C57B1/6 × DBA/2), we inoculated both BDF$_1$ and DBA/2 mice intraperitoneally with varying numbers (5×10^2 to 5×10^5) of tumor cells and observed for development of ascitic tumors. At comparable low cell inocula, BDF$_1$ mice developed fewer ascitic tumors than DBA/2 mice. Moreover, outgrowth of tumors in BDF$_1$ mice occurred much later than in comparably inoculated DBA/2 mice (data not shown). Experiment 1 in Table 3 shows that 7 of 15 BDF$_1$ mice inoculated intraperitoneally with various numbers of L5178Y cells remained clinically normal for many weeks after all comparably inoculated DBA/2 mice had succumbed to the tumor. At least five of these seven dormant mice still harbored residual tumor cells as evidenced by eventual

TABLE 3. *Delayed L5178Y ascitic tumor outgrowth and dormancy in BDF₁ mice*

Day after L5178Y cell inoculation[a]	Tumor outgrowth				
	Experiment #1		Experiment #2		
	BDF₁ *In vivo*	DBA/2 *In vivo*	BDF₁ *In vitro*	BDF₁ *In vivo*	DBA/2 *In vivo*
8			2/5		
16	8	15	5/5	0	4
27	0		4/5	0	1
49	0			1	
61	3			1	
76	1			0	
90	1			0	
Number positive/total	13/15[b]	15/15	11/15	2/5[c]	5/5

[a] Experiment #1 — a summation of tumor production in mice inoculated with 5×10^3 to 5×10^5 L5178Y cells i.p.
Experiment #2 — 5×10^2 L5178Y cells were inoculated i.p.
[b] Two mice alive and clinically normal at day 270.
[c] Three mice alive and clinically normal at day 200.

emergence of ascitic tumors. Serologic testing of the late-emerging tumor cells isolated from the BDF₁ mice showed that they expressed only H-2^d antigenic specificities and thus were progeny of the original L5178Y inoculum and not new tumors arising from BDF₁ host cells.

In a second series of experiments we picked five clinically normal BDF₁ mice from a group that had been inoculated with 500 L5178Y cells and tested them for the presence of residual tumor cells in the peritoneal cavity. On selected days after tumor inoculation peritoneal washout cells were collected and placed in culture and observed for L5178Y cell outgrowth. Tumor cell outgrowth was scored as positive in cultures showing an increase in the number of lymphoblastoid cells which, when transferred to culture vessels containing fresh media, continued to proliferate. As indicated in experiment 2 in Table 3, on day 27, when 100% of DBA/2 mice had overt ascitic tumor, 100% of the BDF₁ mice were clinically normal. However, we were able to isolate and grow out in culture tumor cells from four of the five mice tested. The five remaining clinically normal BDF₁ mice were maintained for long-term observation, and two of these five mice developed ascitic tumors 49 and 61 days, respectively, after inoculation.

These experimental results demonstrate clearly that BDF₁ mice are able to delay L5178Y tumor cell outgrowth and in some instances to maintain a tumor dormant state for considerable periods of time.

DISCUSSION

The three experimental systems described in this chapter are models in which dormancy of viral- and nonviral-induced tumors can be studied. As shown in the three models, different mechanisms may be involved in the establishment and maintenance of dormancy of different tumors. Moreover, the factors responsible for the prevention of tumor outgrowth at the primary tumor site(s) may not necessarily be the same as those responsible for prevention of invasion or metastasis. A feature of all these systems is that they are relatively unstable, in that we cannot predict in any given animal whether the inoculated virus or tumor cells will produce overt neoplasia, be suppressed to a dormant state, or be eradicated from the host. Clearly, the competence of the host's immune and nonspecific tumor defense mechanisms determines the fate of the tumor cell, and these host factors can fluctuate widely from mouse to mouse even within a single age-matched shipment of inbred mice. Given these inherent complexities, it is not surprising that our understanding of tumor dormancy is still at a primitive level.

In the first animal model, an established Friend leukemia virus infection is diverted from a lethal course to one of dormancy by stimulation of both nonspecific and specific immune host defense mechanisms. We have found that stimulation of nonspecific host defenses such as interferon and macrophages is insufficient for tumor suppression (30). Further evidence indicates that restoration of immunocompetence directed against virus-coded antigens is the essential factor for the establishment of the dormant state. However, it is not known whether immune stimulation alone, in the absence of interferon production and macrophage stimulation, would be sufficient for tumor suppression, since in this model system immune stimulation always occurs in combination with stimulation of nonspecific host defenses. Mice with dormant FLV infections are clinically normal and their sera contain antibodies that lyse FLV-transformed cells *in vitro* in the presence of exogenous complement, and that react with virion polypeptides designated gp69/71, gp43, p15, and p12. Our current goals in this model system are to determine if and how these antibodies establish and maintain tumor dormancy. Studies in progress show that sera from animals with dormant FLV infections can cause modulation of virus-induced cell surface antigens. Several other investigators (31,32) have reported the disappearance of tumor-associated membrane antigens after antibody contact and have called this phenomenon antigenic modulation. Further studies in our laboratory will seek to determine whether changes induced by antigenic modulation play a role in tumor dormancy. Finally, we hope to learn whether antibodies against virion polypeptides also react with virus-coded antigens on tumor cells and thereby participate in maintaining tumor dormancy. Special emphasis will be placed on understanding the role of p12 antibody, since this antibody is present in the sera of mice with dormant FLV infections but is absent in sera of mice with overt FLV infections.

Our finding that specifically immunized DBA/2 mice challenged with L5178Y lymphoma cells are capable of harboring tumor cells for prolonged periods of time provides us with the opportunity to investigate the phenomenon of tumor dormancy involving a tumor that exhibits a high degree of compatibility with its host strain of origin. Immunization with mitomycin C-treated tumor cells renders mice resistant to subsequent tumor cell challenge. In some instances rejection of the tumor cell inoculum is incomplete, and in such cases tumor cells appear to persist in a specifically immune environment. A noncytolytic, cytophilic antibody has been detected in the sera of mice immunized and challenged with L5178Y (33). Similarly, peritoneal exudate cells, but not spleen cells, from such mice have been found to be active in a 4-hr "killer assay" using ^{51}Cr-labeled L5178Y cells as targets (K. J. Weinhold et al., *unpublished observation*). The relative contributions of these two responses to the establishment and maintenance of the tumor dormant state are, at present, under investigation. The rapid *in vitro* outgrowth of tumor cells from peritoneal or spleen cell cultures from tumor dormant mice indicates that factors operative in the *in vivo* suppression of tumor cells are lost when these cells are removed from the host.

The observation that some BDF_1 mice suppress or delay the outgrowth of small numbers of L5178Y lymphoma cells demonstrates that the hybrid effect is operative in our system, thereby providing us with a model to study natural mechanisms of tumor suppression. Our recent experimental results indicate that an adherent peritoneal cell with macrophage-like properties is involved in maintaining tumor cells in a dormant state. These adherent peritoneal cells have been found to inhibit incorporation of the DNA precursor ^{3}HTdR in L5178Y cells *in vitro*. Several reports demonstrate that macrophages are capable of inhibiting tumor cell growth by both cytolytic (34–36) and cytostatic (37–40) mechanisms. The techniques that we have thus far employed to demonstrate tumor suppression do not differentiate between cytolytic or cytostatic mechanisms.

Cudkowicz and co-workers (41) have reported that hybrid mice inhibit the growth of parental cells by an immunologic mechanism directed toward parental antigens not expressed by the hybrid mice. However, Oth and Burg (42) suggested that the hybrid effect is due to an enhanced ability to recognize and eliminate cells possessing tumor-associated antigens. Currently we are investigating the mechanism of tumor suppression by BDF_1-adherent peritoneal cells and will determine whether tumor suppression is mediated through recognition of parental antigens, tumor-associated antigens, or both.

During tumor dormancy the tumor cell may persist in a nondividing state, may divide slowly, or may divide at a rate commensurate with cytolysis thereby resulting in a net balance of no tumor outgrowth. It is also possible that all three states can exist in a population of tumor cells during dormancy. A detailed analysis is required of the tumor cell cycle and population kinetics in tumor dormant animals. Such experiments are complicated, however, by the difficulty in locating tumor cells in dormant mice and studying them under controlled conditions. Moreover, introduction of exogenous tumor cells into tumor dormant animals may not provide a suitable model for study of the tumor dormancy since Eccles and Alexander (9) have reported that a secondary tumor cell challenge can be rejected by rats harboring the same type of tumor cells in a dormant state.

In the analysis of tumor dormancy it is important to compare the tumor virus or cell from tumor dormant animals with virus or cells from the original inoculum. Differences in the type and/or amount of tumor-associated antigen displayed on the surface of viruses or tumor cells from tumor dormant animals versus the original inoculum might be the basis for establishment of tumor dormancy. We have performed comparative studies on FLV recovered from dormant FLV-infected mice and the original virus inoculum and have found no serologic or pathogenetic differences. Similar analysis of the L5178Y syngeneic and F_1 hybrid systems remains to be performed. Alexander (43) compared cells emerging in rats from dormant metastases with cells from the original inoculum in a variety of assays and found them to be indistinguishable.

Our current efforts are directed at determining the status of tumor cell populations in tumor dormant animals and identifying the host factors that prevent tumor outgrowth. Our future objective is to find ways to enhance the tumor-suppressive capacity of the host to achieve either complete tumor eradication or at least prolonged tumor dormancy.

ACKNOWLEDGMENT

The research described in this chapter was supported by Public Health Service Grants CA-12461-05 and CA-18995-01.

We would like to acknowledge the excellent technical assistance of Saidee Thompson and Wilhemina G. Marum.

REFERENCES

1. Beckwith, J. B., and Perrin, E. V. (1963): In situ neuroblastomas: A contribution to the natural history of neural crest tumors. *Am. J. Pathol.*, 43:1089.
2. Mortensen, J. D., Woolner, L. B., and Bennett, W. A. (1955): Gross and microscopic findings in clinically normal thyroid glands. *J. Clin. Endocrinol. Metab.*, 15:1270.
3. Ashley, D. J. B. (1965): On the incidence of carcinoma of the prostate. *J. Pathol. Bacteriol.*, 90:217.
4. Munsie, W. J., and Foster, E. A. (1968): Unsuspected very small foci of carcinoma of the prostate in transurethral resection specimens. *Cancer*, 21:692.

5. Green, G. H. (1966): The significance of cervical carcinoma in situ. *Am. J. Obstet. Gynecol.*, 94:1009.

6. Coppleson, M., and Reid, B. (1968): Management of cervical carcinoma-in-situ. *Lancet*, 2:873.

7. Ashley, D. J. B. (1966): The biological status of carcinoma in-situ of the uterine cervix. *J. Obstet. Gynaecol. Br. Commonw.*, 73:372.

8. Fisher, B., and Fisher, E. R. (1959): Experimental evidence in support of the dormant tumor cell. *Science*, 130:918.

9. Eccles, S. A., and Alexander, P. (1975): Immunologically-mediated restraint of latent tumour metastasis. *Nature*, 257:52.

10. Wheelock, E. F., Toy, S. T., Caroline, N. L., Sibal, L. R., Fink, M. A., Beverley, P. C. L., and Allison, A. C. (1972): Suppression of established Friend virus leukemia by statolon. IV. Role of humoral antibody in the development of a dormant infection. *J. Natl. Cancer Inst.*, 48:665.

11. Marx, P. A., and Wheelock, E. F. (1976): Influence of immune stimulators on viral leukemogenesis. *Ann. N.Y. Acad. Sci.*, 276:502.

12. Weislow, O. S., and Wheelock, E. F. (1975): Suppression of established Friend virus leukemia by statolon: Potentiation of statolon's leukemosuppressive activity by chlorite-oxidized oxyamylose. *Infect. Immunol.*, 11:129.

13. Wheelock, E. F., Toy, S. T., Weislow, O. S., and Levy, M. H. (1974): Restored immune and nonimmune functions in Friend virus leukemic mice treated with statolon. Immunology of cancer. *Prog. Exp. Tumor Res.*, 19:369.

14. Ihle, J. N., Yurconic, M., Jr., and Hanna, M. G., Jr. (1973): Autogenous immunity to endogenous RNA tumor virus. *J. Exp. Med.*, 138:194.

15. Hunsman, G., Moennig, V., and Schäfer, W. (1975): Properties of mouse leukemia viruses. IX. Active and passive immunization of mice against Friend leukemia with isolated viral GP_{71} glycoprotein and its corresponding antiserum. *Virology*, 66:327.

16. Old, L. J., Clarke, D. A., Benacerraf, B., and Goldsmith, M. (1960): The reticuloendothelial system and the neoplastic process. *Ann. N.Y. Acad. Sci.*, 88:264.

17. Millian, S. S., and Schaeffer, M. (1960): Antibody production by mice infected with selected murine oncogenic agents. *Cancer*, 21:989.

18. Weislow, O. S., Friedman, H., and Wheelock, E. F. (1973): Suppression of established Friend virus leukemia by statolon. V. Reversal of virus-induced immunodepression to sheep erythrocytes. *Proc. Soc. Exp. Biol. Med.*, 142:401.

19. Snell, G. D. (1958): Histocompatibility genes of the mouse. II. Production and analysis of isogenic resistant lines. *J. Natl. Cancer Inst.*, 21:843.

20. Cudkowicz, G., and Stimpfling, H. H. (1964): Deficient growth of C57B1 marrow cells transplanted in F_1 mice. Association with the histocompatibility-2 locus. *Immunology*, 7:291.

21. Cudkowicz, G. (1971): Genetic control of bone marrow graft rejection. I. Determinant-specific differences of reactivity in two pairs of inbred mouse strains. *J. Exp. Med.*, 134:281.

22. Cudkowicz, G., and Bennett, M. (1971): Peculiar immunobiology of bone marrow allograft. I. Graft rejection by irradiated responder mice. *J. Exp. Med.*, 134:83.

23. Cudkowicz, G., and Bennett, M. (1971): Peculiar immunobiology of bone marrow allografts. II. Rejection of parental grafts by resistant F_1 hybrid mice. *J. Exp. Med.*, 134:1513.

24. Cudkowicz, G., and Lotzova, E. (1973): Hemopoietic cell-defined components of the major histocompatibility complex of mice. Identification of responsive and unresponsive recipients for bone marrow transplants. *Transplant. Proc.*, 4:1399.

25. Lotzova, E., and Cudkowicz, G. (1974): Abrogation of resistance to bone marrow grafts by silica particles. Prevention of the silica effect by macrophage stabilizer poly-2-vinyl pyridine N-oxide. *J. Immunol.*, 113:798.

26. Cudkowicz, G., and Rossi, G. B. (1972): Hybrid resistance to parental DBA/2 grafts; independence from the H-2 locus. I. Studies with normal hemopoietic cells. *J. Natl. Cancer Inst.*, 48:131.

27. Cudkowicz, G., Rossi, G. B., Haddad, J. R., and Friend, C. (1972): Hybrid resistance to parental DBA/2 grafts: Independence from the H-2 locus. II. Studies with Friend virus-induced leukemia cells. *J. Natl. Cancer Inst.*, 48:997.

28. Bennett, M. (1973): Prevention of marrow allograft rejection with radioactive strontium: Evidence for marrow-dependent effector cells. *J. Immunol.,* 110:510.
29. Kumar, V., Bennett, M., and Eckner, R. J. (1974): Mechanisms of genetic resistance to Friend virus leukemia in mice. I. Role of ^{89}Sr-sensitive effector cells responsible for rejection of bone marrow allografts. *J. Exp. Med.,* 39:1093.
30. Levy, M. H., and Wheelock, E. F. (1975): Impaired macrophage function in Friend virus leukemia: Restoration by statolon. *J. Immunol.,* 114:962.
31. Old, L. J., Stockert, E., Boyse, E. A., and Kim, J. H. (1968): Antigenic modulation: Loss of TL antigen from cells exposed to TL antibody. Study of the phenomenon in vitro. *J. Exp. Med.,* 127:523.
32. Joseph, B. S., and Oldstone, M. B. A. (1975): Immunologic injury in measles virus infection. Suppression of immune injury through antigenic modulation. *J. Exp. Med.,* 142:864.
33. Goldstein, L. T., Klinman, N. R., and Manson, L. A. (1973): A microtest radioimmunoassay for noncytotoxic tumor specific antibody to cell-surface antigens. *J. Natl. Cancer Inst.,* 51:1713.
34. Keller, R. (1974): Mechanisms by which activated normal macrophages destroy syngeneic rat tumor cells in vitro. *Immunology,* 27:285.
35. Zembala, M., Dtak, W., and Hanczakowska, M. (1973): The role of macrophages in the cytotoxic killing of tumor cells in vitro. *Immunology,* 25:631.
36. Evans, R., and Alexander, D. (1972): Mechanism of immunologically specific killing of tumour cells by macrophages. *Nature,* 236:168.
37. Krahenbuhl, J., and Remington, J. (1974): The role of activated macrophages in specific and nonspecific cytostasis of tumor cells. *J. Immunol.,* 113:507.
38. Sethi, K. K., and Brandis, H. (1975): Cytotoxicity mediated by soluble macrophage products. *J. Natl. Cancer Inst.,* 55:393.
39. Kirchner, H., Holden, H., and Herberman, R. (1975): Inhibition of in vitro growth of lymphoma cells by macrophages from tumor-bearing mice. *J. Natl. Cancer Inst.,* 55:971.
40. Keller, R. (1973): Cytostatic elimination of syngeneic rat tumor cells in vitro by nonspecifically activated macrophages. *J. Exp. Med.,* 133:625.
41. Shearer, G. M., Cudkowicz, G., Schmitt-Verhulst, A., Rehn, T., Wakoal, H., and Evans, P. (1976): F₁ hybrid anti-parental cell-mediated lympholysis. A comparison with bone marrow graft rejection and with cell-mediated lympholysis to alloantigens. *Cold Spring Harbor Symp. (in press).*
42. Oth, D., and Burg, C. (1967): In: *Symposium on Cell-Bound Immunity with Special Reference to Antilymphocyte Serum and Immunotherapy of Cancer,* pp. 1–12. Tiege les Spa. l'Université de Liege, Liege.
43. Alexander, P. (1976): Dormant metastases which manifest on immunosuppression and the role of macrophages in tumours. In: *Fundamental Aspects of Metastasis,* edited by L. Weiss, pp. 227–239. North-Holland Publishing Co., Amsterdam.

Cancer Invasion and Metastasis: Biologic Mechanisms and Therapy, edited by S. B. Day et al. Raven Press, New York © 1977.

Kinetics of Metastases in Experimental Tumors

L. Simpson-Herren, T. A. Springer, A. H. Sanford, and J. P. Holmquist

Southern Research Institute, Birmingham, Alabama 35205

The goal of combined modality therapy is to reduce the residual tumor cell burden below the number of cells capable of initiating tumor recurrence and yet spare the patient any unnecessary hazard or discomfort as a result of therapy. These are demanding requirements with existing techniques, and success frequently depends on usage of any and all available therapeutic advantages.

Much effort is now directed toward improvement of therapeutic protocols through studies of (a) drug interaction (7,15), (b) relative host and tumor recovery (20,29,30), (c) changes that occur during radiation therapy (28) and (d) cell kinetics (3,21,22,27,30,31). Even with the significant progress made in the last few years, for the forseeable future, surgical removal of the primary tumor mass appears to be a necessary part of a "curative" therapy for many human tumors. Thus, the tumor cells remaining after surgery (either local or metastatic) become the appropriate targets for chemotherapy, immunotherapy, and radiotherapy (23). For scheduling of adjuvant therapy it then becomes necessary to understand the growth kinetics of the residual tumor and metastases rather than the primary tumor.

The Lewis lung (LL) carcinoma in BDF_1 mice, a transplanted tumor system with a high rate of metastasis to lungs and other sites, has been widely used for chemotherapy studies and was used for the kinetic studies reported here.

KINETICS OF PRIMARY AND METASTATIC FOCI

Subcutaneously (s.c.) implanted LL carcinoma (hereafter referred to as the primary tumor) is characterized by an increase in mass doubling time (Fig. 1) and an increase in length of the cell cycle (Tc) from about 17 hr at day 5 to about 25 hr at day 21 (25). The thymidine index (TI) decreases with increasing tumor mass from about 0.50 at 350 mg to less than 0.30 at 4,000 mg (26). Lung metastases are established in 100% of the mice by day 6, and growth of the total tumor mass in the lung is also characterized by an increase in mass doubling time (Fig. 1). The TI of the lung metastases

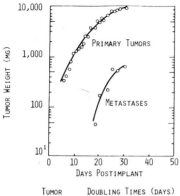

FIG. 1. Gompertz-fitted growth data for primary s.c. LL tumors and spontaneous lung metastases (25). Doubling times were obtained from tangents to the growth curves.

TUMOR WEIGHT (MG)	DOUBLING TIMES (DAYS) PRIMARY	METASTASES
50	1.5	1.1
100	1.7	1.5
500	2.5	6.5
1000	3.1	---
5000	7.7	---

decreases with time, but at any point in time where the TI of primary and metastatic foci could be measured in the same host (Fig. 2), the TI of the lung metastases was significantly higher ($p < 0.0001$) than the TI of the primary tumor. In studies of 75 primary and metastatic human breast tumors, Schiffer et al. (24) have also observed a higher TI (about 0.08) in metastases than in primary tumors (about 0.04).

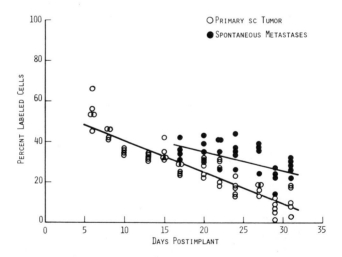

FIG. 2. Observed pulse TIs from primary s.c. LL tumors and spontaneous lung metastases from the same hosts. Lines were obtained from linear regression analysis of the data but do not well represent the data due to the scatter. The difference between TIs of the primary and lung nodules is highly significant ($p < 0.0001$).

Percent-labeled mitoses (PLM) curves for LL tumors, determined at 21 days post-implant, indicated that the median Tc of the primary tumors was about 25 hr compared with 14 hr in the metastatic foci (Fig. 3). At this time the lung metastases might be considered microscopic in size, ranging from a few cells to approximately 1 mm in diameter (estimated 10^5 to 10^6 cells). Necrosis was extensive in the primary tumors but seldom evident in the lung foci at this size.

INTERACTION OF MULTIPLE TUMOR FOCI

Humphreys and Karrer (11) and Mayo et al. (16) were among the early investigators who reported cures of mice bearing metastasized Lewis lung carcinoma when surgical excision of the primary tumor was followed by chemotherapy with cyclophosphamide (NSC-26271) or methyl-CCNU (NSC-94541). No cures were obtained by either surgery or chemotherapy alone after the disease was widespread. Artificial metastases, induced by i.v. implantation of 10^6 counted cells, can be cured by chemotherapy alone even when the disease is moderately advanced (16). Kinetic studies of the artificial lung metastases at day 15 post-implant revealed that the Tc was

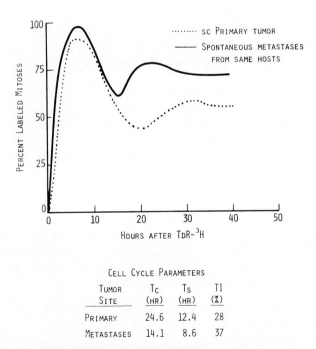

Cell Cycle Parameters			
Tumor Site	Tc (hr)	Ts (hr)	TI (%)
Primary	24.6	12.4	28
Metastases	14.1	8.6	37

FIG. 3. Curves and cell cycle parameters obtained from computer analysis of PLM data for s.c. primary tumors and spontaneous lung nodules at 21 days post-implant from the same hosts (25). (Computer analysis courtesy of Dr. G. G. Steel.)

slightly longer than the Tc found in the spontaneous metastases at day 21 but the TI was approximately 0.50 (compared to 0.37 for spontaneous metastases). The disease was more advanced in the artificial metastases if judged by size and number of lung nodules (up to 3 to 5 mm) that replaced much of the lung tissue. TIs measured from day 5 to day 22 post-implant (past the median day of death) did not decline with time and were apparently independent of size, within the limits of the study (Fig. 4A). This observation raised the question of whether the large growing s.c. tumor might tend to suppress the growth of the metastases as suggested for clinical tumors (2,5,6,19) and experimental tumors (4,8–10).

Tumor fragments were implanted 2 days prior to implantation of the artificial metastases to investigate this possibility, and the results of TI studies with time are shown in Fig. 4B. The results are more variable in this artificial system, and suppression of the TI of the metastases is not as pronounced as seen in the spontaneous metastases (Fig. 4C), but the trend toward a decrease with time is evident and significant ($p < 0.005$). The 2-day interval was arbitrary but was chosen to approximate the natural course of the disease, i.e., establishment of the primary tumor prior to metastasis.

Effects of the time interval between implants on life span are shown in Fig. 5. An s.c. tumor implanted at intervals from 5 days before to 5 days after implant of the artificial metastases resulted in a 1- to 5-day increase in survival time of the doubly implanted mice. This observation would support the conclusion that a large, growing s.c. tumor suppresses the growth rate of lung metastases, either spontaneous or artificial.

These studies are being extended to evaluate the kinetics of brain metastases. We are using an i.c. implant of 10^5 counted Lewis lung cells (artificial brain metastases) as a model system. Life span data (Fig. 6) provide no evidence for any interaction between the artificial brain metastases and tumors growing in other sites.

In one study, TIs of artificial brain and lung metastases growing in the same hosts were similar, with mean values of about 0.55, and no evidence of a decrease with time through day 9 post-implant (Fig. 7). Although the data are very limited at this time, one observation appears to be important. Small foci of Lewis lung carcinoma cells in the brain have a mean pulse TI (approximately 0.55) that equals the maximum value observed for this tumor under any conditions. Additional studies are now in progress to evaluate the effects of a growing s.c. tumor on the TI of brain metastases and to obtain data to, or past, the median day of death.

→

FIG. 4. Observed pulse TIs from mice bearing artificial lung metastases (10^6 cells i.v.), artificial lung metastases (10^6 cells i.v.) implanted 2 days after s.c. tumor implants, and spontaneous lung metastases. Lines were obtained from linear regression analysis of the data but do not well represent the data due to their variability. The TIs for artificial metastases are significantly different from the TIs of spontaneous lung metastases and artificial lung metastases ($p < 0.005$).

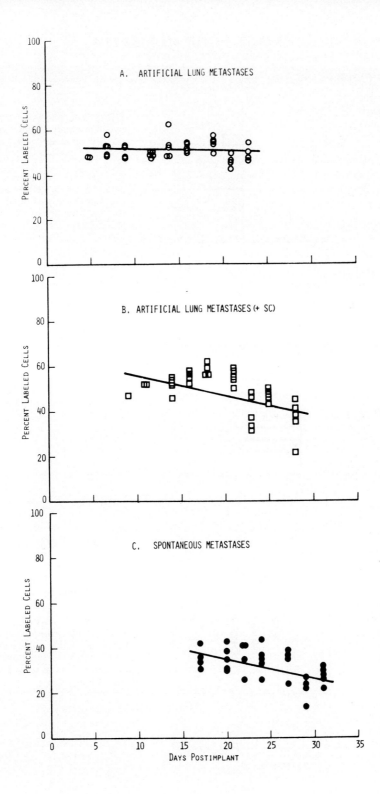

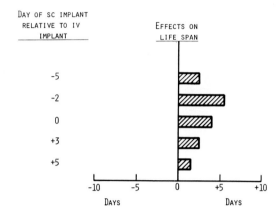

DAY OF SC IMPLANT RELATIVE TO IV IMPLANT

EFFECTS ON LIFE SPAN

FIG. 5. The effects of time between implant of the two tumors on life span of mice bearing both s.c. tumors and artificial lung metastases (10^6 cells i.v.). The median day of death for each group is compared with the median day of death (20.5) for the concurrent i.v. control (10^6 cells, i.v., only).

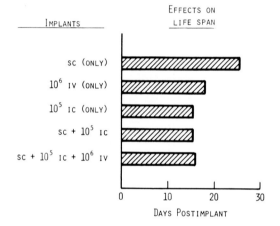

IMPLANTS

EFFECTS ON LIFE SPAN

FIG. 6. Effects of multiple tumor implants on the life span of mice bearing i.c. implants of 10^5 cells.

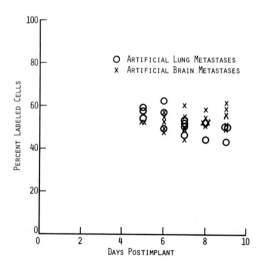

O ARTIFICIAL LUNG METASTASES
X ARTIFICIAL BRAIN METASTASES

FIG. 7. Observed pulse TIs of artificial lung metastases (10^6 cells i.v.) and artificial brain metastases (10^5 cells i.v.) implanted simultaneously in the same hosts as a function of time post-implant.

EFFECTS OF SURGERY ON RESIDUAL TUMOR

If chemotherapy is to be used as an adjuvant to surgery, then knowledge of the kinetic behavior of residual tumor tissue after surgery should provide some indication of the most advantageous times to initiate therapy. The observed increased sensitivity to chemotherapy after surgical excision of the primary Lewis lung tumor (11,16) is consistent with the shorter Tc, the higher TI of the metastatic foci, and the reduced body burden of tumor cells, but it now appears that the surgical procedure may also act to recruit residual tumor cells into proliferation in this system (26).

PLM curves for the lung metastases 96 hr after surgical excision of the primary (3 to 4 g) tumors (day 14) indicate that the surgical procedure produced no lasting effect on the Tc of metastases (Fig. 8). A PLM curve at 48 hr after surgery suggested a small (3.5 hr) increase in the calculated median length of Tc. If this could be attributed to a real change in kinetic parameters rather than to biological variation, then it was apparently of short duration. In contrast, there does appear to be an increase in the TI of metastases; the magnitude of this effect and the length of time that it persists are related to the time and type of surgery.

Surgical excision of the primary s.c. tumor results in an increase in TI of lung metastases, and there is little evidence of a decrease with time post-implant until day 32 (Fig. 9A and C). At this point the mice were cachectic and near death. Thus, it appears that for a period of 12 to 14 days after surgical excision, the lung tumor foci have a mean TI of about 0.55; this value approximates the maximum mean TI that we have observed in

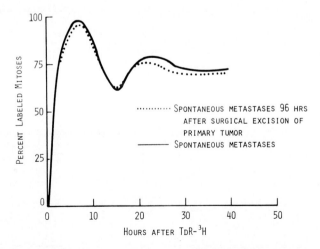

FIG. 8. Curves obtained from computer analysis of PLM data for spontaneous lung metastases in untreated mice and for spontaneous lung metastases 96 hr after surgical excision of the primary s.c. tumor (26).

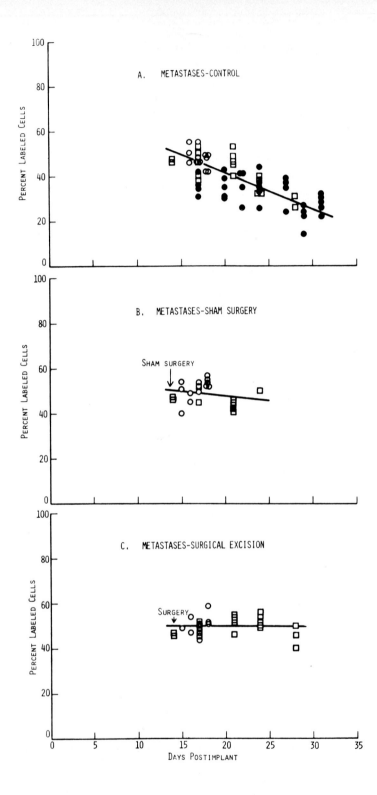

this system, at any stage or condition of growth. The difference in TIs for the control and surgery groups is highly significant ($p < 0.005$). During one of the studies shown in Fig. 9, we also measured the uptake of tritiated thymidine (TdR-^{3}H) into the acid-insoluble fraction of the intestine for the control and surgical excision groups. We found no increase in specific activity of the intestine in contrast to the increased TI of the tumor in the same host.

Preliminary data indicate that the magnitude of increase in TI after surgery depends on the stage of the disease. Surgery performed when the TI of the metastases is about 0.5 produces little increase, but subsequently the TI does not decrease with time as would be expected in untreated mice. Surgery, performed on day 21 (after the TI of the metastases has decreased to about 0.35), causes the observed TI to approach the maximum value (about 0.5). At this time mice are near the median day of death and the period that the TI remains elevated has not yet been defined.

The observed stimulation of cell proliferation might be attributed to one or more of the following factors: (a) effects related to the surgical procedure *per se,* (b) reduction of tumor cell burden, (c) rebound of host immunity with resultant tumor growth stimulation (1,2,6–8,12–14,17,18), or (d) others as yet undefined. The effects of the surgical procedure *per se* were evaluated by a sham procedure similar to surgical excision that left the large s.c. tumor undisturbed. TIs of the lung nodules (Fig. 9) were elevated by 24 hr after sham surgery and remained higher than the control for 7 days or possibly longer. Only one animal survived as long as 10 days after the sham procedure in this experiment, thus limiting the extent of the study. The most unexpected observation was the increase in TI of the primary tumor (Fig. 10). Even though the data are variable, the increase in TI following the sham procedure is significant at the $p < 0.001$ level.

These observations are consistent with and supported by the life span data shown in Fig. 11. Surgical excision of the primary tumor before day 6 results in 10 to 40% cures and a variable but generally beneficial effect on life span of those animals that eventually die of the disease. Surgical excision on day 6 or later produces no cures and a small but consistently detrimental effect on life span of dying mice. Preliminary results of total lung bioassays at 2 and 4 days post-implant of the s.c. tumor indicate that 0/20 animals had sufficient tumor cells in the lungs to be detected by the assay procedure. If we may assume from these data that metastasis from Lewis

FIG. 9. Observed pulse TI for spontaneous metastases in untreated mice, in mice after sham surgery on day 14, and in mice after surgical excision of the primary s.c. tumor on day 14 as a function of time post-implant. Each symbol represents the data from one mouse and different symbols represent different experiments. Lines are obtained from linear regression analysis of the data but do not well represent the variability. Effects of surgery on observed pulse TI is very significant ($p < 0.005$).

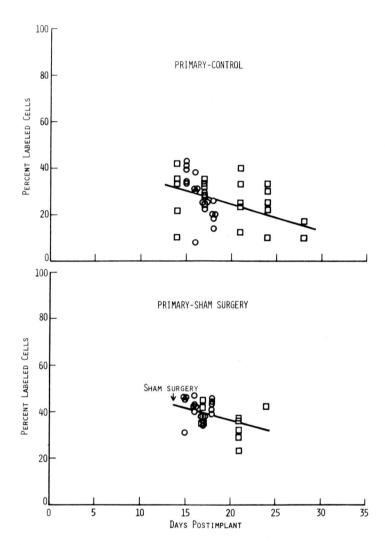

FIG. 10. Observed pulse TIs of primary tumors in untreated mice and in mice subjected to sham surgery on day 14. Different symbols represent different experiments. The increase in TI of primary tumors following sham surgery is significant ($p < 0.001$).

lung usually does not occur before day 5 or 6, then the beneficial effects of early surgery on life span may result from a delay in time to metastasis by surgical reduction of the primary tumor mass. This makes the assumption that metastasis does not occur below some critical size of tumor mass. Those animals that die of the disease after early surgery usually have gross evidence of recurrence at either the site of the incision or regional lymph nodes.

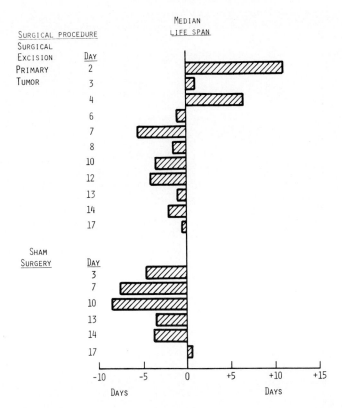

FIG. 11. The effects of a surgical procedure performed at different intervals post-implant on the median life span of the hosts compared with the median life span of concurrent controls (29 days). The surgical excision group contains pooled data from three experiments, and the sham surgery group has pooled data from two experiments. (Each bar represents data from 10 to 40 mice.)

The sham procedure has a more adverse effect on survival time than surgical excision of the tumor based on the life span data. This might be attributed to the increased rate of cell proliferation in the primary tumor that results in an increase in rate of metastasis, although we have no data at present to support this assumption.

RESULTS OF GRAIN COUNT ANALYSIS

The observed increases in TIs after surgery only reflect an increase in the fraction of cells with grains in excess of the background and provide no indication of whether this change might be due to an increase in the fraction of cells engaged in DNA synthesis at a minimal rate. If the latter were true, some question would exist concerning the significance of the increase in TI in relation to chemotherapy. Observation of the autoradiographs used

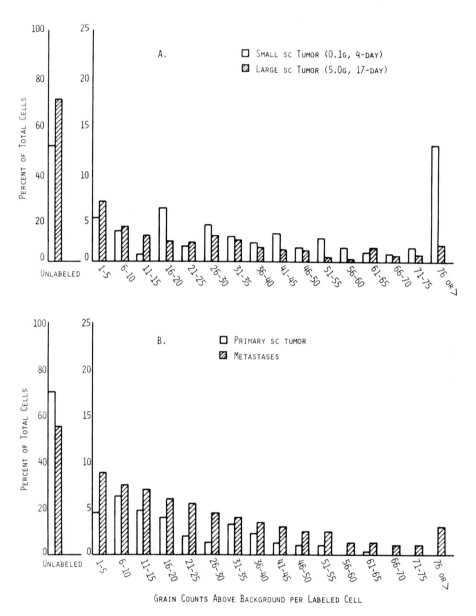

FIG. 12. Grain count distributions for small and large LL s.c. tumors **(A)** and primary s.c. tumors and spontaneous lung metastases in same hosts **(B)** following a pulse exposure to TdR-³H.

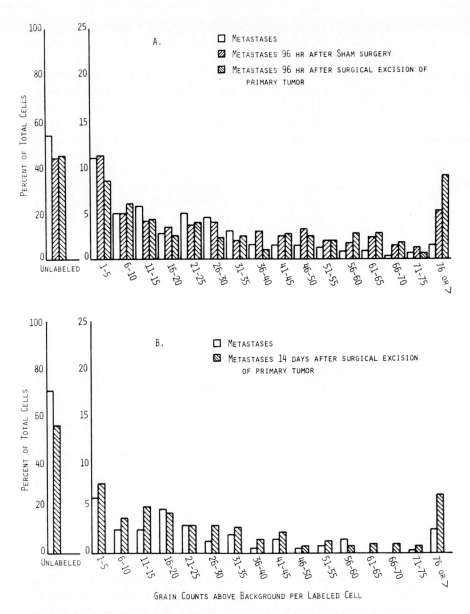

FIG. 13. Grain count distributions for spontaneous lung metastases in control, sham surgery (after 96 hr), and surgical excision (96 hr after removal of s.c. primary tumor) groups **(A)** following a pulse exposure to TdR-³H. **B:** Grain count distributions in spontaneous metastases in control and surgical excision groups at 28 days post-implant and 14 days after surgery following a pulse exposure to TdR-³H. No mice survived in the sham surgery group.

for studies of the TIs indicated that these changes were not due to the presence of lightly labeled cells, nevertheless grain/cell distributions were analyzed to quantitate the observations.

Tissues used for analysis of grain distributions were chosen from those used for TI studies reported above. Autoradiographs, exposed to emulsion for 4 weeks and processed in an identical manner, were analyzed. In each case, where direct comparisons are made, the tissues were from a single experiment and autoradiographs were processed simultaneously. Each distribution contains pooled data from grain counts of 100 cells from one autoradiograph for each of five tissues (when possible). If insufficient tissue (as occasionally occurs in the case of lung nodules) was present, additional counts were made on each of the other autoradiographs to yield a total of 500 cells. A similar procedure was used in the comparison of metastases on day 28 when only two or three animals survived in each group.

The TI of primary LL tumors decreases with time post-implant (Fig. 2), and analysis of the distribution of grain counts indicates (Fig. 12) a general shift toward a lower grain count per cell in the population as well as a decrease in the number of cells scored as labeled. The shift in the distribution may be explained, at least in part, by the increase in the length of the S-phase with tumor growth. If the DNA compliment per cell remains constant, then the same amount of DNA would be synthesized over a longer period of time and at a slower rate, thus incorporating less TdR-^{3}H during a pulse exposure. The slower rate of DNA synthesis would result in a lower specific activity on a per cell basis and a shift in distribution.

Grain count distributions for primary s.c. tumors and lung metastases in the same hosts are consistent with both an increase in the number of labeled cells and the presence of more highly labeled cells in the metastatic cell population (Fig. 12). The length of the S-phase is shorter in the metastases than in the primary tumors and may be responsible, in part, for the observed difference.

Grain count distributions for the lung metastases at 96 hr after surgery (either surgical excision or sham) indicate that more highly labeled cells are found in the surgical excision (Fig. 13A) than in the control group even though the length of the S-phase is identical (Fig. 8). A similar, but possibly less pronounced, change in the grain count distribution for the sham surgical groups is seen. By 14 days after surgery (day 28 post-implant), no mice survived in the sham group, but grain-count distributions in the lung metastases of control and surgical excision groups (Fig. 13B) provide evidence for persistent effects of the surgery.

CONCLUSIONS

The following conclusions may be drawn from these studies:

1. The cell cycle is shorter and the TI higher in the lung metastases than in the s.c. primary LL tumor at any point in time where both could be studied in the same host.

2. The presence of a growing s.c. tumor suppresses the TI of the lung metastases and tends to increase life span.

3. Preliminary results indicate that there is little or no interaction between a growing s.c. tumor or lung metastases on the growth of artificial brain metastases. The TI of the brain metastases is approximately equal to the maximum TI seen in LL under any conditions examined.

4. Surgical excision of a primary tumor results in an increase in TI of the residual lung metastases that persists for 10 to 14 days and a slight, but consistent, adverse effect on life span.

5. Sham surgery that leaves the primary tumor undisturbed also increases the TI of lung metastases and, to a lesser degree, the TI of primary tumors, and the elevation of TI persists for about 7 days after surgery.

6. The most notable difference in grain count distributions of lung metastases 96 hr after surgery is the presence of highly labeled cells; highly labeled cells are apparent, to a lesser extent, 14 days after surgery.

These results with the Lewis lung carcinoma provide strong support for adjuvant chemotherapy after surgery in this system. By 48 hr after surgical removal of the primary tumor, the effects on the TI of metastases were apparent in all studies (at 24 hr the results were variable). In view of the rapid proliferation of the residual tumor cells, chemotherapy should be administered at 48 hr or as soon as possible thereafter to take advantage of the proliferative state and to limit the increase in tumor cell burden.

These conclusions are based on data from one experimental tumor system, but the "outbursts" of metastatic growth after surgery reported for several clinical tumors (5,19) suggest the need for careful reappraisal of clinical data to determine whether surgery may also stimulate cell proliferation in some tumors in man.

ACKNOWLEDGMENTS

We wish to thank Mr. John A. Burdeshaw for the statistical analysis of data. This work was supported by Contract NO1-CM-43756, Division of Cancer Treatment, N.I.H., H.E.W.

REFERENCES

1. Barski, G., and Youn, J. K. (1969): Evaluation of cell-mediated immunity in mice bearing an antigenic tumor. Influence of tumor growth and surgical removal. *J. Natl. Cancer Inst.*, 43:111–121.
2. Belehradek, J., Jr., Barski, G., and Thonier, M. (1972): Evaluation of cell-mediated antitumor immunity in mice bearing a syngeneic chemically induced tumor. Influence of tumor growth, surgical removal and treatment with irradiated tumor cells. *Int. J. Cancer,* 9:461–469.
3. Braunschweiger, P. G., and Schiffer, L. M. (1976): Cell kinetics as a basis for chemotherapy scheduling in solid tumors. *Proc. AACR,* 17:57.

4. DeWys, W. D. (1972): Studies correlating the growth rate of a tumor and its metastases and providing evidence for tumor-related systemic growth-retarding factors. *Cancer Res.,* 32:374–379.
5. Dunphy, J. E. (1950): Some observations on the natural behavior of cancer in man. *N. Engl. J. Med.,* 242:167–172.
6. Gershon, R. K., Carter, R. L., and Kondo, K. (1968): Immunologic defenses against metastases: Impairment by excision of an allotransplanted lymphoma. *Science,* 159:646–648.
7. Goldin, A., Venditti, J. M., and Mantel, N. (1974): Combination chemotherapy: Basic considerations. In: *Antineoplastic and Immunosuppressive Agents I,* edited by A. C. Sartorelli and D. G. Johns, pp. 411–448. Springer-Verlag, Berlin.
8. Greene, H. S. N., and Harvey, E. K. (1960): The inhibitory influence of a transplanted hamster lymphoma on metastasis. *Cancer Res.,* 20:1094–1100.
9. Halleraker, B., and Hartveit, F. (1971): Interaction between subcutaneous and intraperitoneal transplants of Ehrlich carcinoma: The possible role of antitumour antibody. *J. Pathol.,* 105(2):95–103.
10. Hartveit, F., and Halleraker, B. (1971): Effect of subcutaneous transplants of Ehrlich carcinoma on the survival time of mice with intraperitoneal transplants of the same tumour. *J. Pathol.,* 105(2):85–93.
11. Humphreys, S. R., and Karrer, K. (1970): Relationship of dose schedules to the effectiveness of adjuvant chemotherapy. *Cancer Chemother. Rep.,* 54:379–392.
12. Jeejeebhoy, H. F. (1974): Stimulation of tumor growth by the immune response. *Int. J. Cancer,* 13:665–678.
13. Kensey, D. L. (1961): Effects of surgery upon cancer metastasis. *J.A.M.A.,* 18:734–735.
14. Ketcham, A. S., Wexler, H., and Mantel, N. (1961): Studies on the effects of surgery on transplanted animal tumors and their metastases. *J. Natl. Cancer Inst.,* 27:1311–1319.
15. Maugh, T. H., II (1976): Cancer chemotherapy: An unexpected drug interaction. *Science,* 194:310.
16. Mayo, J. G., Laster, W. R., Jr., Andrews, C. M., and Schabel, F. M., Jr. (1972): Success and failure in the treatment of solid tumors. III. "Cure" of metastatic Lewis lung carcinoma with methyl-CCNU (NSC-95441) and surgery-chemotherapy. *Cancer Chemother. Rep.,* 56:183–195.
17. Paranjpe, M. S., and Boone, C. W. (1974): Kinetics of the antitumor delayed hypersensitivity response in mice with progressively growing tumors: Stimulation followed by specific suppression. *Int. J. Cancer,* 13:179–186.
18. Prehn, R. T. (1972): The immune reaction as a stimulator of tumor growth. *Science,* 176:170–171.
19. Price, C. H. G., and Jeffree, G. M. (1973): Metastatic spread of osteosarcoma. *Br. J. Cancer,* 28:515–524.
20. Rosenoff, S. H., Bull, J. M., and Young, R. C. (1975): The effect of chemotherapy on the kinetics and proliferative capacity of normal and tumorous tissues *in vivo. Blood,* 45:107–118.
21. Schabel, F. M., Jr. (1969): Cellular kinetics and its implication in cancer chemotherapy. In: *Neoplasia in Childhood,* pp. 61–78. (The University of Texas M. D. Anderson Hospital and Tumor Institute.) Year Book Medical Publishers, Chicago.
22. Schabel, F. M., Jr. (1969): The use of tumor growth kinetics in planning "curative" chemotherapy of advanced solid tumors. *Cancer Res.,* 29:2384–2389.
23. Schabel, F. M., Jr. (1975): Concepts for systemic treatment of micrometastases. *Cancer,* 35:15–24.
24. Schiffer, L., Braunschweiger, P., and Dobrosielski-Vergona, K. (1976): Analyses of human and animal breast tumor cell kinetics and utilization for treatment. *The Cancer Letter,* October 1.
25. Simpson-Herren, L., Sanford, A. H., and Holmquist, J. P. (1974): Cell population kinetics of transplanted and metastatic Lewis lung carcinoma. *Cell Tissue Kinet.,* 7:349–361.
26. Simpson-Herren, L., Sanford, A. H., and Holmquist, J. P. (1977): Effects of surgery on the cell kinetics of residual tumor. Proceedings of Cell Kinetics and Chemotherapy Meeting in Annapolis, Maryland, Nov. 4–6, 1975. *Cancer Treatment Rep.,* 60:1749–1760.
27. Skipper, H. E., Schabel, F. M., Jr., Mellett, L. B., Montgomery, J. A., Wilkoff, L. H., Lloyd, H. H., and Brockman, R. W. (1970): Implications of biochemical, cytokinetic,

pharmacologic, and toxicologic relationships in design of optimal therapeutic schedules. *Cancer Chemother. Rep.,* 54:431–450.

28. Tolmach, L. J., and Hopwood, L. E. (1974): Radiation research: Survival kinetics. In: *Antineoplastic and Immunosuppressive Agents I,* edited by A. C. Sartorelli and D. G. Johns, pp. 489–506. Springer-Verlag, Berlin.

29. Young, R. C. (1973): The effect of methyl CCNU (NSC-95441) on the cellular kinetics of normal and leukemic murine tissues *in vivo. Cell Tissue Kinet.,* 6:35–43.

30. Young, R. C., Goldberg, D., and Grotzinger, K. R. (1976): Alterations in ^{3}H-thymidine incorporation into DNA induced by methyl-CCNU [1-(2-chloroethyl)-3-(4-methyl cyclohexyl)-1-nitrosourea] in normal and tumorous tissues *in vivo. Cell Tissue Kinet.,* 9:325–332.

31. Young, R. C., Goldberg, D., and Schein, P. S. (1973): Enhanced antitumor effect of cytosine arabinoside given in a schedule dictated by kinetic studies *in vivo. Biochem. Pharmacol.,* 22:277–280.

Cancer Invasion and Metastasis: Biologic Mechanisms and Therapy, edited by S. B. Day et al. Raven Press, New York © 1977.

Release of Tumor Cells

*J. Kleinerman and **L. Liotta

* Department of Pathology, Division of Pathology Research, Saint Luke's Hospital, Cleveland, Ohio 44104; and ** Laboratory of Pathology, National Cancer Institute, National Institutes of Health, Bethesda, Maryland 20014

The metastatic process begins with the release of tumor cells from the primary tumor. A small proportion of these liberated tumor cells ultimately survives to initiate distant metastasis. The concept that hematogenous tumor cell release is a consequence of vascular invasion was first proposed in the 1800s. Cruveilhier in 1829 (1) associated primary tumor invasion of local blood vessels with the development of remote metastases. He suggested that a "cancerous juice" traveled in the circulation to produce metastasis.

Lomer in 1883 (2) was the first to recognize that metastases were initiated by circulating free tumor cells or emboli. Since that time there have been few insights into the factors that determine the onset, mechanism, and time course of tumor cell release.

We have been working with a system of tumor transplantation and perfusion which allows quantitation of tumor cells and clumps in the tumor venous drainage. Using this model we have been studying: (a) the relationship of tumor growth and vascularization to tumor cell release (3); (b) the significance of hematogenous tumor cell clumps in the metastatic process (4); and (c) the effect of BCG immunotherapy on the rate of tumor cell release (5).

This model allows the collection of metastasizing tumor cells. We have recently evaluated the proteolytic properties of these tumor cells with regard to basement membrane degradation *in vitro* and compared them with the majority of the tumor cells in the primary mass (6).

MATERIALS AND METHODS

The syngeneic T241 fibrosarcoma-C57B1 murine system with a femoral growth site was chosen because of its rapid and reproducible metastatic behavior to the lungs (7). The rapid exponential increase in the number of macroscopic pulmonary metastases following tumor transplantation is shown in Fig. 1. Macroscopic metastases were counted by transilluminating lungs fixed by tracheal perfusion with neutral buffered formalin (3). Metastases greater than 0.5 mm are identified by this method (3). Additional

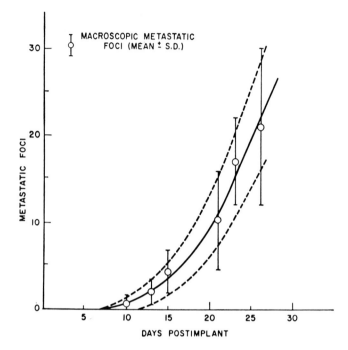

FIG. 1. Increase in numbers of metastatic foci with days after implantation. (Modified from Liotta et al., ref. 10.)

studies of microscopic pulmonary metastases were done by serial section-ing lung lobes and expressing microscopic metastases per unit area of lobe section (5). The rate of entry and clump size distribution of hematogenous tumor cells were quantified by perfusing the tumor vascular bed (3). As shown in Fig. 2, all the venous effluent from a pressure-controlled perfusion is immediately collected through a nucleopore filter. Tumor cells are identi-fied among the cells collected on the filter by the use of quantitative morpho-logic criteria. The criteria were developed from histograms of cell size and nuclear:cytoplasmic ratio for tumor cells, lymphoblasts, and macrophages as shown previously (3). Tumor cells collected on the filter usually impacted over filter pores and were found in single-cell and clump form. In any given experiment clumps were found in a size ranging from 2 to 12 cells. Perfused tumor vessels were identified by a low-viscosity crystal violet stain solution (8). Vessels were then counted and sized in tumor sections.

The effect of BCG on metastases in this system was studied by trans-planting tumors in admixture with BCG or spleen cells from BCG-exposed donors. The rate of tumor cell release and the number of pulmonary metas-tases were quantitated following these treatments.

Basement membrane is a major barrier to penetration of vascular endo-thelium by tumor cells. In order to study the mechanism of this penetration,

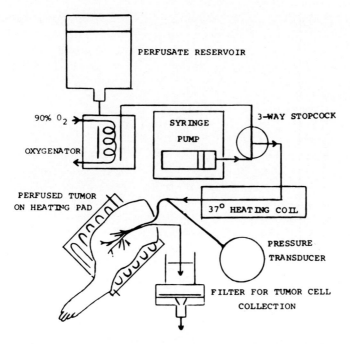

FIG. 2. Diagram of perfusion circuit. (From Liotta et al., ref. 3.)

we cultured tumor cells on an isolated pulmonary basement membrane substrate (9). The substrate was proven to contain type IV collagen by amino acid analysis (6). The degradation of basement membrane was measured by determining the solubilized hydroxyproline and hexose glyoprotein from the substrate (6).

RESULTS

The time course of the release of tumor cells into the circulation is shown in Fig. 3. Tumor cell concentration in the tumor venous effluent rises exponentially following day 4 post-implant. The first appearance of tumor cells in the venous effluent corresponds directly with the first microscopic evidence of tumor neovascularization. From these data the estimated total number of tumor cells released per day rises from 10^3 cells on day 5 to 10^5 cells on day 15. This release rate can be mathematically related to the accumulation of pulmonary metastatic foci (10).

The clump size distribution of the released tumor cells shown in Fig. 4 is relatively stationary in time. Our experimental studies (4) as well as those of Fidler (11) have shown that clumps survive longer in the lung vessels and consequently initiate more metastases per tumor cell than the same number of single cells.

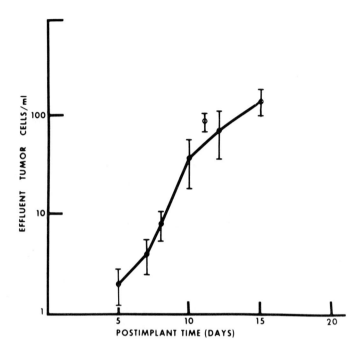

FIG. 3. Semilog plot of the total number of tumor cells in tumor venous effluent vs. post-implant time. Means ±SD are plotted. (From Liotta et al., ref. 3.)

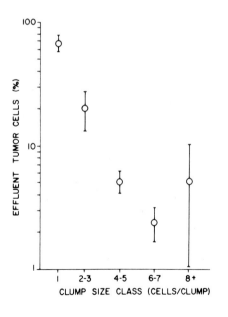

FIG. 4. Clump size distribution combined for all time periods. (From Liotta et al., ref. 4.)

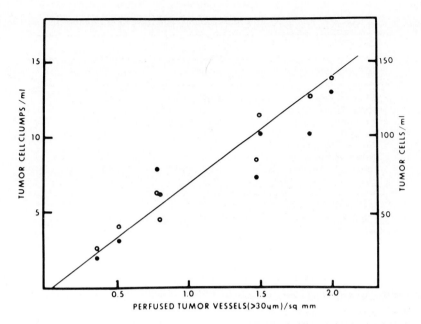

FIG. 5. Relationship of number of perfused tumor vascular channels greater than 30 μm, concentration of total tumor cells (*filled circles*) and tumor cell clumps (2 cells or more; *open circles*) observed in the tumor venous effluent. The regression line (0.97) represents the best least-squares fit of cell clumps as a function of tumor vessels 30 μm and larger. Note the intersection of the regression line near zero. (From Liotta et al., ref. 3.)

A direct relationship (Fig. 5) was found between the concentration of effluent tumor cells and the density of perfused tumor vessels for tumors compared at the same postimplant time.

A direct relationship was also noted between clump size distribution and vessel size (diameter) distribution (3). Our model system can be used to study the effects of treatments on the release of tumor cells.

As shown in Table 1, transplantation of the tumor in admixture with

TABLE 1. *BCG and tumor venous effluent*[a]

Treatment	No.	Tumor cells/ml	Tumor cell clumps	Associated macrophages
BCG	6	$16.0 \pm 5.9^{b,c}$	13.0 ± 7.0^{c}	0.18 ± 0.05^{c}
Control	5	38.0 ± 6.1	43.0 ± 4.0	0.04 ± 0.02

[a] Effects of 1×10^{6} BCG organisms transplanted in admixture with the tumor cells on the (a) concentration of venous effluent tumor cells, (b) percentage of effluent tumor cells in clump form, and (c) proportion of tumor cells in intimate contact with macrophages.
[b] Mean ±SE.
[c] Significantly different; $p < 0.05$.
From Liotta et al., ref. 5.

TABLE 2. *Ability of tumor cells to degrade basement membrane*

Cell population (No.)[a]	Solubilized hydroxyproline (μg $\times 10^{-6}$/cell)	Solubilized protein-bound hexose (μg $\times 10^{-4}$/cell)
1. Effluent tumor cells (7)	2.49 ± 1.33[b]	4.19 ± 1.27[b]
2. Primary tumor cells (5)	0.21 ± 0.12	2.30 ± 0.35
3. Effluent leukocytes (from perfusion of muscle implanted with dead tumor cells) (3)	0.06 ± 0.03	1.10 ± 0.41

[a] Number of tumors studied.
[b] Significantly different $p < 0.01$ from groups 2 and 3 by Student's *t*-test.

BCG reduced the concentration of effluent tumor cells and clumps. In addition, BCG treatment resulted in more effluent tumor cells attached to macrophages (5).

The enzymatic ability of tumor cells collected in the tumor venous drainage to degrade isolated whole pulmonary basement membrane is shown in Table 2.

Tumor cells collected in the venous drainage of perfused muscle bearing the T241 fibrosarcoma had the ability to solubilize basement membrane *in vitro* at neutral pH following 18 hr in culture. The tumor cell activity was significantly greater than that of cultured effluent leukocytes collected from a control perfusion of muscle implanted with dead tumor cells. In addition, tumor cells collected in the venous drainage solubilized basement membrane to a significantly greater extent than tumor cells taken from the primary

TABLE 3. *Collagenase activity of tumor cells cultured with purified human collagen*

Cell population (No.)[a]	Solubilized hydroxyproline (μg $\times 10^{-6}$/cell)
1. Venous effluent tumor cells (4)	1.39 ± 0.40[b]
2. Primary tumor cells (4)	0.48 ± 0.44
3. Effluent leukocytes[c] (4)	0.52 ± 0.30
4. Spleen cells (2)	0.33 ± 0.14
5. Liver cells (2)	0.16 ± 0.10

[a] Number of animals studied.
[b] Significant difference from groups 3, 4, 5, and 6, $p < 0.05$ by Student's *t*-test.
[c] From perfusion of muscle implanted with dead tumor cells.

TABLE 4. *Greatest activity of the tumor cell "collagenase" occurred at pH 7.5 for effluent tumor cells*

Assay pH	Hydroxyproline liberated (μg $\times$ 10^{-6}/cell)[a]
8.0	0.90
7.5	1.2
6.0	0.5
4.0	0.2

[a] Mean of 3 assays.

tumor. Activity was not detected when tumor cells were incubated with substrate at 4°C.

In separate experiments populations were incubated with purified dura type I collagen and the solubilized hydroxyproline quantitated. Effluent tumor cells were found to solubilize hydroxyproline to a significantly greater level than primary tumor cells, effluent leukocytes, spleen cells, or liver cells (Table 3).

As shown in Table 4, the greatest solubilization of hydroxyproline for effluent tumor cells occurred at pH 7.5.

A linear relationship was found between the amount of solubilized hydroxyproline and the number of cells per assay. Incubation for 48 hr instead of 18 hr increased the yield of hydroxyproline by a factor of greater than two for the effluent tumor cells.

DISCUSSION

It has been recognized that tumor angiogenesis is a necessary prerequisite for progressive tumor growth (12). Tumor vascularization is the first step in the hematogenous metastatic process. The present results demonstrate that tumor cells are first seen in the tumor venous effluent following neovascularization and that their concentration is related to the number and size of tumor vessels present. These data indicate that the majority of newly formed tumor vessels are involved in tumor cell release. This conclusion is contrary to the previously held view that only a small number of large venules at the tumor periphery are the site of tumor cell release (13).

The mechanism by which tumor cells penetrate the vascular wall to enter the circulation may be related to intrinsic defects coupled with the invasive propensity of tumor cells. We can postulate that there may be a relationship between the integrity of the new vessels induced by a tumor and its ability to release tumor cells.

A number of investigators have postulated that tumor cell proteases (14–16), and possibly collagenase (17), play a role in malignant invasion.

Vascular invasion is one component of the hematogenous metastatic process, involving both the entry of tumor cells into the circulation (18) and the initiation of metastases (19). Generally, to traverse the vascular wall tumor cells must penetrate the endothelial basement membrane (19). Although electron microscopic studies have shown defects in basement membrane, adjacent to invading tumor cells (20), a tumor enzyme which degrades a basement membrane substrate has not previously been identified. Therefore a major objective of this study was to examine the ability of tumor cells from a metastasizing fibrosarcoma to degrade isolated pulmonary basement membrane *in vitro.*

In this study tumor cells collected in the tumor venous effluent showed a significantly greater ability to break down basement membrane and purified collagen than did tumor cells taken from the primary tumor mass. Tumor cell populations are now recognized to be heterogeneous with respect to various biological and immunogenic properties (21). This may be pertinent to the metastatic process because tumor cells that form metastases may be part of a subpopulation of tumor cells having special properties. This hypothesis is consistent with the work of Fidler (22), who showed that tumor cells injected intravenously could be selected out based on their ability to form metastases. Differences in the tumor cell populations studied here may be due to differences in their intrinsic qualities. However, it is also possible that tumor cells entering the circulation were conditioned by their environment. Humoral factors, absence of cell crowding, and maximum access to blood-borne nutrients may have all played a part in affecting the behavior of intravascular tumor cells.

REFERENCES

1. Cruveilhier (1829–1842): *Anatomic Pathologique du Corps Humain.* Bailliere, Paris.
2. Lomer, E. (1883): Zur Frage der Heilbarkeit des Carcinoms. *Z. Geburtsh. Gynaek.,* 9:277.
3. Liotta, L. A., Kleinerman, J., and Saidel, G. M. (1974): Quantitative relationships of intravascular tumor cells, tumor vessels, and pulmonary metastases following tumor implantation. *Cancer Res., 34:997–1004.*
4. Liotta, L. A., Kleinerman, J., and Saidel, G. M. (1976): The significance of hematogenous tumor cell clumps in the metastatic process. *Cancer Res., 36:889–894.*
5. Liotta, L., Kleinerman, J., and Saidel, G. (1976): Mechanism of BCG induced suppression of metastases in a poorly immunogenic fibrosarcoma. *Cancer Res., 36:3255–3259.*
6. Liotta, L., Kleinerman, J., Catanzaro, P., and Rynbrandt, D. (1977): Degradation of basement membrane by murine tumor cells. *J. Natl. Cancer Inst. (in press).*
7. Wexler, H., Orme, K. S., and Ketcham, A. S. (1968): Biological behavior through successive transplant generations of transplantable tumors derived originally from primary chemically-induced and spontaneous sources in mice. *J. Natl. Cancer Inst.,* 40:513.
8. Liotta, L., Oldham, E., and Kleinerman, J. (1976): Identification of functional tumor vessels by resorcin-crystal violet stain infusion. *Stain Technol.,* 51:99–102.
9. Kefalides, N. A., and Denduchis, B. (1969): Structural components of epithelial and endothelial basement membranes. *Biochemistry,* 8:4613–4621.
10. Liotta, L., Saidel, G., and Kleinerman, J. (1976): Stochastic model of metastases formation. *Biometrics,* 32:535–550.

11. Fidler, I. J. (1973): The relationship of embolic homogeneity, number, size and viability to the incidence of experimental metastasis. *Eur. J. Cancer*, 9:223.
12. Folkman, J. (1974): Tumor angiogenesis factor. *Cancer Res.*, 34:2109–2113.
13. Griffiths, J. D., and Salsbury, A. J. (1965): *Circulating Cancer Cells*. Charles C Thomas, Springfield, Ill.
14. Sylven, B., and Bois-Svensson, I. (1960): Protein content and enzymatic assays of interstitial fluid from some normal tissues and transplanted mouse tumors. *Cancer Res.*, 20: 831–836.
15. Koono, J., Ushijima, K., and Hayashi, H. (1974): Studies on the mechanisms of invasion in cancer. III. Purification of a neutral protease of rat ascites hepatoma cell associated with production of chemotactic factor for cancer cells. *Int. J. Cancer*, 13:105–115.
16. Florey, H. W. (1970): *General Pathology*, pp. 656–660. W. B. Saunders Co., Philadelphia.
17. Dresden, M. H., Heilman, S. A., and Schmidt, J. D. (1972): Collagenolytic enzymes in human neoplasms. *Cancer Res.*, 32:993–996.
18. Coman, D. R. (1953): Mechanisms responsible for the origin and distribution of bloodborne tumor metastases: A review. *Cancer Res.*, 13:397–404.
19. Warren, B. A., and Vales, O. (1972): The adhesion of thromboplastic tumor emboli to vessel walls in vivo. *Br. J. Exp. Pathol.*, 53:301–311.
20. Kellner, B., and Sugar, J. (1967): Morphological factors accompanying growth and invasion. In: *Endogenous Factors Influencing Host-Tumor Balance*, edited by R. W. Wissler, T. L. Dao, and S. Wood, Jr., pp. 239–248. University of Chicago Press, Chicago.
21. Killion, J. J., and Kollmorgen, G. M. (1976): Isolation of immunogenic tumour cells by cell-affinity chromatography. *Nature*, 259:674–676.
22. Fidler, I. J. (1973): Selection of successive tumour lines for metastasis. *Nature [New Biol.]*, 242:148–149.

Cancer Invasion and Metastasis: Biologic Mechanisms and Therapy, edited by S. B. Day et al. Raven Press, New York © 1977.

Metastasis and Chemotherapy, with Reference to Permeability of the Microcirculation System

Haruo Sato and Maroh Suzuki

Department of Oncology, Research Institute for Tuberculosis, Leprosy and Cancer, Tohoku University, Sendai, Japan

Expecting effective treatment in cancer, investigators have tested various combination treatments according to several concepts and working hypotheses. It is considered that at least three factors govern the effectiveness of cancer chemotherapy. The first one is the drug sensitivity of cancer cells. Each strain of the rat ascites hepatoma has its own sensitivity to various chemotherapeutic drugs (9). Presumably, each type of human cancer cell might have individual drug sensitivity, but there is no definite way to determine the most sensitive drug for the target cells of human cancer prior to the practical use.

The second factor relating to the effective result is the number of tumor cells. In animal experiments using tumor cells sensitive to a drug, the drug is more effective when it is administered in an early stage of tumor growth after transplantation. No effect can be expected in either the cure or longevity of tumor-bearing animals when the drug is given in the end stage of tumor growth even if the drug is sensitive to the tumor cells.

The third factor is delivery of a sufficient quantity of drug to the site where tumor cells are growing. This concept has been initiated from a series of studies on the mechanism of metastasis formation, particularly early growth patterns in hematogenous metastasis. Thus, for example, metastatic foci in blood-borne metastasis are initiated in the extravascular spaces around venules and capillaries, and further growth is extended in the interstitium. This explains a result of i.v.-i.v. experiments (tumor cells are transplanted intravenously and drug is administered intravenously) in which no effect of chemotherapy was obtained, despite the use of a sensitive combination of tumor cells and drugs which was examined by i.p.-i.p. experiment (tumor cells are transplanted intraperitoneally and drug is administered intraperitoneally). Therefore, it is suggested that enhanced delivery of the amounts of drug to the site of tumor growth might promote the effect of chemotherapy for either primary or metastatic cancer.

In this chapter model experiments on brain metastases, particularly for treatment of meningeal leukemia, which is hardly curable in human cases, are described and the enhanced effect of chemotherapy is reported by increasing the blood pressure with angiotensin. Also discussed is the role of the blood-brain (or blood-cerebrospinal fluid) barrier in delivery of drug to the site where tumor cells proliferate.

EXPERIMENTAL MODEL OF BRAIN METASTASIS AND MENINGEAL LEUKEMIA

Suzuki (6) reported that typical meningeal carcinomatosis can be produced by transplanting some strains of tumor cells of the rat ascites hepatomas into the carotid artery. This series of transplantable tumors is well known as they possess their own individual characteristics either in morphological or biological phenotypes (9). For example, the ascitic feature of each strain is different, i.e., tumor cells are completely free and separated in some strains, whereas various sizes of cell complexes—small to large—are seen in the ascites in others. These clusters are called "hepatoma

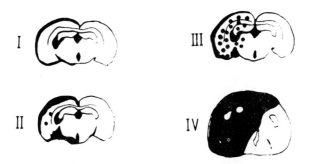

FIG. 1. Four types of brain metastases formed by transplantation of tumor cells from various strains of rat ascites hepatomas.
Type 1: Metastasis is formed diffusely in the meninges and choroid plexus of the ventricles. No metastasis is formed in the brain parenchyma. Tumor cells which form this type of metastasis are those of AH66F, AH7974F, AH13, AH13M, AH13R, and GV (a subline of Yoshida sarcoma), and occasionally AH210A. All of these are single cells in ascites.
Type II: Besides metastases in the meninges and choroid plexus, a few metastatic foci are formed in the brain parenchyma. Meningeal metastasis is diffuse, sometimes slightly nodular, and invasive growth from meninges to the brain parenchyma is seen occasionally. Tumor strains of this type are AH210A, AH41C, AH225A, AH109A, AH21, AH272, AH66, AH63, AH127, and AH7974. This type is seen in AH130, AH60C, and AH601 occasionally. The ascitic picture of these strains is a mixed type of single cells and small islands (of 2–10 cells) with a few large islands of more than 10 cells.
Type III: As in type II, multiple metastases are seen in the brain parenchyma. Tumor strains of this type are AH130, AH127, AH60C, AH601, and AH65C. In the ascitic picture, the number of large islands is increased.
Type IV: Large nodular metastasis is seen, such as occupying the hemisphere of the brain. Tumor strains are AH173 and AH108A, occasionally AH127. In the ascitic picture, these tumors are mainly large islands with a few single cells.

islands." The population of single cells and islands is inherited and characteristic in each strain of the rat ascites hepatoma. Correlation between the types of brain metastases and ascitic features of tumor strains, the cells of which were transplanted into the carotid artery of rats, is summarized in Fig. 1. It was noted that diffuse and widespread metastasis could be induced in the meninges and choroid plexus of the ventricles, but not at all in the brain parenchyma when free single-cell type of tumor was inoculated into the carotid artery. Later it was found that diffuse meningeal carcinomatosis can be produced by direct transplantation of these tumors in the meninges. Moreover, a model of meningeal leukemia (8) could be formed in rats by direct inoculation of cells of DBLA-6 tumor, which is a transplantable ascites leukemia established by Odashima (3,4). Invasive growth of leukemia cells spreads diffusely in the dura mater, subarachnoid space or ventricles involving choroid plexus, and finally into the brain parenchyma.

CHEMOTHERAPY FOR MENINGEAL LEUKEMIA

Using the above-mentioned experimental system, we investigated the therapeutic effect of daunomycin on meningeal leukemia in rats. When 10^6 DBLA-6 cells which were sensitive to daunomycin (1,2) were inoculated directly on the brain through the skull, the animals usually died around 12 days after transplantation. In this series of experiments the cells were transplanted on day 0, then daunomycin was administered three times a day (1 mg each time in the first through third days; 2 mg each time in the second through fourth days). The animals were sacrificed on the sixth day to examine the growth of leukemia cells in various sites of the brain microscopically. After daunomycin was given, it was noted that the growth of leukemia cells was inhibited markedly in the dura mater, but not in the subarachnoid space. It was assumed that the existence of the so-called blood-cerebrospinal fluid barrier might inhibit the delivery of the drug to the tumor cells growing in the interstitial tissues of the subarachnoid space.

BLOOD-CEREBROSPINAL FLUID BARRIER DYSFUNCTION IN ANGIOTENSIN-INDUCED HYPERTENSION

By using a technique of fluorescein cineangiography reported by Rosenblum (5), it was clearly demonstrated that there was no barrier in the dura mater, although the blood-cerebrospinal fluid barrier was present in the subarachnoid space. In this series of observations, the dural and pial microcirculation was investigated in live animals and filmed in a 16-mm movie. The above-described difference in chemotherapeutic results between the dura mater and the subarachnoid space might be attributed to presence or absence of the blood-cerebrospinal fluid barrier. Suzuki et al. (7) reported that extravasation of fluorescein sodium from the dilated arterioles as well as capillaries and venules was seen and recorded in fluorescein cineangiography in a series of experiments of acute angiotensin-induced hypertension of rats. In our observation, lesions of the blood-cerebrospinal fluid barrier were found in rats in which the mean arterial pressure was sustained for 2.5 min or longer at a level of 75% or more above normal.

CHEMOTHERAPY FOR MENINGEAL LEUKEMIA WITH ACUTE ANGIOTENSIN-INDUCED HYPERTENSION

In this series of experiments, the effect of blood-cerebrospinal fluid barrier dysfunction on chemotherapy for meningeal leukemia was investigated. It was confirmed that the blood pressure of rats (about 90 mm Hg) is increased approximately 100% by administering 60 μg/kg of angiotensin intravenously for 3 min (20 μg/kg for 1 min). Treatment with daunomycin followed that with angiotensin in the rats in which DBLA-6 cells were transplanted directly in the brain. The treatment was carried out 24 or 48 hr after transplantation and repeated three times either in the first through third or second through fourth days, respectively. The animals were sacrificed on the seventh day and examined microscopically. The growth of DBLA-6 leukemia cells was inhibited markedly not only in the dura mater but also in the subarachnoid space and brain (Table 1). From these findings, a role of the blood-brain (or blood-cerebrospinal fluid) barrier is suggested in effective chemotherapy in meningeal leukemia.

TABLE 1. *Metastatic growth of DBLA-6 (leukemia) cells in various sites of brain and effect of chemotherapy with reference to breaking the blood-brain barrier with angiotensin*

| | | | Site and grade of metastasis (%) | | | | | |
| | | | Dura | | | Subarachnoid | | |
Experiment	No. of animals	Amount of drug	−	+	++	−	+	++
Control[a]	6		17	67	17	17	50	33
Daunomycin[b]	16	1–2 mg/kg × 3	63	38	0	31	25	44
Daunomycin and angiotensin[c]	16	1–2 mg/kg × 3 60 μg/kg/3 min/day	100	0	0	88	12	0

[a] DBLA-6 cells were inoculated on the brain directly.
[b] The drug was administered i.v.
[c] Angiotensin was given 3 times in either the 1st–3rd or 2nd–4th days in 8 rats, respectively.

SUMMARY

General treatment such as chemotherapy is indispensable when considering the properties of cancer such as dissemination of cancer cells and spread of metastasis. Immunology might be a great help also from a view-point of general treatment of cancer. In cancer chemotherapy several points should be noted, such as the sensitivity of cancer cells to the drug adminis-tered and the amount of drug delivered to cancer tissue. The specificity in physiopathology of host and tumor should be noted to obtain an enhanced effect of cancer chemotherapy. As an example, a result in experimental meningeal leukemia was reported suggesting a correlation between the blood-brain barrier and delivery of chemotherapeutic drug to tumor cells growing outside blood vessels.

REFERENCES

1. Aoshima, M., and Sakurai, Y. (1972): Sensitivity of transplantable rat leukemia, DBLA-6, to antitumor agents. *Gann,* 63:281–290.
2. Aoshima, M., Ishidate, M., Jr., and Sakurai, Y. (1971): Comparative studies on biological characteristics of transplantable rat leukemia, DBLA lines. *Gann,* 62:95–106.
3. Odashima, S. (1970): Leukemogenesis of N-nitrosobutylurea in the rat. I. Effect of various concentrations in the drinking water to female Donryu rats. *Gann,* 61:245–253.
4. Odashima, S., and Fuei-Chang Wang (1970): Establishment of four lines of transplantable rat leukemia induced by N-nitrosobutyl urea in Donryu rats. *Gann,* 61:597–600.
5. Rosenblum, W. I. (1970): Effects of blood pressure and blood viscosity on fluorescein transit time in cerebral microcirculation in the mouse. *Circ. Res.,* 27:825–833.
6. Suzuki, M. (1968): Studies on metastasis XXIV. Experiments on the brain metastasis of the rat ascites hepatoma cells. *Kosankinbyo-Kenkyu Zasshi,* 20:181–194 (in Japanese).
7. Suzuki, T., Tominaga, S., Strandgaard, S., and Nakamura, T. (1975): Fluorescein cine-angiography of the pial microcirculation in the rat in acute angiotensin-induced hyper-tension. In: *Blood Flow and Metabolism in the Brain,* edited by A. M. Harper et al., pp. 58–59. Churchill Livingstone, Edinburgh.
8. Thomas, L. B., Chirigos, M. A., Humphreys, S. R., and Goldin, A. (1962): Pathology of the spread of L1210 leukemia in the central nervous system of mice and effect of treatment with cytoxan. *J. Natl. Cancer Inst.,* 28:1355–1389.
9. Yoshida, T. (1971): Comparative studies of ascites hepatoma. *Meth. Cancer Res.,* 6:95–157.

ADDENDUM

A part of this work was reported in detail as follows: Suzuki, M., and Sato, H. (1977): Experimental studies on local penetration of anticancer drugs in tumor tissue (in Japanese). *Cancer and Chemotherapy,* 4(Suppl.): 97–102.

Cancer Invasion and Metastasis: Biologic Mechanisms and Therapy, edited by S. B. Day et al. Raven Press, New York © 1977.

Hemostasis and Experimental Cancer Dissemination

Maria Benedetta Donati, Andreina Poggi, Luciana Mussoni, Giovanni de Gaetano, and Silvio Garattini

Laboratory for Hemostasis and Thrombosis Research, Istituto di Ricerche Farmacologiche "Mario Negri," Milan, Italy

The hemostatic system, with the complexity of its various components, comprises a number of activities which, it has been suggested, may play a role in tumor growth and metastasis formation. All the steps leading to cancer cell dissemination and implantation in distant organs, such as detachment from the primary tumor, local invasion and penetration into capillaries, transport in blood or lymph, reentry and lodgment in target tissues, invasion, and growth, appear to be possibly influenced by factors derived from platelets and/or from the coagulation/fibrinolysis system.

BLOOD PLATELETS

Circulating blood platelets may be activated by contact with cancer cells and consequently aggregate, as shown both *in vitro* and *in vivo* (12,21,37, 62); aggregation of circulating tumor cells with other cells such as platelets, lymphocytes, and vascular endothelial cells is thought to be important in determining the arrest and survival of malignant cells (18,37). In addition, activated platelets are the source of substances such as prostaglandins, which might be important in the control of tumor cell growth (52).

Platelets can also stimulate the growth of fibroblasts and smooth muscle cells (50,51). The platelet release reaction leads to liberation of serotonin and of other amines active on vascular permeability (27,36), which may influence cell transit toward extravascular districts.

BLOOD COAGULATION

Blood coagulation is an amplified enzymatic process which may be started in several ways by introduction into the circulation of tissue thromboplastin (a protein-phospholipid complex whose presence is increased in some cancer and leukemia cells) (23,31,57); or by intrinsic activation of the so-called contact factor (factor XII or Hageman factor) (47) (Fig. 1). Factor

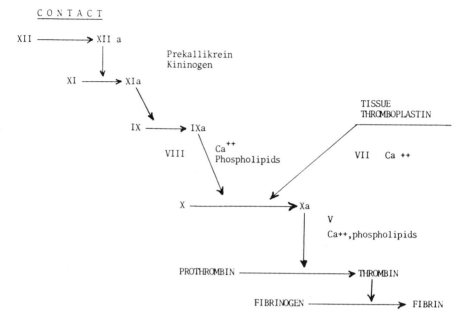

FIG. 1. Schematic representation of the coagulation system.

XII may be activated by a variety of stimuli: endothelial lesions, collagen-like substances, antigen-antibody complexes, particulate material, proteolytic enzymes, and activated complement fractions. Once activated, it plays a key role in triggering several enzymatic cascades, leading not only to thrombin and fibrin formation, but also to fibrinolysis and complement activation and to formation of kinins active on vascular permeability, chemotaxis, and cell growth (47,63). However, it has been recently reported that malignant tissue produces a serine protease capable of starting coagulation by directly activating factor X (22).

Thrombin, both product and catalyst of the clotting cascade, acts in turn as a potent stimulator of cell growth (11), possibly by specific proteolytic attack of cell surface protein(s), the lack of which would trigger renewed cell proliferation (59). Due to its serine protease activity, thrombin can also specifically split actin (35) and activate contractile proteins in cancer cells (16). The increase of contractile proteins recently found in tumoral tissues might be a factor favoring invasiveness and loss of growth control in malignant cells (20). When forming fibrin, thrombin splits from fibrinogen two peptides which are chemotactically active (29). Fibrin itself can be deposited at the tumor periphery, thus providing a structure along which cancer cells may grow; moreover, fibrin could act as a stimulus to mesodermal cells, promoting development and organization of granulation tissue in association with advancing cancer tissue (1,3). It may be relevant to recall that normal mesodermal cells, such as fibroblasts, have been shown to interact with fibrin *in vitro* and to cause fibrin clot retraction (13,39).

This property is lost in aged and in transformed cells (13,38) and in cultured fibroblasts from patients with abnormal wound healing (15,48); the loss of fibrin clot retractile activity by fibroblasts has recently been proposed as a phenotypic indicator of oncogenic transformation in fibroblasts from cancer patients (4,13).

FIBRINOLYSIS

Fibrinolysis is closely linked to blood coagulation, kinin formation, and complement activation and may not only result from activation of an enzymatic cascade of plasmatic factors, but may also be associated with cellular elements (41) (Fig. 2).

Increased production and release of a protein that converts the inactive precursor (plasminogen) to the active fibrinolytic enzyme (plasmin) have been observed in transformed and tumor cells as well as in activated macrophages and other actively migrating cells such as the cells from ovarian follicles shortly before ovulation (5,40,49,61). Plasminogen activator released in human ovarian carcinoma tissue culture has been found immunologically identical to human urokinase (2).

Plasmin itself is a potent mitogen and stimulator of cell migration (46); its proteolytic action on substrates such as fibrinogen or fibrin generates several peptides active on vascular permeability, chemotaxis, and possibly cell growth (8,58).

In summary, activation of fibrinolysis and/or of other proteolytic activities associated with malignant cells may contribute to cohesive failure in solid tumors resulting in the release of cancer cells into the bloodstream and lymph; platelet aggregates and tumor procoagulant activities (leading to

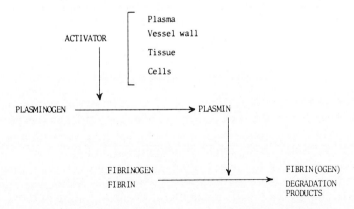

FIG. 2. Schematic representation of the fibrinolytic system.

fibrin formation) may facilitate the arrest of tumor cell clusters within the microcirculation. Endothelial damage and changes in vascular permeability may be provoked by platelet aggregates or substances derived from either platelets or the coagulation/fibrinolysis system. Once lodgment has taken place, fibrin formation and dissolution are probably accelerated (due to stasis and hypoxia) in the tortuous, newly formed vascular network of metastatic foci (1,19).

EXPERIMENTAL MODELS

This proposed theoretical scheme of the sequence of the events linking hemostasis and cancer dissemination has, over the past 20 years, received some experimental support, although indirect.

Treatment of animals with antiaggregating, anticoagulant, or fibrinolytic agents can reduce the number of circulating cancer cells and/or their persistence in the blood [for review, see Hilgard and Thornes (26)]; however, both the suitability of the various models and the benefits of this therapeutic approach have been questioned (26,44,55).

Several long-term experiments were carried out with allogeneic tumors, therefore leaving open the possibility that uncontrolled immunological factors may have influenced the results. Metastasis formation has been followed in many studies after abrupt intravenous injection of huge amounts of cancer cells; this is a highly artificial system, since the injected animals usually have none of the biological changes (e.g., in the plasma protein pattern) associated with the growth of a primary tumor. This model could, however, represent the dissemination process that occurs in some clinical conditions, such as following surgical removal of solid tumors.

In addition, antithrombotic treatments have usually been evaluated without taking into account the possible changes in hemostatic parameters in tumor-bearing animals; then, too, the multiplicity of pharmacological actions of many of these agents (e.g., their effects on other functions of the host or directly on the tumoral cells) makes it difficult to interpret the experimental results to date.

Lewis Lung Carcinoma Model

We have therefore studied the role of the hemostatic system in cancer dissemination using the Lewis lung carcinoma (3LL), an experimental model in which spontaneous metastasis to the lungs can be reliably obtained and measured in syngeneic conditions (28,53,54).

Accelerated labeled fibrinogen turnover has been observed during development of the 3LL tumor, in the absence of any overt hemorrhagic diathesis or any marked signs of disseminated intravascular clotting (43–45). Radiolabeled fibrin accumulated both in the primary tumor and in the lungs.

Thrombocytopenia, with a normal platelet survival time and low platelet turnover, developed progressively during the dissemination phase; these findings, together with a reduction in bone marrow megakaryocytes, suggested that platelet production was impaired in 3LL-bearing mice.

As in some cases of human malignancy (7) and other experimental tumors (25), microangiopathic hemolytic anemia was also found in this model and interpreted as due to erythrocyte damage during passage through small vessels partially occluded by localized fibrin deposits and/or by cancer cells.

Suspensions of 3LL cells were found *in vitro* to have marked procoagulant activity on normal plasma (9); this activity did not require any of the factors of the intrinsic pathway of blood coagulation and only partially the presence of factor VII (9,14). When injected intravenously into C57B1 mice, 3LL cells induced an acute consumption coagulopathy syndrome, characterized by an abrupt and marked fall in platelet count and fibrinogen concentration and by a slower rise in soluble fibrin monomer complexes and fibrin(ogen) degradation products (45).

Thrombocytopenia could be prevented by pretreating the animals not only with antiaggregating agents (32,33), but also with an oral anticoagulant (warfarin) (42). This suggests that the drop in platelet count observed in this model was mainly due to thrombin-induced aggregation of blood platelets.

The platelet count decrease was directly related to the number of cells injected; however, dead cells and cell fragments (from other experimental tumors) induced a similar drop in circulating platelets in acute experiments reported by Hilgard (24).

The different mechanisms of thrombocytopenia observed after i.m. or i.v. injection of 3LL cells underline the difficulties of drawing conclusions about the role of platelets or fibrin in metastasis formation from (acute) short-term experiments in which cancer cells are injected intravenously at high concentrations.

Markedly different hemostatic changes have been found during metastatic growth of 3LL in three different experimental systems, i.e., spontaneous metastasis with and without removal of the primary tumor, and blood-borne tumor emboli. Only when the primary tumor was present were thrombocytopenia, anemia, and hyperfibrinogenemia observed (Table 1).

TABLE 1. *Hematological changes occurring during metastasis growth of 3LL tumor in different experimental systems*

System	Intramuscular implantation	Intramuscular implantation + amputation	Intravenous injection
Red cells	Decreased	Unchanged	Unchanged
Platelets	Decreased	Unchanged	Unchanged
Fibrinogen	Increased	Unchanged	Unchanged

SOME PHARMACOLOGICAL APPROACHES

Both the number and weight of spontaneous lung metastases were significantly lower in 3LL-bearing mice anticoagulated with racemic sodium warfarin (coumadin, Crinos, Villaguardia, Italy) during the whole tumor development period (prothrombin complex activity around 20%). This treatment had less effect on the primary tumor. The antimetastatic effect was slightly greater after larger doses of warfarin, which lowered the prothrombin complex activity to less than 5% (42). Continuous anticoagulation protected the animals from pulmonary growth of blood-borne tumor emboli following intravenous injection of 3LL cells (42).

These data confirm and extend previous observations on the antimetastatic effect of coumarin anticoagulants (27); however, there is some question of how relevant these results are as an indication of the role of fibrin in metastatic formation, since warfarin could reduce metastasis formation by several other mechanisms, such as a direct cytotoxic effect, inhibition of tumor cell motility, and mitotic activity mechanisms (10,30,60). In our experimental conditions, however, the antimetastatic effect of warfarin seemed closely associated with its anticoagulant activity. Experiments using the racemic form of warfarin and each of its resolved enantiomers showed that R-warfarin had almost no anticlotting activity in mice and did not modify the metastatic growth of 3LL; the opposite was true for S-warfarin (17) (Table 2).

Lung metastasis growth was increased in mice kept defibrinogenated during the whole period of tumor development by treatment with batroxobin (Defibrase®, Pentapharm, Basel, Switzerland); this is a substance extracted from *Bothrops moojeni* snake venom, which acts on fibrinogen much the same way as thrombin but without activating any other coagulation factor or platelets. This drug removes fibrinogen from the circulation without inducing intravascular clotting (6,56).

In mice kept defibrinated only during the period of metastasis growth, with or without surgical removal of the primary tumor, metastasis formation

TABLE 2. *Lung weight and metastasis number at day 17 after intravenous injection of 3LL cells (2×10^5)[a]*

	Metastasis no.	Lung weight (mg)
Control	21.0 ± 2.8	740 ± 70
RS-warfarin	4.2 ± 1.0[b]	300 ± 20[b]
R-warfarin	19.2 ± 6.8	770 ± 90
S-warfarin	2.0 ± 0.5[b]	370 ± 40[b]

[a] Daily treatment with warfarin (2.5 mg/l drinking water) was started 2 days before injection and continued until the end of the experiment.
[b] $p < 0.01$ at Duncan's new multiple range test.

was slightly decreased (34). This suggests that fibrin may play different roles in the various phases of metastatic spreading of the same tumor, such as release of cells from the primary tumor (which is possibly decreased by the presence of fibrin within the tumor) and, on the other hand, arrest and growth in the lung (a process which may be facilitated by the presence of fibrin as a guideline).

The presence of fibrin around cancer cells within the primary tumor or in metastatic foci could also modify the access to cancer cells of drugs used for chemotherapy or immunological defense mechanisms. It is therefore conceivable that new combined approaches to treatment of metastases might associate anticoagulation or defibrination with chemotherapy or immuno-stimulation.

We have obtained preliminary results with the combination of *Corynebacterium parvum* and warfarin showing these treatments potentiate each other's effect in reducing spontaneous metastases of 3LL tumors.

CONCLUSION

In conclusion, there is now sufficient experimental evidence that fibrin and platelets may interact with cancer cells *in vitro*. The results obtained *in vivo* with drugs active on hemostasis in various experimental models of dissemination are difficult to interpret in view of the multiplicity of the models and of the range of pharmacological effects of the drugs used.

Hemostatic changes certainly occur during development of the Lewis lung carcinoma, and the results obtained with anticoagulation and defibrination in this tumor in various experimental conditions suggest that fibrin may well have various roles in different phases of the metastatic spread.

ACKNOWLEDGMENTS

The authors' work reported in this chapter was supported by grants NIH PHRB-1 RO1 CA 12764–01 and CNR (Italian Research Council) 73.00400.04. The authors gratefully acknowledge the assistance of Judith Baggott, Graziella Scalvini, and Gigliola Brambilla in preparing the manuscript.

REFERENCES

1. Ambrus, J. L., Ambrus, C. M., Pickern, J., Soldes, S., and Bross, I. (1975): Hematologic changes and thromboembolic complications in neoplastic disease and their relationship to metastasis. *J. Med. (Basel)*, 6:433–458.
2. Åstedt, B., and Holmberg, L. (1976): Immunological identity of urokinase and ovarian carcinoma plasminogen activator released in tissue culture. *Nature*, 261:595–597.
3. Astrup, T. (1968): Blood coagulation and fibrinolysis in tissue culture and tissue repair. *Biochem. Pharmacol.*, 17:241–257.
4. Azzarone, B., Pedullà, D., and Romanzi, C. A. (1976): Spontaneous transformation of human skin fibroblasts derived from neoplastic patients. *Nature*, 262:74–75.

5. Beers, W. H., Strickland, S., and Reich, E. (1975): Ovarian plasminogen activator: Relationship to ovulation and hormonal regulation. *Cell,* 6:387–394.
6. Blombäck, B., Blombäck, M., and Nilsson, I. M. (1957): Coagulation studies on "Reptilase," an extract of the venom from "Bothrops jararaca." *Thromb. Diath. Haemorrh.,* 1:76–81.
7. Brain, M. C., Azzopardi, J. G., Baker, L. R. I., Pineo, G. F., Roberts, P. D., and Dacie, J. V. (1970): Microangiopathic haemolytic anaemia and mucin-forming adenocarcinoma. *Br. J. Haematol.,* 18:183–193.
8. Buczko, W., de Gaetano, G., Franco, R., and Donati, M. B. (1976): Biological properties of dialysable peptides derived from plasmin digestion of bovine fibrinogen preparations. *Thromb. Haemost.,* 35:651–657.
9. Cattan, A., and Bresson, M. L. (1976): Murine tumor cell activity on in vitro hemostasis. *Biomedicine,* 25:252–254.
10. Chang, J. C., and Hall, T. C. (1973): In vitro effect of sodium warfarin on DNA and RNA synthesis of mouse L1210 leukemic cells and Walker tumor cells. *Oncology,* 28:232–237.
11. Chen, L. B., and Buchanan, J. M. (1975): Mitogenic activity of blood components. I. Thrombin and prothrombin. *Proc. Natl. Acad. Sci. U.S.A.,* 72:131–135.
12. Copley, A. L., and Witte, S. (1976): On physiological microthromboembolization as the primary platelet function: Elimination of invaded particles from the circulation and its pathogenic significance. *Thromb. Res.,* 8:251–262.
13. Dolfini, E., Azzarone, B., Pedulla, D., Ottaviano, E., de Gaetano, G., Donati, M. B., and Morasca, L. (1976): Characterization of human fibroblasts from cancer patients: Loss of fibrin clot retractile activity after "in vitro" spontaneous transformation. *Eur. J. Cancer,* 12:823–825.
14. Dolfini, E., Mussoni, L., Poggi, A., Morasca, L., and Donati, M. B. (1977): On the procoagulant activity of Lewis lung carcinoma cells: An in vitro and in vivo study (*in preparation*).
15. Donati, M. B., Balconi, G., Remuzzi, G., Borgia, R., Morasca, L., and de Gaetano, G. (1977): Skin fibroblasts from a patient with Glanzmann's thrombasthenia do not induce fibron clot retraction. *Thromb. Res.,* 10:173–174.
16. Donati, M. B., Dolfini, E., Morasca, L., and de Gaetano, G. (1976): Fibrin clot retraction by a rat rhabdomyosarcoma cell line. *Thromb. Res.,* 8:707–711.
17. Donati, M. B., Poggi, A., Mussoni, L., Kornblitt, L., and Garattini, S. (1977): On the antimetastatic effect of warfarin in an experimental tumor (3LL): Studies with warfarin enantiomers (*in preparation*).
18. Fidler, I. J. (1975): Biological behavior of malignant melanoma cells correlated to their survival "in vivo." *Cancer Res.,* 35:218–244.
19. Folkman, J., Merler, E., Abernathy, C., and Williams, G. (1971): Isolation of a tumor factor responsible for angiogenesis. *J. Exp. Med.,* 133:275–287.
20. Gabbiani, G., Csank-Brassert, J., Schneeberger, J.-C., Kapanci, Y., Trenchev, P., and Holborow, E. J. (1976): Contractile proteins in human cancer cells. *Am. J. Pathol.,* 83: 457–466.
21. Gasic, G. J., Gasic, T. B., Galanti, N., Johnson, T., and Murphy, S. (1973): Platelet-tumor-cell interactions in mice. The role of platelets in the spread of malignant disease. *Int. J. Cancer,* 11:704–718.
22. Gordon, S. G., Franks, J. J., and Lewis, B. (1975): Cancer procoagulant A: A factor X activating procoagulant from malignant tissue. *Thromb. Res.,* 6:127–137.
23. Gralnick, H. R., and Tan, H. K. (1974): Acute promyelocytic leukemia. A model for understanding the role of the malignant cell in hemostasis. *Hum. Pathol.,* 5:661–673.
24. Hilgard, P. (1973): The role of blood platelets in experimental metastases. *Br. J. Cancer,* 28:429–435.
25. Hilgard, P., Hohage, R., Schmitt, W., and Köhle, W. (1973): Microangiopathic haemolytic anaemia associated with hypercalcaemia in an experimental rat tumour. *Br. J. Haematol.,* 24:245–254.
26. Hilgard, P., and Thornes, R. D. (1976): Anticoagulants in the treatment of cancer. *Eur. J. Cancer,* 12:755–762.
27. Holmsen, H., Day, H. J., and Stormorken, H. (1969): The blood platelet release reaction. *Scand. J. Haematol. [Suppl.],* 8:3–26.

28. Karrer, K., Humphreys, S. R., and Goldin, A. (1967): An experimental model for studying factors which influence metastasis of malignant tumors. *Int. J. Cancer,* 2:213–223.
29. Kay, A. B., Pepper, D. S., and Ewart, M. R. (1973): Generation of chemotactic activity for leucocytes by the action of thrombin on human fibrinogen. *Nature [New Biol.],* 243:56.
30. Kirsch, W. M., Schulz, D., Van Buskirk, J. J., and Young, H. E. (1974): Effects of sodium warfarin and other carcinostatic agents on malignant cells: A study of drug synergy. *J. Med. (Basel),* 5:69–82.
31. Mussoni, L., Bertoni, M. P., Curatolo, L., Poggi, A., and Donati, M. B. (1977): In vitro interactions of L5222 and BN-M-L leukemia cells with fibrin. A preliminary report. *Leukemia Res. (in press).*
32. Mussoni, L., Poggi, A., de Gaetano, G., and Donati, M. B. (1977): Effects of ditazole — an inhibitor of platelet aggregation — on a metastasizing tumour in mice. *Haemostasis (submitted for publication).*
33. Mussoni, L., Poggi, A., Donati, M. B., and de Gaetano, G. (1977): Ditazole and platelets. III. Effect of ditazole on tumour-cell induced thrombocytopenia and on bleeding time in mice. *Hemostasis (in press).*
34. Mussoni, L., Poggi, A., Donati, M. B., and Garattini, S. (1977): Growth and metastatization of the Lewis lung carcinoma in mice defibrinated with Defibrase® *(in preparation).*
35. Muszbek, L., and Laki, K. (1974): Cleavage of actin by thrombin. *Proc. Natl. Acad. Sci. U.S.A.,* 71:2208–2211.
36. Nachman, R. L., Weksler, B., and Ferris, B. (1972): Characterization of human platelet vascular permeability-enhancing activity. *J. Clin. Invest.,* 51:549–556.
37. Nicolson, G. L., Winkelhake, J. L., and Nussey, A. C. (1976): An approach to studying the cellular properties associated with metastasis: Some in vitro properties of tumor variants selected in vivo for enhanced metastasis. In: *Fundamental Aspects of Metastasis,* edited by L. Weiss, pp. 291–303. North Holland, Amsterdam.
38. Niewiarowski, S., and Goldstein, S. (1973): Interaction of cultured human fibroblasts with fibrin: Modification by drugs and aging in vitro. *J. Lab. Clin. Med.,* 82:605–610.
39. Niewiarowski, S., Regoeczi, E., and Mustard, F. (1972): Adhesion of fibroblasts to polymerizing fibrin and retraction of fibrin induced by fibroblasts. *Proc. Soc. Exp. Biol. Med.,* 140:199–204.
40. Ossowski, L., Quigley, J. P., Kellerman, G. M., and Reich, E. (1973): Fibrinolysis associated with oncogenic transformation. Requirement of plasminogen for correlated changes in cellular morphology, colony formation in agar, and cell migration. *J. Exp. Med.,* 138:1056–1064.
41. Plow, E. F., and Edgington, T. S. (1975): An alternative pathway for fibrinolysis. I. The cleavage of fibrinogen by leucocyte proteases at physiologic pH. *J. Clin. Invest.,* 56:30–38.
42. Poggi, A., de Gaetano, G., Mussoni, L., Donati, M. B., and Garattini, S. (1977): Effect of anticoagulation with warfarin on Lewis Lung carcinoma in mice *(in preparation).*
43. Poggi, A., Donati, M. B., Polentarutti, N., de Gaetano, G., and Garattini, S. (1976): On the thrombocytopenia developing in mice bearing a spontaneously metastasizing tumor. *Z. Krebsforsch.,* 86:303–306.
44. Poggi, A., Polentarutti, N., Donati, M. B., de Gaetano, G., and Garattini, S. (1975): Fibrinogen, platelet and red cell kinetics in mice bearing an experimental tumor. *Thromb. Diath. Haemorrh.,* 34:946–947.
45. Poggi, A., Polentarutti, N., Donati, M. B., de Gaetano, G., and Garattini, S. (1977): Blood coagulation changes in mice bearing Lewis Lung carcinoma, a metastasizing tumor. *Cancer Res.,* 37:272–277.
46. Pollack, R., and Rifkin, D. (1975): Actin-containing cables within anchorage-dependent rat embryo cells are dissociated by plasmin and trypsin. *Cell,* 6:495–506.
47. Ratnoff, O. D. (1974): Some recent advances in the study of hemostasis. *Circ. Res.,* 35: 1–14.
48. Remuzzi, G., Marchesi, E., de Gaetano, G., and Donati, M. B. (1977): Abnormal tissue repair in Glanzmann's thrombasthenia. *Lancet,* 1:374–375.
49. Rifkin, D. B., Loeb, J. N., Moore, G., and Reich, E. (1974): Properties of plasminogen activators formed by neoplastic human cell cultures. *J. Exp. Med.,* 139:1317–1328.
50. Ross, R., Glomset, J., Kariya, B., and Harker, L. (1974): A platelet-dependent serum factor

that stimulates the proliferation of arterial smooth muscle cells "in vitro." *Proc. Natl. Acad. Sci. U.S.A.,* 71:1207–1210.

51. Rutherford, R. B., and Ross, R. (1976): Platelet factors stimulate fibroblasts and smooth muscle cells quiescent in plasma serum to proliferate. *J. Cell Biol.,* 69:196–203.

52. Santoro, M. G., Philpott, G. W., and Jaffe, B. M. (1976): Inhibition of tumour growth *in vivo* and *in vitro* by prostaglandin E. *Nature,* 263:777–779.

53. Schabel, F. M., Jr. (1975): Concepts for systemic treatment of micrometastases. *Cancer,* 35:15–24.

54. Simpson-Herren, L., and Lloyd, H. H. (1970): Kinetic parameters and growth curves for experimental tumor systems. *Cancer Chemother. Rep.,* 54:143–174.

55. Spreafico, F., and Garattini, S. (1974): Selective antimetastatic treatment—current status and future prospects. *Cancer Treatment Rev.,* 1:239–250.

56. Stocker, K., and Egberg, N. (1973): Reptilase as a defibrinogenating agent. *Thromb. Diath. Haemorrh. [Suppl.],* 54:361–370.

57. Svanberg, L. (1975): Thromboplastic activity of human ovarian tumours. *Thromb. Res.,* 6:307–313.

58. Takaki, A., Yamaguchi, T., and Ohsato, K. (1974): Kinin-like activities of the synthetic low molecular weight fragments of fibrinogen degradation products. *Thromb. Diath. Haemorrh.,* 32:350–355.

59. Teng, N. N. H., and Chen, L. B. (1976): Thrombin-sensitive surface protein of cultured chick embryo cells. *Nature,* 259:578–580.

60. Thornes, R. D., Edlow, D. W., and Wood, S., Jr. (1968): Inhibition of locomotion of cancer cells in vivo by anticoagulant therapy. I. Effects of sodium warfarin on V₂ cancer cells, granulocytes, lymphocytes and macrophages in rabbits. *Johns Hopkins Med. J.,* 123: 305–316.

61. Unkeless, J. C., Gordon, S., and Reich, E. (1974): Secretion of plasminogen activator by stimulated macrophages. *J. Exp. Med.,* 139:834–850.

62. Warren, B. A. (1974): Tumor metastasis and thrombosis. *Thromb. Diath. Haemorrh. [Suppl.],* 59:139.

63. Whitfield, J. F., MacManus, J. P., and Gillan, D. J. (1970): Cyclic AMP mediation of bradykinin-induced stimulation of mitotic activity and DNA synthesis in thymocytes. *Proc. Soc. Exp. Biol. Med.,* 133:1270–1274.

Cancer Invasion and Metastasis: Biologic
Mechanisms and Therapy, edited by S. B. Day
et al. Raven Press, New York © 1977.

Discussion Summary: The Process
of Metastatic Spread

Peter Alexander

*Division of Tumor Immunology, Chester Beatty Research Institute,
Belmont, Sutton, Surrey, England*

All of the chapters in this section attracted much interest, and the discussion could usefully have been extended. Much of the time was devoted to tumor angiogenesis and its possible link with the phenomenon of tumor dormancy.

In response to questions, Dr. Folkman said (a) that tumor angiogenesis factor (TAF) was not species specific, and (b) that a comparable angiogenesis factor was not released from any of a large number of normal tissues which he had studied except the salivary gland and at sites of a graft-versus-host reaction; however, in the latter case the active principle did not exactly mimic TAF. Dr. Gullino felt that the association between neoplasia and TAF production was exemplified in the genesis of mouse mammary carcinoma, in which preneoplastic lesions did not release TAF but early neoplastic nodules did. Dr. Folkman's experience was that different tumor cells when grown *in vitro* produced TAF at similar rates.

The possible occurrence of a circulating TAF antagonist which inhibited TAF-induced angiogenesis as does the factor in cartilage was referred to by several speakers. Dr. Vaage asked if immune reactivity influenced angiogenesis and if ischemic death might be an important mechanism in the immunological destruction of a metastatic focus. Even though a graft-versus-host reaction caused angiogenesis, Dr. Borsos thought an anti-TAF principle might be elaborated by cells of the immune system.

The discussion then turned to a possible link between TAF and the phenomenon of dormancy, which Dr. Wheelock had elegantly documented by suitably manipulating the host prior to inoculating tumor cells. The latter initially failed to grow but all the injected tumor cells were not killed because (a) there was a frequent late occurrence of tumor, and (b) viable tumor cells could be recovered by culture *in vitro*. A related phenomenon had been encountered by Eccles and Alexander who found that the late occurrence of distant metastasis following removal of the primary tumor was promoted by immune suppression given several weeks after surgery. Dr. Alexander said that the available evidence was consistent with the hypothesis that the dormant foci contained dividing tumor cells without a blood supply. This could come about because of an anti-TAF activity released by inflammatory cells within the dormant lesion. Immune suppression reduces the inflammatory infiltrate and this turns the balance of factors in favor of angiogenesis and results in the appearance of clinical metastases. This, however, is unlikely to be the whole story, and Dr. Kleinerman's work, in which he had found that the tumor cells within the lung metastases were a distinct subpopulation with greater potential for degrading pulmonary basement membrane, raised the whole question of the role of cell variants in metastasis. Although the appearance on selection of such variants is not in doubt, it is far from clear whether the populations of the primary tumor and of the metastasis always differ.

Dr. Dominique-Vassetti's hypothesis of a causal link between invasion and the increased production of plasminogen activator, which occurs when normal cells are transformed to the malignant state, requires that the parallel increase of plasminogen activator release by cells of the mononuclear phagocytic series following treatments that do not result in malignancy also renders these normal cells invasive. The macrophages at sites of inflammation produce increasing amounts of plasminogen activator, and this Dr. Dominique-Vassetti saw as an example of plasminogen activator facilitated invasion. Others, however, felt that the more usual interpretation could not be dismissed, namely, that blood monocytes extravasate to sites of inflammation because of a chemotactic stimulus, that the changes leading to increased plasminogen activator synthesis occur after the cells have extravasated, and that extravasation of monocytes and invasion cannot usefully be linked.

Dr. Donati's excellent summary of the complexity of the relationship between hemostasis and cancer dissemination was amplified by several discussants. Most speakers shared Dr. Donati's view that the available information was inadequate to manipulate anticoagulation so as to reduce metastasis in a clinical setting. Such factors as optimum timing and suitability of different tumor types remained to be elucidated. Dr. Gullino expressed the view that this approach holds promise but is not yet ready to be applied.

Cancer Invasion and Metastasis: Biologic Mechanisms and Therapy, edited by S. B. Day et al. Raven Press, New York © 1977.

Cell Surfaces and Blood-Borne Tumor Metastasis

Garth L. Nicolson

Department of Developmental and Cell Biology, University of California, Irvine, California 92717

The spread or metastasis of tumors by blood-borne route is a multistep process dependent on both host and tumor properties (6,16,42,58,66). Metastasis usually begins when a primary tumor mass extends or invades surrounding tissues [local or primary invasion (42)], and this loss of proper cell positioning and tissue-cell interaction characterizes the malignant state (39). Eaves (10) has proposed that tumor invasion occurs because of mechanical pressure on the growing, expanding tumor mass and that extension of the tumor follows pathways of mechanical weakness in the surrounding tissue. Alternatively, actively expanding tumors are known to contain large concentrations of degradative enzymes which are released and break down normal tissue matrix (7,33,57).

During primary invasion neoplastic cells can detach from the original tumor mass. The detachment process is an important event during tumor spread, allowing tumor cells to take up residence near or even at locations distant from the primary site (62). Once invasion has proceeded to the point where tumor entry into the lymphatics, circulatory system, or coelomic cavities is imminent, cell detachment can result in a change of tumor cell emboli to various parts of the host (6,16,42,66). When tumor cells gain entry into a major transportation channel such as the bloodstream and are released, they are rapidly disseminated, but their ultimate fate is still uncertain. Malignant tumors invading blood vessels (usually the thin-walled veins) can grow at the site of invasion and plug the vessel, but they often detach and circulate. However, the mere presence of free tumor cells or their emboli in the blood does not necessarily indicate that subsequent blood-borne metastases will form (36,50). Salsbury (50) has examined the clinical data on the presence of tumor cells in the blood. It was concluded that blood-borne cancer cells are necessary but not sufficient to cause distant metastases, and their presence does not necessarily indicate a worse prognosis than their absence. Most tumor cells die rapidly in the circulation, and only a few actually survive to form secondary tumors (5,11,16,50). Fidler (11) found that less than 1% of intravenously injected B16 melanoma cells survived within 24 hr, but those that did survive had a high probability of later forming gross metastases.

Tumor cells in the blood undergo cellular interactions with circulating and noncirculating host cells, soluble blood components, and other tumor cells. The interactions of tumor cells with platelets (4,28,61), lymphocytes (17), and possibly other yet unidentified host blood cells lead to enhanced tumor cell arrest in the capillaries. This probably occurs because of heterotypic (nonself) cell adhesion resulting in larger circulating tumor-host cell emboli. It has been found experimentally that the larger the circulating embolus, the greater the rate of arrest and survival to form more secondary tumors (12). Larger cell clumps or emboli are more effectively trapped in the capillaries than are single cells or small groups of cells. Homotypic (self) adhesion of metastatic tumor cells to form clumps may also be important during their circulation (12,43,44,64). Also, due to the high thromboplastic activities of many tumor cells, they can be coated with fibrin and perhaps other deposits in the circulation which alter their arrest in the capillaries (2,4,61,65). Thus, purely mechanical factors such as emboli size and emboli as well as capillary deformability (51,67) should be important in metastatic tumor cell arrest by increasing the chance of lodgment in the first capillary bed encountered.

Nonspecific trapping of large tumor cell emboli can occur. However, Zeidman (67) has provided evidence showing that the rates at which tumor cells and emboli pass through capillaries are related not to their size, but instead to their ability to be deformed while traversing the small capillaries. When injected intravenously, many malignant tumor cells pass easily through the first capillary bed encountered and do not form secondary tumors at these sites (19,20,22,56,68).

In several experimental metastatic systems the sites of gross metastases are nonrandom and do not correlate with simple trapping in the first capillary bed suggesting that factors other than emboli trapping are involved. There have been several reports on the organ specificity of circulating tumor cells such as plasmacytoma (47), histiocytoma (9), melanoma (42), reticulum cell sarcoma (46), and others (9). The heterotypic adhesive properties of metastatic tumor cells have been proposed to be important in determining their localization and arrest patterns. Recognition of unique capillary vascular endothelial cell surface determinants by circulating malignant cells could result in arrest and implantation at specific sites (21,40–44).

Once specific arrest has occurred, diapedesis, extravasation, or secondary invasion by tumor cells through the capillary endothelium (and often underlying basement membrane) seems to be the usual next step in the metastatic process. Soon after tumor cell or emboli arrest, these cells appear in many cases to be quickly trapped in a fibrin matrix (4,65). However, this is often not the case (22,35). If fibrinization of the arrested tumor cells occurs (4,28), they must escape from this matrix by fibrinolysis and dissolution of the thrombus (4,52,65). Invasion of the endothelial cell layer can also occur by diapedesis where tumor cells enter gaps left by white cells or where the endothelial cells contract. Chew et al. (4) have noted that the endothelium and underlying basement membranes can be literally destroyed at multiple sites by extravascularizing malignant cells. Cell surface or secreted enzymes (3,7,33,34,54,57,65a) and other released chemotactic factors (45) probably aid in secondary as well as in primary invasion. Once in the extravascular tissue, tumor cells can proliferate, but their growth seems to be limited unless they can be vascularized (25,26,29).

The vascularization of secondary tumors allows them to grow into gross metastases. Vascularization after tissue damage or in the presence of malignant cells seems to be stimulated by tumor angiogenesis factor (24–27), a glycoprotein secreted by malignant tumor cells and also some types of normal host cells (27).

At every step during the pathogenesis of metastasis, malignant cells must escape host defenses which can be nonimmune or immune in nature (16). Immunological surveillance against neoplasms (53) can account for inhibition of tumor growth and spread in some systems (1,37,59) but is woefully inadequate or even stimulatory in others (8,14,15,18,21,48).

The uniqueness of the malignant tumor cell surface appears to be an important property in determining the ultimate fate and location of secondary tumors. In a variety of studies enzymatic manipulation of malignant cells has been shown to modify the distribution, arrest, and subsequent survival of metastatic cells. For example, protease treatment of malignant melanoma cells by Hagmar and Norrby (31) before intravenous injection into mice increased their extrapulmonary arrest and survival to form gross metastases. Use of other tumor cell surface-modifying enzymes such as neuraminidase before intravenous administration enhances tumor cell extrapulmonary localization (63). Modification of cell surface anionic groups with polyanions or polycations can also alter the number, size, and location of experimental metastases (32,54,55).

MODELS FOR STUDYING BLOOD-BORNE METASTASIS

Selection of variant tumor cell lines with enhanced ability to form successful experimental pulmonary metastases in syngeneic hosts was used by Fidler (13) to obtain evidence that unique tumor cell properties may determine the outcome of metastasis. In these experiments viable B16 melanoma cells were injected into the tail veins of C57BL/6 mice, and 3 weeks later the visible (pigmented) melanoma nodules were removed from lungs, and the cells adapted to tissue culture. The B16 melanoma cells that grew out in culture to form gross pulmonary tumors (first *in vivo* selection) were established as a continuous cell line and were called B16-F1. These cells (B16-F1) were injected intravenously back into new syngeneic animals, and 3 weeks later a new group of lung tumor colonies was removed and put into culture (B16-F2). With each succeeding cycle *in vivo* the ability of the selected B16 lines to implant, survive, and form lung tumors increased (13,17). This process was repeated ten times to obtain line B16-F10, which forms significantly more experimental pulmonary metastases than line B16-F1 after intravenous or intracardiac injection (19).

ORGAN SELECTIVITY OF BLOOD-BORNE METASTATIC VARIANT LINES

When the organ distribution of ^{125}I-iodo-2'-deoxyuridine (^{125}IUDR)-labeled B16-F1 and B16-F10 was examined following tail vein injection into C57BL/6 mice, approximately 60% and 99% of the injected F1 and F10 cells, respectively, were found in the lungs within 2 min (17). Although most of the viable cells in the lungs died or left the lungs within 1 day, few extrapulmonary metastases were found. It could be argued that after intravenous injection the B16 cells destined to form pulmonary growths entered the lung capillary bed first, were nonspecifically trapped, and never recirculated. Alternatively, cells from B16 lines selected for increased lung metastasis may possess unique properties that determine their distribution and subsequent survival and growth independent of the route of cell entry into the circulation. To answer this we injected 50,000 viable B16 cells into C57BL/6 mice by intravenous tail vein and by left ventricle heart puncture. We confirmed that the intracardiac route was through the left side of the heart by determining the quantitative distribution of ^{125}IUDR-labeled tumor cells immediately after injection. In all of our control experiments, greater than 9/10 animals were injected intracardially into the left side of the heart as judged by the high concentration of tumor cells in the blood and extrapulmonary organs. Next, 50,000 viable B16-F1 and -F10 cells were injected intravenously or intracardially into syngeneic recipients, and 2 weeks later the average number of experimental metastases was counted.

The number of pulmonary colonies in intravenously or intracardially injected animals was the same within experimental error. However, intravenous or intracardiac injection of B16-F10 line yielded eight to ten times as many lung tumors as B16-F1 (19). In this experiment intracardiac injection of B16-F1 resulted in extrapulmonary tumors in 4/8, 3/5, and 6/10 test animals, whereas no extrapulmonary metastases were found in mice injected intracardially with F10 cells (19).

The tissue distribution of ^{125}IUDR-labeled B16-F1 and B16-F10 was assessed after intravenous or intracardiac injection of a viable single-cell suspension. Within 2 min after intravenous injection of B16-F1, approximately 60 to 70% of the cells were found in the lungs compared to 25 to 30% after 2 min following intracardiac injection. By 1 to 3 hr after intravenous injection, the number of viable tumor cells in the lungs declined, whereas the number of viable cells increased in the lungs during the same period after intracardiac injection. Similar kinetic distributions were obtained with B16-F10. Initially (2 min post-injection) 99% and approximately 30% of the B16-F10 cells were arrested after intravenous or intracardiac injection, respectively, but during the interval of 1 to 3 hr post-injection the number of viable cells in the lungs decreased in animals intravenously injected with B16-F10 and increased in mice injected intracardially. One day after injection animals receiving B16 melanoma cells by intracardiac or intravenous routes had the same number of viable tumor cells in the lungs, and fourteen days after injection the same numbers of gross pulmonary metastases were found, indicating that nonspecific tumor cell trapping in the first organ capillary bed encountered does not influence the final outcome of metastasis (19). The selected B16 melanoma cells must be capable of traversing non-target capillaries and homing to pulmonary capillaries where they arrest, survive, and form lung tumors.

SELECTION OF OTHER BLOOD-BORNE METASTATIC VARIANT LINES

Another test of organ specificity of metastasizing tumors is to ask whether tumor cell lines which metastasize preferentially to one organ can be re-targeted to other organs using *in vivo* selection techniques. In the case of the selected B16 melanoma lines, Fidler (13,17) selected for lung implantation, survival, and growth after tail vein injection. Since the lung capillary beds are the first encountered using this selection scheme, we have used instead the left cardioventricular route for introducing once-selected (lung) B16-F1 cells into C57BL/6 mice and recovering the rare brain tumors when they were found. Theoretically any route of tumor cell entry into the circulation should eventually result in tumor cell dissemination; however, in practice we failed to find brain tumors after tail vein injection of B16-F1. This could have been due to lower concentrations of melanoma cells in the blood after tail vein compared to left ventricle administration (19). Alternatively, the melanoma cells destined to form successful tumors may implant more effectively, leaving other less successful cells to recirculate. Once the tumor cells reach the lungs, these more successful cells do not recirculate (20).

The B16-F1 brain tumor nodules obtained after left ventricle injection were dispersed, and the cells cultured *in vitro* in the usual manner. When enough brain-selected melanoma cells (B16-B1) were obtained from *in vitro* growth, these were injected intracardially back into new C57BL/6 recipients to obtain B16-B2. After three to four selections we found that the tail vein injection route could be used for selection. By eight selections all of the mice, if injected intracardially, had brain tumors, and the number of B16-B8 tumor colonies was approximately >12 times greater in brain and

TABLE 1. *Selection for organ-homing metastatic variants of B16 melanoma in C57BL/6 mice*

B16 melanoma line	No. of *in vivo* selections (organ site)	Average No. of tumors per mouse organ[a] (range)	
		Brain	Lung
B16-F1	1 (lung	<1 (0–1)	29 (11–46)
B16-F10	10 (lung)	0	168 (139–203)
B16-F1B6	6 (brain)	4 (1–7)	20 (9–33)
B16-F1B8	8 (brain)	12 (5–23)	13 (5–19)

[a] Mice were injected with 100,000 viable B16 cells in the left side of the heart and sacrificed 2 weeks later. Pigmented tumor colonies were scored with the aid of a dissecting microscope. Data from Nicolson and Brunson (38).

less in lung compared to line B16-F1 cells (Table 1) (38,43). The location of B16-B8 colonies in the brains of C57BL/6 mice is also interesting. The tumor line seems to form colonies almost exclusively in the ventricle brain regions, suggesting not only organ preference but also regional preference within that organ. These results, although preliminary, suggest that further selection of B16-B8 could lead to a tumor cell line which will form only brain colonies and perhaps only brain colonies in specific brain regions.

In continuing these studies we have selected for two apparently different types of brain-homing melanoma cell lines in the B16-B series. One type (Bn) seems to home to the forward ventricle brain regions, form small multiple lesions, and cause neurological disorders in animals consisting of loss in equilibrium, staggering gait, and other symptoms suggestive of neuromotor impairment. The other type of brain homing tumor (Bb) seems to form fewer but larger lesions, and these appear to be localized in the dorsal cerebral brain regions. Animals bearing B16-B9Bb brain tumors apparently do not display the types of neurological symptoms described above for Bn malignant melanomas (K. W. Brunson and G. L. Nicolson, *in preparation*).

ENZYMATIC AND INVASIVE PROPERTIES OF BLOOD-BORNE METASTATIC VARIANT LINES

Using the B16-F system Bosmann et al. (3) reported that the more metastatic B16 variants produce higher levels of trypsin-like and cathepsin-like enzymes in tissue culture; however, these differences were found only when the melanoma lines were replated at low cell densities. In addition, glycosidases such as N-acetyl-β-D-glucosaminidase, β-L-fucosidase, and β-galactosidase were more active in the highly metastatic cell lines, but again, these differences were observed only at low cell densities. We have examined the trypsin-like and cathepsin-like activities of line B16-F1 and the more metastatic variant B16-F10 in tissue culture. These assays were performed using soluble or insolubilized ^{125}I-labeled protein substrates such as gammaglobulin, casein, and bovine serum albumin. The release of ^{125}I-peptides in the presence of B16 melanoma cells was taken as an estimate of the activities of cell surface-associated and -secreted proteolytic enzymes. This assay can reproducibly detect protease activities as low as 10 mg/ml trypsin-equivalent units per hour at 37°C.

Cultured B16 melanoma cell lines of differing metastatic potentials *in vivo* do not show significant differences in protease levels *in vitro* under a variety of growth conditions. However, the situation may be quite different *in vivo* where the involvement of host serum components and histiocytes, as well as the presence of dead and dying tumor and host cells, all contribute enzymes to the extracellular environment of the tumor. In this regard, many transformed cells produce high levels of plasminogen activator, a serine protease released from cells that converts plasminogen to plasmin, which in turn hydrolyzes fibrin (for review, see 49). When we examined the release of plasminogen activator by the B16 variants, we found no significant differences between the various melanoma lines of differing metastatic potentials. These assays were performed *in vitro* using several different serum sources: calf, dog, syngeneic mouse, and serum from B16 melanoma-bearing syngeneic animals (44). Enhanced fibrinolysis should reduce fibrin deposition in the tumor area after implantation, and hence it might be inhibitory rather than enhancing for metastasis. Enhanced implantation seems to be related to fibrin deposition around the arrested tumor cells (30). This is consistent with the well-known observation that inhibition of blood clotting actually reduces implantation in many systems (23).

Enzymatic differences between the B16 melanoma lines of differing metastatic potentials, although undetected *in vitro* in our preliminary experiments, might be important in local tumor invasion. The highly metastatic B16 lines are known to be more invasive *in vivo* (17) and also *in vitro* (43). The latter assay was performed by measuring the ability of B16 melanoma cells to invade the multicell layer of the chick chorioallantoic membrane (CAM) in tissue culture. In this assay purely mechanical and host immunological factors are eliminated and should not contribute to invasion. B16-F1 and B16-F10 were allowed to adhere to the surfaces of CAM in cultures, and at various times samples were removed and fixed for histological examination. Our results showed that only the highly metastatic B16 cells invaded into the CAM within 12 hr, and the invasion of B16-F10 seemed to be accompanied by widespread CAM destruction. We are currently investigating the possibilities that cell surface (as opposed to secreted) enzymes or other cytotoxic secretory products might be involved in CAM destruction.

ADHESIVE PROPERTIES OF BLOOD-BORNE METASTATIC VARIANT LINES

Once malignant tumor cells have gained entry into the circulation, their cell detachment and cell interactions during transport are of importance in determining the extent and location of secondary colonization. Using the B16 melanoma system the homotypic or heterotypic rates of adhesion (B16 to B16 cells or B16 to other cells) that could be important during blood-borne transport have been examined using *in vitro* assays. The quantitative rates of single-cell B16 capture by homotypic B16 monolayers were assayed using the techniques of Walther et al. (60). In these assays the rates of attachment of the more metastatic B16 variants were always higher than the rates of homotypic attachment of B16-F1 to B16-F1 (the relative rates of homotypic adhesion are B16-F13 > B16-F10 > B16-F5 > B16-F1) (44,64). Similarly, the heterotypic rates of monolayer attachment of the more metastatic B16 variants to cultured endothelial cells were also higher (relative rates of heterotypic adhesion: B16-F13 > B16-F10 > B16-F5 > B16-F1) (44,64). Using the same B16 melanoma system Gasic et al. (28) found that highly metastatic B16-F10 heterotypically aggregated with platelets at faster rates compared to B16-F1. These results indicate that modifications in adhesive behavior accompany selection of highly metastatic variants. These modifications in adhesive properties may aid in blood-borne tumor arrest and trapping of multicell emboli that form in the circulation.

The organ (lung) specificity of B16-F10 (19) and similar lines was mimicked by an *in vitro* gyration-aggregation assay (21,42,44,63). In this assay a partly purified, viable, single-organ cell suspension was mixed with B16 melanoma cells of differing metastatic potentials (B16-F1, -F5, -F10, and -F13) (see 21, 42, or 44 for details). Within minutes the highly metastatic B16-F13 line aggregated lung cells into a single heterotypic clump at 22°C, whereas B16-F1 cells caused only slight lung cell aggregation. Other suspended organ cells from nontarget tissues such as kidney, spleen, and liver were not aggregated by the B16 cells above control homotypic levels during the assays. These results suggest that target organ recognition may occur during tumor cell transport in the blood resulting in cell adherence and implantation at specific tissue and organ locations. The fact that virtually all lung cells (endothelial, epithelial, fibroblast, etc.) were aggregated into a single clump by the B16-F13 line suggested that all the suspended organ cells possessed determinants recognized by the melanoma cells. That these "determinants" are exposed on vascular endothelial cells *in situ* and are responsible for organ-specific implantation remains to be demonstrated, but the possibility is intriguing.

Although few actual biochemical differences have been documented on B16 melanoma cells of differing metastatic potentials, certain cell surface properties such as adhesion, invasion, and angiogenesis are dissimilar and correlate with actual metastatic properties *in vivo*. Future work will undoubtedly focus more on the actual biochemical events responsible for the physiological differences between metastasizing and nonmetastasizing tumor cells in syngeneic hosts and less on simply cataloging cell surface properties. Using *in vivo* selected malignant cell lines of differing metastatic potentials and secondary site preferences, we should ultimately gain insight into the important molecular events involved in tumor metastasis.

ACKNOWLEDGMENTS

This work was supported by U.S. National Cancer Institute contract NO1-CB-33879 and grants from the American Cancer Society (BC-211) and the U.S. Public Health Service (CA-15122).

REFERENCES

1. Baldwin, R. W., and Pimm, M. V. (1974): B.C.G. Suppression of pulmonary metastases from primary rat hepatomata. *Br. J. Cancer,* 30:473.
2. Baserga, R. and Saffiotti, U. (1955): Experimental studies on histogenesis of blood-borne metastasis. *Arch. Pathol.,* 59:26.
3. Bosmann, H. B., Bieber, G. F., Brown, A. E., Case, K. R., Gersten, D. M., Kimmerer, T. W., and Lione, A. (1973): Biochemical parameters correlated with tumour cell implantation. *Nature,* 246:487.
4. Chew, E. C., Josephson, R. L., and Wallace, A. C. (1976): Morphologic aspects of the arrest of circulating cancer cells. In: *Fundamental Aspects of Metastasis,* edited by L. Weiss, p. 121. North-Holland, Amsterdam.
5. Cliffton, E. E., and Agostino, D. (1962): Factors affecting the development of metastatic cancer. Effect of alterations in clotting mechanism. *Cancer,* 15:276.
6. Coman, D. R. (1953): Mechanisms responsible for the origin and distribution of blood-borne tumor metastases: A review. *Cancer Res.,* 13:397.
7. Dresden, M. H., Heilman, S. A., and Schmidt, J. D. (1972): Collagenolytic enzymes in human neoplasms. *Cancer Res.,* 32:993.
8. Duff, R., Doller, E., and Rapp, F. (1973): Immunologic manipulation of metastasis due to Herpesvirus transformed cells. *Science,* 180:79.
9. Dunn, T. B. (1954): Normal and pathologic anatomy of the reticular tissue in laboratory mice, with a classification and discussion of neoplasms. *J. Natl. Cancer Inst.,* 14:1281.
10. Eaves, G. (1973): The invasive growth of malignant tumors as a purely mechanical process. *J. Pathol.,* 109:233.
11. Fidler, I. J. (1970): Metastasis: Quantitative analysis of distribution and fate of tumor emboli labeled with ^{125}I-5-iodo-2'-deoxyuridine. *J. Natl. Cancer Inst.,* 45:775.
12. Fidler, I. J. (1973): The relationship of embolic homogeneity, number, size and viability to the incidence of experimental metastasis. *Eur. J. Cancer,* 9:22.
13. Fidler, I. J. (1973): Selection of successive tumor lines for metastasis. *Nature [New Biol.],* 242:148.
14. Fidler, I. J. (1974): Immune stimulation-inhibition of experimental cancer metastasis. *Cancer Res.,* 34:491.
15. Fidler, I. J. (1974): Inhibition of pulmonary metastasis by intravenous injection of specifically activated macrophages. *Cancer Res.,* 34:1074.
16. Fidler, I. J. (1975): Mechanisms of cancer invasion and metastasis. In: *Biology of Tumors: Surfaces, Immunology and Comparative Pathology, Vol. 4, Cancer: A Comprehensive Treatise,* edited by F. F. Becker, p. 101. Plenum Press, New York.
17. Fidler, I. J. (1975): Biological behavior of malignant melanoma cells correlated to their survival *in vivo. Cancer Res.,* 35:219.

18. Fidler, I. J., Gersten, D. M., and Riggs, C. W. (1977): Relation of host immune status to tumor cell arrest, distribution and survival in experimental metastasis. *Cancer (in press)*.
19. Fidler, I. J., and Nicolson, G. L. (1976): Organ selectivity for implantation, survival and growth of B16 melanoma variant tumor lines. *J. Natl. Cancer Inst.*, 57:1199.
20. Fidler, I. J., and Nicolson, G. L. (1977): The fate of recirculating B16 melanoma metastatic variant cells in parabiosed syngeneic recipients. *J. Natl. Cancer Inst. (in press)*.
21. Fidler, I. J., and Nicolson, G. L. (1977): Tumor cell and host properties affecting the implantation and survival of blood-borne metastatic variants of B16 melanoma. *Israel J. Med. Sci. (in press)*.
22. Fisher, B., and Fisher, E. R. (1967): The organ distribution of disseminated ^{51}Cr-labeled tumor cells. *Cancer Res.*, 27:412.
23. Fisher, B., and Fisher, E. R. (1967): Anticoagulants and tumor cell lodgment. *Cancer Res.*, 27:421.
24. Folkman, J. (1974): Tumor angiogenesis. *Adv. Cancer Res.*, 19:331.
25. Folkman, J. (1975): Tumor angiogenesis. In: *Biology of Tumors: Cellular Biology and Growth, Vol. 3, Cancer: A Comprehensive Treatise*, edited by F. F. Becker, p. 355. Plenum Press, New York.
26. Folkman, J., and Hochberg, M. (1973): Self regulation of growth in three dimensions. *J. Exp. Med.*, 138:745.
27. Folkman, J., Merler, E., Abernathy, C., and Williams, G. (1971): Isolation of a tumor factor responsible for angiogenesis. *J. Exp. Med.*, 133:275.
28. Gasic, G. J., Gasic, T. B., Galanti, N., Johnson, T., and Murphy, S. (1973): Platelet-tumor cell interaction in mice. The role of platelets in the spread of malignant disease. *Int. J. Cancer*, 11:704.
29. Gospodarowicz, D., and Moran, J. S. (1976): Growth factors in mammalian cell culture. *Annu. Rev. Biochem.*, 45:531.
30. Hagmar, B. (1972): Defibrination and metastasis formation: Effects of arvin on experimental metastases in mice. *Eur. J. Cancer*, 8:17.
31. Hagmar, B., and Norrby, K. (1970): Evidence for effects of heparin on cell surfaces influencing experimental metastases. *Int. J. Cancer*, 5:72.
32. Hagmar, B., and Norrby, K. (1973): Influence of cultivation, trypsinization and aggregation on the transplantability of melanoma B16 cells. *Int. J. Cancer*, 11:663.
33. Hashimoto, K., Yamanishi, Y., and Dabbous, Y. (1972): Electron microscopic observations of collagenolytic activity of basal cell epithelioma of the skin *in vivo* and *in vitro*. *Cancer Res.*, 32:2561.
34. Koono, M., Ushijima, K., and Hayashi, H. (1974): Studies on the mechanisms of invasion in cancer. III. Purification of a neutral protease or rat ascites hepatoma cell associated with production of chemotactic factor for cancer cells. *Int. J. Cancer*, 13:105.
35. Ludatsher, R. M., Luse, S. A., and Suntzeff, V. (1967): An electron microscopic study of pulmonary tumor emboli from transplanted Morris hepatoma 5123. *Cancer Res.*, 27:1939.
36. Malmgren, R. A. (1967): Studies of circulating tumor cells in cancer patients. In: *Mechanisms of Invasion of Cancer*, edited by P. Derick, p. 108. Springer-Verlag, New York.
37. Milas, L., Hunter, N., Mason, K., and Withers, H. R. (1974): Immunological resistance to pulmonary metastases in C3Hf-Bu mice bearing syngeneic fibrosarcoma of different sizes. *Cancer Res.*, 34:61.
38. Nicolson, G. L., and Brunson, K. W. (1977): Organ specificity of malignant B16 melanomas: *In vivo* selection for organ preference of blood-borne metastasis. *Gann*, 20:15.
39. Nicolson, G. L., and Poste, G. (1976): The cancer cell: Dynamic aspects and modifications in cell-surface organization. *N. Engl. J. Med.*, 295:197 (Part I); 295:253 (Part II).
40. Nicolson, G. L., and Winkelhake, J. L. (1975): Organ specificity of blood-borne tumour metastasis determined by cell adhesion? *Nature*, 255:230.
41. Nicolson, G. L., and Winkelhake, J. L. (1976): An experimental approach to studying organ specificity of pulmonary tumor metastasis. In: *Cell Surfaces and Malignancy*, Fogarty Int. Center Proc. No. 24, edited by P. T. Mora, p. 271. U.S. Government Printing Office, Washington, D.C.
42. Nicolson, G. L., Birdwell, C. R., Brunson, K. W., and Robbins, J. C. (1976): Cellular interactions in the metastatic process. *Membranes and neoplasia: New approaches and strategies. J. Supramol. Struct. [Suppl.]*, 1:237.

43. Nicolson, G. L., Birdwell, C. R., Brunson, K. W., Robbins, J. C., Beattie, G., and Fidler, I. J. (1977): Cell interactions in the metastatic process: Some cell surface properties associated with successful blood-borne tumor spread. In: *Cell and Tissue Interactions*, edited by M. M. Burger and J. Lash. Raven Press, New York (*in press*).

44. Nicolson, G. L., Winkelhake, J. L., and Nussey, A. C. (1976): An approach to studying the cellular properties associated with metastasis: Some *in vitro* properties of tumor variants selected *in vivo* for enhanced metastasis. In: *Fundamental Aspects of Metastasis*, edited by L. Weiss, p. 291. North-Holland, Amsterdam.

45. Ozaki, T., Yoshida, K., Ushijima, K., and Hayashi, H. (1971): Studies on the mechanisms of invasion in cancer. II. *In vivo* effects of a factor chemotactic for cancer cells. *Int. J. Cancer*, 7:93.

46. Parks, R. C. (1974): Organ-specific metastasis of a transplantable reticulum cell sarcoma. *J. Natl. Cancer Inst.*, 52:971.

47. Potter, M., Rahey, J. L., and Pilgrim, H. I. (1957): Abnormal serum protein and bone destruction in transmissible mouse plasma cell neoplasm (multiple myeloma). *Proc. Soc. Exp. Biol. Med.*, 94:327.

48. Prehn, R. T., and Lappé, M. A. (1971): An immunostimulation theory of tumor development. *Transplant. Rev.*, 7:26.

49. Roblin, R., Albert, S. O., Gelb, N. A., and Black, P. H. (1975): Cell surface changes correlated with density-dependent growth inhibition. Glycosaminoglycan metabolism in 3T3, SV3T3, and Con A selected revertant cells. *Biochemistry*, 14:347.

50. Salsbury, A. J. (1975): The significance of the circulating cancer cell. *Cancer Treatment Rev.*, 2:55.

51. Sato, H., and Suzuki, M. (1976): Deformability and viability of tumor cells by transcapillary passage, with reference to organ affinity of metastasis in cancer. In: *Fundamental Aspects of Metastasis*, edited by L. Weiss, p. 311. North-Holland, Amsterdam.

52. Sindelar, W. F., Tralka, T. S., and Ketcham, A. S. (1975): Electron microscopic observations on formation of pulmonary metastases. *J. Surg. Res.*, 18:137.

53. Smith, R. T., and Landy, M. (1971): *Immune Surveillance*, Academic Press, New York.

54. Strauch, L. (1972): The role of collagenases in tumor invasion. In: *Tissue Interactions in Carcinogenesis*, edited by D. Tarin, p. 399. Academic Press, New York.

55. Suemasu, K., and Ishikawa, S. (1970): Inhibitive effect of heparin and dextran sulfate on experimental pulmonary metastases. *Gann*, 61:125.

56. Sugarbaker, E. D. (1952): The organ selectivity of experimentally induced metastasis in rats. *Cancer*, 5:606.

57. Sylvén, B. (1973): Biochemical and enzymatic factors involved in cellular detachment. In: *Chemotherapy of Cancer Dissemination and Metastasis*, edited by S. Garattini and G. Franchi, p. 129. Raven Press, New York.

58. Tarin, D. (1976): Cellular interactions in neoplasia. In: *Fundamental Aspects of Metastasis*, edited by L. Weiss, p. 151. North-Holland, Amsterdam.

59. Vaage, J., Chen, K., and Merrick, S. (1971): Effect of immune status on the development of artificially induced metastases in different anatomical locations. *Cancer Res.*, 31:496.

60. Walther, B. T., Öhman, R., and Roseman, S. (1973): A quantitative assay for intercellular adhesion. *Proc. Natl. Acad. Sci. U.S.A.*, 70:1569.

61. Warren, B. A. (1973): Environment of the blood-borne tumor embolus adherent to vessel wall. *J. Med.*, 4:150.

62. Weiss, L. (1967): The cell periphery, metastasis and other contact phenomena. In: *Frontiers of Biology, Vol. 7*, edited by A. Neuberger and E. L. Tatum. North-Holland, Amsterdam.

63. Weiss, L., Glaves, D., and Waite, D. A. (1974): The influence of host immunity on the arrest of circulating cancer cells, and its modification by neuraminidase. *Int. J. Cancer*, 13:850.

64. Winkelhake, J. L., and Nicolson, G. L. (1976): Determination of adhesive properties of variant metastatic melanoma cells to BALB/3T3 cells and their virus-transformed derivatives by a monolayer attachment assay. *J. Natl. Cancer Inst.*, 56:285.

65. Wood, S., Jr. (1964): Experimental studies of the intravascular dissemination of ascitic V2 carcinoma cells in the rabbit, with special reference to fibrinogen and fibrinolytic agents. *Bull. Schweiz. Akad. Med. Wiss.*, 20:92.

65a. Yamanishi, Y., Maeyens, E., Dabbous, M. K., Ohyama, H., and Hashimoto, K. (1973):

Collagenolytic activity in malignant melanoma: Physicochemical studies. *Cancer Res.,* 33:2507.

66. Zeidman, I. (1957): Metastasis: A review of recent advances. *Cancer Res.,* 17:157.

67. Zeidman, I. (1961): The fate of circulating tumor cells. I. Passage of cells through capillaries. *Cancer Res.,* 21:38.

68. Zeidman, I., and Buss, J. M. (1952): Transpulmonary passage of tumor cell emboli. *Cancer Res.,* 12:731.

Cancer Invasion and Metastasis: Biologic Mechanisms and Therapy, edited by S. B. Day et al. Raven Press, New York © 1977.

Early Arrest of Circulating Tumor Cells in Tumor-Bearing Mice

Dorothy Glaves and Leonard Weiss

Department of Experimental Pathology, Roswell Park Memorial Institute, Buffalo, New York 14263

In many experimental animals of known immunogenetic background, antigens associated with transplantable tumors may cause modification of the response of the host to its tumor. We have been particularly interested in the interactions between the host immune system and the various components of the metastatic cascade (10,23).

In this chapter we will consider whether in the mouse, host sensitization by tumor bearing affects the initial arrest patterns of circulating cancer cells, and whether any such alterations are immunospecific. It must be emphasized that initial arrest of tumor cells is only one part of an exceptionally complex metastatic process as discussed in this volume and elsewhere (20–22), and as indicated in Fig. 1.

We have examined two murine tumor systems: a methylcholanthrene-induced fibrosarcoma, maintained by serial transplantation in syngeneic C3H/HeHa mice, and the estradiol-induced 6C3HED lymphosarcoma which was serially passaged in syngeneic C3H/StHa hosts.

Both tumor types evoked humoral and cell-mediated immune responses upon subcutaneous injection into their respective hosts. The presence of humoral antibody in the circulation of fibrosarcoma- and lymphosarcoma-bearing mice was demonstrated by indirect membrane immunofluorescence assays. Sera from animals with fibrosarcomas gave a mean fluorescence index of 0.59, and those from lymphosarcoma-bearing mice, 0.34 (25). Lymphocyte-mediated immune responses to these tumors were detected using peritoneal exudate cell migration tests. The migration of peritoneal exudate cells from fibrosarcoma-bearing mice was inhibited by 54 to 55% compared with that in normal mice, after exposure of exudates to tumor cells. In the case of the lymphosarcoma, migration of exudate cells was specifically inhibited by 57 to 63% (25).

In order to determine early arrest patterns, we injected tumor-bearing and normal mice intravenously with ^{125}iodo-deoxyuridine (IudR)-labeled ascites variants of the fibrosarcoma and lymphosarcoma. Arrest patterns were

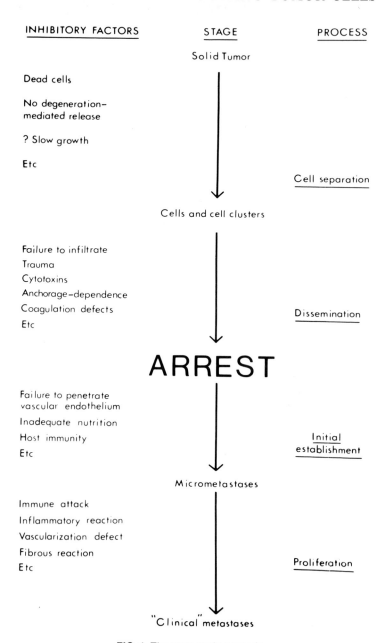

FIG. 1. The metastatic cascade.

assessed 1 hr after injection of 4×10^6 radiolabeled tumor cells and the results are shown in Figs. 2 and 3.

From these histograms it can be seen that arrest patterns in fibrosarcoma-bearing mice (Fig. 2) are markedly altered compared with those in normal, non-tumor-bearing animals. The percentage of injected radioactivity recovered in the lungs was much less in tumor-bearing animals, and that in the liver much greater. Even in organs from which much lesser amounts

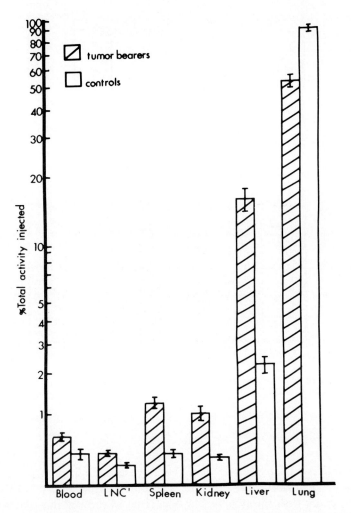

FIG. 2. Localization of [125]IudR-labeled fibrosarcoma cells in fibrosarcoma-bearing and normal mice (from ref. 25).

[1] Axillary, mesenteric, and cervical.

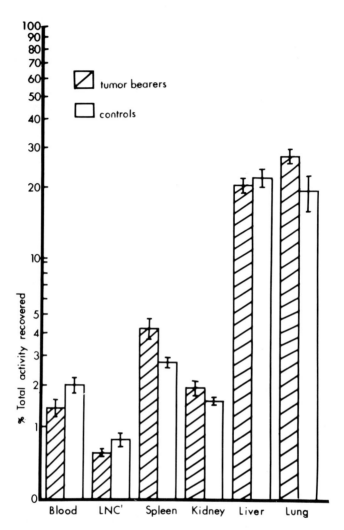

FIG. 3. Localization of [125]IudR-labeled lymphosarcoma cells in lymphosarcoma-bearing and normal mice (from ref. 25).

[1] Axillary, mesenteric, and cervical.

of radioactivity were recoverable, there were statistically significant differences in localization between fibrosarcoma bearers and controls.

Experiments with the lymphosarcoma (Fig. 3) showed that shifts of early arrest patterns in lymphosarcoma-bearing mice compared with controls were detectable, but that these alterations were neither comparable in magnitude nor direction with those in fibrosarcoma bearers. There was a tendency toward greater localization of radiolabeled cells in the lungs of lymphosarcoma bearers and less clear-cut differences in arrest in the liver. Of the other organs examined, the spleens and kidneys of lymphosarcoma bearers showed differences in localization, changes which paralleled those in the fibrosarcoma system.

It would appear from these results that the early arrest patterns of injected tumor cells are indeed influenced by the presence of a tumor to which the host is sensitized. These shifts in patterns of localization may have been due to specific factors associated with immune responses or, alternatively, to nonspecific pharmacologic and inflammatory factors which accompany, or are part of, immunologically mediated defense reactions (2,3). The mere presence of a growing tumor will also alter host physiology, not necessarily involving host defense mechanisms, including, for example, changes in vascular hemodynamics and plasma components (1,14).

The fact that the alterations in early arrest patterns of both tumor types examined were demonstrable in non-tumor-bearing but hyperimmunized animals (25) tends to implicate immunologic/defense reactions as a basis for these alterations. In order to evaluate this hypothesis, we planned experiments in which mice bearing tumors to which they were sensitized would be injected with a second tumor of different etiology and subsequent early arrest patterns determined.

The fibrosarcoma and lymphosarcoma were again used in this study. Initial experiments were made to determine possible cross-reacting antigens on these tumors, and peritoneal exudate cell migration assays were performed as previously described (25). Peritoneal exudate cells from lymphosarcoma-bearing mice were assayed against fibrosarcoma cells and vice versa, using appropriate syngeneic normal mice as controls. Migration of exudate cells from lymphosarcoma bearers was specifically inhibited by 64% in the presence of lymphosarcoma cells compared with a nonsignificant 16% upon exposure to fibrosarcoma cells. In the reverse experiments, the migration of exudate cells from fibrosarcoma bearers was inhibited by only 1% when exposed to lymphosarcoma cells.

Having established this lack of antigen cross-reactivity between the two tumor types, we conducted localization studies. Groups of 10 mice bearing fibrosarcomas, and normal mice of the same strain, were injected with ^{125}IudR-labeled fibrosarcoma or lymphosarcoma cells and arrest patterns determined. The results (Fig. 4) show that the shifts in arrest patterns obtained with fibrosarcoma cells were not demonstrable after injection of lymphosarcoma cells into fibrosarcoma bearers. The parallel experiments, in which lymphosarcoma bearers received lymphosarcoma or fibrosarcoma cells, gave comparable results (Fig. 5). Arrest patterns were altered only following injection of the homologous tumor type; arrest patterns of the unrelated tumor were not affected in either set of experiments.

These findings show that the shifts in patterns of localization in tumor-

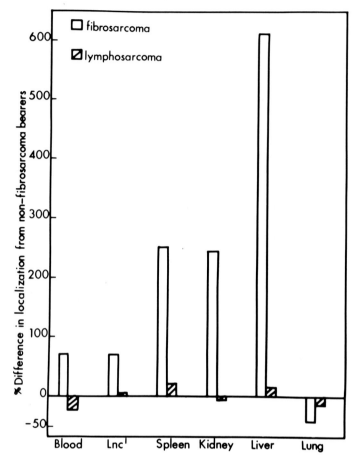

FIG. 4. Localization of [125]IudR-labeled fibrosarcoma and lymphosarcoma cells in fibrosarcoma-bearing and normal mice (from ref. 24).

[1] Axillary, mesenteric, and cervical.

bearing mice originally observed were indeed mediated by host defense reactions.

We have followed the initial distribution patterns of radiolabeled tumor cells injected intravenously into tumor-bearing and non-tumor-bearing mice as a model for the early arrest of circulating tumor cells in metastasis. In common with all other models of parts of the metastatic process, the model does not yield analytic data on all of the complex mechanisms involved in metastasis formation, some of which are discussed in depth elsewhere (21). It is pertinent to consider the relevance of observations of this type to metastasis. Although there is general agreement that hematogenous metastases arise from arrested circulating tumor cells, the relative quantitative

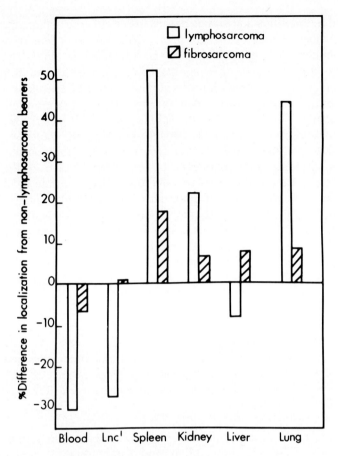

FIG. 5. Localization of [125]IudR-labeled fibrosarcoma and lymphosarcoma cells in lympho-sarcoma-bearing and normal mice (from ref. 24).

[1] Axillary, mesenteric, and cervical.

aspects of arrest and metastasis formation are not clear. This partly reflects the low overall efficiency of the metastatic cascade as revealed in many observations indicating that in experimental animals, in many but not all cancers, many viable tumor cells must be injected intravenously to produce few hematogenous "metastases" (7,11).

It is currently impossible to assess the efficiency of the metastatic process in man, where clinical measurements of primary tumor size and growth rate do not allow discrimination between cancer cell loss by cell death and loss by dissemination (19), and where detection of the end-product is neither ethically nor technically feasible in the case of micrometastases. It should also be noted that in man, even the correlation between the presence of circulating cancer cells and metastasis is uncertain since many of the papers published in the fifties and sixties describing circulating malignant cells were in error; most of these cells are now recognized as megakaryocytes and other nonmalignant cells, particularly in a degenerate state. The fact that metastases are present in the majority of patients with most solid tumors, if sufficient time elapses without treatment (26), may be taken to indicate the cumulative results of many cancer cells continuously entering the metastatic cascade. This concept is strongly supported by Butler and Gullino's (4) demonstration that in the rat, 10^6 cells per gram of adenocarcinoma are released into the blood per 24-hr period. The size of the potential cell reservoir and the magnitude of release can be appreciated from the common observation that the viable parts of solid tumors may contain 10^8 to 10^9 cells per cm^3. In spite of the lack of quantitation, the general feeling, with which we concur, is that the establishment of metastases is a statistically uncommon event, and that each hematogenous, secondary deposit of clinical dimensions represents but a small fraction of a large number of circulating cancer cells, most of which perished.

Only those circulating cancer cells which survive mechanical damage (18) and exposure to various cytotoxic humoral (15) and cellular (12) factors are able to form metastases after arrest. This background of trauma dictates the apparently short survival time of circulating malignant cells. On following the arrest patterns of isotopically labeled circulating cancer cells, it is clear from the work of Fidler (7) and others that many of the initially arrested cells die, with the subsequent appearance of isotope in the urine. There may subsequently be a significant release of temporarily arrested cells into the bloodstream, where they are again subjected to trauma and where many perish. In a well-documented study of the fate of 200,000 ^{125}IudR-labeled B16 melanoma cells injected intravenously into non-tumor-bearing mice, Fidler (7) showed that after 1 min 136,000 viable cells were present in the lungs; the number, based on radioisotope counts, fell to 108,000 after 1 hr, 5,500 after 12 hr, and 355 after 14 days. If low counts of radioactivity after 14 days can be extrapolated to cell numbers in comparison with high counts after 1 hr, then these results indicate how few of the injected and initially arrested cells remain in the lungs. In another paper, Fidler (6) notes that 14 days after an initial injection of only 100,000 melanoma cells, approximately 400 pulmonary metastases were visible with a dissecting microscope. It could therefore be argued that, in the absence of outside recruitment, each of the cells retained in the lungs for 14 days grew into at least one overt metastasis. This implies a remarkable degree of selection among the original malignant cell population in terms of virulence (i.e., in excess of 100% takes) and resistance of the final pulmonary B16 population, which now comprises only 0.07% of those originally arrested at this site.

From what has been said, the question of metastatic variants within a cell population is of relevance in the present considerations. Thus, Foulds (9) postulated progressive development in tumor cell populations toward increased malignancy and associated metastasis, and Yamada et al. (27) showed that in a number of human tumors the karyotype of metastatic cells differed in general from that of their primary lesions. Fidler (7) has described the selection of metastatic sublines of B16 melanoma, and, using similar techniques, Nicolson et al. (16) have selected for variants of B16 populations showing specific organ arrest patterns. Thus, regardless of the mechanisms involved, there is a distinct possibility that subpopulations of cells from primary tumors generate metastases. It could therefore be argued that data on the initial arrest patterns of ostensibly nonselected populations of injected cells are irrelevant to the ensuing "metastatic" process. Although this is true in an absolute numerical sense, we take the viewpoint that in similar cell/host situations, with similarly sized inocula of malignant cells, the numbers of potentially metastasis-forming cells delivered to an organ will bear some fairly constant relationship to the total number of the "unselected" population initially arrested in them. In tumor-bearing experimental animals, the acquired immunity demonstrated by us may inhibit or enhance the subsequent development of metastases from the arrested cells, and immunoselective pressures may impose additional restrictions on the type of cell found in the metastases which do develop. These and other interactions between the arrested cells and their environment will determine whether a metastasis ultimately develops. Thus, although in defined and comparable circumstances, it is expected that the greater the number of cells initially arrested at a particular site, the greater the number of metastases that develop. Most previous studies by others on tumor cell arrest have usually involved the intravascular injection of cancer cells into normal, non-tumor-bearing animals (e.g., 5,8,13,17). The results presented here indicate that this may well be an unrealistic model for the study of arrest patterns. The precise numerical relationships between the two distinct but interrelated phenomena of arrest and subsequent metastasis development are extremely complex. In spite of these complexities, the fact remains that when metastasis occurs as part of the natural history of cancer, it is always in a tumor-bearing patient.

ACKNOWLEDGMENT

This work was supported by Grant CA-14993 from the National Institutes of Health.

REFERENCES

1. Apffell, C. A. (1976): Nonimmunological host defenses: A review. *Cancer Res.*, 36:1527–1537.
2. Becker, E. L. (1971): Nature and classification of immediate-type allergic reactions. *Adv. Immunol.*, 13:267–313.

3. Becker, E. L., and Henson, P. M. (1973): In vitro studies of immunologically induced secretion of mediators from cells and related phenomena. *Adv. Immunol.*, 17:93–193.
4. Butler, T. P., and Gullino, P. M. (1975): Quantitation of cell shedding into efferent blood of mammary adenocarcinoma. *Cancer Res.*, 35:512–516.
5. Fidler, I. J. (1970): Metastasis: Quantitative analysis of distribution and fate of tumor emboli labeled with ^{125}I-5-iodo-2'-deoxyuridine. *J. Natl. Cancer Inst.*, 45:773–782.
6. Fidler, I. J. (1973): The relationship of embolic homogeneity, number, size and viability to the incidence of experimental metastasis. *Eur. J. Cancer*, 9:223–227.
7. Fidler, I. J. (1976): Patterns of tumor cell arrest and development. In: *Fundamental Aspects of Metastasis*, edited by L. Weiss, pp. 275–290. North Holland, Amsterdam.
8. Fisher, B., and Fisher, E. R. (1967): The organ distribution of disseminated ^{51}Cr-labelled tumor cells. *Cancer Res.*, 27:412–420.
9. Foulds, L. (1969): *Neoplastic Development*. Academic Press, London.
10. Glaves, D., and Weiss, L. (1976): Initial arrest patterns of circulating cancer cells: Effects of host sensitization and anticoagulation. In: *Fundamental Aspects of Metastasis*, edited by L. Weiss, pp. 263–273. North Holland, Amsterdam.
11. Griffiths, J. D., and Salsbury, A. J. (1965): *Circulating Cancer Cells*, p. 109. Charles C Thomas, Springfield, Ill.
12. Herberman, R. B. (1974): Cell-mediated immunity to tumor cells. *Adv. Cancer Res.*, 19:207–263.
13. Hofer, K. G., Prensky, W., and Hughes, W. L. (1969): Death and metastatic distribution of tumor cells in mice monitored with ^{125}I-iododeoxyuridine. *J. Natl. Cancer Inst.*, 43:763–773.
14. Mershey, C. (1974): Pathogenesis and treatment of altered blood coagulability in patients with malignant tumors. *Ann. N.Y. Acad. Sci.*, 230:289–293.
15. Nairn, R. C., Nind, A. P. P., Guli, E. P. G., Muller, H. K., Rolland, J. M., and Minty, C. C. J. (1971): Specific immune responses in human skin carcinoma. *Br. Med. J.*, 4:701–705.
16. Nicolson, G. L., Winkelhake, J. L., and Nussey, A. C. (1976): An approach to studying the cellular properties associated with metastasis: Some in vitro properties of tumor variants selected in vivo for enhanced metastasis. In: *Fundamental Aspects of Metastasis*, edited by L. Weiss, pp. 291–303. North Holland, Amsterdam.
17. Parks, R. C. (1974): Organ-specific metastasis of a transplantable reticulum cell sarcoma. *J. Natl. Cancer Inst.*, 52:971–973.
18. Sato, H., and Suzuki, M. (1976): Deformability and viability of tumor cells by transcapillary passage, with reference to organ affinity of metastasis in cancer. In: *Fundamental Aspects of Metastasis*, edited by L. Weiss, pp. 311–317. North Holland, Amsterdam.
19. Steel, G. G. (1968): Cell loss from experimental tumors. *Cell Tissue Kinet.*, 1:193–207.
20. Weiss, L. (1967): *The Cell Periphery, Metastasis and Other Contact Phenomena*. North Holland, Amsterdam.
21. Weiss, L. (Ed.) (1976): *Fundamental Aspects of Metastasis*. North Holland, Amsterdam.
22. Weiss, L. A. (1977): Pathobiologic overview of metastasis. *Semin. Oncol. (in press)*.
23. Weiss, L., and Glaves, D. (1977): Immunity and metastasis. Handbook of Cancer/Immunology. *Int. J. Cancer*, 18:774–777.
24. Weiss, L., and Glaves, D. (1977): The immunospecificity of altered arrest patterns of circulating cancer cells in tumor-bearing mice. *Int. J. Cancer (in press)*.
25. Weiss, L., Glaves, D., and Waite, D. A. (1974): The influence of host immunity on the arrest of circulating cancer cells and its modification by neuraminidase. *Int. J. Cancer*, 13:850–862.
26. Willis, R. A. (1952): *The Spread of Tumours in the Human Body*. Butterworths, London.
27. Yamada, K., Takagi, N., and Sandberg, A. A. (1966): The chromosomes and causation of human cancer and leukemia. II. Karyotypes of human solid tumors. *Cancer*, 19:1879–1890.

Cancer Invasion and Metastasis: Biologic Mechanisms and Therapy, edited by S. B. Day et al. Raven Press, New York © 1977.

Blood-Borne Tumor Emboli and Their Adherence to Vessel Walls

B. A. Warren, W. J. Chauvin, and J. Philips

Department of Pathology, University of Western Ontario, London, Ontario, Canada

Blood-borne tumor emboli represent a specific phase of the biology of certain malignancies. In such tumors they are a stage in the development of metastases, although the majority of individual emboli do not accomplish this end. Blood-borne tumor cells reach the circulation by active invasion, intravasation, passive movement, and growth down the lumen of vessels.

Attempts can be made to correlate observations on the biology of certain categories of tumors which give rise to blood-borne emboli with artificially constructed segments of this type of metastatic process using experimental tumors (12,13). One of the difficulties in this approach is that the application of information from the experimental model to the human situation must be made with considerable care. Specific observations on the continuing biology of the blood-borne metastatic process in man are incidental to the demands of diagnosis and therapy. There are, however, specimens of tumors and autopsies which can provide useful insights into the process of the blood-borne tumor metastasis and adhesion of circulating tumor emboli to vessel walls in man.

The structures of the two surfaces involved, viz., the tumor embolus and the vessel wall itself, are pivotal in a consideration of the nature of the adhesive process. The scanning electron microscope promises to do for surface topography what the transmission electron microscope did for the examination of thin sections. In this chapter we present the results of observations by scanning electron microscopy correlated with light microscopy on blood-borne tumor emboli in a case of mammary adenocarcinoma with metastases.

MATERIALS AND METHODS

Case History

A 38-year-old woman presented for diagnosis of a mass in the left breast which had been present for 8 months. A radical mastectomy was performed following the diagnosis of an infiltrating duct carcinoma. During subsequent follow-up, chest X-ray was clear but a bone scan showed multiple metastases in the thoracolumbar spine. Irradiation of the ovaries was performed. Three weeks before her final admission she became confused without localizing signs. There was no evidence of local recurrence or of enlargement of the supraclavicular or axillary lymph nodes, nor was there abnormality on brain scan. Hepatomegaly of 2 cm below the costal margin was found. Significant laboratory results were a serum calcium of 18.5 mg%, white cell count of 2,200/cu mm, platelet count of 40,000/cu mm, and a hemoglobin of 8.6 g%. Under conservative treatment the calcium returned to normal. She developed diarrhea, began vomiting bile, and died in pulmonary edema 2 months after initial presentation.

Autopsy Report

The larynx and trachea contained frothy blood-stained fluid. The lungs were heavy (right 565 g, left 620 g) and had scattered small tumor nodules over the pleural surfaces. The average diameter of the deposits was 2 mm. The cut surfaces were mottled, and fairly large areas of collapse were noted. Numerous metastatic nodules of varying sizes were present throughout the liver. Some of these were necrotic. Secondary tumor nodules were found in both adrenal glands. Small nodules of about 1 mm in diameter were found in both kidneys. Necrotic tumor tissue was found in the vertebral bodies of the lumbar spine. Acute ulceration of the ileum was noted. No significant abnormalities were found in other organs and the brain appeared normal.

Histological examination confirmed the presence of tumor deposits throughout the lung fields, in the adrenal glands and liver, and in several enlarged lymph nodes near the porta hepatis and bone. Extramedullary hemopoiesis was found in the spleen.

Comment

Sections of the lung showed numerous small vessels which contained tumor emboli together with various stages of metastatic development in the extravascular space.

Scanning electron microscopy (SEM) of these sections was carried out. These were sections of tissues prepared in a standard fashion for paraffin sections commencing with buffered formalin.

SEM of Histopathology Slides

Following examination and photography in the light microscope, selected slides were placed in xylene until the coverslips came free. While in xylene the slides were scored to appropriate areas and sizes with a diamond stylus and broken. The glass slivers were first washed in two changes of absolute alcohol followed by two changes of absolute acetone. The sections were then critical point dried from liquid CO_2, mounted on aluminum stubs, sputter coated with gold, and examined in a Hitachi HHS-2 scanning electron microscope.

RESULTS

One problem in examining processes by SEM which occur in the lumen of vessels is fixation of the plasma proteins. The fixed plasma proteins are opaque on scanning electron microscopy and interfere with observation of fine structure at the endothelial surface. One method to avoid this is to flush the lumen with balanced salt solution. This, of course, would be injurious to the phenomenon of adherence. The SEM of light microscopy

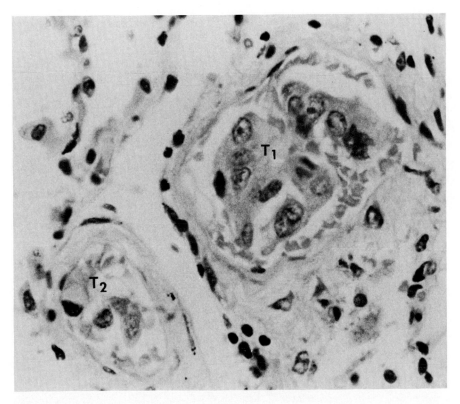

FIG. 1. Photomicrograph of two tumor emboli (T_1 and T_2) in small vessels in the lung of a woman who died with widespread metastases from a mammary adenocarcinoma. Hematoxylin and eosin stained section ($\times$ 700).

sections avoids this difficulty. A further advantage is that interpretation is facilitated by previous observation of the tissue section by light microscopy. Because of its distinctive structure, the lung permits ready localization of vessels. The red cell provides the specific marker for vessels by SEM.

Sections of lung observed by light microscopy revealed numerous small blood vessels which contained tumor emboli (Fig. 1) from the adenocarcinoma of the breast. There had been evidently a showering of the lung fields with tumor cells which were, at the time of death, in groups of 5 to 35 as emboli within the microcirculation of the lung. A form of circulation around these partially adherent tumor emboli was evident in the arrangement of the red cells within the remaining lumen of the vessels. The vessels containing emboli appeared "bloated" and had lost the symmetrical circular profile of normal pulmonary vessels. A puckering of the vessel wall was evident at several points in the circumference of such arteries. The tumor cells themselves were arranged in a haphazard fashion in the embolus but

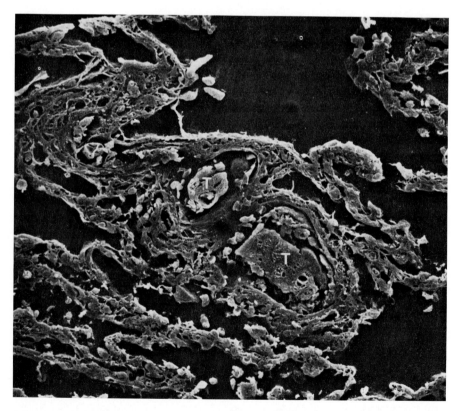

FIG. 2. Scanning electron micrograph of two tumor emboli (T) in a serial section to the one shown in Fig. 1 (× 500).

did exhibit clefts between groups of cells. Some of these may have been due to fixation procedures.

Scanning electron microscopy of approximately 8-μ sections of lung disclosed emboli within the vessels (Fig. 2). SEM allows the connective tissue framework of the alveolar septae to appear prominent. Macrophages were prominent in the alveolar spaces and the structures of the alveolar walls were thrown into relief. At higher power on SEM the sectioned surface is seen with various enclosures possibly due to diverse cytoplasmic structures (Fig. 3). The surfaces defining the emboli were irregular and frequently contained considerable indentations and clefts (Fig. 4). In other regions of the lung there were small pulmonary arteries which contained a mixture of partially organized thrombus on which fibrin was deposited (Fig. 5). The lumen of such vessels was reduced to a half-moon. In some instances sections of associated branches contained tumor emboli (Fig. 5). It appeared that the peripheral branches of the main artery had been occluded by tumor

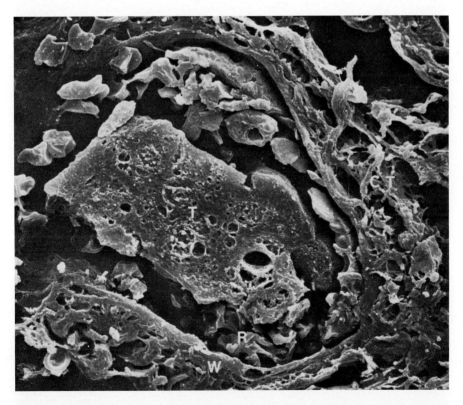

FIG. 3. Higher power view of one of the emboli seen in Fig. 2. Red cells (R) are present between the embolus (T) and the vessel wall (W). The collagen framework of the adjacent tissue (CT) is shown beyond the vessel wall ($\times$ 1,400).

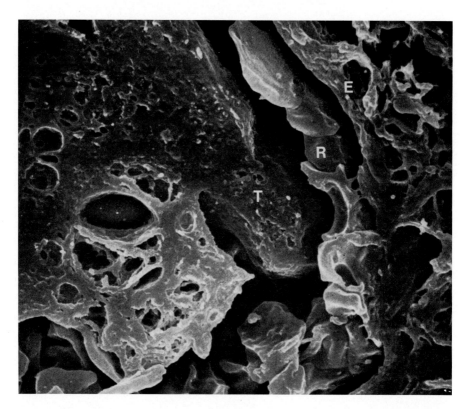

FIG. 4. SEM of the edge of the tumor embolus (T) which can be seen projecting downward into the specimen. Several flattened red cells (R) are present between the embolus and the endothelium (E). This shows detail of the edge of the embolus in Fig. 3 (× 3,500).

emboli, and retrograde thrombosis had ensued. The remaining lumen probably supplied branches that had escaped occlusion by emboli. The usefulness of the technique incorporating a combination of SEM and sectioning at about 8 μ is illustrated in Figs. 6 and 7. Figure 6 shows a pulmonary artery with its contained cells and a microthrombus. This small collection of fibrin strands and enmeshed red cells is seen at higher power in Fig. 7. Soluble plasma proteins have been washed out in the preparative stages. Individual fibrin strands are seen to the level where they have been sectioned. The clarity of the image of the fibrin strands in this field suggests that fibrin at this structural level was not formed around the tumor emboli. Profiles of cells of appropriate size to be tumor cells were detected impacted in pulmonary capillaries (Fig. 8). Dispersed stubby microvilli were present on the surface of these cells similar to those found on adenocarcinoma cells in solid adenocarcinomas.

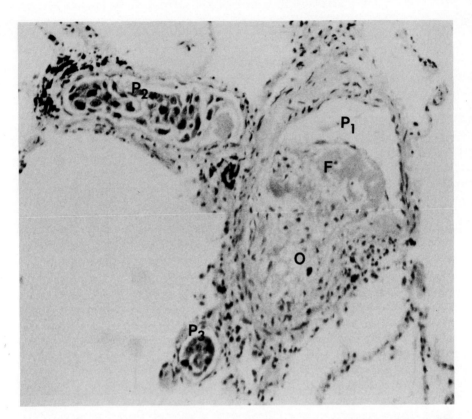

FIG. 5. Photomicrograph of a section of lung showing profiles of 3 pulmonary arteries. The larger vessel (P_1) contains an organized thrombus (O) on which fibrin (F) is laid down. The two smaller vessels (P_2 and P_3) contain tumor emboli from a mammary adenocarcinoma. H & E stained section ($\times$ 180).

DISCUSSION

The case presented here exemplifies some of the difficulties associated with human material. Platelet consumption as a result of multiple tumor emboli could have resulted in the greatly lowered platelet count. This in turn renders it less likely that platelets would be found associated with the emboli. Winterbauer et al. (17) examined 366 patients with various forms of carcinoma, predominantly adenocarcinoma (namely, carcinoma of breast or stomach, renal cell adenocarcinoma, hepatoma, and choriocarcinoma). Of these, 26% had some degree of embolization, and histological examination of material from this series of patients confirmed an association of tumor emboli with thrombus material, although this did not occur in the majority of cases. The fibrin was seen in the center with tumor cells around

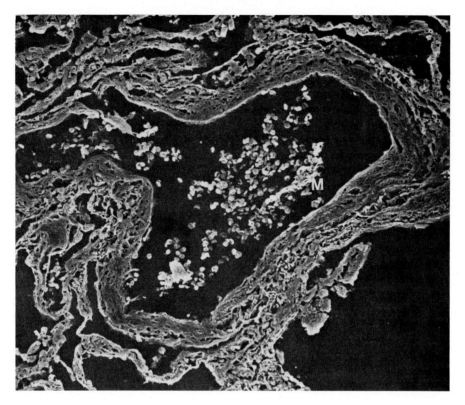

FIG. 6. SEM of a pulmonary artery. The endothelial layer, red cells, and a microthrombus (M) are clearly represented (× 350).

the periphery of the embolus. Certainly in the case here thrombosis was induced in the pulmonary tree (Fig. 5) and probably occurred in association with tumor cells.

Platelet-tumor adhesion appears to differ from the platelet-fibrin or platelet-platelet aggregation.

Abrahamsen (1) found shortened survival and increased consumption of labeled platelets in 20 patients with metastatic cancer. Patients with metastatic cancer appear to have a permanent shortening of platelet survival. Platelet aggregation inhibitors such as acetylsalicylic acid and dipyridamole in doses known to inhibit platelet aggregation had no effect on platelet consumption (2). In 51 patients with cancer, Peck and Reiquam (9) reported the results of coagulation tests including platelet count, factor V assay, fibrinogen-fibrin split products, and serial thrombin time. They concluded that cancer patients have a delicately balanced coagulation mechanism and that chronic disseminated coagulation may be induced or made worse by a number of stimuli including radiation and chemotherapy.

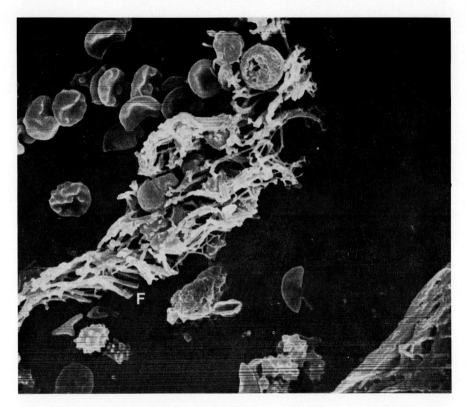

FIG. 7. Higher power SEM of the microthrombus. The individual fibrin strands are readily discernible. They are cut squarely at the termination of the section at about 8 μ (F). Red cells are present both enmeshed in the microthrombus and free in the lumen of the vessel. Some show crenation ($\times$ 2,000).

Changes in platelet count have also been noted in animal tumor systems. For example, Gasic et al. (6) found that thrombocytopenia reduced the number of metastases produced by a wide variety of murine tumors. Many tumors were found to aggregate platelets *in vitro* and/or produce thrombocytopenia *in vivo*. They noted that tumors with platelet-aggregating capacities usually produced lung metastases whereas those devoid of such property showed more widespread distribution.

Roberts (11) reviewed in considerable depth many aspects of the dissemination of cancer via the vascular system. In one part of his review he listed the processes leading to the intravascular death of cancer cells as being (a) the intravascular formation of a thrombus, (b) the organization of the thrombus, and (c) the complete destruction of cancer cells. He emphasized that organization of the thrombus which surrounds tumor cells does not occur at sites of survival of cancer cells (15).

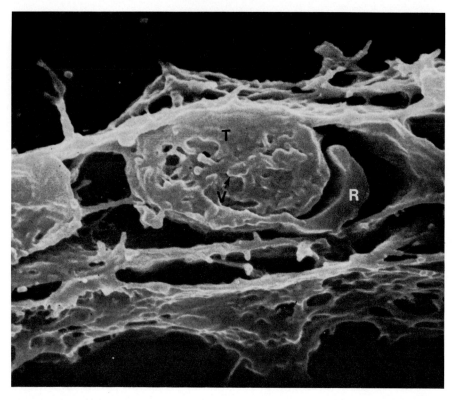

FIG. 8. SEM of pulmonary capillary with an impacted cell, probably a tumor cell (T), within its lumen. The large cell possesses short microvilli (V). A red cell (R) is shown in section (× 7,700).

The initial adherence of tumor cells to endothelium *in vivo* in Wood's studies (18–20) was thought to be independent of such factors as rate of flow, capillary diameter, leukocyte sticking, and vasomotion. The importance of endothelial injury to the progression of the adherent tumor embolus to metastasis formation was emphasized in this work since leukocytes preceded cancer cells through the vessel wall.

We have reported experiments in which the inferior venae cavae of mice and rats were injured by crushing with forceps and suspensions of an ascitic form of thymic lymphoma in mice and Walker 256 carcinoma in rats were injected intravenously (14). In the damaged segments two types of adherent tumor emboli could be distinguished depending on the integrity of the endothelial layer (types I and II). Where there was intact endothelium (type I), tumor cells and platelets formed a tumor-platelet body. This was surrounded by a "boundary" layer of fibrin with little fibrin being present in the embolus itself. Adhesion to the endothelial plasmalemma was by pseudopodia of the component tumor cells. In areas where the endothelial layer was damaged or completely destroyed (type II), fibrin (apparently in a low polymeric form) constituted the principal bond between the tumor cells and the vessel wall. There appeared in such cases to be few barriers to the progression of tumor cells through the fibrin to the basement membrane, in contrast to the case where there was an intact endothelial layer.

It would thus appear that it is easier for the tumor cell to gain firm attachment to the vessel wall if (a) the endothelium is damaged or contains gaps, or (b) there is less than complete investment of endothelium around the lumen of the vessel. Bennett et al. (3) distinguished three types of endothelium in capillaries: capillary type 1—continuous, nonfenestrated endothelium, e.g., in heart, skeletal muscle, and lung; capillary type 2—endothelium containing intracellular fenestrations, e.g., in kidney, intestine, stomach, and many endocrine glands; capillary type 3—endothelial lining which contains many large gaps between endothelial cells, e.g., in liver, spleen, and bone marrow. It may be that this variation in normal structure plays some part in the capacity of circulating tumor emboli to adhere firmly to the vessel wall.

Thus a number of factors tend toward firmer adhesion than would occur normally, and these are listed in Fig. 9.

The other half of the equation is the nature of the tumor cell embolus itself and the periphery of the tumor (16). Work on the changes associated with malignancy and the nature of the malignant cell periphery has recently

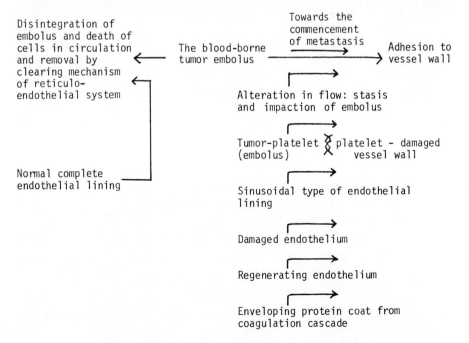

FIG. 9. Possible fates of the blood-borne tumor embolus.

been extensively reviewed (7,10). Scanning electron microscopy of the changes in the cell surface that occur on transformation to malignancy have been described by Malick and Langenbach (8). They found that, although the control nontumorigenic cell line of C3H mouse embryo cells was polygonal in shape, extensively flattened with smooth surfaces, the cell lines derived from it by treatment *in vitro* with carcinogens showed marked alterations in surface topography from this. Cell lines were derived from the control by treatment with 7,12-dimethylbenz(a)-anthracene (DMBA) and 3-methylcholanthrene (MCA). The *in vitro* transformants were thicker than the control cells, were pleomorphic in shape, and lacked contact inhibition.

Small marginal ruffles and microvilli of variable lengths were characteristic surface alterations of the MCA-transformed cells. Inoculation of the DMBA-transformed cells into C3H mice and reestablishment of cells from one of the subsequent fibrosarcomas in culture showed increased numbers of microvilli on the surface of the cells.

Alterations in the coagulation cascade and in the layer of blood protein coat enveloping the tumor embolus may aid in adhesion. Fibrin has been demonstrated around tumor cells in the early stages of experimental metastases in the lungs of rats following intravenous injection of Walker 256 carcinoma cells (4,5). An alternative method for the passage of the tumor cell from the intravascular compartment to the extravascular situation is described by these workers (4). They suggest that once the tumor embolus is fixed in the small vessel or capillary, erosion of the surrounding endothelium and vessel wall may take place resulting in the destruction of the previous existing structures and, in parallel, the advent of the tumor cells into extravascular space.

In summary, then, it appears that the adhesion of the blood-borne tumor embolus to the vessel wall is influenced by:

1. Alteration in the coagulation cascade and in the layer of blood protein coat enveloping the tumor embolus and/or the adhesion of platelets. These changes may be associated with changes in the cell periphery consequent upon malignant transformation.
2. Alteration in the endothelial lining of the vessel wall, e.g.,
   (a) damaged and/or regenerating endothelium,
   (b) variation in endothelial structure in various organs.
3. Alteration in blood flow such as stasis of flow and impaction of the embolus in the capillary bed.

ACKNOWLEDGMENT

The support of the National Cancer Institute of Canada is gratefully acknowledged.

REFERENCES

1. Abrahamsen, A. F. (1972): The effects of acetylsalicylic acid and dipyridamole on platelet economy in metastatic cancer. *Scand. J. Haematol.,* 9:562.
2. Abrahamsen, A. F. (1976): Platelet turnover in metastatic cancer and the effect of platelet aggregation inhibitors. *Z. Krebsforsch.,* 86:109.
3. Bennett, H. S., Luft, J. H., and Hampton, J. C. (1959): Morphological classification of vertebrate blood capillaries. *Am. J. Physiol.,* 196:381.
4. Chew, E. C., Josephson, R. L., and Wallace, A. C. (1976): Morphologic aspects of the arrest of circulating cancer cells. In: *Fundamental Aspects of Metastasis,* edited by L. Weiss, p. 121. North Holland Publishing Co., Amsterdam.
5. Chew, E. C., and Wallace, A. C. (1976): Demonstration of fibrin in early stages of experimental metastases. *Cancer Res.,* 36:1904.
6. Gasic, G. J., Gasic, T. B., Galanti, N., Johnson, T., and Murphy, S. (1973): Platelet-tumor-cell interactions in mice. The role of platelets in the spread of malignant disease. *Int. J. Cancer,* 11:704.
7. Glick, M. C. (1976): Cell surface changes associated with malignancy. In: *Fundamental Aspects of Metastasis,* edited by L. Weiss, p. 9. North Holland Publishing Co., Amsterdam.
8. Malick, L. E., and Langenbach, R. (1976): Scanning electron microscopy of *in vitro* chemically transformed mouse embryo cells. *J. Cell Biol.,* 68:654.
9. Peck, S. D., and Reiquam, C. W. (1973): Disseminated intravascular coagulation in cancer patients: Supportive evidence. *Cancer,* 31:1114.
10. Poste, G., and Weiss, L. (1976): Some considerations on cell surface alterations in malignancy. In: *Fundamental Aspects of Metastasis,* edited by L. Weiss, p. 25. North Holland Publishing Co., Amsterdam.
11. Roberts, S. S. (1961): Spread by the vascular system. In: *Dissemination of Cancer, Prevention and Therapy,* edited by W. H. Cole, G. O. McDonald, S. S. Roberts, and H. W. Southwick, p. 61. Appleton-Century-Crofts, New York.
12. Warren, B. A. (1973): Environment of the blood-borne tumor embolus adherent to vessel wall. *J. Med.,* 4:150.
13. Warren, B. A. (1976): Some aspects of blood borne tumor emboli associated with thrombosis. *Z. Krebsforsch.,* 87:1.
14. Warren, B. A., and Vales, O. (1972): The adhesion of thromboplastic tumor emboli to vessel walls *in vivo. Br. J. Exp. Pathol.,* 53:301.
15. Warren, S., and Gates, O. (1936): The fate of intravenously injected tumor cells. *Am. J. Cancer,* 27:485.
16. Weiss, L. (1967): *The Cell Periphery, Metastasis and Other Contact Phenomena.* North Holland Publishing Co., Amsterdam.
17. Winterbauer, R. H., Elfenbein, I. B., and Ball, W. C. (1968): Incidence and clinical significance of tumor embolization to the lungs. *Am. J. Med.,* 45:271.
18. Wood, S., Jr. (1958): Pathogenesis of metastasis formation observed *in vivo* in the rabbit ear chamber. *A.M.A. Arch. Pathol.,* 66:550.
19. Wood, S., Jr. (1964): Experimental studies of the intravascular dissemination of ascitic V2 carcinoma cells in the rabbit, with special reference to fibrinogen and fibrinolytic agents. *Bull. Schweiz. Akad. Med. Wiss.,* 20:92.
20. Wood, S., Jr., Holyoke, E. D., and Yardley, J. H. (1961): Mechanisms of metastasis production by blood borne cancer cells. *Canadian Cancer Conference,* 4:167.

Cancer Invasion and Metastasis: Biologic Mechanisms and Therapy, edited by S. B. Day et al. Raven Press, New York © 1977.

Biochemical Criteria of Metastatic Growth in Human Cancer

Oscar Bodansky

Memorial Sloan-Kettering Cancer Center, New York, New York 10021

There are many potential biochemical criteria of metastatic growth and regression in cancer patients. Tables 1 and 2 show a partial list. These criteria have usually been employed as indicators of the presence of cancer, but in most of the reports no mention is made concerning the presence of metastases. The reader is left to presume that, in advanced cases at least, metastases do exist.

To establish a biochemical parameter as a reliable criterion of metastatic

TABLE 1. *Serum (plasma) biochemical criteria of metastatic cancer*

1. Alkaline phosphatase activity
2. 5'-Nucleotidase activity
3. Acid phosphatase activity
4. Aspartate and alanine aminotransferase activities
5. Phosphohexose isomerase activity
6. Lactic dehydrogenase activity
7. Other serum enzyme activities
8. Glycoprotein concentration
9. Carcinoembryonic antigen concentration
10. α-Fetoprotein concentration
11. Polyamine concentration
12. Ectopic hormone concentration
13. Other biochemical components

TABLE 2. *CSF and uninary criteria of metastatic growth*

Cerebrospinal fluid criteria
   1. Glucose concentration
   2. Protein concentration
   3. Other components
Urinary biochemical criteria
   1. Calcium excretion
   2. Hydroxyproline excretion
   3. Polyamine excretion

growth or regression, it is first necessary to conduct detailed studies in a group of patients in which the level of this parameter, almost always in serum and sometimes in urine, is correlated sequentially and frequently in each of the individual patients with other parameters, such as other bio-chemical and hematological determinations, physical examination, X-rays, nuclear scans, administration or withdrawal of therapy, operative pro-cedures, and symptomatology during a period of at least several months. As will be seen later, few studies in the literature meet these standards.

INCIDENCE OF METASTASES

Table 3 shows the distribution by site of origin of 1,000 consecutive autopsied cases of carcinoma (1). In spite of certain factors intrinsic in any series of autopsies, such as the inability to perform autopsies in all deaths in a hospital and the interests of the various members of the hospital, the distribution of the sites of origin in the series of Abrams et al. (1) is not too different from the distribution of estimated new cases of primary sites for the year 1974 (28).

Table 4 shows the incidences of metastatic involvement at various sites in 1,000 consecutive autopsies for all primary types of tumors studied and also for various of these types as, for example, carcinoma of the breast. The distribution of metastases in patients with cancer depends on the frequency of the primary site of cancer and the frequency of metastatic involvement

TABLE 3. *Comparison of percent incidence of primary sites of cancer in 1,000 autopsied cases[a] and in 655,000 estimated new cases and 355,000 estimated deaths for 1974[b]*

Site of origin	1,000 autopsies (%)	Estimated new cases (%)	Estimated mortality (%)
Total	100.0	100.0	100.0
Breast	16.7	13.7	9.2
Lung	16.0	12.6	21.1
Stomach	11.9	3.6	4.1
Colon	11.8	10.3	10.5
Rectum	8.7	4.7	3.3
Ovary	6.4	2.6	3.3
Kidney	3.4	2.2	1.7
Pancreas	3.2	3.1	5.4
Corpus uteri	2.5	4.1	1.0
Cervix	1.3	2.9	2.2
Prostate	1.9	8.3	5.0
Bladder	1.9	4.3	2.6
Unknown and other primary sites	2.6	3.9	6.1

[a] Abrams et al. (1).
[b] Silverberg and Holleb (28).

TABLE 4. *Site of metastatic involvement in percent of 1,000 consecutive autopsied cases and in various types of primary cancer*

Site of metastatic involvement	In 1,000 consecutive autopsies (%)	In 167 cases of primary breast cancer (%)	In 160 cases of primary lung cancer (%)	In 118 cases of primary colon cancer (%)
Abdominal nodes	50	44	29	59
Liver	49	61	40	65
Lungs	47	77	47	37
Mediastinal nodes	42	67	83	14
Pleura	28	65	28	14
Bone	27	73	33	9
Adrenal	27	54	36	14
GI tract	27	15	11	27
Diaphragm	20	25	16	11
Brain (cerebral)	18	9	43	–

at various sites. For example, according to Table 3, the frequency of carcinoma of the breast as a primary site is 16.7%, and the frequencies of metastatic involvement in the liver and bone due to breast cancer are, respectively, 61% and 73% (not shown in table). One can say, therefore, that of every 1,000 autopsies, the liver will have metastases in 167 × 61% or 102 cases. Since there were few cases of prostatic carcinoma, 1.9%, in the series of Abrams et al. (1), no data were given on the site and frequency of metastatic involvement. However, other studies show that metastases to bone and liver occur in about 80% and 20%, respectively (12,34). Accordingly, of every 1,000 autopsies, the liver will have metastases in 19 × 20%, or four cases of carcinoma of the prostate and the skeleton will have metastases in 19 × 80% or 15 cases of carcinoma of the prostate. If we took a more liberal estimate of the incidence of carcinoma of the prostate in new cases of cancer (28), namely, 54,000 out of 655,000, or about 8.3%, then the number of liver metastases due to prostatic carcinoma in the country at large would be 54,000 × 20% or 10,800, and that of skeletal metastases would be 54,000 × 80% or 43,200. For breast cancer, the numbers of liver and skeletal metastases are 90,000 × 61% or 54,900, and 90,000 × 73% or 65,700 cases. Similarly, values can be determined for cancer with other primary sites.

Tables 1 and 2 contain a list of biochemical criteria of metastatic cancer. We shall describe the role of some of these briefly here and, in a subsequent section, discuss sequential determinations in illustrations of three of these criteria as indicators of the growth or regression of metastases in individual patients.

SERUM PHOSPHOHYDROLASES

The best known and some of the oldest of these biochemical procedures are, of course, alkaline phosphatase, studied in the twenties and thirties

(4,22), and acid phosphatase, discovered in the thirties (16,19). As is well appreciated, the determination of serum alkaline phosphatase activity has proved to be a useful and durable aid in the diagnosis and management of neoplastic disease involving the skeletal and hepatobiliary systems, and acid phosphatase has proved equally useful in the diagnosis and management of carcinoma of the prostate. Serum 5'-nucleotidase activity is elevated in hepatobiliary disease but not in skeletal disorders (10). Hence, when serum alkaline phosphatase activity is elevated, the determination of serum 5'-nucleotidase activity can be used to differentiate between metastatic disease in the liver and that in the skeleton.

The ectopic production of a placental-like isoenzyme of alkaline phosphatase (13) is present in the serum in about 3.3% of cases of metastatic cancer (30), and another isoenzyme that cannot hydrolyze S-substituted phosphate esters has been reported as constituting up to 100% of serum alkaline phosphatase in patients with acute or chronic lymphatic leukemia (24) and as being absent from the serum of normal persons. Its presence in metastatic carcinoma has not been studied.

POLYPEPTIDE HORMONES: HUMAN CHORIONIC GONADOTROPIN

We may also mention briefly at this time two of the more recently developed biochemical criteria. The secretion of polypeptide hormones by neoplasms (ectopic humoral syndrome) has been known for about 50 years. The development of more sophisticated and sensitive techniques has revealed the presence in serum and urine of very low levels. Human chorionic gonadotropin (HCG) has been the most useful of these various polypeptide hormones in revealing the presence of metastatic cancer. The minimal value for positive results corresponds to 1 ng or 5 mIU of immunologic activity of HCG/ml relative to the Second International Standard for HCG. No positive results were obtained in controls consisting of 321 serum samples from 8 cycling women, 127 samples from 75 postmenopausal women, and in sera from each of 147 patients with nonneoplastic disease. In contrast, 14 positive results (2.7%) were obtained in a group of 541 patients with lymphomas, sarcomas, and various neoplastic conditions of the hemopoietic system. The incidence was higher in other types of malignant neoplasms: breast carcinoma (11%), bronchogenic carcinoma (7%), gastrointestinal carcinoma (21%), and testicular tumors (59%). Although no data are given concerning the presence and extent of metastases in the tumors, the likelihood is that most of these cases were advanced and had metastases. According to a more recent survey (33), the incidence of elevated HCG values in serum ranged from 17 to 40% in selected tumor types. In a variety of tumors, the tissue extract, serum, and urine contained not only HCG but either or both subunits of HCG (32). A few rare tumors have had only free alpha or free beta subunits present (26,35).

Recently, several studies have appeared on the correlation between clinical status and serial determinations of the serum levels of the parameters HCG, placental lactogen (HPL), and α-fetoprotein (20,23,25). These will be described in greater detail in the section Serum Human Chorionic Gonadotropin . . . , p. 209.

POLYAMINES

The existence of polyamines (putrescine, cadaverine, etc.) in connection with living matter has been recognized for many years, usually in association with the process of putrefaction. In 1967 Cohen and Raina (9) emphasized that, because of their polycationic nature, polyamines have a strong affinity for nucleic acids *in vivo* and *in vitro* and that these compounds may have a role in the control of rRNA metabolism. Other investigators (8,11) found that polyamine synthesis and accumulation were markedly elevated early after tissue stimulation.

The concentration of polyamines was found to be elevated in the sera and the urinary excretion increased in patients with cancer (2,31). These procedures were grossly nonspecific; within the past few years more refined and specific methods, availing themselves of automated amino acid analyzer procedures, gas-liquid chromatography, and thin-layer chromatography, have been applied to the assay of polyamines. With the use of these techniques, Russell et al. (27) found that the urinary excretions of putrescine were only moderately elevated, whereas those of spermine and spermidine were substantially elevated. Of the 26 patients studied in this series, 22 had metastases. Increased urinary excretions of polyamines in patients with cancer have also been reported by Fleisher and Russell (14) and by Lipton et al. (21). The cases considered by the former were advanced and most probably had metastases. Lipton et al. (21) definitely showed a relation between the level of 24-hr excretion of urinary polyamines and metastatic spread in 24 patients with gastrointestinal tumors. The concentration of polyamines in the serum of patients with cancer is also elevated to varying degrees above the normal level, sometimes considerably so (3). Again, the patients studied are advanced cases of cancer and, although no information is given, the presumption is that they have metastases.

CORRELATIONS BETWEEN BIOCHEMICAL PARAMETERS AND METASTATIC GROWTH

As was indicated earlier, some of the criteria have been studied sequentially in individual patients so as to obtain correlations between the changes in the level of the criterion's parameter in the serum and the growth or regression of metastases in various organs of the patient. Illustrative of such studies are those of serum acid and alkaline phosphatase following treatment of patients with metastatic carcinoma of the prostate by orchiectomy or estrogen administration (18) and those of Griboff et al. (15) on the inverse relationship between changes in serum calcium of patients with metastatic carcinoma of the breast and serum alkaline phosphatase levels. In the latter study, as the patients were followed, decreases in the latter parameter frequently heralded the onset of hypercalcemia and exacerbation of the disease. In the following sections, three biochemical parameters will be illustrated in individual patients so as to demonstrate the relationship between changes in these parameters and the course of metastatic disease.

SERUM PHOSPHOHEXOSE ISOMERASE AS CRITERION OF METASTATIC GROWTH

L. G., a 41-year-old white married woman, first came for examination in January, 1947, because of a small nodule in the breast, but she did not return for further study until March, 1953, when examination revealed a hard, 8-cm tumor in the right breast. Simple right mastectomy with modified axillary dissection was performed and pathological examination showed infiltrating duct carcinoma, grade III, metastatic to the nodes. Skeletal X-rays were negative. Within 2 months she developed pain in the left side of the neck, shoulder, anterior chest, and lumbosacral region, and X-rays showed osteolytic metastases to the skull. The serum alkaline phosphatase activity was elevated to 29.7 and 55.2 Bodansky (B) units, as compared with a normal range of 1.6 to 4.2 units.

Phosphohexose isomerase (PHI) studies were begun on June 1, 1953, and were frequently performed until the patient's death on October 28 (Fig. 1). Until June 12, when oöphorectomy was performed, the isomerase, already elevated at the beginning of the study, increased from 88 units to about 180 units. (The mean value is 21 units and the upper limit of normal is 40 units.) These elevated values paralleled excessive calcium excretion, up to 990 mg/day (as compared with a normal excretion of 50 to 150 mg/day); elevated serum calcium concentrations, ranging from 11.2 to 15.1 mg/100 ml; elevated serum alkaline phosphatase activity up to 89 B units on June 9; enlarged liver and increased bromsulfalein retention and slight elevations of serum bilirubin concentration. The first period was characterized, therefore, chiefly by involvement of skeletal functions and, to some extent also, of hepatic functions.

Oöphorectomy was performed on June 12, and metastases to the liver, spleen, and ovaries were visible. Symptomatic improvement occurred. Although the serum PHI activity and bilirubin concentration continued at elevated levels, the concentration of serum calcium and the excretion of urinary calcium began to decrease. It seemed, therefore, that oöphorectomy had affected chiefly the growth of the skeletal metastases.

On June 24, cortisone administration was begun at an oral dose of 300

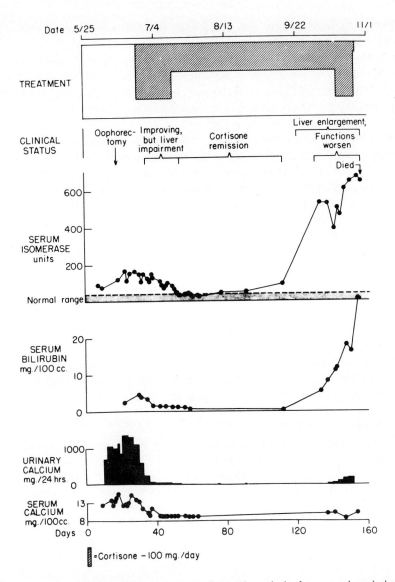

FIG. 1. Sequential determinations during a 5-month period of serum phosphohexose isomerase levels in a female patient with metastatic mammary carcinoma of skeleton and liver. Comparison with other biochemical parameters and with clinical status (5,6).

mg/day for the first 20 days, then 225 mg for the next 2 days, and 150 mg for the next 2 months. Clinical remission set in. This remission lasted until September 14 although cortisone administration continued beyond that date, as characterized by decreased pain and increased appetite. Not only was there clinical improvement, but the serum PHI declined from a level of 153 units immediately preceding institution of cortisone therapy (June 24) to normal levels on July 28. The serum bilirubin concentration and the size of the liver decreased and the cephalin-flocculation tests became negative. Similarly, and perhaps more impressive, the concentration of serum level of calcium and the daily urinary excretion of calcium promptly returned to normal levels. These findings were manifestations of the halt of metastatic growth in the liver and skeletal system.

The fourth and final, fatal subperiod began about September 14, although slightly elevated levels of serum PHI activity, namely, 52 units on August 10 and 50 units on August 24, could be considered as heralds of an impending worsening of the patient's condition. On September 14 the patient was seen in the outpatient clinic and her serum PHI activity was now substantially elevated to 97 units, the highest in 2 months. Her clinical condition still seemed satisfactory. One week later, on September 21, her liver had enlarged to 9 cm below the costal margin. On October 5 she was symptomatically much worse, complaining of episodes of nausea and of right subcostal pain radiating to the back. The urinary calcium excretion for that 24-hr period was still low, 52 mg. But the bilirubin concentration had now risen to 6.8 mg/100 ml. The serum PHI activity rose to the remarkably high level of 532 units. The clinical condition of the patient deteriorated rapidly and she was admitted on October 8.

During the next 3 weeks, objective evidence of increasing parenchymal liver damage and bile duct obstruction manifested itself with the serum bilirubin rising progressively to a level of 30 mg/100 ml, the total serum cholesterol to 889 mg/100 ml (normal, 150 to 250 mg/100 ml), and the serum PHI to a level of 676 units. Although the serum calcium level was normal, the urinary calcium excretion increased slightly. During this final period the patient became increasingly jaundiced, had episodes of pain and drowsiness, went into coma, and died on October 28.

This case illustrates a striking parallelism between, on the one hand, elevation of serum PHI activity and, on the other hand, clinical and other biochemical manifestations for the growth of metastatic tumor in the skeleton and/or liver. The levels of PHI activity seemed to be the most sensitive reflector of the activity of the patient's disease. This case was fairly representative of 10 cases of metastatic carcinoma of the breast which were studied in similar detail (5,6).

SERUM GLYCOPROTEIN

The patient (A.B.) to be discussed as an illustration of this parameter was one of a group with advanced cancer. Although insufficient clinical and pathological information is given, it is to be presumed that most had metastatic disease. This is very probable for A.B., who, because of the extensiveness of his disease, carcinoma of the lung, had a partial resection. As may be seen from Fig. 2, drawn from values reported by Harshman et al. (17), the first determination of plasma glycoprotein was done about 2 weeks after surgery and showed a decrease from a preoperative level of 180 mg/100 ml to one of 104 mg/100 ml. At 1.4 months after surgery, the level had dropped further to 78 mg/100 ml, well within the normal range. By 2.5 months after surgery, the level rose to 172 mg/100 ml and remained at that level until the sixth postoperative month when he was given cobalt therapy. This produced a rapid but transient decrease in the serum concentration of glycoprotein to normal levels, but then the concentration began to rise again to progressively higher levels until it reached, at the beginning of the 19th month, the highest level so far attained, namely, 224 mg/100 ml. Nitrogen mustard was then administered for 1 month. This therapy produced both subjective improvement in the patient and objective improvement in that obstruction in the superior vena cava was diminished. Paralleling the treatment and these signs of improvement was a decrease in the concentration of serum glycoprotein to a level of 166 mg/100 ml. There was no further treatment and the patient died 31 months after surgery.

Although this report by Harshman et al. (17) did not have detailed clinical, X-ray, pathological, or biochemical observations, it shows an impressive parallelism between the concentration of serum glycoprotein and the institution of various therapeutic measures, namely, surgery itself, cobalt radiation, and administration of nitrogen mustard in a patient with lung carcinoma having metastatic disease.

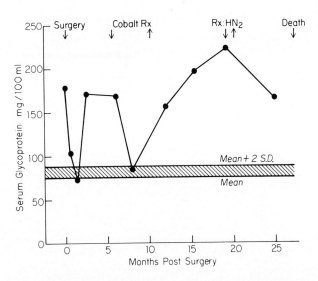

FIG. 2. Sequential determinations of serum glycoprotein levels during 25-month treatment period following partial surgical resection of lung in male patient with metastatic lung carcinoma. Calculated from data for patient A.B. (17).

CARCINOEMBRYONIC ANTIGEN IN SERUM

This parameter as a measure of metastatic growth is illustrated by the following study (29). A 51-year-old woman was seen in November, 1971, with primary cancer of the right breast and skeletal pain. Radiographic examination revealed bony metastases, and a radioisotope scan indicated possible spotty liver metastases. Her initial carcinoembryonic antigen (CEA) level was 14.9 ng/100 ml, as compared with an upper normal limit of 2.5 mg/100 ml (Fig. 3). A simple mastectomy was performed to remove the primary cancer, and the CEA concentration fell after operation to 7.7 and < 1 ng/ml/100 ml at 7 and 10 days, respectively. Adrenalectomy and oöphorectomy were performed at 10 days and she had a good clinical response. However, the CEA levels increased to 2.7 ng/ml at 11 days and 3.6 ng/ml at 39 days after the combined adrenalectomy and oöphorectomy. In August, 1972, about 9 months after she was first seen, she developed bone pain and was given a course of irradiation followed by fluoxymesterone (Halotestin®), chlorambucil, and prednisone. This temporarily relieved her pain, and the concentrations of serum CEA remained only slightly elevated as, for example, 3.5 ng/ml in December, 1972. Symptoms again improved with the administration of dimethyl testosterone, 50 mg q.i.d., but unfortunately no CEA determinations were done for the next several months. In May, 1973, the concentration was found to be elevated to 11.5 ng/ml. Nor were any detailed clinical observations reported for this period. The patient died in September, 1973, about 20 months after she was first seen.

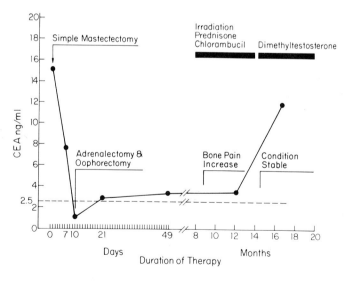

FIG. 3. Sequential determinations of serum carcinoembryonic antigen levels during 20-month treatment period following simple mastectomy in female patient with metastatic scirrhous breast cancer. After Fig. 7 of Steward et al. (29).

This case shows some parallelism between therapy, clinical condition, and CEA levels, particularly after the initial mastectomy. But, as indicated, the sequential determinations of CEA levels and the accompanying clinical observations were not done at sufficiently short intervals during most of the patient's course to reveal either the existence or absence of close parallelism between the CEA parameter and the growth of metastases.

SERUM HUMAN CHORIONIC GONADOTROPIN, HUMAN PLACENTAL LACTOGEN, AND α-FETOPROTEIN

As was previously noted, these parameters are more specific for cancer and, indeed, for certain types of cancer than the three parameters we have just illustrated. As was also previously noted, several studies have recently appeared on the relationship between clinical status and sequential determinations of the parameters of HCG, HPL, and α-fetoprotein.

Muggia et al. (23) have described four cases of cancer in whom sequential determinations of the serum levels of the above parameters were done and correlated with the clinical status, particularly metastatic growth or regression. The course of one of these can be described in detail. The patient, a 46-year-old male union executive, had a history of heavy smoking and sought medical attention because of a 2-month history of increasing cough, dyspnea, and breast enlargement. Physical examination revealed facial plethora, slight exophthalmos, right jugular vein distention, and decreased breath sounds and dullness at the right base. Roentgenography showed a large right paratracheal mass and multiple lung nodules. Venography revealed a mass narrowing the lumen of the superior vena cava. The source of the primary site of the neoplasm could not be determined. On admission, the serum HCG was elevated to about 1,000 ng/ml, as estimated from a figure presented by Muggia et al. (23) and as compared with a value in normal men of less than 1 ng/ml. During an initial period of 18 days without therapy, the serum HCG rose to about 2,500 ng/ml.

To ameliorate symptoms, particularly of increasing venous pressure and obstruction of the superior vena cava, the patient received 3,600 rads between days 18 and 41 of his hospitalization and, in addition, chemotherapy consisting of dactinomycin, cyclophosphamide, and vincristine at various scheduled times. The levels of serum HCG decreased to normal or very low levels by the 30th day of hospital admission and remained there until the 40th day. Because of peripheral neuropathy, chemotherapy was temporarily interrupted and then given intermittently. The serum HCG slowly began to rise, although a roentgenogram taken on day 60 showed a marked decrease in the transverse diameter and size of the metastatic lesion in the left lung. After day 60, the serum HCG levels rose further, oscillating between about 2,500 and 3,500 ng/ml, until day 98 when the chest X-ray showed marked increase in the size of the metastatic lesions. Hepatomegaly had also become manifest and liver biopsy confirmed the infiltration of the liver by an undifferentiated carcinoma. Thereafter, the serum HCG rose rapidly, reaching a level of between 50,000 and 60,000 ng/ml on day 120. The size of the metastatic lesions in the lung also increased considerably as shown by X-ray. Progressive obtundation and respiratory embarrassment led to death on the 132nd day. At autopsy, the anterior mediastinum, pleura, lungs, and mediastinum and paraortic lymph nodes were replaced by tumor. Metastases were also present in the jejunal mucosa, liver, kidneys, spleen, left adrenal, meninges, pituitary stalk, cerebral cortex, and cerebellum.

SUMMARY

The various considerations and illustrations that have been presented show that several biochemical parameters may serve as aids in following the growth or regression of metastases in patients with cancer. The value of each of these parameters has to be demonstrated by preliminary studies on several patients with each type of cancer in which the serum level or urinary excretion is determined sequentially at frequent intervals and is correlated with alterations in the clinical condition and physical examination, X-rays, nuclear scans, and other biochemical parameters. It would appear that this has been done most thoroughly for the nonspecific parameter phosphohexose isomerase, and less so for glycoprotein and for carcinoembryonic antigen. It is hoped that detailed sequential studies will be done for these last two parameters as well as for others mentioned in this chapter. In this connection, the more specific parameters — HCG, human placental lactogen, and α-fetoprotein — are of particular interest.

REFERENCES

1. Abrams, H. L. (1950): Metastases in carcinoma. Analysis of 1000 autopsied cases. *Cancer,* 3:74–85.
2. Bachrach, U., and Robinson, E. (1965): Occurrence of spermine in sera of cancer bearing individuals. *Israel J. Med. Sci.,* 1:247–250.
3. Bartos, D., Campbell, R. A., Bartos, F., and Grettie, D. (1975): Direct determination of polyamines in human serum by radioimmunoassay. *Cancer Res.,* 30:2056–2060.
4. Bodansky, A. (1933): Phosphatase studies. II. Determination of serum phosphatase. Factors influencing the accuracy of the determination. *J. Biol. Chem.,* 101:93–104.
5. Bodansky, O. (1954): Serum phosphohexose isomerase in cancer. II. As an index of tumor growth in metastatic carcinoma of the breast. *Cancer,* 7:1200–1226.
6. Bodansky, O. (1965): Biochemical changes of clinical significance in cancer. In: *Proceedings of the Fifth National Cancer Conference,* pp. 687–703. J. B. Lippincott and Co., Philadelphia.
7. Braunstein, G. D., Vaitukitis, J. L., Carbone, P. P., and Ross, G. T. (1973): Ectopic production of human chorionic gonadotropin by neoplasms. *Ann. Intern. Med.,* 78:39–45.
8. Caldarera, C. M., Barbiroli, B., and Moruzzi, G. (1965): Polyamines and nucleic acids during development of the chick embryo. *Biochem. J.,* 97:84–88.
9. Cohen, S. S., and Raina, A. (1967): Some interrelations on natural polyamines and nucleic acids in growing and various infected bacteria. In: *Organizational Biosynthesis,*

edited by H. J. Vogel, J. V. Lampen, and V. Bryson, pp. 157–182. Academic Press, New York.

10. Dixon, T. F., and Purdom, M. (1954): Serum 5'-nucleotidase. *J. Clin. Pathol.*, 7:341–343.

11. Dykstra, W. J., Jr., and Herbst, E. J. (1965): Spermidine in regenerating liver: Relation to rapid synthesis of ribonucleic acid. *Science*, 149:428–429.

12. Elkin, M., and Mueller, H. O. (1954): Metastases from cancer of the prostate; autopsy and roentgenological findings. *Cancer*, 7:1246–1248.

13. Fishman, W. H. (1969): Immunologic and biochemical approaches to alkaline phosphatase isoenzymes: The Regan isoenzyme. *Ann. N.Y. Acad. Sci.*, 166:745–759.

14. Fleisher, J. H., and Russell, D. H. (1975): Estimation of urinary diamines and polyamines by thin layer chromatography. *J. Chromatogr.*, 110:335–340.

15. Griboff, S. I., Hermann, J. B., Smelin, A., and Moss, J. (1954): Hypercalcemia secondary to bone metastases from carcinoma of the breast. I. Relationship between serum calcium and alkaline phosphatase values. *J. Clin. Endocrinol.*, 14:378–388.

16. Gutman, A. B., and Gutman, E. B. (1938): An "acid" phosphatase occurring in the serum of patients with metastasizing carcinoma of the prostate gland. *J. Clin. Invest.*, 17:473–478.

17. Harshman, S., Patikas, P. T., Dayani, K., and Reynolds, V. H. (1967): Serum mucoid levels in patients with cancer and the effect of surgical treatment. *Cancer Res.*, 27:1286–1295.

18. Huggins, C., and Hodges, C. V. (1941): Studies on prostatic cancer. I. Effect of castration, of estrogen and of androgen injection on serum phosphatases in metastatic carcinoma of the prostate. *Cancer Res.*, 1:293–297.

19. Kutscher, W., and Wörner, A. (1936): Prostataphosphatase. 2. Mitteilung. *Hoppe-Seyler's Z. Physiol. Chem.*, 239:109–126.

20. Lange, P. H., McIntire, R., Waldmann, T. A., Hakala, T. R., and Fraley, E. E. (1976): Serum alpha fetoprotein and human chorionic gonadotropin in the diagnosis and management of nonseminomatous germ-cell testicular cancer. *N. Engl. J. Med.*, 295:1237–1240.

21. Lipton, A., Sheehan, L., and Harvey, H. A. (1975): Urinary polyamine levels in patients with gastrointestinal malignancy. *Cancer*, 36:2351–2354.

22. Martland, M., Hansman, F. S., and Robison, R. (1924): The phosphoric-esterase of blood. *Biochem. J.*, 18:1152–1160.

23. Muggia, F. M., Rosen, S. W., Weintraub, B. C., and Hansen, H. H. (1975): Ectopic placental proteins in nontrophoblastic tumors. Serial measurement following chemotherapy. *Cancer*, 36:1327–1337.

24. Neumann, H., Moran, E. M., Russell, R. M., and Rosenberg, I. H. (1974): Distinct alkaline phosphatase in serum of patients with lymphatic leukemia and infectious mononucleosis. *Science*, 186:151–153.

25. Perlin, E., Engeler, J. E., Edson, M., et al. (1976): The value of serial measurement of both human chorionic gonadotropin and alpha-fetoprotein for monitoring germinal cell tumors. *Cancer*, 37:215–219.

26. Rosen, S. W., and Weintraub, B. D. (1974): Ectopic production of the isolated alpha subunit of the glycoprotein hormones. *N. Engl. J. Med.*, 290:1442–1447.

27. Russell, D. H., Levy, C. C., Schimpf, S. C., and Hawk, I. A. (1971): Urinary polyamines in cancer patients. *Cancer Res.*, 31:1555–1558.

28. Silverberg, E., and Holleb, A. I. (1974): Cancer statistics, 1974 — Worldwide epidemiology. *CA*, 24:2–21.

29. Steward, A. M., Nixon, D., Zamcheck, N., and Aisenberg, M. (1974): Carcinoembryonic antigen in breast cancer patients: Serum levels and disease progress. *Cancer*, 33:1236–1252.

30. Stolbach, L. L. (1969): Clinical application of alkaline phosphatase isoenzyme analysis. *Ann. N.Y. Acad. Sci.*, 166:760–774.

31. Tokuoku, S. (1950): Spermine reaction of serum for the diagnosis of cancer. *Acta Sch. Med. Univ. Kioto*, 27:241–247.

32. Vaitukitis, J. L. (1973): Immunologic and physical characterization of human chorionic gonadotropin (hCG) secreted by tumors. *J. Clin. Endocrinol. Metab.*, 37:505–514.

33. Vaitukitis, J. L. (1976): Peptide hormones as tumor markers. *Cancer*, 37:567–572.

34. Vest, S. A. (1954): Prostatic malignancy. *Ciba Clin. Symp.*, 6:93–103.

35. Weintraub, B. D., and Rosen, S. W. (1973): Ectopic production of the isolated beta subunit of human chorionic gonadotropin. *J. Clin. Invest.*, 52:3135–3142.

Cancer Invasion and Metastasis: Biologic
Mechanisms and Therapy, edited by S. B. Day
et al. Raven Press, New York © 1977.

Current Status of Alternative Selective Antimetastatic Therapy

Federico Spreafico, Giovanni Mistrello, Maria Luisa Moras,
and Monica Cairo

Department of Cancer Chemotherapy and Immunology, Istituto di Ricerche Farmacologiche "Mario Negri," Milan, Italy

In the distribution of tasks for this volume we have been given that of discussing the current status of alternative and selective antimetastatic treatments, i.e., of those treatment approaches which aim to reduce cancer dissemination and metastasis formation not relying solely on the use of the traditional antineoplastic strategies such as radiotherapy or chemotherapy.

The rationale for the search for agents capable of selectively influencing cancerous dissemination has been presented elsewhere and will not be discussed in detail, the interested reader being referred to other recent publications on this topic (5,17). Briefly, as repeatedly emphasized by others in this volume, the formation of tumor secondaries can rightly be considered as the cornerstone of clinical malignancy since with current therapeutic possibilities, by far the majority of tumorous patients succumb because of metastasis rather than as a direct consequence of the primary tumor. Secondly, although certain types of normal cells can occasionally migrate from the solid organ of their origin and establish deposits in other parenchyma (20), the tendency to invade and disseminate is a property practically exclusive of neoplastic elements. Accordingly, agents capable of selectively interfering with this characteristic of tumor cells could represent a useful new addition to the available antineoplastic armamentarium with compounds having, at least in principle, the advantage of specificity.

If the sequence of events including cell separation from the primary tumor and local invasion, dissemination, establishment in normal tissues, and subsequent proliferation can be accepted as a general scheme of the main phases leading ultimately to the formation of a "clinical" metastasis, it is also obvious that each of these major steps has in turn to be divided into a series of interconnected substeps and that at the level of each of them there most probably occurs a complex interplay of factors, pertaining to the tumor or to the host, either promoting or inhibiting dissemination or metastasis formation.

In principle, this very complexity of the process should offer a whole series of possible levels at which pharmacological manipulation could be exerted (Table 1) through a variety of mechanisms, many of which would not involve a direct reduction of the cell reproductive integrity, thus overcoming the intrinsic limit of available cytotoxic antitumorals deriving from their limited specificity for the neoplastic elements. In practice, however, current possibilities for influencing tumor cell dissemination and metastatic establishment are still limited to only some of the steps in this complex chain of events, and the possible mechanisms of interference so far explored are still very restricted in number. An in-depth analysis of the results so far obtained in the attempts to pharmacologically control neoplastic spreading is beyond the limits of this chapter. Suffice here to say that the search for selective antidisseminative or, more in general, of nondirectly cytotoxic antimetastatic compounds is still in its infancy and has been conducted more on a pragmatic than on a rationalized basis, owing to the still large ignorance of many basic events and mechanisms of cancerous spreading. Indeed, it seems fair to say that for most of the compounds investigated for such an activity, the main intent was not so much to develop therapeutic agents but rather to use them as tools in the dissection of the metastatization process and to establish the principle that a selective pharmacological manipulation of neoplastic dissemination and metastasis establishment (as distinct from metastatic growth) is in fact possible.

Although other approaches have also been explored as previously reviewed (17), most of the experimental attempts toward a selective reduction of metastasis formation appear to have centered on the use either of agents acting more or less specifically on the coagulative-anticoagulative equilibrium or of polymeric substances. For the latter, a representative but probably not exhaustive list is presented in Table 2. The rationales for the use of the second group of substances were often mixed in view of their frequently complex biological activities, a common denominator appearing, however, to have been the attempt to influence membrane properties of neoplastic cells believed to play a role in dissemination such as surface charge, adhesiveness, deformability, and aggregability. Although changes in adhesiveness, homo- and heterotypic aggregability, mobility, etc. have been described, for many of these agents the evidence for a selective antimetastatic activity *in vivo* is either contradictory or very much dependent

TABLE 1. *Possible targets for antimetastatic manipulation*

Cellular adhesiveness (homotypic and heterotypic)	Influx and activity of attacker cells
Cellular motility	Quality and quantity of neovessels
Cellular invasiveness	Embolic size
Cellular plasticity	Arrest and filtering capacity
Cellular immunogenicity	Tumor dormancy
Tumor micromilieu	Regrowth

TABLE 2. *Polymers investigated for antimetastatic activity*

Polyanions:	dextran sulfate, hyaluronic acid, polymetha-crylic acid, polyacrylic acid, chondroitin sulfate, polyethylene sulfonate, heparin
Polycations:	DEAE-dextran, DEAE-polyacrilate, polyethylenimine, polypropylenimine, polyvinylamine, chitosan, protamine sulfate, polyamidoamines, betaines
Nonionic:	Tritons

on the experimental conditions employed. It should be noted in fact that many of these substances were investigated only in systems of artificial metastasis as obtained with i.v. injections of tumor cells, thus making it difficult to evaluate their potential in conditions of more physiological, continuous dissemination.

More cogent is the demonstration for a number of these molecules of a direct cytotoxic capacity [e.g., heparin (14), DEAE-dextran (22), polyethyleneimine (12)], thus raising doubts on the real mechanisms at the basis of the observed reductions in artificial or spontaneous metastasis formation. In the same direction, the possibility that a major determinant in the tumor inhibitory effect of some polymers is played by changes in cell immunogenicity (8,13), possibly through interactions with surface glycoproteins, cannot be discounted.

For other polymeric compounds, results obtained have been more suggestive for a potential exploitation as antimetastasis agents. We would tend to place in this category Triton WR 1339 (TWR 1339), a nonionic detergent inactive *in vivo* on several tumors and not cytotoxic *in vitro* even at high concentrations, with a long half-life in the circulation, which is capable of reducing the number of metastases in various (but not all) experimental systems of spontaneous or simulated dissemination. As shown in Table 3 for the C57B1/6 mouse Lewis lung (3LL) carcinoma, the antimetastatic effect of TWR 1339 (most probably exerted by a combined activity on the host and the tumor cell) is obtained without detectable modification of the primary tumor growth rate, and this dichotomy of activities is a useful preliminary yardstick of the search for selective antimetastatic compounds.

As examples of other molecules investigated by us for a selective antimetastatic activity, we could mention polyaminoamides (Table 4) (4) and polymethacrylic acid (PMAA) (Table 5). The latter compound was originally described as a mobilizer of malignant and normal cells from their tissue deposits (23), thus it is possible that, at least in part, its effects are mediated by the immune system.

According to the definition presented above, a drug such as ICRF 159 (K. Hellmann, *this volume*) should not be classified among selective anti-

TABLE 3. Antimetastatic effect of TWR 1339 on 3LL carcinoma

Exp. group	Dose (mg/kg i.p.)	Days of treatment	MST[a] (days)	Primary tumor weight (g)	Lung metast. weight (mg)	No. lung metast. (±SE)	% mice with metast.
Control	—	—	28.7 ± 1.5	5.8 ± 0.4	213 ± 18	41 ± 3	100
TWR 1339	500	0–10	30.5 ± 1.7	6.1 ± 0.6	94 ± 15	9 ± 3	80
	500	0–25	31.4 ± 1.3	5.7 ± 0.3	50 ± 9	7 ± 4	50
	500	15–25	29.7 ± 1.0	5.8 ± 0.4	87 ± 15	31 ± 6	100
	200	0–10	29.4 ± 1.5	5.2 ± 0.5	101 ± 12	14 ± 5	75
	200	0–25	27.8 ± 2.3	5.4 ± 0.7	33 ± 7	11 ± 4	65
	200	15–25	30.2 ± 0.9	6.0 ± 0.4	126 ± 20	22 ± 5	100
	50	0–25	31.3 ± 1.1	6.1 ± 0.3	69 ± 20	15 ± 3	90

[a] MST, median survival time.
C57B1/6 mice were transplanted with 2.10^5 3LL cells i.m. on day 0.

metastatic compounds. In fact, although this agent can markedly reduce metastasis at doses having no apparent effect on the primary tumor, the drug also possesses a clear direct cytotoxic activity. The bases for expecting a greater sensitivity to cytotoxic chemotherapy for secondary outgrowths in respect to primary, larger neoplasms have been discussed elsewhere (15,18). However, the capacity of this drug to act on tumor vasculature (6), which allegedly could contribute to its inhibition of tumor spreading, is just one

TABLE 4. Antimetastatic effects of polyaminoamides[a] in 3LL carcinoma

Code no.	Structure	Dose (mg/kg i.v.)	% of control No. metast.	% of control Weight metast.
G 3	$R = (CH_2)_2OH$ (70%) $(CH_2)_{11}CH_3$ (30%)	10	45	20
G 14		200	35	15

Treatment was on days 0, 4, 7, 11, 14, and 18; evaluation on day 25 after the i.m. transplant of 2.10^5 3LL cells in C57B1/6 mice.

TABLE 5. *Antimetastatic effects of polymethacrylic acid in 3LL carcinoma*

Exp. group	Dose (mg/kg)	Schedule	Primary tumor weight (g)	No. lung metast.
Control	—	—	6.8 ± 0.5	23 ± 2
PMAA	40, i.v.	q. 5 d., 0–20	7.1 ± 0.3	9 ± 2^a
	40, s.c.	q. 5 d., 0–20	6.6 ± 0.4	17 ± 3
	40, os	q. 5 d., 0–20	7.0 ± 0.6	20 ± 3
	40, i.p.	q. 5 d., 0–20	6.7 ± 0.2	8 ± 2^a
	10, i. p.	q. d., 0–20	6.1 ± 0.3	5 ± 2^a
	10, i.p.	q. 2 d., 0–20	6.3 ± 0.3	8 ± 2^a
	5, i.p.	q. 2 d., 0–20	6.7 ± 0.4	15 ± 3

^{a} $p < 0.05$.
C57B1/6 mice were transplanted i.m. with 2.10^5 3LL cells and sacrificed on day 25.

example of the many still open levels at which interference with tumor progression and dissemination could be aimed.

The fact that agents such as TWR 1339 appear not to influence the growth of already established secondaries but only to act on earlier phases of metastasis, as for instance indicated by the absence of metastasis reduction when drug treatment is initiated after the surgical removal of the primary disseminating tumor (Table 6), would seem to restrict the potential practical exploitability of this type of antidisseminative compound to only a relatively small number of clinical conditions. These substances could in principle be of interest, for instance, in cases of not surgically resectable, disseminating primary neoplasms, or in those conditions in which the disease is already systemic at diagnosis and has a high tendency to widely disseminate as might be represented by Hodgkin's lymphoma. In addition to their possible prevention of dissemination to anatomical sanctuaries difficult to attack with chemotherapy, a larger area of potential use would be found for this type of compound if it is shown that metastases can in turn metastasize, a problem still not satisfactorily solved. In this context and considering that

TABLE 6. *Effects of surgery plus TWR 1339 on 3LL carcinoma*

Exp. group	Dose (mg/kg i.p.)	Schedule	MST (days)	% cures	No. lung metast.
Control	—	—	25	0	36 ± 6
Surgery	—	10	30	0	27 ± 4
Surgery + TWR 1339	200	q. d., 0–10	41^a	20	18 ± 2^a
Surgery + TWR 1339	200	q. d., 11–25	32	0	24 ± 3

^{a} $p < 0.05$.
Surgery was performed 10 days after the i.m. transplant of 2.10^5 3LL cells.

even if selective antimetastatic treatments of the types discussed will ever be developed to a clinical stage they will be employed as adjunct to classic antitumoral approaches, it is noteworthy that for at least a number of anti-metastatic compounds it has been shown that they can successfully be employed in conjunction with conventional chemotherapeutic agents as exemplified by the data of Table 7.

One may thus conclude that although the objective of a selective pharma-cological manipulation of metastasis formation is not the subject of pure speculation, it is also clear that the available active agents are too few and are unsatisfactory in a number of aspects, and that the levels so far investi-gated for possible control of this process are still very limited. Substantial progress in this area and thus the development of newer, more "on target" agents for a noncytotoxic interference with metastasis will be dependent on better elucidation of: (a) the specific cellular and subcellular characteristics enabling a malignant cell to invade, disseminate, and establish in new sur-roundings and (b) the local and systemic mechanisms favoring or opposing these phenomena.

Another not yet traditional approach to metastasis control, i.e., immuno-therapy, should now be briefly considered. A discussion of the role of immunity in cancerous spreading as well as of the basis which renders this approach especially suitable for attack on limited numbers of tumor cells is beyond the scope of this chapter. In addition to the chapters in this volume dealing with this topic, an excellent review of the subject has recently ap-peared (1). We will thus only summarize some of our more recent experience in this field concentrating on the use of nonspecific immunomodulators, i.e., of the type of immunotherapeutic intervention at the present time most commonly employed in the clinic. The objective is to give a few indications from experimental systems of the potential of this type of treatment and to

TABLE 7. *Effects of polymethacrylic acid or Triton WR 1339 in combination with cyclo-phosphamide on 3LL carcinoma*

Exp. group	Dose (mg/kg i.p.)	Schedule	Primary tumor weight (g)	Lung metast. weight (mg)	No. lung metast.
Control	—	—	7.7 ± 0.4	158 ± 25	32 ± 6
Cyclophosphamide	155	7, 14	4.8 ± 0.3^a	64 ± 9^a	13 ± 5
PMAA	40	q. 5 d., 0–20	7.5 ± 0.6	55 ± 7^a	10 ± 3^a
Cyclophosphamide +	125	7, 14			
PMAA	40	q. 5 d., 0–20	4.2 ± 0.4^a	12 ± 4^b	3 ± 1
TWR 1339	200	q. d., 0–20	6.9 ± 0.5	31 ± 8^a	7 ± 3^a
Cyclophosphamide +	125	7, 14			
TWR 1339	200	q. d., 0–20	3.8 ± 0.3^a	14 ± 2^b	2 ± 1^b

[a] $p < 0.05$ vs controls.
[b] $p < 0.05$ vs cyclophosphamide.

discuss aspects of its application that may have direct relevance for a more logical and effective clinical exploitation.

That tumor secondaries can be more sensitive than the primary to nonspecific immunotherapy is illustrated by the data of Table 8 obtained in a system of low antigenicity such as the 3LL carcinoma. The nonmodification of survival time in these conditions depends on the fact that in this model system the extent of pulmonary metastasis is not a prime determinant of the time of death (see Table 6), except when the primary tumor has been removed. These results show not only that for some agents this effect is seen even when the treatment is applied after the primary neoplasm has already amply disseminated, but also that new compounds are being added in these years to the list of active immunostimulants, for instance, NSC 208828 [3-(p-chlorophenyl)-2,3-dihydro-3-hydroxythiazolo(3,2-a)-benzimidazole], a recently developed drug possessing interesting properties.

Table 9 shows that better therapeutic results can be obtained when combinations of immunostimulants are employed instead of single agents, although the choice of drugs and the treatment schedule can be critical for observing synergism or additive effects. The latter type of therapeutic approach has not yet been systematically explored even in experimental systems, whereas it may hold considerable practical promise especially when agents having different and complementary activities on the various antitumoral immune effector mechanisms are employed.

With the exception of some selected conditions, e.g., malignant melanoma, it is uncommon for nonspecific immunotherapy to be clinically applied alone, more frequent being its use following cytoreductive treatments such as surgery or chemotherapy. This practice is based on a large body of experimental evidence indicating that host reactivity can be antitumorally curative only when confronting a relatively limited tumor load, generally estimated to be of the order of 10^7 to 10^8 cells, although reliable quantitative estimates are often difficult to obtain, especially in the case of solid neoplasms. The

TABLE 8. Antimetastatic effects of different immunomodulators on 3LL carcinoma

Exp. group	Dose (mg/kg i.p.)	Day of treatment	Primary tumor weight (g)	No. lung metast.	% mice with metast.
Control	—	—	7.3 ± 0.5	34 ± 4	100
C. parvum	1.4^a	0	6.1 ± 0.3	8 ± 2^b	60–70
	1.4^a	14	6.7 ± 0.4	13 ± 3^b	90–100
NSC 208828	50	1	6.7 ± 0.3	18 ± 2^b	100
	150	1	6.2 ± 0.5	10 ± 1^b	60–70
Pyran	40	1–8	5.9 ± 0.2	15 ± 4^b	70–80

[a] Dose i.v. per mouse.
[b] $p < 0.05$.
C57BL/6 mice were sacrificed 25 days after the i.m. transplant of 2.10^5 3LL cells.

TABLE 9. *Antimetastatic activity on 3LL carcinoma of combinations of immunostimulants*

Exp. group	Day of treatment	Lung metast. weight (mg)	No. lung metast.
Control	—	184 ± 35	31 ± 6
C. parvum	15	87 ± 18	16 ± 3
Levamisole	16–19	121 ± 21	22 ± 5
Pyran	1–8	95 ± 13	18 ± 4
C. parvum + Levamisole	15 16–19	12 ± 7^a	6 ± 2^a
Pyran + Levamisole	1–8 16–19	43 ± 10^a	10 ± 1^a

[a] $p < 0.05$ vs the single agents.
The doses were 0.7 mg/mouse i.v. for *C. parvum*, 20 mg/kg i.p. for pyran, and 3 mg/kg i.p. for levamisole. C57Bl/6 mice were sacrificed 25 days after the i.m. inoculum of 2.10^5 3LL cells.

potential of combining chemotherapy with nonspecific immunostimulation is illustrated in Table 10, both treatments being initiated on a quite advanced tumor in order to simulate the frequently encountered clinical condition of a neoplasm already metastasized at the time of first diagnosis of the disease.

Table 11 shows that the triple combination surgery-chemotherapy-immunotherapy can obviously give better therapeutic results than either of the binary treatments, as shown not only by the proportion of mice with tumor secondaries at sacrifice which was markedly lower than seen with any of the other treatments, but also by the increase in survival which was approximately doubled in respect to untreated controls. Moreover, with this

TABLE 10. *Combination chemoimmunotherapy for advanced 3LL carcinoma*

Exp. group	Day of treatment	% of mice with metast.	Primary tumor weight (g)	Lung metast. weight (mg)	No. lung metast.
Control	—	100	7.6 ± 0.6	126 ± 24	28 ± 3
Adriamycin	14	80	6.1 ± 0.5	31 ± 13^a	9 ± 3^a
C. parvum	18	90	6.3 ± 0.6	62 ± 26^a	16 ± 3^a
Adriamycin + *C. parvum*	14 18	$20^{a,b}$	4.9 ± 0.4^a	11 ± 3^a	6 ± 2^a
BCG	18	100	7.9 ± 0.7	141 ± 36	27 ± 2
Adriamycin + BCG	14 18	80	5.8 ± 0.3	40 ± 10^a	8 ± 2^a

[a] $p < 0.05$ vs controls.
[b] $p < 0.05$ vs adriamycin.
C57B1/6 mice were sacrificed 23 days after the i.m. transplant of 2.10^5 3LL cells. Adriamycin: 10 mg/kg i.v.; *C. parvum:* 0.7 mg i.v.; BCG: 1 mg i.v.

TABLE 11. *Effect of the triple combination surgery-chemotherapy-immunotherapy on 3LL carcinoma*

Exp. group	Day of treatment	MST[a] (days)	% mice[b] metast.	Primary tumor[b] weight (g)	Lung metast.[b] weight (mg)
Control	—	24	100	8.7 ± 0.4	98 ± 16
Adriamycin	11	28	80	5.4 ± 1.0^c	23 ± 1^c
C. parvum	15	29	100	5.9 ± 0.7^c	42 ± 9^c
Adriamycin + C. parvum	11 15	$35^{c,d}$	$40^{e,f}$	4.4 ± 0.5^c	9 ± 1^f
Surgery	9	30^c	90	—	95 ± 44
Surgery + Adriamycin	9 11	36^c	50	—	8 ± 1^f
Surgery + C. parvum	9 15	34^c	70	—	58 ± 13
Surgery + Adriamycin + C. parvum	9 11 15	$46^{f,g,h}$	$20^{f,g,h}$	—	3 ± 1^f

[a] Median survival time.
[b] C57B1/6 sacrificed 23 days after the i.m. transplant of 2.10^5 3LL cells. Adriamycin: 10 mg/kg i.v.; *C. parvum:* 0.7 mg/mouse i.v.
[c] $p < 0.05$.
[d] $p < 0.05$ vs surgery.
[e] $p < 0.05$ vs adriamycin.
[f] $p < 0.01$ vs controls.
[g] $p < 0.05$ vs surgery + *C. parvum.*
[h] $p < 0.05$ vs surgery + adriamycin.

triple treatment a low (20 to 30%) but consistently observable proportion of animals was cured. These data, in conjunction with similar ones obtained by others in this and different systems also employing other chemotherapeutic and immunostimulatory compounds (2,11,21), thus appear to provide a clear rationale for suggesting the usefulness of adding immunotherapy to the current combined modality of surgery-chemotherapy in the treatment of various solid human malignancies such as breast carcinoma.

It is well known that various factors (staging of the tumor, its antigenicity, the respective sequence and scheduling of the two treatments, etc.) can markedly influence the effectiveness of combined chemoimmunotherapy. Of critical importance in determining the therapeutic outcome can, however, be the appropriate choice of the drugs employed in the chemoimmunotherapeutic combination, a fact not surprising considering that immunomodulators differ in their effects on the various immunocyte subpopulations (Table 12) and that cancer chemotherapeutic agents can vary significantly both quantitatively and qualitatively in their immunosuppressive activity (16).

A practical and sensitive experimental model for investigating the importance of pairing of agents in chemoimmunotherapy was found to be the L 1210 leukemia, and Table 13 shows the marked differences in therapeutic effectiveness observable when an optimal dose of adriamycin is combined

TABLE 12. *Effects of different immunomodulators on various immune parameters*

Parameter	C. parvum	BCG	Levamisole	Pyran
T-lymphocyte function	−	+	+	?
B-lymphocyte function	+	+	0	+
Macrophage function	++	++	±	++
ADCC[a]	++	++	0	+
CMC	+	+	0	?
Spleen cellularity	++	++	0	++
T-suppressor activity	−−	−	+	?

[a] ADCC, antibody-dependent cellular cytotoxicity; CMC, cell-mediated cytotoxicity.

with optimal treatments of different immunostimulants or (Table 14) when one immunostimulant is combined with different antitumorals administered in equiactive doses. Similar results have been obtained in other nonleukemic neoplasms (see Table 10). Although the mechanisms of the observed synergism between adriamycin and *Corynebacterium parvum* are still being investigated, present evidence supports our hypothesis (19) that an important if not crucial factor is played by complementarity in the mode of action of the two agents at the immunocyte subpopulations level. Synergism between these agents could in fact have been expected on the basis of previous demonstrations that after adriamycin treatment, and at variance with what was seen with other antitumorals (e.g., daunomycin), macrophage activity and antibody-dependent cellular cytotoxicity (ADCC) were relatively spared (10); both these mechanisms play a major role in the antitumoral effect of *C. parvum* (9).

Recent data to be detailed elsewhere have in fact shown that the tumor

TABLE 13. *Antileukemic effects of adriamycin combined with different immunomodulators on L 1210 leukemia*

Day of administration of				% ILS[a]	% cures
Adriamycin	C. parvum	BCG	Levamisole		
1	−	−	−	61	0
−	6	−	−	0	0
−	−	6	−	0	0
−	−	−	6–9	0	0
1	6	−	−	187	80
1	−	6	−	130[b]	0
1	−	−	6–9	92[b,c]	0

[a] Increase in lifespan over untreated controls.
[b] $p < 0.05$ vs adriamycin.
[c] $p < 0.05$ vs adriamycin-BCG.
10^5 L 1210 Ha cells were transplanted i.p. on day 0 in CD_2F_1 mice. The dose of *C. parvum* was 0.7 mg i.v.; those of BCG and levamisole 1 mg i.v. and 3 mg/kg i.p., respectively; adriamycin 10 mg/kg i.v.

TABLE 14. *Effect of various antitumorals combined with* C. parvum *on L 1210 leukemia*

Drug	Dose (mg/kg)	Day of treatment	% ILS[a]	% cures
Adriamycin	7.5	1	32	0
Adriamycin	10	1	70	0
Cyclophosphamide	55	1	65	0
5-FU	200	1	75	0
Daunomycin	10	1	35	0
Adriamycin +	10	1	120	90[b]
C. parvum	0.7	6		
Daunomycin +	10	1	37	0
C. parvum	0.7	6		
Cyclophosphamide +	55	1	140	40[b,c]
C. parvum	0.7	6		
5-FU +	200	1	67	0
C. parvum	0.7	6		

[a] Increase in lifespan over untreated controls.
[b] $p < 0.01$ vs controls.
[c] $p < 0.05$ vs Adriamycin = C. parvum.
10^5 L 1210 Ha cells were transplanted i.p. on day 0 in CD_2F_1 mice.

cytotoxic capacity of macrophages after combined adriamycin-*C. parvum* treatment is as high, if not better, than after injections of the immunostimulant alone. Similarly, the increased activity of ADCC-mediating cells induced by *C. parvum* is not reduced by previous administration of this chemotherapeutic agent. The importance of ADCC as an immune effector mechanism has recently been substantiated (7,25), and the role of macrophages in the control of malignant growth and in metastasis formation has been discussed in this volume and in previous publications by Alexander and by others (3,24).

If immunotherapy, even in the relatively crude form currently employed, seems thus to be an effective form of antimetastatic treatment employed either alone in certain specialized conditions (e.g., melanoma, pleural effusions) or more frequently as an adjuvant to surgery-chemotherapy, it is nevertheless clear that much still remains to be done before its full potential is defined, also through the development of more rationalized modes of its application, for instance, along the above-described lines of "complementary level" chemoimmunotherapy.

ACKNOWLEDGMENT

This work was supported by grant no. 5RO1 CA12764-05, National Institutes of Health, NCI, Bethesda, Md.

REFERENCES

1. Baldwin, R. W., and Pimm, M. V. (1977): Immunological aspects of metastasis. In: *The Secondary Spread of Cancer,* edited by R. W. Baldwin. Academic Press, New York (*in press*).

2. Bogden, A. E., Esber, H. J., Taylor, D. J., and Gray, J. H. (1974): Comparative study on the effects of surgery, chemotherapy, and immunotherapy, alone and in combination, on metastasis of the 13762 mammary adenocarcinoma. *Cancer Res.,* 34:1627–1631.
3. Eccles, S. A., and Alexander, P. (1974): Macrophage content of tumors in relation to metastatic spread and host immune reaction. *Nature,* 250:667–669.
4. Ferruti, P., Danusso, F., Franchi, G., Polentarutti, N., and Garattini, S. (1973): Effects of a series of new synthetic high polymers on cancer metastases. *J. Med. Chem.,* 16:496–499.
5. Garattini, S., and Franchi, G. (Eds.) (1973): *Chemotherapy of Cancer Dissemination and Metastasis.* Raven Press, New York.
6. Hellmann, K., and Burrage, K. (1969): Control of malignant metastases by ICRF 159. *Nature,* 224:273–275.
7. Hersey, P. (1973): New look at antiserum therapy of leukaemia. *Nature [New Biol.],* 244:22–24.
8. Larsen, B. (1973): Tumor toxic effect of polybases depending on molecular size. In: *Chemotherapy of Cancer Dissemination and Metastasis,* edited by S. Garattini and G. Franchi, pp. 235–243. Raven Press, New York.
9. Mantovani, A., Tagliabue, A., Vecchi, A., and Spreafico, F. (1976): Effect of "Corynebacterium parvum" on cellular and humoral antitumoral immune effector mechanisms. *Eur. J. Cancer,* 12:113–123.
10. Mantovani, A., Tagliabue, A., Vecchi, A., and Spreafico, F. (1976): Effects of adriamycin and daunomycin on spleen cell populations in normal and tumor allografted mice. *Eur. J. Cancer,* 12:381–387.
11. Martin, D. S., Hayworth, P. E., and Fugmann, R. A. (1970): Enhanced cures of spontaneous murine mammary tumors with surgery, combination chemotherapy and immunotherapy. *Cancer Res.,* 30:709–716.
12. Moroson, H. (1971): Polycation-treated tumor cells "in vivo" and "in vitro." *Cancer Res.,* 31:373–380.
13. Moroson, H. (1973): Tumor growth inhibiting effects of the polycations PEI, PPI and PVA. In: *Chemotherapy of Cancer Dissemination and Metastasis,* edited by S. Garattini and G. Franchi, pp. 245–252. Raven Press, New York.
14. Norrby, K. (1973): Effect of heparin on cell proliferation and kinetics "in vitro." An outline of a drug-testing scheme. In: *Chemotherapy of Cancer Dissemination and Metastasis,* edited by S. Garattini and G. Franchi, pp. 269–277. Raven Press, New York.
15. Schabel, F. M., Jr. (1975): Concepts for systemic treatment of micrometastases. *Cancer,* 35:15–24.
16. Spreafico, F., and Anaclerio, A. (1977): Immunosuppressive agents. In: *Immunopharmacology,* edited by J. W. Hadden, R. G. Coffey, and F. Spreafico. Raven Press, New York *(in press).*
17. Spreafico, F., and Garattini, S. (1974): Selective antimetastatic treatment—current status and future prospects. *Cancer Treatment Rev.,* 1:239–250.
18. Spreafico, F., and Garattini, S. (1977): Principles of the chemotherapy of metastases. In: *The Secondary Spread of Cancer,* edited by R. W. Baldwin. Academic Press, New York *(in press).*
19. Tagliabue, A., Polentarutti, N., Vecchi, A., Mantovani, A., and Spreafico, F. (1977): Combination chemoimmunotherapy with adriamycin in experimental tumor systems. *Eur. J. Cancer (in press).*
20. Tarin, D. (1976): Cellular interactions in neoplasia. In: *Fundamental Aspects of Metastasis,* edited by L. Weiss, pp. 151–190. North Holland, Amsterdam.
21. Thompson, R. B., Alberola, V., and Mathé, G. (1972): Evaluation of surgery, chemotherapy and immunotherapy on Lewis lung tumour. *Rev. Eur. Etud. Clin. Biol.,* 17:900–902.
22. Thorling, E. B., and Larsen, B. (1969): Inhibition effect of DEAE-dextran on tumour growth. (2). A). Effect of DEAE-dextran in vivo on the transplantable ascites tumour JBI in C3H/A mice. B). Action of dextran sulphate administered after inoculation of DEAE-dextran inhibited tumour cells. *Acta Pathol. Microbiol. Scand.,* 75:237–246.
23. Van Bekkum, D. W., and Ross, W. M. (1973): Mobilization of normal and malignant cells by polymethacrylic acid and other polyanions. In: *Chemotherapy of Cancer Dissemination*

and Metastasis, edited by S. Garattini and G. Franchi, pp. 195–204. Raven Press, New York.

24. Wood, G. W., and Gillespie, G. Y. (1975): Studies on the role of macrophages in regulation of growth and metastasis of murine chemically induced fibrosarcomas. *Int. J. Cancer,* 16:1022–1029.

25. Zighelboim, J., Bonavida, B., and Fahey, J. L. (1974): Antibody-mediated in vivo suppression of EL4 leukemia in a syngeneic host. *J. Natl. Cancer Inst.,* 52:879–881.

Cancer Invasion and Metastasis: Biologic
Mechanisms and Therapy, edited by S. B. Day
et al. Raven Press, New York © 1977.

Inhibitory Effect of a Primary Tumor on Metastasis

*Everett V. Sugarbaker, †Jerry Thornthwaite, and
†Alfred S. Ketcham

*·†Division of Oncology, Department of Surgery, University of Miami School of
Medicine, Miami, Florida 33152; and *Veterans Administration Research Hospital,
Miami, Florida 33152

Many locally advanced human cancers are resected for apparent "cure" after the usual systemic work-up for metastases proves negative. However, explosive metastatic recurrence after such resection for advanced disease is not an uncommon clinical observation. Figure 1 illustrates this type of systemic disease explosion after wide excision and grafting of an apparently localized malignant melanoma of the scalp. In other patients palliative or partial tumor resection is sometimes followed by accelerated metastatic disease progression. Upon observation of such patients, questions invariably arise as to the biologic mechanisms involved. The theoretic considerations include possible stimulation of systemic micrometastases by surgical trauma and stress, the immunosuppressive effects of surgery and/or anesthesia, blood hypercoagulability induced by surgery, mechanical dissemination of tumor by the surgical procedure, and possible release of an inhibitory effect which the primary tumor has over disseminated tumor cells (23). Although explanations for a given clinical observation may well include all of the above possibilities, a significant body of evidence supports at least involvement of the latter mechanism.

As a background for further studies, it seems relevant to review the data related to this putative inhibitory effect of a primary tumor on metastases. The mechanism of such an inhibitory effect on metastases might be a therapeutically exploitable mechanism in tumor biology and possibly useful as an adjuvant to surgical resection. This chapter will attempt three things. First, we will examine the experimental evidence related to the inhibitory effect of a primary tumor on metastases. Second, we will review parallel experimental observations demonstrating an inhibitory effect of an established tumor on other implanted tumors or on itself. Likewise, an inhibitory effect on tumor cell growth is apparent in expanding ascites or tissue culture

227

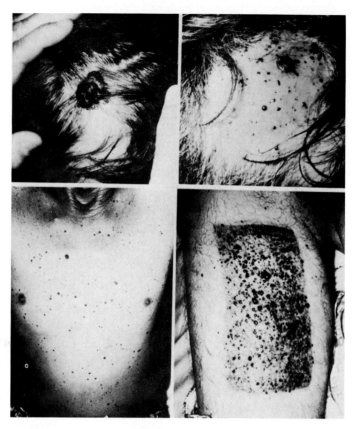

FIG. 1. This 26-year-old male presented with an invasive malignant melanoma of the scalp. The disease was clinically localized and evaluation revealed no disseminated metastases. A wide excision and graft was performed. Six weeks postoperatively, numerous subcutaneous nodules as well as visceral metastases appeared. Notably, metastases were concentrated beneath the donor site of his skin graft. Such a clinical observation suggests an inhibitory influence of the primary tumor on disseminated tumor cells.

tumor populations. These parallel observations suggest that an inhibitory effect of a primary on metastases is a generalized phenomenon, related to the total systemic tumor mass. Third, we will review the possible mechanisms for this type of tumor inhibition.

EXPERIMENTAL DATA DEMONSTRATING INHIBITORY EFFECT OF THE PRIMARY TUMOR ON METASTASIS

The process of metastasis is a complex, multifaceted event as is apparent from recent reviews of this subject (23). In briefest description, tumor cells (a) enter a vascular conduit, (b) circulate to a distant organ, and (c) become arrested, migrate outside the vascular conduit, and initiate a new focus of tumor growth—a metastasis. The inhibitory effect of a primary tumor on metastasis can be demonstrated only after steps a and b have occurred. Therefore, the central focus of this chapter is on factors controlling the growth of disseminated tumor rather than on the events which initiated the metastasis.

Early Observations

Some of the earliest observations in experimental tumor biology relate to factors controlling metastatic tumor dissemination. In 1910 Clunet (quoted by Tyzzer) (27) compared the incidence of spontaneous metastasis in mice dying of a transplanted primary tumor to that in mice undergoing surgical resection of the primary. Few metastases were observed with an intact primary, but resected mice had many metastases. However, survival time was prolonged in mice having surgical resection possibly contributing to the results. Tyzzer (27) queried: "In patients in which metastasis has already occurred will the growth of secondary masses be accelerated by the removal of primary tumors. . . . Do . . . surgical operations increase or diminish the incidence of metastases?"

In studies of tumor metastasis in a transplantable murine tumor system, Tyzzer showed that the size of the primary, surgical trauma (massage), and survival duration all influenced pulmonary metastasis. He designed experiments controlling these variables and clearly demonstrated that partial or complete removal of the primary tumor, after metastases had occurred, resulted in much larger pulmonary metastases than if the primary remained intact. Tyzzer (27) believed that the better nutritional status of the tumor-amputated mice versus the cachexia of tumor-bearing mice explained these results. Alternatively stated, the primary inhibited the growth of metastases by consuming most of the nutritional foodstuffs. In 1924 Tadenuma and Okonogi (24) also demonstrated increased size of metastases after partial excision of the primary tumor. None of these studies, however, used controls for the effects of surgical trauma or anesthesia. In 1948 Kaplan and Murphy (12) demonstrated an increase in experimental metastasis after partial or complete irradiation of the primary tumor.

More Recent Studies

Schatten (20) later explored this subject in carefully controlled experiments. Using the DBA sarcoma 49 and the S91 Cloudman melanoma, he inoculated mice with a standard tumor dose. Twenty-one days later tumors reached 1.5 cm size, a size known to produce pulmonary metastases. Mice were then divided into three equal groups: Tumors in group 1 were amputated by using atraumatic technique, and a venous tourniquet was employed to prevent systemic escape of tumor cells. No anesthesia was used. Tumors in group 2 remained intact. Group 3 tumors remained intact and the non-tumor-bearing leg was amputated as a control for surgical trauma.

Twenty-one days later (42 days after initial primary tumor inoculation as the tumor-bearing mice began to die) all mice were sacrificed, lungs examined for numbers of metastases, and metastasis sized by comparison to measured standards. The striking finding was the significant increase in size of the metastases in tumor-amputated mice compared to tumor-bearing mice. Amputation of the non-tumor-bearing leg had no effect on size or numbers of metastases (Fig. 2). Schatten (20) also noted increased numbers of metastases from the DBA-49 sarcoma in amputated mice. However, as has been pointed out subsequently (13–15), this result was probably an artifact of the direct visual examination of the lung for metastases. When special methods are used to produce contrast between the metastases and adjacent normal pulmonary parenchyma, very small metastases are identified. This conclusion is supported by the lack of a significant increase in numbers of metastases after amputation of the S91 melanoma in his study (20). In this tumor system "contrast" for identification is provided by the black pigmented metastases themselves. Many other investigations, although confirming the increased size of metastases after tumor ablation, have not demonstrated any increase in numbers of metastases (12–15,21,28).

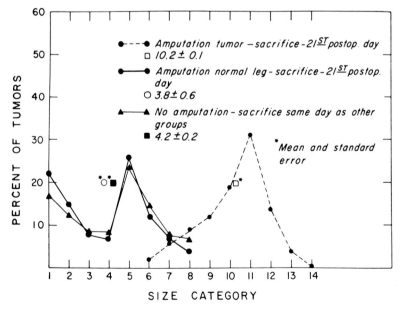

FIG. 2. Amputation of the S91 melanoma released an inhibitory influence of the primary tumor on metastases. As is demonstrated, metastatic size 21 days after amputation was significantly increased in amputated vs tumor-bearing mice. [Taken from Schatten (20); reproduced with permission of author and publisher.]

In subsequent experiments, Schatten (20) sacrificed groups of S91 melanoma-bearing and tumor-amputated mice at two intervals, 21 and 28 days after amputation. The metastases in tumor-amputated mice showed progressive enlargement during this 7-day period while metastases in tumor-bearing mice remained static in size although increasing in number (Fig. 3). Ketcham et al. (13,14) more extensively studied the progressive growth of established metastases in tumor-amputated mice versus the static size (while they were increasing in numbers) of metastases in tumor-bearing mice. Studies in five spontaneously metastasizing murine tumor systems all confirmed the larger size of pulmonary metastases in tumor-amputated versus tumor-bearing mice and the more rapid growth of established metastases after amputation of the primary (Fig. 4). Kinsey (15), likewise, added additional confirmatory data, as did Lewis and Cole (18), although appropriate controls for surgical trauma are lacking in the latter report. In all studies in spontaneously metastasizing murine tumor systems definitive acceleration of the growth rate of established pulmonary metastases occurred after surgical resection of the primary tumor. Schatten (20) and

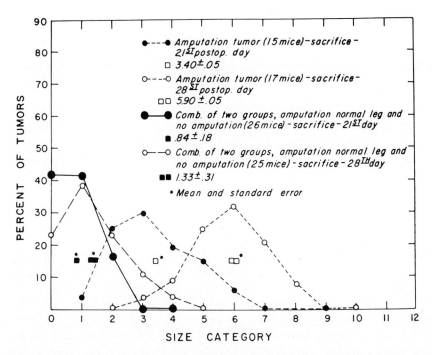

FIG. 3. As taken from Schatten (20), amputation of S91 melanoma-bearing mice was performed at two intervals and comparisons made with tumor-bearing mice. The established metastases in tumor-bearing mice remained static in size while a rapid progressive growth was noted in amputated mice. (Reproduced with permission of author and publisher.)

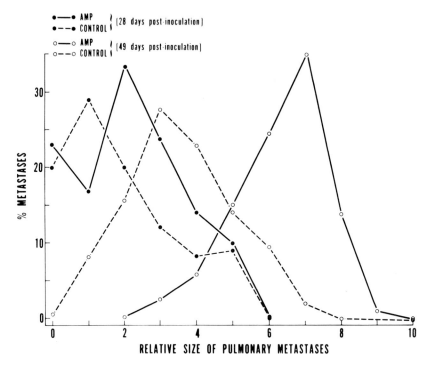

FIG. 4. Additional confirmation of progressive growth of pulmonary metastases in amputated vs tumor-bearing mice in the S91 melanoma system. [Taken from data presented by Ketcham et al. (13).]

Ketcham et al. (13,14) hypothesized the presence of an inhibitory effect of the primary tumor on the growth of metastases.

Another graphic example of the inhibitory effect of a primary tumor on metastases is found in the work of Greene and Harvey (10). Their studies utilized a lymphoblastic hamster lymphoma which only rarely spontaneously metastasized before death caused by the primary tumor. Despite the rarity of gross metastases, bioassays of the blood and most organs demonstrated the presence of viable circulating tumor cells by 7 days after tumor inoculation. Importantly, if the primary was excised 7 or more days after inoculation, i.e., after these viable tumor cells began to enter the circulation, diffuse gross metastases occurred. Operative stress, tumor manipulation, tumor incision, and time of observation were all excluded as the cause of these experimental observations. Additionally, the connective tissue stroma of the tumor-bearing host would not react to disseminated tumor cells, thus the tumor cells remained dormant until the primary was removed. Greene and Harvey (10) theorized that the inhibitory effect of the primary tumor on metastases was mediated through an inhibitory effect on host stromal tissues. Similarly, Van den Brenk and Sharpington (28) showed that irradia-

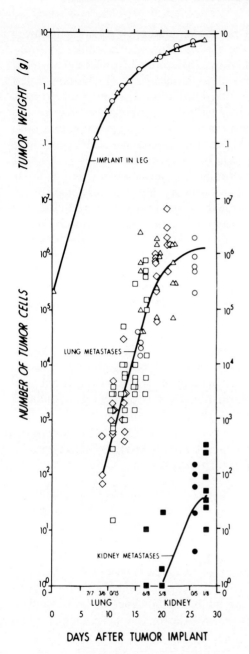

FIG. 5. Using a quantitative bioassay technique, DeWys (6) noted a synchronous slowing of metastases in lung and kidney with the primary tumor (as measured by serial tumor diameters). (Reproduced with permission of author and publisher.)

tion ablation of the primary p388 rat sarcoma stopped additional cancer cell dissemination, but stimulated the growth of metastases already established in regional lymph nodes and lungs. Sheldon and Fowler (21) using a spontaneously metastasizing murine lymphosarcoma also demonstrated that nodal metastatic rate was faster after irradiation ablation of the primary tumor. DeWys (6,7) has extensively studied this inhibitory effect of the primary on metastasis using the early metastasizing, aggressive, and non-immunogenic Lewis lung carcinoma. He used a bioassay technique which quantitated the number of tumor cells present in metastases in lung or kidney. The growth of the primary tumor was measured by serial tumor diameters. Early after implantation the primary and its early metastases grew exponentially. Later, as the growth of the primary slowed, a nearly synchronous slowing of the growth in metastases was demonstrated (Fig. 5).

In all these studies, the common observation is that the growth rate of disseminated tumor cells is stimulated by the surgical removal or irradiation ablation of the primary tumor. The converse of this statement generates the hypothesis that the primary tumor has an inhibitory influence on disseminated tumor cells. The relative strength of this putative inhibitory influence would seem to vary from tumor system to tumor system and with the volume of tumor present (10). In the studies reported by Ketcham et al. (13,14), Kinsey (15), Schatten (20), and Van den Brenk and Sharpington (28), apparently the inhibition pertained only to established metastases for no increased numbers of metastases were demonstrated. However, in the system studied by Greene et al. (10), dormant cells were apparently stimulated to macroscopic growth after removal of the primary tumor.

OTHER PARALLEL OBSERVATIONS OF TUMOR INHIBITION OF TUMOR GROWTH

Other observations in tumor biology suggest that the inhibitory influence of a primary tumor on metastasis is not necessarily a property of the primary-metastases axis, but more likely a generalized inhibitory influence of expanding tumor mass on itself. These parallel observations have demonstrated: (a) the inhibitory influence of one transplanted tumor on a second tumor transplant; (b) the inhibitory influence of metastases, when they develop from small primary tumors with great biologic aggressiveness, on the growth rate of a primary tumor; and (c) the inhibitory influence of an expanding solid tumor mass on its own growth, and the inhibitory influence of an expanding ascites or tissue culture population of tumor cells on itself.

Inhibitory Influence of a Primary Tumor on a Second Tumor Transplant

Tyzzer (27) studied this phenomenon. Mice were inoculated with tumor. Thirty-one days later, mice were divided into two groups. The first had most of the tumor excised. In the second group, this tumor was undisturbed. On the same day, second tumors were inoculated at distant sites into mice of both groups. Forty-nine days later, both groups were killed and the second tumor transplants excised and weighed. The second implants in mice with partial excision weighed nearly two times those with the initial tumor intact. Goodman (9) also specifically studied the effect of an established tumor on the growth rate of a second transplant. He reported a size-dependent inhibition of the second transplant growth rate by the first. Final total tumor mass at death was the same regardless of whether the animal bore one or two tumors. These findings might also be explained by concomitant tumor immunity (5) as this aspect of tumor growth was not studied in Goodman's report. However, DeWys (6), using the nonimmunogenic Lewis lung carcinoma in C57 BL/6 mice, also investigated the effect of a growing tumor on a second tumor implant. The first tumor was initiated by inoculation of 2×10^5 cells. Eight and fifteen days later, a second inoculation of 2×10^5 cells was made into the opposite leg. Using a bioassay technique which quantitated the number of cells present, DeWys found that the growth rates during the preclinical and the palpable range of tumor growth were inhibited by the established growing tumor. Amputation of the first tumor resulted in the reversal of this inhibition and rapid increase in the number of cells. Goodman's (9) studies likewise demonstrated that the smaller second tumor implant influences the growth rate of the established larger tumor.

Inhibition of Primary Growth by Development of Early Metastases

If a second tumor implant can slow the growth rate of the primary, it would readily seem possible for metastases to have the same effect in slowing primary growth rate. Yuhas and Pazmiño (29) have in fact studied the effect of artificial metastases (i.e., inoculations of tumor cell suspensions) in slowing the growth rate of the primary tumor. Using an alveolar cell carcinoma in Balb/C mice, they injected live or dead tumor cells intravenously at the same time as subcutaneous tumor inoculation. Twenty-one days later, the subcutaneous tumors in mice with the artificially produced metastases were significantly smaller than controls or those injected with dead tumor cells. Other data from this series of experiments showed early spontaneous metastasis and smaller primary tumors after an immunosuppressive dose of total body radiation. They concluded that the large volume of pulmonary metastasis caused by the immunosuppressive effects of total body irradiation inhibited the growth of the primary tumor.

Inhibitory Effect of an Expanding Solid Tumor, an Ascites Tumor, or a Tumor Tissue Culture Population on Itself

Other parallel observations in tumor biology have established an inhibitory effect of increasing tumor mass on itself. This effect is apparent in a growing solid tumor or ascites cell population. The grossly measured growth rate of solid tumors in animals is best described by the gompertzian equation.

Simply stated, this equation demonstrates an exponential slowing of tumor growth rate with increasing tumor size (16).

Kinetic studies have established a progressive decrease in the thymidine labeling index of solid tumors with increasing tumor size. Using the Lewis lung carcinoma, Simpson-Herren et al. (22) demonstrated a steady decline in mean tritiated-labeling index from 50 to 33 to 11% in 5, 21, and 31 days post-tumor implant. The cell cycle time (T_c) showed only a minor increase over this period from $T_c = 22$ hr at 5 days to 26 hr at 21 days. Frindel et al. (8) likewise have documented the slowing of a grossly measured solid tumor growth rate in an experimental fibrosarcoma of C3H mice. They also studied tumor cell kinetics using autoradiographic methods. With progressive tumor growth the proportion of cells engaged in the cell cycle (growth fraction) diminished. T_c was relatively unchanged. Therefore, the exponential slowing was explained by a diminished growth fraction and possibly increased cell death. Transplantation of small pieces of large tumors to normal animals reverses this growth retardation and rapid growth proceeds until large tumor volumes are again attained (7). The strength of this tumor inhibition is proportional to tumor mass as empirically observed and as predicted by the gompertz equation (7,8). Parallel studies of growth of this fibrosarcoma in tissue culture gave identical results, that is, constancy in T_c with progressive decrease in the growth fraction with increasing cell population (8).

Many observations in several ascites tumor systems have likewise documented a diminished growth fraction as total cell mass increased (2,3,8,11). The gompertzian equation also describes this retardation in ascites systems (2,3,11). Kinetically, this retardation of growth has been shown due to a diminished growth fraction (more cells in G_1-G_0) and to a lesser extent by lengthening of T_c (3,11).

Summary on Inhibitory Interactions of Tumor Masses One on Another

As reviewed, the evidence supporting an inhibitory influence of a primary tumor on the growth of metastasis is significant and compelling. However, the other observations reviewed above suggest that this phenomenon is one manifestation of a more generalized phenomenon in tumor biology (Table 1), i.e., an inhibitory influence of an expanding total tumor mass on itself. Other manifestations of this phenomenon include the inhibitory influence of one tumor mass on a second tumor implant (6,9,27), the inhibitory influence of early-appearing metastases on the primary tumor growth (28), the inhibitory influence of a primary tumor on itself (6,8,16,17), and the inhibitory influence of an ascites cell or tissue culture population on further growth (2,3,8,11). This phenomenon would, therefore, seem to be a negative feedback mechanism in otherwise "uncontrolled" tumor growth. As demonstrated, the intensity or strength of this negative feedback mechanism increases with expanding tumor mass.

TABLE 1. *Demonstrated inhibitory effect of total tumor mass*

1. Primary solid tumor on itself.
2. Primary tumor on metastases.
3. Primary tumor implant on second implant.
4. Second implant on primary tumor implant.
5. Metastases on primary tumor.
6. Ascites cell population on itself.
7. Tissue culture population on itself.
8. Primary tumor on host tissues?
   Host cachexia ↓ body weight.

POSSIBLE MECHANISMS OF THE INHIBITORY EFFECTS ON TUMOR GROWTH

Local Inhibitory Factors

Although internal autoregulation or inhibition is a possible explanation for the gompertzian growth of solid primary tumors, a systemic effect must be hypothesized for observations in categories 2 through 8 in Table 1. Both local and systemic mechanisms may be important in solid tumors for it has been demonstrated that the distance from effective capillary perfusion affects the labeling index, growth fraction, and development of histologic necrosis in solid tumors (25,26). Therefore, distance from arterially supplied nutrition clearly is important in primary solid tumor biology. It is also possible that systemic effects may be elaborated once necrosis or anoxia develops at one focus of tumor growth.

Systemic Inhibitory Mechanisms

Immunologic and nutritional mechanisms are unlikely explanations. Despite the probability that local nutrition, perfusion, and Po_2 gradients affect solid tumor growth, local inhibitory mechanisms clearly cannot explain the systemic effects apparently active in phenomena 2 through 8 in Table 1, the intensity of which increases with expanding total tumor mass. Since concomitant tumor immunity disappears at the upper limits of tumor mass (5), a stage of tumor growth in which the inhibitory effect on growth is maximally expressed, and since such inhibitory influences are obvious in nonimmunogenic tumor systems such as the Lewis lung carcinoma (6,7), tumor-specific immunologic reactions could not play a critical role. Total body competition for nutrition, an application of the theory of athrepsia (1), was suggested by Tyzzer (27) to explain his observations. However, as has been emphasized by Laird (16), the gradual decline in growth rate is totally different from the abrupt cessation of cell division observed when an *E. coli* culture expends essential nutrients. Additionally, in studies of expanding ascites cell populations, Harris et al. (11) have correlated cyclic AMP concentration and lactic dehydrogenase (LDH) concentration during the transition from aerobic to anaerobic growth conditions. Although LDH increases greatly as Po_2 falls and the thymidine labeling index (of the growth fraction) falls as this transition to anaerobic growth occurs, there is no change in intracellular AMP concentrations. These data suggest that the energy substrate is not insufficient as ascites cell growth slows, and mechanisms other than nutritional deficiencies must be found.

Systemic Mitotic Inhibitors: Specific (Chalones) and Nonspecific

DeWys (6,7) hypothesized the presence of a nonspecific systemic inhibitor of tumor growth which also might have an inhibitory effect on host tissues, explaining the host cachexia observed with advanced tumor growth. Bullough (4) has demonstrated the presence of tissue-specific mitotic inhibitors (chalones) in neoplastic tissues. Based on his findings, he concludes that tumors produce chalones as do normal tissues, but that these substances readily leak into the systemic circulation. Therefore, only a low intracellular tumor concentration of chalones develops. His theory states that as a tumor grows, secreting large amounts of chalones into the systemic circulation, an inhibitory systemic concentration eventually develops which retards the primary growth rate and produces the effect documented in Table 1. Specificity is the key difference in his hypothesis from that of DeWys, for chalones by definition are tissue specific.

Mitotic inhibitors have been studied in expanding ascites cell populations by Bichel et al. (3). These investigators found that ultrafiltrate ($< 50,000$ daltons) of ascites fluid from plateau-phase ascites tumor temporarily arrested the growth of tumor cells at the G_1-S border of the cell cycle. Contradictory data and an alternate mechanism, however, have been proposed by Harris et al. (11). In studies of ascites cell populations, specific tumor inhibitors could not be demonstrated; however, only crude ascites fluid was used for testing. Importantly, they showed a sharp increase in ornithine decarboxylase (ODC) just before tumor cells enter S phase. They hypothesized that this enzyme through its effect on polyamine synthesis may be important in directing cellular traffic from G_0-G_1 into S phase. Therefore, another possible mechanism includes changes in concentration of polyamines, substances shown to be important in the growth of other cell systems (19). Studies employing newly developed flow microfluorometric (FMF) techniques due to their ease, accuracy, and rapidity should enable prompt resolution of these apparently conflicting theories regarding mechanisms and allow better quantitative delineation of "inhibitor strength."

THERAPEUTIC IMPLICATIONS OF MITOTIC INHIBITION

Adjuvant chemotherapy attempts to exploit quantitative differences between the kinetics of a primary tumor and that of micrometastases, i.e., the greater growth fraction of these small systemic deposits. Importantly, the above discussion indicates that the bulky primary tumor must be removed before such a differential in growth fraction becomes apparent. Secondly, if such inhibitors could be extracted or produced in sufficient quantity, they might be utilizable as adjuvants to immunotherapy. In this application, these mitotic inhibitors might arrest tumor cell division. This use would enable host defenses to overcome the overwhelming kinetic advantage often cited as the reason for failure of host reactivity to eradicate a neoplastic disease process.

SUMMARY

In human and many experimental tumor systems, metastasis is a function of tumor size and the time of tumor growth. Once viable tumor cells are present in the circulation and reach distant organs, the data reviewed suggest that the primary tumor can exert an inhibitory influence on metastases. Other parallel observations indicate that a tumor exhibits an inhibitory effect on a second tumor transplant, that metastases can inhibit a primary tumor if they reach significant proportions early in the disease course, and that expanding tumor populations of solid tumors, ascites tumors, or tissue culture systems inhibit further growth.

In some tumor systems, the strength of this inhibition results in dormancy of metastasis as has been described by Greene (10). In others, the growth rate of established metastases is impaired (7,13–15). It is conceivable that in other systems yet to be studied, such inhibitory influences will not be found. With removal of the primary tumor, an accelerated growth is observed in experimental metastatic foci, and this observation may explain the explosive postoperative metastases sometimes seen by the clinician. The obvious therapeutic implication of these findings is that large primary tumors may have to be removed before the higher growth fraction of micrometastases can be exploited by adjuvant chemotherapy. Several mechanisms for tumor inhibition, including nonspecific systemic mitotic inhibitors, tumor chalones, and polyamine metabolism, have been discussed. Additional studies using FMF techniques should allow rapid and quantitative study of this important phenomenon.

ACKNOWLEDGMENT

This work was supported in part by a Faculty Fellowship to one author (E.V.S.) (JFCF #373) from the American Cancer Society and by the Comprehensive Cancer Center of the state of Florida, CCC grant #NCI CA14395 and 1PO1CA-1932101.

REFERENCES

1. Apolant, H. (1911): The question of athrepsia. *J. Exp. Med.*, 3:316–321.
2. Baserga, R. (1965): The relationship of the cell cycles to tumor growth and control of cell division: A review. *Cancer Res.*, 25:581–595.
3. Bichel, P., Barfod, N. M., and Jakobsen, A. (1975): Employment of synchronized cells

and flow microfluorometry in investigations on the JB-1 tumour chalones. *Virchows Arch.* [*Zellpathol.*], 19:127–133.
4. Bullough, W. S. (1975): Mitotic control in adult mammalian tissue. *Biol. Rev.,* 50:99–127.
5. Deckers, P. J., Pardridge, D. H., Wang, B. S., and Mannick, J. A. (1976): The specificity of concomitant immunity at large tumor volumes. *Cancer Res.,* 36:3690–3694.
6. DeWys, W. D. (1972): Studies correlating the growth rate of a tumor and its metastases and providing evidence for tumor-related systemic growth-retarding factors. *Cancer Res.,* 32:374–379.
7. DeWys, W. D. (1972): A quantitative model for the study of the growth and treatment of a tumor and its metastases with correlation between proliferative state and sensitivity to cyclophosphamide. *Cancer Res.,* 32:367–373.
8. Frindel, E., Malaise, E. P., Alpen, E., and Tubiana, M. (1967): Kinetics of cell proliferation of an experimental tumor. *Cancer Res.,* 27:1122–1131.
9. Goodman, G. J. (1957): Effects of one tumor upon the growth of another. *Proc. Am. Assoc. Cancer Res.,* 2:207.
10. Greene, H. S. N., and Harvey, E. K. (1960): The inhibitory influence of a transplanted hamster lymphoma on metastasis. *Cancer Res.,* 20:1094–1100.
11. Harris, J. W., Wong, Y. P., Kehe, C. R., and Teng, S. S. (1975): The role of adenosine triphosphate, chalones, and specific proteins in controlling tumor growth fraction. *Cancer Res.,* 35:3181–3186.
12. Kaplan, H. S., and Murphy, E. D. (1948): The effect of local roentgen irradiation on the biological behavior of a transplantable mouse carcinoma I. Increased frequency of pulmonary metastasis. *J. Natl. Cancer Inst.,* 407–413.
13. Ketcham, A. S., Kinsey, D. L., Wexler, H., and Mantel, N. (1961): The development of spontaneous metastases after the removal of a primary tumor. *Cancer,* 14:875–881.
14. Ketcham, A. S., Wexler, H., and Mantel, N. (1959): The effect of removal of a "primary" tumor on the development of spontaneous metastases. I. Development of a standardized experimental technique. *Cancer Res.,* 19:940–944.
15. Kinsey, D. L. (1961): Effects of surgery upon cancer metastasis. *J.A.M.A.,* 178:734–735.
16. Laird, A. K. (1964): Dynamics of tumor growth. *Br. J. Cancer,* 18:490–502.
17. Lala, P. K., and Patt. H. M. (1968): A characterization of the boundary between cycling and resting states in ascites tumor cells. *Cell Tissue Kinet.,* 1:137–146.
18. Lewis, M. R., and Cole. W. H. (1958): Experimental increase of lung metastases after operative trauma. *Arch. Surg.,* 77:621–626.
19. Russell, D. H., and Stambrook, P. J. (1975): Cell cycle specific fluctuations in adenosine 3'5'-cyclic monophosphate and polyamines of Chinese hamster cells. *Proc. Natl. Acad. Sci. U.S.A.,* 72:1482–1486.
20. Schatten, W. E. (1958): An experimental study of postoperative tumor metastases. *Cancer,* 11:455–459.
21. Sheldon, P. W., and Fowler, J. F. (1973): The effect of irradiating a transplanted murine lymphosarcoma on the subsequent development of metastases. *Br. J. Cancer,* 28:508.
22. Simpson-Herren, L., Holmquist, J. P., and Sanford, A. H. (1973): Further studies of the population kinetics of primary and metastatic Lewis lung carcinoma in BDF mice. *Proc. Am. Assoc. Cancer Res.,* 14:27.
23. Sugarbaker, E. V., and Ketcham, A. S. (1977): Mechanism and prevention of cancer dissemination. *Semin. Oncol.* (*in press*).
24. Tadenuma, K., and Okonogi, S. (1924): Experimentelle Untersuchugen uber Metastasen bei Mausecarcinom. *Z. Krebsforsch.,* 21:168–172.
25. Tannok, I. F. (1968): The relation between cell proliferation and the vascular system in a transplanted mouse mammary tumor. *Br. J. Cancer,* 22:258–273.
26. Tomlinson, R. H., and Gray, L. H. (1955): The histologic structure of some human lung cancers and the possible implications for radiotherapy. *Br. J. Cancer,* 9:539–549.
27. Tyzzer, E. E. (1913): Factors in the production and growth of tumor metastases. *J. Med. Res.,* 28:309–332.
28. Van den Brenk, H. A. S., and Sharpington, C. (1971): Effect of local X-irradiation of a primary sarcoma in the rat on dissemination and growth of metastases: Dose-response characteristics. *Br. J. Cancer,* 25:812–830.
29. Yuhas, J. M., and Pazmiño, N. H. (1974): Inhibition of subcutaneously growing line 1 carcinomas due to metastatic spread. *Cancer Res.,* 34:2005–2010.

Cancer Invasion and Metastasis: Biologic
Mechanisms and Therapy, edited by S. B. Day
et al. Raven Press, New York © 1977.

Discussion Summary: Establishment
and Distribution of Metastasis

Martin G. Lewis

Cancer Unit, McGill University, Montreal, Quebec, Canada

In general terms, most of the speakers and discussants were faced with the same difficulty and problems, namely, an attempt to focus on the small aspects of what is clearly a complicated and dynamic interplay among many factors. Almost every speaker commented on this dilemma but quite rightly then had to attempt to focus attention on details, which was not always easy to interpret on the whole.

Some of the chapters addressed themselves to the problems of factors that determine how and where metastases occur with particular reference to organ specificity. One approach advocated by Nicolson was the use of cells with high and low metastatic rates, some of which then were shown to have particular specificity against different target organ sites, so that variants of the B_{16} melanoma could be chosen for lung specificity or brain specificity in their metastatic spread. This was further studied using a cell aggregation technique where aggregation of tumor cells to various cells of specific organs was noted to be related to the ability of the tumors to metastasize.

Warren pointed out that one of the most important factors was the adherence of tumor cells to the endothelium of blood vessels and that the types of blood vessels in the capillary beds differed so that nonfenestrated, fenestrated, and intercellular fenestrated varieties could be seen, and also that different types of fibrin were involved in the initial interaction between tumor cells, endothelium, and the coagulation system. Glaves pointed out that the ability of tumor cells derived from different tumor types to become arrested in different organs after intravenous injection might be affected by immunological factors.

The question of endothelial cells was brought up several times during the discussion. For instance, is the specificity leveled at the endothelial cell or the parenchymal cell of the organ concerned, and how does the status of the tumor-bearing animal in terms of immune reactions affect this?

There was also considerable discussion concerning the problems of identifying the distribution of tumor cells, particularly using labeled cells with the detachment of the label, and the subsequent recirculation or further spread of tumors having lodged in certain organ sites. The site of injection obviously became a critical point.

The question of selective pressures in the clonal differentiation of cells used in several of experiments was raised, particularly whether the *in vitro* and *in vivo* conditions would not in fact alter the ability of cells not only to grow but to adhere to endothelium and become metastatic; it became clear that the growth rate and metastatic rate of cells were not necessarily related.

There was some suggestion that although organ specificity may be important in the establishment of metastases, the situation of dormancy of tumor cells in particular organs might also be of considerable importance.

Further presentations emphasized the patterns of metastatic spread as reported by Robert Golbey, and clinical experience points toward a series of potential experimental situations; emphasis was placed on observing the situation in man and designing one's models appropriately. A sentiment echoed several times during the session was that although few animal models were appropriate, at least the best ones were based on the particular aspect of the human problem being studied. Bodansky then extensively reviewed the biochemical criteria that might be important in metastasis from the point of view of assessing the phenomenon. He concluded that although over the years numerous serum factors, metabolic products, and ectopic hormones have been studied, few gave reliable enough information to be of any great importance. It was clear that further or detailed analytical procedures were necessary, particularly in sequential studies.

Questions were raised as to the use of biochemical approaches in the diagnosis of cancer when the primary tumor is not known. Although numerous examples are available, none of them is 100% reliable. Spreafico summarized some of the approaches using chemotherapeutic agents and immune regulators in the control of metastases, pointing out that certain agents could selectively prevent metastatic spread without altering the growth of the primary tumor. In addition, he mentioned the drug Levamisole and its effect in combination with *Corynebacterium parvum* and other agents in being effective against experimental metastases.

Sugarbaker pointed out the sometimes explosive metastases that follow surgical excision in certain individuals. He developed the theme of the inhibitory effect of the primary tumor on metastatic spread, indicating that nutritional, blood supply, immunological, and humoral metastatic inhibitor effects may be relevant. However, it was pointed out during the discussion that this phenomenon was certainly not a uniform or reproducible one, since the opposite was seen in some tumor systems. The question of inhibitor substances released by the primary tumor versus inhibition of the macrometastases by a large growing tumor by means of nutritional competition was raised. The additional factor of relative immunogenicity of primary and secondary tumors in the systems studied was not known. It was clear, however, that the primary tumor can have profound effects on metastatic spread, but not necessarily in one particular direction, and that multiple factors were involved. The question finally centered on the speed with which metastasis may occur since it was pointed out that multiple showering of metastases may occur in some tumor systems. Warren estimated that it takes a week or more for tumor cells to go through the process of adherence to endothelium and become established metastases, whereas others mentioned that 1 to 2 days may be all that is necessary. It was clear that the different types of tumor vessel and fibrin interplay plus the many other factors considered, both in the coagulation system and in the immune system, may alter or modify the speed with which such tumor cells become established metastases.

In summary, therefore, a rather diverse approach to the mechanisms of metastasis formation resulted in discussion of a complicated series of mechanisms, more than one of which may interfere with the ability of the cancer cell to circumvent blood vasculature and establish independent existence. Once a metastasis has established itself in the extravascular tissues, other selective factors obviously determine whether the tumor cell will survive in that particular environment, remain dormant, or be completely destroyed.

Cancer Invasion and Metastasis: Biologic
Mechanisms and Therapy, edited by S. B. Day
et al. Raven Press, New York © 1977.

Humoral Immune Factors in Metastasis in Human Cancer

M. G. Lewis, T. M. Phillips, G. Rowden, and L. M. Jerry

McGill University Cancer Research Unit, Montreal, Quebec H3G 1Y6, Canada

REASONS FOR STUDYING HUMORAL IMMUNITY

There are numerous reasons for attempting to study the role of immunity in malignancy, and these have been extensively reviewed in recent years (12,18,35). In this chapter it is proposed to deliberately concentrate on the role of humoral immunity, including positive and negative aspects in relationship to two modes of metastatic spread in human tumors, namely, blood borne and via regional lymph nodes.

It is proposed first to briefly review some of the key reasons why one should look for humoral immune reactions under these circumstances and to give some rational basis for why these studies were initiated.

Natural History of Human Tumors

Many of the thoughts and ideas in the field of tumor immunology have been influenced and largely dominated by concepts evolved in studies of transplantation phenomena. Attention has therefore often been directed toward rejection of tumors as if they represented grafted tissues, so that tumor-specific transplantation antigens and T cell-mediated responses have been strongly emphasized.

Had parallels been sought, however, in the fields of infectious disease or host-parasite relationships, a somewhat different perspective viewpoint would have arisen. In these circumstances, organisms can be combatted by the host defenses both in the tissues and in the body fluids, particularly the bloodstream. In the latter the real danger to the whole being occurs, in that septicemia, viremia, and parasitemia are often lethal. Grafts do not metastasize, but dissemination of tumor cells—particularly through the bloodstream—makes cancer in most instances a killing disease.

Antibodies have been clearly shown to be of considerable importance in limiting blood-borne spread of infectious microorganisms, and it would be strange if similar relationships did not exist in malignancy.

Certain features during the evolution of cancer in man might suggest a role of antitumor antibody. In some human tumors the variations in the ability of tumors to progress in local areas yet disseminate with different degrees of intensity are well known (12). Perhaps one of the classic examples is the removal of an intraocular malignant melanoma with the appearance of widespread metastasis many years later, and at the time of removal of the eye no residual tumor was present in the orbit. Since the eye has no lymphatic drainage, the tumor cells must have been released into the circulation, which is their only route for dissemination.

Studies of malignant melanoma in Africa (26) clearly showed that a tumor could remain localized and yet still grow on the sole of the foot for months or years with no widespread dissemination. Yet other individuals with identical primary tumors had widespread metastasis in a matter of weeks or months. It seemed that the key to the difference in these individuals was the ability in one instance for the tumor to successfully disseminate through the blood vessel, whereas in the other it remained localized for long periods of time. In both instances, however, the primary tumors continued to grow, and therefore it seemed reasonable to search for a cause for these differences in the bloodstream and look for circulating antibodies (21).

Circulating Cancer Cells

Perhaps one of the best reasons for investigating circulating antibody is the potential role played by circulating cancer cells in patients with malignancy. The concept that malignancy may spread by disseminating individual cells through the bloodstream was argued eloquently by Virchow in lectures given in 1858 (51), and since that time this theory has been investigated extensively (11,44). Some of the most elegant experiments of Sumner Wood (56,58) resulted in a clear statement that the ability of tumor cells to survive in the bloodstream and adhere to the endothelium of blood vessels was the prerequisite for successful metastasis. This has subsequently been discussed in fuller detail by others (54).

White and Griffiths (55), in a recent review of extensive studies carried out by these authors, also point to some interesting and apparently paradoxical relationships between circulating tumor cells and subsequent behavior of the tumor as judged by prognosis. In a series of 62 patients with colonic carcinoma, the best 10-year survivals (58%) were seen in those in which it was easy to detect circulating tumor cells after operation. The group with the worst 10-year survival figure (30%) showed few or no free circulating tumor cells. The explanation suggested was that in the first group, cells failed to adhere to the vascular endothelium and were therefore seen free in the circulation, whereas in the second group adherence of tumor cells was rapid. White and Griffiths (55) relate their findings to the importance of the fibrinolytic system in metastasis (55). One could, however, equally argue a role for antibody in preventing adherence of circulating tumor cells to the endothelium in the first instance, thus preventing the initial and probably critical phase of metastasis formation.

ADDITIONAL REASONS FOR STUDYING HUMORAL IMMUNITY IN PATIENTS WITH MALIGNANT TUMORS

Studies of humoral immunity, even if they do not answer the immediate problem of metastasis, are likely to result in the better understanding of the whole interplay between the immune system and the tumor. Evidence will also be presented to show the usefulness of such studies in terms of determining factors responsible for derangements in malignancy which might point to some of the reasons why the immune system fails to control metastatic dissemination of tumors. This discussion is divided, therefore, into three sections: (a) identification of and evidence suggesting that antitumor antibodies may have a positive role in the control of blood-borne metastasis; (b) evidence that antibodies directed against different tumor antigens of the same tumor may have opposite functions in regional lymph node metastasis; (c) discussion of the role played by both positive and negative aspects of humoral immunity in immune derangement as a central phenomenon in the underlying failure of control of metastatic spread.

Antitumor Antibodies

Using a multitude of methods, many investigators have reported the presence of antibody directed against human tumor antigens, and this has been extensively reviewed elsewhere (4,22,23,35). This section will concentrate on studies which distinguish different antibody responses against distinct components of the tumor cells in the same individual. The original serum factor detected in our studies of malignant melanoma was shown to be a complement-dependent cytotoxic antibody (21,25). This was first described in an attempt to explain the difference in behavior of melanoma in Ugandans. Serum plus complement from patients with localized tumors prevented the adherence of autologous tumor cells to glass coverslips, whereas serum from patients with rapidly disseminated disease had no such effect when it was tested against their own or other tumor cells. The antibody appeared to be individually specific, that is, not cross-reacting with the cells of other patients, and had as its main effect the prevention of adhesion of tumor cells to glass coverslips in Pulvertaft culture chambers (14). If the cells were attached in advance to the coverslips, the antibody had little or no effect, suggesting it is not a conventional cytotoxic or cytolytic antibody.

Subsequent studies by immunofluorescence using the same sera showed that the antibody was an IgG in most instances and it could produce discrete surface fluorescence. Once again, the pattern was noted predominantly in autologous situations in that this was seen more often and at higher titers in autologous rather than allogeneic sera (25,29,37–39). In recent unpublished observations, we have also demonstrated that the antibody can alter the adherence of tumor cells to endothelial cells. In attempts to further define the effects of antibody on tumor cell adherence, we performed the following experiments.

A goat was immunized with an established melanoma cell line (designated M40) and an antiserum produced which was absorbed with a variety of normal human tissues and unrelated tumors. This antiserum, normal goat serum (preimmunized serum from the same goat), and human AB serum as a source of complement were tested against the M40 cell line in Pulvertaft culture chambers (43). The various sera, complement, and media were added to the melanoma cells and then the mixture added to the chambers and coverslips placed on top. The rings were then placed coverslip down and incubated at 37°C for 48 hr, and subsequently placed coverslip upwards and examined for adherence of cells to the coverslip surface. The procedures and results are diagrammatically represented in Fig. 1. The coverslips were then removed and any cells which had detached and were found lying in the medium or on the bottom of the chamber were removed and examined for viability by trypan blue exclusion and also by immunofluorescence.

The results indicate that antibody reacting with the surface of tumor cells in the absence of complement can prevent adherence of the cells, but it

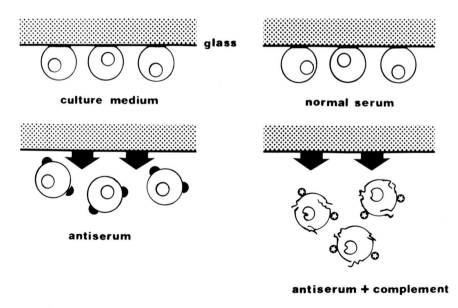

FIG. 1. Diagrammatic summary of effects of antitumor antibodies on adherence of melanoma cells to glass surfaces.

cannot produce lysis. The presence of complement, however, may result in both nonadherence and subsequent lysis.

Further reports of antibodies in the sera of patients with melanoma and other tumors showing individual specificity have been recently published (6,50,52). Using immunofluorescence and more recently an enzyme-linked immunoassay and immunoelectron microscopy (9), we have also been able to demonstrate the presence of antigens within the cytoplasm of tumor cells (41) which show a much higher degree of cross-reactivity. These antigens, however, may well be shared with normal tissue antigens and would explain some of the high background on so-called false-positive reactions that numerous investigators have reported (57). For the sake of clarity, the main emphasis will be on the distinction between antimembrane (individually specific) and anticytoplasmic (group specific) antibody/antigen reactions, realizing that there are many other specificities both on the membrane and in the cytoplasm which are both individually specific and group specific.

Relationship Between the Natural History of the Tumor and Antitumor Antibody

We have been able, in company with other investigators (25), to demonstrate some degree of relationship between the stage of the disease and the presence of some form of humoral immunity. In this case, the antimembrane antibody appears to be the most clearly related to the stage of the disease in that it is largely confined to the early premetastatic phase of malignant melanoma. The antibody to cytoplasmic or internal antigens has been shown to vary independently of the stage of the disease and often persists into the metastatic phase of malignancy (28). This particular antibody system will be looked at more closely in the section on regional lymph node metastasis. It has been possible to separate by affinity chromatography and electrophoresis the different antibodies described above (29). Detailed analysis of sequential studies of large numbers of individual patients with malignant melanoma shows that the fluctuation in the antimembrane antibody appears to be independent of the size of the tumor or the tumor burden of the individual at the time (28). This result has recently been confirmed by another group (6).

There is, however, as mentioned before, a clear relationship to the stage of the disease so that independent of size, if the tumor is localized, the antibody is more likely to be present and vice versa. We have consistently detected a fall in the titer of the antimembrane antibodies prior to the clinical appearance of metastasis, and this has been a very striking phenomenon in our studies (49) (Fig. 2). Studies to determine whether, despite the lack of correlation with tumor size, this is due to soaking up by tumor revealed that tumor cells were not the cause of this fall of antimembrane antibody. The

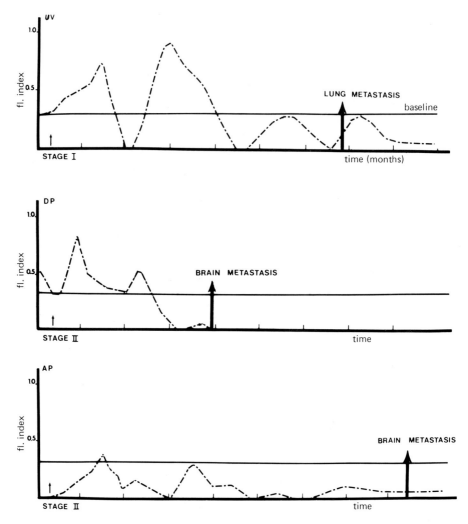

FIG. 2. Sequential studies of antimembrane antibody in serum of patients showing fall in titer preceding clinical appearance of new metastatic deposits. (From ref. 49 with permission.)

small amounts of immunoglobulin detectable by direct fluorescence on the surface of melanoma cells from subcutaneous nodules were independent of the level of the antibody in the serum at that time. In addition to instances in which antibody was present were those in which demonstrable plasma cells, lymphocytes, and monocytes were seen within the tumor (33,45). It seems reasonable, therefore, to explore other explanations for this fall in antimembrane antibody, and these are discussed in the section Humoral Immunity and Failure . . . , p. 253.

Humoral Immunity and Regional Lymph Node Metastasis

It has been known for some time that lymph nodes draining tumors behave abnormally, and in some respects they exhibit a form of paralysis (2,3,42). Lymph nodes have also been the subject of a number of morphological studies showing a variety of reactive changes including germinal center hyperplasia, sinus histiocytosis, and paracortical activity.

In several instances, authors have noted an apparent increase in germinal center hyperplasia and B cell content of the lymph nodes with progressive involvement of the nodes by tumor cells (15). In an extensive recent study we have been able to confirm both of these observations. As the lymph nodes of patients with melanoma become progressively involved in tumor, germinal center hyperplasia increases and analysis of the lymph node cells clearly shows some increase in the proportion of the immunoglobulin-positive cells. There is also a reciprocal drop in peroxidase-positive cells of the monocyte/macrophage series during this time. We have attempted to elute the immunoglobulin from the regional nodes in various stages of the malignancy to determine if such changes may be reflected either qualitatively or quantitatively in the antitumor antibody levels. It has been possible to obtain immunoglobulin by elution from regional nodes and to relate this to the histological and cytological features.

There are indications that as the tumor cells progressively involve the node, the increase in B cell activity is to a large extent due to the production of antibody against cytoplasmic antigen with a concomitant fall in levels of antibody against any membrane antigen in the same nodes (32) (Figs. 3 and 4). Therefore, this picture is similar to that seen in peripheral blood during the same time period and suggests that the liberation of cell debris, as suggested by Hunter and his colleagues (15), might be a crucial factor in con-

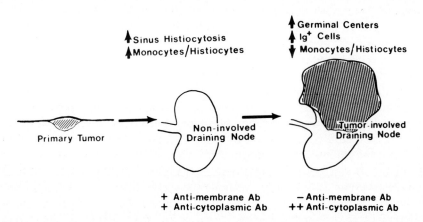

FIG. 3. Schematic summary of changes occurring in regional lymph nodes in patients with various degrees of tumor involvement.

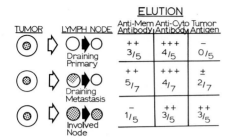

TUMOR	LYMPH NODE	ELUTION		
		Anti-Mem Antibody	Anti-Cyto Antibody	Tumor Antigen
⊚	⇨ ○◗○ Draining Primary	++ 3/5	+++ 4/5	– 0/5
⊚	⇨ ⊚◗○ Draining Metastasis	++ 5/7	+++ 4/7	± 2/7
⊚	⇨ ⊚◗⊚ Involved Node	– 1/5	++ 3/5	++ 3/5

FIG. 4. Proportions and relative amounts of antitumor antibodies and tumor antigen eluted from regional lymph nodes in patients with melanoma at different stages of invasion. (From ref. 24 with permission.)

trolling the response in the node. In a sense, the response may also be regarded as being inappropriate at this stage.

Thus we suggest that the regional nodes responding to disrupted and liberated cell contents have diverted their attention and response to an antigen which is in greater quantity, but the response to which provides no protective function against the growing tumor and could therefore be at least in part responsible for the lack of immunological control of malignancy. Certainly, it may also provide a perfect situation for the production of immune complexes which have also been detected in the serum (16) and in the reticuloendothelial system and the vessels, particularly in the kidneys (27,46).

The concept of liberation from cells of large amounts of internal antigens, i.e., those not usually expressed on the cell surface, producing a subsequent diversion of the immune response, has also been suggested in parasitic infections. For instance, in amebiasis, the host produces antibodies against the internal components of the amoeba at high levels, but few or no anti-surface membrane antibodies are evident, and the organisms thus invade and metastasize (36). If one argues that all cells contain in their cytoplasm normally unexpressed antigenic material, so that the cytoplasm is a "privilege site," then liberation of such cytoplasmic contents might be expected to result in autoantibody production. Numerous examples can be put forward to support this contention, for instance, the antimyocardial antibodies following infarction; anti-smooth muscle antibodies in biopsies in liver disease; and antithyroid antibodies in thyroiditis. The question naturally arises as to why this does not occur continually as cells age and die. This has been answered recently by the demonstration of a phenomenon termed apoptosis (17,59), in which cells proceed through a gradual stage of atrophic change with condensation of their nuclear and cytoplasmic contents, with resulting shrinkage in size and phagocytosis. This process overcomes the need for cell destruction during aging without excessive liberation of cytoplasmic contents. Many human tumors exhibit significant degrees of apoptosis, whereas other cell loss involves classic coagulative necrosis. These variations might provide a reasonable explanation for the differing levels of anticytoplasmic antibody levels detected at different stages of the disease in different individuals.

Humoral Immunity and Failure of Control of Metastasis. Anti-Antibodies and Immune Complexes

In the course of earlier attempts to account for falling antimembrane antibody levels in the circulation, individuals were immunized with their own irradiated tumor cells. Antimembrane antibody responses which were significantly blocked by mixture with the preimmunized negative serum from the same individuals were regularly achieved. This was subsequently shown to be an immunoglobulin reaction directed against immunoglobulin (30). In more detailed studies, we demonstrated that this involves an auto-anti-idiotypic antibody (31). In recent years, this subject has become of considerable interest to a number of immunobiologists, since it appears to be central to the concept of immune regulation (5,7,10,19,20,40,48). We have demonstrated the presence of similar auto-anti-antibodies in tumors other than melanoma, including colon, prostate, and renal cell carcinoma. The exact mechanism of their production and how they operate in bringing about the fall of antimembrane antibody have yet to be determined, but it has been shown that anti-idiotypic antibodies in small quantities can completely shut down the immune response against the particular antigen (10,47). Therefore, we feel that it is not unreasonable to suggest that auto-anti-idiotypic antibodies are one mechanism involved in the failure of antibody control of blood-borne metastasis. In making this proposal, we are aware that many other factors, such as circulating antigen or immune complexes present, may be important. This has led to a search for other anti-antibodies and has resulted in the detection of antibodies against a number of different components of the immunoglobulin G molecule in the sera of cancer patients (16). All of these serum factors seem to increase with the stage of disease, but observed fluctuations in their titers during the disease led us to postulate that they were directed against different types of tumor antibody.

The anti-F(ab)$'_2$ antibody, first described as a serum agglutinator, has also been shown to be present in high titers in serum of patients with chronic gram-positive infections (53). Such antibodies have been detected in the serum of patients with chronic parasitic infections and autoimmune disease (24). In some instances, patients with melanoma and other tumors showed very high titers and these anti-F(ab)$'_2$ antibodies appeared to be related to anticytoplasmic antibodies (13). Furthermore, by attaching both the anti-F(ab)$'_2$ and anticytoplasmic antibodies on affinity columns, we have been able to identify antibody/anti-antibody combinations and distinguish them (24). Fragments of IgG have been demonstrated on the surface of leukemic cells, and the presence of antiproteases was also demonstrated. These studies may indicate a method for the production of anti-antibodies (8).

Rheumatoid-like factors or anti-Fc anti-antibodies have also been seen in the serum of patients with a number of different malignancies (16). The exact nature of these anti-Fc antibodies and their roles are as yet to be determined. Since, however, in a number of circumstances they have been shown to be directed against immune complexes, this is an area of obvious future investigation. These studies have therefore led us to postulate that certain classes of antitumor antibodies have a beneficial effect in respect to the prevention of blood-borne metastasis, which appears to be counteracted by anti-antibodies. Particularly in this category are the anti-membrane antibody and the corresponding anti-idiotypic antibody, summarized diagrammatically in Fig. 5.

There are also anti-antibodies directed against anticytoplasmic antibodies, and they appear to persist late into the progression of the disease. This class of factors is postulated as being inappropriate. This anti-antibody response may be an attempt to clear the system of persistent antibody directed against internal cellular antigens. The anti-Fc antibodies, in keeping with other situations in which rheumatoid-like factors occur, may be a response to immune complex formation.

All of these points led us to develop the concept that some form of immune derangement, central or peripheral, occurs in patients with malignancy, leading to a triad of anergy, anti-antibodies, and immune complexes.

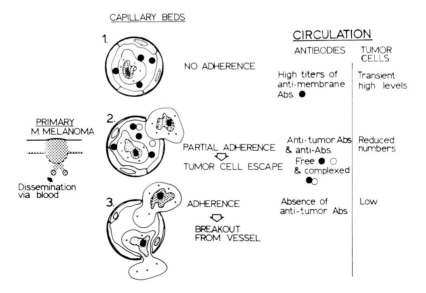

FIG. 5. Proposed relationship between antimembrane antitumor antibodies and anti-idiotypic antibodies in control of blood-borne metastases. (From ref. 24 with permission.)

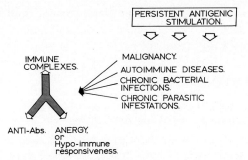

FIG. 6. Summary of concept of immune derangement resulting from persistent antigenic stimulation in cancer and other chronic diseases. (From ref. 24 with permission.)

All three factors have been demonstrated in malignancy. Significantly, this triad is also operative in a number of unrelated disorders in which chronic antigenic stimulation is the single common factor (Fig. 6).

In recent studies of the immune complexes in patients with malignancy, we have detected not only the presence of antibody-antigen complexes as predicted and shown by others, but in addition the presence of anti-antibody complexes. This is illustrated in Fig. 7, in which antimembrane antibody initially identified in the serum of an individual patient suddenly became undetectable. The decline in levels of antitumor antibody was associated with a sharp rise and subsequent fall in the C1q assay for immune complexes (1,16). The complexes were shown to contain among other factors anti-idiotypic antibody and antimembrane antibody. It is not being overenthusiastic to consider that the study of humoral immunity in relation to metastasis might not only lead to an understanding of why the immune system fails to control metastasis. In addition, it may also explain how the persistence of

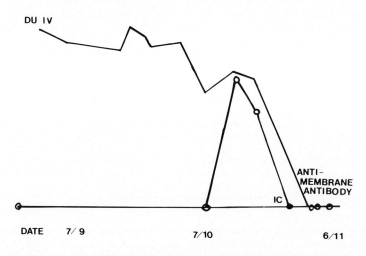

FIG. 7. Fall in antitumor antibody (antimembrane) with concomitant transient rise in circulating immune complexes as measured by C1q deviation assay.

tumor antigen in its various forms produces immune derangement, and might lead to a more fruitful approach to unravelling the fundamental question of regulation of the immune response in general.

REFERENCES

1. Agnello, V., Winchester, R. J., and Kunkel, H. G. (1970): Precipitin reactions of the C1q component of complement with aggregated γ-globulin and immune complexes in gel diffusion. *Immunology,* 19:909.
2. Alexander, P., Bernsted, J., and Delorme, E. J. (1969): The cellular immune response to primary sarcomata in rats. II. Abnormal responses of nodes draining the tumour. *Proc. R. Soc. Lond. [Biol.],* 3:174:237.
3. Alexander, P., Delorme, E. J., and Hall, J. G. (1966): The effect of lymphoid cells from the lymph of specifically immunized sheep on the growth of primary sarcomata in rats. *Lancet,* 1:1186.
4. Baker, M. A., and Taub, R. N. (1973): Immunology of human cancer. *Prog. Allergy,* 17:227.
5. Beatty, P. G., Kim, B. S., Rowley, D. A., and Coppleson, L. W. (1976): Antibody against the antigen receptor of a plasmacytoma prolongs survival of mice bearing the tumor. *J. Immunol.,* 116:1391.
6. Bodurtha, A. J., Chee, D. O., Laucius, J. F., Mastrangelo, M. J., and Prehn, R. T. (1975): Clinical and immunological significance of human melanoma cytotoxic antibody. *Cancer Res.,* 35:189.
7. Cosenza, H., and Kohler, H. (1972): Specific suppression of the antibody response by antibodies to receptors. *Proc. Natl. Acad. Sci. U.S.A.,* 69:2701.
8. Cotropia, J. P., Gutterman, J. U., Hersh, E. M., Granatek, C. H., and Mavugit, G. M. (1976): Antigen expression and cell surface properties of human leukaemic blasts. *Ann. N.Y. Acad. Sci.,* 276:146.
9. Deutsch, G. F., and Rowden, G. (1976): Immuno-ultrastructural localization of cytoplasmic tumor antigens in malignant melanoma. *Proc. Microscop. Soc. Can.,* 3:130.
10. Eichmann, K., and Rajewsky, K. (1975): Induction of T and B cell immunity by anti-idiotypic antibody. *Eur. J. Immunol.,* 5:661.
11. Engle, H. C. (1959): Cancer cells in the blood; a five to nine year follow up study. *Ann. Surg.,* 149:457.
12. Hamilton-Fairley, G. (1969): Immunity to malignant disease in man. *Br. Med. J.,* 2:467.
13. Hartmann, D. L., Lewis, M. G., Proctor, J. W., and Lyons, H. (1974): In vitro interactions between anti-tumor antibodies and anti-antibodies in malignancy. *Lancet,* 2:1481.
14. Humble, J. G., Jane, W. H. W., and Pulvertaft, R. J. V. (1956): Biological interaction between lymphocytes and other cells. *Int. J. Haematol.,* 2:283.
15. Hunter, R. L., Ferguson, D. J., and Coppleson, L. W. (1975): Survival with mammary cancer related to the interaction of germinal center hyperplasia and sinus histiocytosis in axillary and internal mammary lymph nodes. *Cancer,* 36:528.
16. Jerry, L. M., Rowden, G., Cano, P. O., Phillips, T. M., Deutsch, G. F., Capek, A., Hartmann, D., and Lewis, M. G. (1976): Immune complexes in human melanoma: A consequence of deranged immune regulation. *Scand. J. Immunol.,* 5:86.
17. Kerr, J. F. R., Wyllie, A. M., and Currie, A. R. (1973): Apoptosis: A basic biological phenomenon with wide ranging implications in tissue kinetics. *Br. J. Cancer,* 26:239.
18. Klein, G. (1975): The Bartne Foundation Memorial Award Lecture: Immunological surveillance against tumors. *M. D. Anderson 26th Annual Symposium on Fundamental Cancer Research (1973),* p. 21. Williams & Wilkins Co., Baltimore.
19. Kohler, H. (1975): The response to phosphorycholine: Dissecting an immune response. *Transplant. Rev.,* 27:24.
20. Kunkel, A. G., Mannik, M., and Williams, R. C. (1963): Individual antigenic specificity of isolated antibodies. *Science,* 140:1218.
21. Lewis, M. G. (1967): Possible immunological factors in human malignant melanoma. *Lancet,* 2:921.

22. Lewis, M. G. (1972): Circulating humoral antibodies in cancer. *Med. Clin. North Am.*, 56:481.
23. Lewis, M. G., Avis, P. J. G., Phillips, T. M., and Sheikh, K. M. A. (1973): Tumor associated antigens in human malignant melanoma. *Yale J. Biol. Med.*, 46:661.
24. Lewis, M. G., Hartmann, D., and Jerry, L. M. (1976): Antibodies and anti-antibodies in human malignancy: An expression of deranged immune regulation. *Ann. N.Y. Acad. Sci.*, 276:316.
25. Lewis, M. G., Ikonopisov, R. L., Nairn, R. C., Phillips, T. M., Hamilton-Fairley, G., Bodenham, D. C., and Alexander, P. (1969): Tumor specific antibodies in human malignant melanoma and their relationship to the extent of the disease. *Br. Med. J.*, 3:547.
26. Lewis, M. G., and Kiryabwire, J. W. M. (1968): Malignant melanoma in Uganda: Aspects of behaviour and natural history. *Cancer*, 21:876.
27. Lewis, M. G., Loughbridge, L. W., and Phillips, T. M. (1971): Immunological studies on a patient with the nephrotic syndrome associated with malignancy of non-renal origin. *Lancet*, 2:134.
28. Lewis, M. G., McCloy, E., and Blake, J. (1973): The significance of circulating antibodies in the localization of human malignant melanoma. *Br. J. Surg.*, 60:443.
29. Lewis, M. G., and Phillips, T. M. (1972): The specificity of surface membrane immunofluorescence in human malignant melanoma. *Int. J. Cancer*, 10:105.
30. Lewis, M. G., Phillips, T. M., Cook, K. B., and Blake, J. (1971): Possible explanation for loss of detectable antibody in patients with disseminated malignant melanoma. *Nature*, 232:52.
31. Lewis, M. G., Phillips, T. M., Rowden, G., and Jerry, L. M. (1977): Auto-anti-idiotypic antibodies in failure of immune control of human malignancy (*in preparation*).
32. Lewis, M. G., Phillips, T. M., Rowden, G., and Shibata, H. (1977): Anti-tumor antibodies in regional lymph nodes of patients with malignant melanoma. *Lancet* (*submitted for publication*).
33. Lewis, M. G., Proctor, J. W., Thomson, D. M. P., Rowden, G., and Phillips, T. M. (1976): Cellular localization of immunoglobulin within human malignant melanomata. *Br. J. Cancer*, 33:260.
34. Mastrangelo, M. J., Berd, D., and Bellet, R. E. (1976): Critical review of previously reported clinical trials of cancer immunotherapy with non-specific immunostimulants. *Ann. N.Y. Acad. Sci.*, 277:94.
35. Mastrangelo, M. J., Laucius, J. F., and Outzen, H. C. (1974): Fundamental concepts in tumor immunology: A brief review. *Semin. Oncol.*, 1:291.
36. McLaughlin, J., and Meerovitch, E. (1975): Immunochemical studies of the surface and cytoplasmic membranes of entamoeba invadens. *Can. J. Microbiol.*, 16:493.
37. Morton, D. L., Malmgren, R. A., Holmes, E. C., and Ketcham, A. S. (1968): Demonstration of antibodies against human malignant melanoma by immunofluorescence. *Surgery*, 65:233.
38. Mukherji, B., Nathanson, L., and Clark, D. A. (1973): Studies of humoral and cell mediated immunity in human melanoma. *Yale J. Biol. Med.*, 46:681.
39. Muna, N. M., Marcus, S., and Smart, C. (1969): Detection by immunofluorescence of antibodies specific for human malignant melanoma cells. *Cancer*, 23:88.
40. Oudin, J. (1966): The genetic control of immunoglobulin synthesis. *Proc. R. Soc. Lond.* [*Biol.*], 166:207.
41. Phillips, T. M., and Lewis, M. G. (1977): The use of an enzyme-linked immunoassay in detection of antibody against human bladder carcinoma (ELISA) (*in preparation*).
42. Pihl, E., Nairn, R. C., Nind, A. P., Muller, H. K., Hughes, E. S. R., Cuthbertson, A. M., and Rollo, A. J. (1976): Correlation of regional lymph nodes' in vitro antitumor immunoreactivity histology with colorectal carcinoma. *Cancer Res.*, 36:3665.
43. Pulvertaft, J. R. V. (1959): The examination of pathological tissues in a fresh state. In: *Modern Trends in Pathology*, edited by D. H. Collins. Butterworth, London.
44. Ritchie, A. C., and Webster, D. R. (1961): Tumor cells in the blood. In: *Proceedings of the Fourth Canadian Cancer Research Conference, June 1960, Vol. 4*, p. 225. Academic Press, New York.
45. Roberts, M. M., Bass, E. M., Wallace, I. W. J., and Stevenson, A. (1973): Local immunoglobulin production in breast cancer. *Br. J. Cancer*, 27:269.

46. Rowden, G., MacFadden, D. K., Phillips, T. M., Deutsch, G. F., and Lewis, M. G. (1976): Immune complex depositis in the kidney in relation to malignant disease. *Proc. Microscop. Soc. Can.,* III:132.
47. Rowley, D. A., Fitch, F. W., Stuart, E. P., Kohler, H., and Consenza, H. (1973): Specific suppression of immune responses. *Science,* 181:1133.
48. Scott-Rodkey, L. (1974): Studies of idiotypic antibodies. Production and characterization of auto-anti-idiotypic antisera. *J. Exp. Med.,* 139:712.
49. Shibata, H. R., Jerry, L. M., Lewis, M. G., Mansell, P. W. A., Capek, A., and Marquis, G. (1976): Immunotherapy of human malignant melanoma with irradiated tumor cells, oral BCG and Levamisole. *Ann. N.Y. Acad. Sci.,* 277:355.
50. Shiku, H., Takahashi, T., Oettgen, H. F., and Old, L. J. (1976): Cell surface antigens of human malignant melanoma. *J. Exp. Med.,* 144:873.
51. Virchow, R. (1858): *Cellular Pathology,* Lecture X, p. 252. Translated from 2nd German Ed. by Frank Chance. Dover Publications, New York (1971).
52. Wainberg, M. A., Markson, Y., Weiss, D. W., and Doljansky, F. (1974): Cellular immunity against Rous sarcoma of chickens. Preferential reactivity against autochthonous target cells are determined by lymphocyte adherence and cytotoxicity in vitro. *Proc. Natl. Acad. Sci. U.S.A.,* 71:3565.
53. Waller, M., and Dumar, R. J. (1972): Increased antibody to IgG fragments: Correlation with infection due to gram positive bacteria. *J. Infect. Dis.,* 125:45.
54. Warren, B. A. (1973): Environment of the blood-borne tumor embolus adherent to vessel wall. *J. Med.,* 4:150.
55. White, H., and Griffiths, J. D. (1976): Circulating malignant cells and fibrinolysis during resection of colorectal cancer. *Proc. R. Soc. Med.,* 69:467.
56. Wood, S. J. (1958): Pathogenesis of metastasis formation observed in vivo in the rabbit ear chamber. *A.M.A. Arch. Pathol.,* 66:550.
57. Wood, S. J., and Barth, R. F. (1974): Immunofluorescent studies of the serological reactivity of patients with malignant melanoma against tumor associated cytoplasmic antigens. *J. Natl. Cancer Inst.,* 53:309.
58. Wood, S. J., Holyoke, E. D., and Yardley, J. H. (1961): Mechanisms of metastasis production by blood borne cancer cells. *Proceedings of the Fourth Canadian Cancer Research Conference, Vol. 4,* p. 167. Academic Press, New York.
59. Wyllie, A. H. (1973): Death in normal and neoplastic cells. *J. Clin. Pathol. [Suppl. 7],* 27:35.

Cancer Invasion and Metastasis: Biologic
Mechanisms and Therapy, edited by S. B. Day
et al. Raven Press, New York © 1977.

Innate Host Resistance to Malignant Cells Not Involving Specific Immunity

Peter Alexander

*Division of Tumour Immunology, Chester Beatty Research Institute,
Belmont, Sutton, Surrey, England*

The aim of this chapter is to interpret experimental observations on the role of immunity on both the genesis and the subsequent biological behavior of malignant tumors on the basis of the diverse mechanisms, "nonspecific" and specific lymphocyte dependent, that are known to contribute to resistance to bacterial and parasitic infection. In addition to clinical findings which suggest that the progress of malignant disease may sometimes be subject to restraint by the host and to pathological observations in man of noninvolved tumor-draining nodes, which suggest a reaction to the tumor by the mononuclear phagocytic system, there are a number of experimental observations which indicate the existence of host resistance to malignant cells.

First, the frequency of transformation of cells *in vitro* (spontaneously, by X-rays, or by carcinogens) is not consistent with the relative rarity and length of latent periods for tumors arising *in vivo*. For example, 1 in 500 of the cells in a culture of fibroblasts is transformed by 50 r of X-rays (1). If there are no mechanisms by which X-ray-induced neoplastic cells are eliminated *in vivo*, then the carcinogenicity of X-rays should be immensely greater than that actually observed.

Second, in most cases to achieve a transplant, many tumor cells must be inoculated into the syngeneic host and the large majority of these inoculated tumor cells are rapidly destroyed (2). Transplants from less than 10 viable tumor cells are seen only with tumors that have undergone frequent passage.

Several investigators, and notably Burnet (3), advanced the hypothesis that this host resistance is due to the existence of membrane-associated tumor antigens which induce specific immunity, requiring the participation of T lymphocytes, and that surveillance is caused by a process akin to the rejection of allografts. However, definitive animal experiments have disproved this concept in that animals depleted of T cells (either as the result of a genetic defect or by experimental manipulation) which permanently accept allografts do not have a higher incidence of spontaneous tumors (4) or a greater susceptibility to chemically induced carcinogenesis. It is interesting that "surveillance" by T lymphocytes could be detected neither for tumors which are highly immunogenic (i.e., those induced by chemical

TABLE 1. *Effect of depletion of T lymphocytes by prolonged (6 day) draining of thoracic duct lymphocytes on distant metastatic spread of the chemically induced sarcoma (HSBPA) implanted into the leg of syngeneic rats*

Experimental protocol		Rats dying from distant metastases within 1.5 yr after removal of tumor
Day 0 to 6 Thoracic duct draining	(a) No thoracic duct draining	8/60 (13%)
Day 7 Tumor implanted		
Day 21 Tumor surgically removed	(b) Thoracic duct draining	21/40 (52%)
Day 0 Tumor implanted		
Day 14 Tumor surgically removed		
Days 15–21 Thoracic duct draining		9/17 (53%)
Days 21–27 " "		7/16 (44%)
Days 30–37 " "		6/16 (37%)
Not drained		8/79 (10%)

carcinogens) nor for the much less immunogenic tumors which occur spontaneously. The only carcinogenic stimuli to which immunosuppressed animals are more susceptible are some DNA oncogenic viruses (5).

Yet once experimental tumors have become clinically recognizable, reactions requiring T lymphocytes may determine their subsequent growth pattern. First, distant metastatic spread of established autochthonous or syngeneic transplanted tumors is facilitated by deprivation of the host of T lymphocytes. Table 1 summarizes a series of experiments (6,7) in which removal of T lymphocytes unassociated with changes in bone marrow function or hemostasis promotes the occurrence of distant metastases. Second, some tumors transplanted into immunologically compromised hosts are less responsive to chemotherapy or radiotherapy (8). Third, the growth of autochthonous chemically induced sarcomata in rats can be retarded by procedures involving specific immunity such as the injection of immune thoracic duct lymphocytes (9) or the specific stimulation of distant lymphoid organs by tumor antigen (10,11).

Taken together, these observations suggest that although surveillance by T lymphocytes requiring mechanisms may not be involved in the initial stages of tumorigenesis, such mechanisms come into play once a tumor has arisen and determine its biological behavior.

IMMUNITY—SELECTIVE AND SPECIFIC

This complex pattern of T-lymphocyte involvement in host resistance to cancer may be understood if it is considered in the light of resistance to infection, which in mammals is effected by two classes of reactions: the first and second line of defense.

The first line of defense (selective but not specific immunity) consists of processes that come into play immediately, do not require induction, and have no memory, i.e., there is no enhanced secondary response. The principal effectors are the phagocytic cells. This class of defense stems from the primitive mechanisms developed in invertebrates to combat infection and parasitism. Circulating factors with receptors capable of discriminating between self and non-self are known to exist in invertebrates (12), but these differ not only structurally from conventional immunoglobulin but also in their general pattern of appearance, in that they are not produced in response to a "non-self" macromolecule but are an intrinsic component of the organism.

The second line of defense (specific immunity) is characterized by the need for its effectors to be induced (i.e., there is an interval of several days before these come into play) and by a memory response (i.e., the response to a second infection with the same organism is faster and more pronounced). The genesis of specific immunity requires first an interaction between the immunogenic molecule (antigen) and specific lymphocyte receptors and subsequently amplification by cell division leading to the generation of antibodies and cytotoxic cells. Specific immunity is an evolutionarily advanced form of defense characteristic of vertebrates.

The reasons for referring to these two types of immunity as the first and second line of defense, respectively, are that following most bacterial infections specific immunity is important only if the capacity of the phagocytic cells to deal with the organisms has been overwhelmed. If the first line cannot cope because either the number of pathogens is too great or the organisms have succeeded in avoiding destruction by the phagocytic cells, then specific immunity takes over; thus mammals deprived of T lymphocytes are not necessarily more susceptible to infection and can, in fact, survive for long periods especially in sheltered environments. Absence of lymphocytes does not constitute a clinical emergency as does granulocytopenia, which is immediately life threatening. A deficit of lymphocytes causes concern for the long-term but is not immediately critical. The first line of defense against virus infection is less well understood. It is not certain whether some viruses are dealt with by the selective (nonspecific) phagocytic processes and some virus infections are facilitated by phagocytosis. Protection of a nonspecific type is no doubt provided by interferon, but on the whole it would appear that the T-cell-requiring second line of defense is called into play more frequently following exposure to viruses than to microorganisms, since the earliest and most common consequences of a T-cell deficit are virus infections.

SELECTIVE RECOGNITION OF CELLS BY MACROPHAGES[1]

I now wish to review the evidence that the first line of defense against malignant cells is by cells of the mononuclear phagocyte series which have

---

[1] Ascribing to macrophages a "first-line defense" function that is selective but not specific does not imply that macrophages do not play an important role in specific immunity. It is quite

the capacity to recognize surface properties characteristic of transformation to the malignant state. Alexander (13) proposed that this process can deal only with small numbers of tumor cells at any one site and that it is unable to restrain an established tumor mass or clusters of cells shed from it — if they are to be combated, these require specific T-cell-mediated immunity. Since metastatic spread occurs predominantly via clusters rather than by single cells, then as has been found experimentally (6), deprivation of T cells should facilitate spread and nonimmunogenic tumors would be expected to be inherently more metastatic.

It is tempting to link the selective recognition of tumor cells by macrophages with the role of the mononuclear phagocyte system in eliminating some "self" components for which there are no lymphocyte receptors and which do not engender specific immunity. The mononuclear phagocyte system is capable of distinguishing between proteins which are intended to circulate (e.g., normal serum proteins) and those which have been released from cells but which have no physiological function in the circulation. The best known of the latter are intracellular enzymes such as lactic dehydrogenase and hydrolytic enzymes released when the liver is traumatized. The specific immune system does not, of course, recognize as foreign these soluble proteins which need to be removed from the circulation unless there is a pathological autoimmune condition. Yet these are cleared from the circulation within a few hours, and sometimes even more rapidly, and build up only when the reticuloendothelial system is impaired, the best example of this being infection with the Riley virus (14). The diagnostic test for the latter is that the level of lactic dehydrogenase in the serum is greatly elevated. This occurs not because more of the enzyme is synthesized or released but because it is cleared less effectively.

The other principal function of the mononuclear phagocyte system is to remove effete (aged) autochthonous red cells and leukocytes. Although it has been suggested that removal of senescent cells by human macrophages (15) involves coating by antibody directed against an altered membrane surface, this cannot be the only or, indeed, the principal mechanism by which the mononuclear phagocyte system recognizes and removes these cells because this process occurs normally in immunosuppressed individuals or in individuals who are agammaglobulinemic. In any case the same process of clearing effete cells is found for hemocytes of invertebrates.

SELECTIVE CYTOTOXICITY OF "ACTIVATED" MACROPHAGES

The hypothesis that macrophages can be made to recognize and then kill transformed cells derives from experiments in which macrophages were

---

clear that they are involved in the initial recognition step whereby the immunogenic macromolecule is bound to a lymphocyte receptor and also that they play a part as a specific effector cell by being armed with immunologically specific moieties such as cytophilic antibodies or antigen-specific T-cell products.

shown to become cytotoxic to a range of sarcoma and lymphoma cells following exposure either *in vitro* or *in vivo* to endotoxin or double-stranded RNA at very low concentrations (16). More recently, peptoglycans extracted from bacterial cell walls (17) and injection *in vivo* of *Corynebacterium parvum* (18) were found to produce the same effect. Lymphocytes are not involved in this reaction, and macrophages from T-cell-deprived mice that are unable to mount specific immune reactions can be rendered cytotoxic to tumor cells by such treatments. Hibbs (19) showed that the cytotoxic activity of endotoxin-treated macrophages was much greater for transformed cells than for their untransformed counterparts. Such tumoricidal macrophages were referred to by us as being "activated" (16), but this was an unfortunate terminology since it had previously been applied also to macrophages treated by procedures that had stimulated their metabolic activity without necessarily rendering them cytotoxic.

Confusion arises because macrophages can also be rendered selectively cytocidal for tumor cells in a nonspecific way by processes which require T-cell-mediated immunity as an intermediary. This occurs (a) when macrophages from suitably immunized animals are brought into contact with the antigen to which they have become sensitized (20), or (b) when macrophages are treated with lymphokines released when allergized lymphocytes meet the specific antigen (21). Thus macrophages of animals immunized, for example, with BCG become cytotoxic when they are exposed to PPD; or when lymphocytes from animals immunized with BCG are treated with PPD they release a factor that renders macrophages tumoricidal. Consequently, animals with a normal specific immune system which have become infected with an organism that gives rise to a persistent infection have macrophages which are tumoricidal because the allergized macrophage encounters the antigen *in vivo* (22).

As yet, almost nothing is known of either the cytotoxic mechanism by which a suitably "activated" macrophage kills tumor cells or the surface characteristic which allows macrophages to distinguish between normal and malignant cells. It is also not clear whether nonactivated macrophages can distinguish between normal and malignant cells and that "activation" is needed to induce the formation of a "toxin." On the other hand, "activation" may be due to a product, cell bound or released, which is selective. The primary event in the killing of tumor cells by "activated" macrophages requires the cells to be in contact or at least in close proximity, and phagocytosis of the tumor cells is a late reaction which occurs only after the target cell has sustained irreversible damage (23). There is a conflict of evidence whether the toxin (e.g., a hydrolytic enzyme) is released by the "activated" macrophage or whether it is fixed within its membranes. Currie and Basham (24) have obtained from endotoxin-treated macrophages a soluble factor that is selectively cytotoxic for malignant cells, whereas other workers find that macrophages kill only when in direct physical contact with the target tumor cell. These contradictory findings might be resolved if there is an antagonist to the toxin in the serum, and therefore the range of action of the toxin is limited. The situation could be similar to that associated with the transmission of nerve impulses by acetylcholine, which was for a long period in dispute because of the rapid destruction of the mediator by circulating cholinesterase.

WHAT CHARACTERISTIC OF THE MALIGNANT CELL DOES THE MACROPHAGE RECOGNIZE?

The nature of the recognition signal which allows the "activated" macrophage to kill selectively is also still obscure. It could reside either in a selective susceptibility to a toxin or in a selective binding to the macrophage or to both. Recognition might be linked to some other surface changes which have been associated with the malignant transformation, such as a low microviscosity and high cholesterol content (25), changes in membrane-associated microtubules (26), ease of agglutination by concanavalin A, control of nuclear division (27), or incomplete synthesis of glycoproteins as instanced for blood group substances in human adenocarcinomas (28). It may be relevant that when soluble glycoproteins are treated with neuraminidase such that a terminal sialic acid group is lost and a galactosyl group appears as a terminal residue, this results in the rapid removal of such a molecule from the circulation (30). The recognition process may also be linked to the greater turnover of certain membrane components by malignant as opposed to normal cell membranes (29). This was shown for the histocompatibility antigens on mouse lymphoma cells and also for the release from the membrane of immune complexes formed between such antigens and specific antibody (31). If the malignant transformation is associated with greater membrane instability, then this could cause the incomplete synthesis of glycoproteins in that the glycosyl transferases may not be able to complete their reactions.

When considering the mechanism involved in the selective killing by "activated" macrophages of cells that have undergone a malignant transformation, it must be borne in mind that this discrimination may not be absolute as macrophages which have acquired the capacity to kill tumor cells are also able to stop DNA synthesis, at least *in vitro*, of normal lymphocytes that have been transformed by phytohemagglutinin (PHA) (32). Thus the failure of leukocytes taken from individuals that have been treated with *C. parvum* to transform with PHA is not due to a defect in their T lymphocytes but is caused by the powerful "activation" of macrophages by *C. parvum*, which then inhibit DNA synthesis of the treated lymphocytes. When leukocytes from individuals treated with *C. parvum* are freed of macrophages, they transform normally with PHA. Thus the recognition signal which allows "activated" macrophages to distinguish between normal and cancer cells appears to be associated with the malignant transformation but is not unique to it. A further complication is that the nature of the cytotoxic event seems to vary for different cell types. Sometimes the cytotoxic action of "activated" macrophages is predominantly cytostatic, lysis and phagocytosis of the "sterilized" tumor cell being a late event, whereas for other tumor cells there may be rapid lysis.

INFLAMMATORY CELLS OTHER THAN MACROPHAGES INVOLVED IN NONSPECIFIC HOST RESPONSE TO TUMORS

We (20) found that macrophages separated from the cells present in the peritoneal cavity of mice which had been immunized with BCG became cytotoxic to tumor cells when exposed to PPD either *in vitro* or *in vivo*. More recently, Parr *et al.* (33) found that the lymphocytes present in these peritoneal washings showed similar properties. Cells from the peritoneal cavities of BCG-treated mice having been rid of macrophages and of the majority of B lymphocytes by passage through a nylon column became highly cytotoxic for tumor cells on the addition of PPD and lysed sarcoma cells within 48 hr at a ratio of 1:1. These T cells (being susceptible to anti-θ serum) showed no tumoricidal activity before the addition of PPD (Table 2). Similar cells from mice that had not been immunized with BCG showed no antitumor activity after exposure to PPD.

It was of particular interest that these "activated" lymphocytes were highly effective in the Winn-type assay in which tumoricidal action is measured by mixing tumor cells with the putative killer cells *in vitro,* injecting

TABLE 2. *Immunologically nonspecific cytotoxicity of stimulated T lymphocytes[a] from the peritoneal cavity of mice immunized with BCG*

Treatment of peritoneal T lymphocytes			Cytotoxicity assayed	
Source	Treated with PPD[b]	Ratio of lymphocytes to tumor cells in test	In vitro % cells killed	In vivo % animals with tumor after inoculation of a mixture of 10^5 syngeneic sarcoma cells and lympho-cytes
Normal	No	10:1	18	100
	Yes	10:1	24	100
BCG	No	10:1	19	100
Immunized	Yes	10:1	81	0
		5:1	—	0
		2:1	—	10
		1:1	—	40

[a] Prepared by fractionation of peritoneal exudate cells on nylon wool columns; 90% lysed by anti-θ serum and complement.
[b] 2 μg (*in vitro*) and 5μg (*in vivo*) PPD added to lymphocytes prior to cytotoxicity assay.

the mixture into animals, and assaying cytotoxicity by growth inhibition of the tumor *in vivo*. In this test the "activated" lymphocytes were much more effective than "activated" macrophages (compare refs. 33 and 34). The relationship of the T lymphocytes of BCG-treated mice which became almost immediately cytotoxic on the addition of PPD to the *in vitro* toxicity of lymphocytes that had been transformed with PHA (35) remains to be established. These experiments show, however, that nonspecific immunity directed against tumor cells may also be mediated by lymphocytes, and when interpreting the results presented in the next section it must be borne in mind that the antitumor effects seen at sites of inflammation may be due in part to lymphocytes which are nonspecifically tumoricidal.

IN VIVO RELEVANCE OF RECOGNITION OF TUMOR CELLS BY INFLAMMATORY CELLS

Depletion of Macrophages

The decisive test to evaluate the role of macrophages in surveillance of tumor cells *in vivo* requires animals which do not have macrophages. This, however, is impossible since extensive and prolonged depletion of macrophages and polymorphs is incompatible with life. Also, no mutants which are severely depleted of phagocytic cells exist, i.e., there is no counterpart to the T-deprived nude mouse. Attempts to kill macrophages *in vivo* using silica are difficult to interpret since administration of large amounts of silica leads to gross damage of lymphoid organs, as can readily be recognized by hemorrhage in lymph nodes and the presence of red blood cells in the thoracic duct lymph. However, even in such animals macrophage depletion is at best partial and only short-lived.

A possible link between macrophage function and susceptibility to tumors comes from the study of Lurie (36) who developed several strains of rabbits which differed widely in their susceptibility to tuberculosis. He showed that this difference was related to the functional activity of the monocytes. Rabbits which had monocytes that rapidly killed tubercle bacilli intracellularly were resistant, whereas those that were susceptible had monocytes which lacked the capacity for killing tubercle bacilli. Detailed necropsy data showed an inverse correlation between susceptibility to tuberculosis and the age-associated incidence of carcinoma in the different strains of rabbits (Fig. 1). Also, neonates, which Argyris (37) showed to have functionally immature macrophages, grow tumors from smaller inocula of syngeneic cells than do adults.

DESTRUCTION OF TUMOR AT SITES OF INFLAMMATION AND OF DELAYED HYPERSENSITIVITY RESPONSES

Both in man and in experimental animals, local tumors—in the skin, the peritoneal cavity, or the pleura—can sometimes be eradicated by inducing

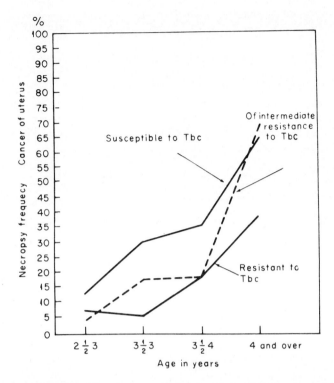

FIG. 1. Relation of cancer of the uterus and native resistance to tuberculosis in the Phipps rabbit colony, 1931–1961.

an inflammatory reaction (38,39). The most effective way of doing this is to sensitize the host to an antigen such as dinitrochlorobenzene and then paint this antigen on the tumor site. This induces an intense delayed hypersensitivity reaction, during which many tumors are totally eradicated. Figure 2 shows that this effect can be readily demonstrated within the peritoneal cavity. This local antitumor action of inflammation or of delayed hypersensitivity is consistent with the *in vitro* data that suitably activated macrophages and lymphocytes are tumoricidal. Macrophages and lymphocytes of this type would be present at the site of a delayed hypersensitivity reaction.

Injection of endotoxin into the peritoneal cavity protects the animals against a subsequent challenge with tumor cells, but unlike the induction of inflammation endotoxin does not retard the growth of an established tumor (34) (Table 3). This suggests that the tumoricidal properties of endotoxin-treated peritoneal cells and of cells present at sites of delayed hypersensitivity may differ.

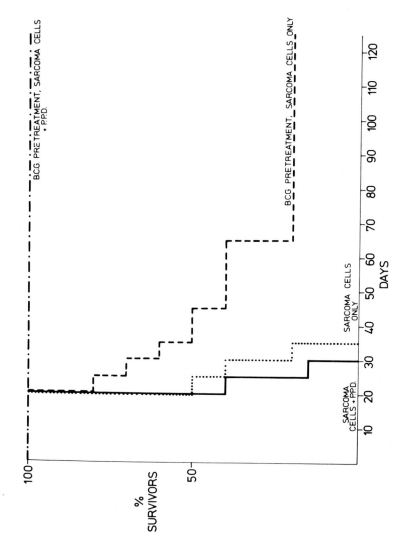

FIG. 2. Effect of PPD on the growth of FS6 fibrosarcoma (benzpyrene induced) injected i.p. into syngeneic mice (C57B1) presensitized with BCG (300 μg/mouse injected i.p. 14 days before tumor challenge). PPD (4 μg/ml) was mixed with sarcoma cells (prepared by trypsinization of the solid tumor) just before the injection of 4×10^6 cells/mouse in 0.5 ml. (From Parr et al., ref. 33.)

TABLE 3. *Effect of endotoxin given i.p. on growth of i.p. inoculated 10^4 syngeneic L5178Y lymphoma cells in DBA/2 mice*

Treatment	% mice alive at:		
	30 days	40 days	50 days
None	0	—	—
10 μg endotoxin 7 days before transplant	60	40	20
,, ,, 3 ,, ,,	100	50	30
,, ,, 1 ,, ,,	0	—	—
,, ,, 1 ,, after	0	—	—
,, ,, 7 ,, ,,	0	—	—

Destruction of Circulating Tumor Cells in the Lung

There is a large body of evidence which indicates that many types of tumor cells are rapidly destroyed within the lung following intravenous inoculation (40). The tumor cells tend to be lysed within about 24 hr (41). The principal mechanism responsible is independent of specific immunity as the extent of trapping and destruction is only slightly greater in animals that have been preimmunized with tumor (42). The mechanism responsible for the lysis is not known, but whole-body irradiation and other procedures which damage the bone marrow decrease the effectiveness of destruction of tumor cells lodged in the lung (43). Nonmalignant cells injected intravenously are, of course, also trapped in the lung, but in general they are destroyed to a much lesser extent even when they are quite large, such as macrophages or immunoblasts. A striking example of this phenomenon is the finding that even in leukemias which give rise to high levels of leukemic cells in the blood there is extensive destruction of the circulating malignant cells in the lung and liver (44) (Fig. 3).

It is tempting to associate the destruction of the trapped cells with the presence in the lung of activated interstitial macrophages. Not only aveolar but possibly also interstitial macrophages in the lung might be activated because they are continually meeting antigens to which the animal has previously been sensitized. This phenomenon may be linked to the protection of the peritoneal cavity following the injection of endotoxin or double-stranded RNA (Table 3), which induces "activated" macrophages (33).

Tumor Macrophages and Monocytosis

Another reason for suspecting that macrophages may exert *in vivo* some control over the dissemination of tumors is that the macrophage content of experimental and possibly also human tumors is inversely related to their capacity to metastasize to distant sites. This observation (6) was first made

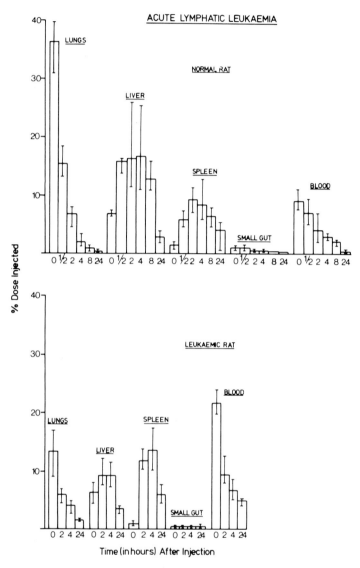

FIG. 3. Distribution of radioactivity in the organs of normal August rats, as a percentage of the injected dose, at various times after they had received an i.v. injection of 5×10^7 ^{125}IUDR-labeled syngeneic myelogenous leukemia cells. Each histogram represents the mean value from 5 recipients; the bar indicates the range of results. The zero time point represents dose within 2–3 min of injection. (From Sadler and Alexander, ref. 44.)

with a variety of chemically induced sarcomata in rats (Table 4), but more recently there are suggestions that this may extend also to human tumors (45). In mice lymphomas which do not metastasize contain fewer cells that on culture mature into macrophages than do lymphomas that metastasize

TABLE 4. *Macrophage content, incidence of metastases, and immunogenicity of chemically induced rat fibrosarcomata transplanted into syngeneic recipients*

Tumor	Mean % macrophages (and range)	Incidence of metastases (%)	Immunogenicity
MC-3	8 (2–12)	100	$<10^3$
HSH	12(10–15)	100	10^3–2×10^4
ASBPI	22(18–26)	50–55	10^5
MCI-M	38(36–42)	20–30	10^6
HSN	40(34–44)	30–35	5×10^6–10^7
HSBPA	54(42–63)	10–12	10^7–5×10^7

The incidence of metastases was measured after excision of tumors which had been growing i.m. in hind limbs for 14 days. Immunogenicity was assessed as the number of cells required for tumor growth in rats immunized by excision of i.m. tumors 14 days previously.

readily. That the growth of tumors in rats (46), mice (47), and in some instances man (48,49) is associated with monocytosis is also indicative of a response of the host to tumors that involves mononuclear phagocytes (Fig. 4).

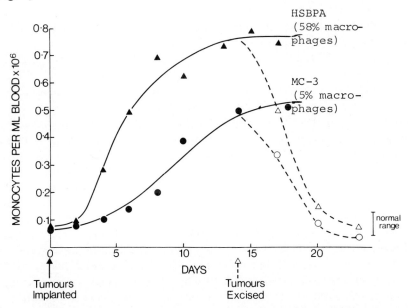

FIG. 4. Number of peripheral blood monocytes in tumor-bearing male hooded rats assayed at intervals during tumor growth by the EA rosette method. (▲) HSBPA tumor-bearing rats; (●) MC-3 tumor-bearing rats; (△) postexcision HSBPA tumor; (○) post-excision MC-3 tumor. Each point represents the mean value from 5 animals, and the vertical bars show the range for the group. The 2 tumors grew at approximately equal rates, attaining average weights of 4.2 g on day 7, 10.4 g on day 10, 15 g on day 14, and 22.5 g on day 18. (From Eccles et al., ref. 46.)

RELATIVE CONTRIBUTIONS OF SPECIFIC AND SELECTIVE (OR NONSPECIFIC) IMMUNITY TO METASTATIC SPREAD

The starting point for the hypothesis discussed in this chapter was the finding made in many laboratories that specific immunity requiring the participation of T lymphocytes determines in part at least the metastatic behavior of tumors. This was concluded from three types of investigation: In the first type, removal of T cells caused sarcomata which do not metastasize normally to disseminate. The restraint imposed by specific immunity could be due to the destruction by specifically immune processes of shed tumor cells, or to reactions which prevent growth but do not kill disseminated "dormant" tumor cells. The second type of investigation revealed the inverse correlation (6) (Table 4) between the capacity of different tumors to induce a state of immunity in the host and the capacity of the tumor to metastasize in an immunologically normal host. Finally, support for linking the effectiveness of specific immunity with metastasis comes from experiments related to the shedding of tumor antigens. Soluble tumor-specific antigens released from the surface of malignant cells reduce the effectiveness as assayed *in vitro* of the immunologically specific host reaction to the tumor antigens situated within the membranes of the tumor cells (50). In animals (51,52) there is a correlation between the rate at which tumor antigens are shed from the membrane and (a) the degree of immunity that can be achieved *in vivo* and (b) the metastatic potential of the tumor.

On the other hand, there is no compelling evidence which suggests that innate (possibly macrophage-mediated) immunity to malignant cells distinguishes between those tumors which are capable of giving rise to distant metastases and those which are not. The limited data do not show a correlation between the effectiveness of innate immunity to a particular type of tumor and its capacity to metastasize. Clearly, some tumors, and indeed some infective organisms, are less vulnerable than others to control by innate immune mechanisms. These tumors which can be transplanted by an inoculum containing only a few tumor cells may be characterized by the capacity to avoid destruction by innate immunity more effectively than those which require a large inoculum to produce a tumor. However, there is no correlation between the minimum number of cells needed to produce a tumor and the capacity of the resulting tumor to metastasize. In some series the two are inversely related, but there are many tumors which can be transplanted from very low numbers of cells which yet do not metastasize. It must be stressed that tumors which can be transplanted from very low numbers of cells are both rare and are seen only after long periods of passage (2). The increase in virulence of bacteria on passage may be analogous. Moreover, in general, tumors can be transplanted only from very low numbers by the intraperitoneal route, and the same type of tumor requires more cells to induce a tumor when inoculated subcutaneously or intravenously.

RELATIVE FUNCTIONS OF INNATE AND SPECIFIC IMMUNITY IN THE TUMOR-HOST RELATIONSHIP—A UNIFYING HYPOTHESIS

The available data suggest that cells involved in nonspecific (or innate) immunity control incipient neoplastic cells which arise sporadically, either as a result of carcinogens or for unknown reasons. This process is effective against isolated cells, and therefore surveillance against induction of cancer can occur in the absence of specific immunity, i.e., in animals that cannot mount a specific immune response. On the other hand, large masses of tumors or tumors released into the circulation as clusters or conglomerates of tumor cells, which remain after radio- or chemotherapy, are relatively invulnerable to the innate mechanisms of immunity and require the processes of specific immunity if they are to be controlled. Therefore, metastatic spread and curability by chemo- or radiotherapy are determined in part by the magnitude of the specific host response.

A corollary to this hypothesis is that one of the reasons why dissemination from single cells gives rise to metastases much less effectively than does the release of clusters is that the mechanisms of innate immunity are relatively ineffective against the latter but do control the former. One may speculate that when cells are released from primary tumors either as single cells or as very small clusters, they are highly vulnerable to destruction by the innate mechanisms of immunity, and that this explains the well-established experimental findings that metastatic spread occurs predominantly from the dissemination of relatively large clusters or emboli of tumor cells. Control of such clusters of circulating tumor cells has to be exercised by the specific immune processes.

ACKNOWLEDGMENTS

The work described in this chapter is supported by a program grant from the Medical Research Council. It is a pleasure to acknowledge many fruitful discussions with Drs. Suzanne Eccles and Graham Currie which contributed greatly to the formulation of these ideas.

REFERENCES

1. Borek, C., and Hall, E. J. (1974): Effect of split doses of X-rays on neoplastic transformation of single cells. *Nature,* 252:499.
2. Hewitt, H. B., Blake, E. R., and Walder, A. S. (1976): A critique of the evidence for active host defence against cancer, based on personal studies of 27 murine tumours of spontaneous origin. *Br. J. Cancer,* 33:241.
3. Burnet, M. (1970): *Immunological Surveillance.* Pergamon Press, London.
4. Sanford, B. H., Kohn, H. I., Daly, J. J., and Soo, S. F. (1973): Long-term spontaneous tumor incidence in neonatally thymectomized mice. *J. Immunol.,* 110:1437.
5. Law, L. W. (1972): Influence of immune suppression on the induction of neoplasms by the leukaemogenic virus MLV and its variant MSV. In: *The Nature of Leukemia. Proceedings of the International Cancer Conference, Sydney, Australia, 1972,* edited by P. C. Vincent, pp. 29–31. VCN Blight Printer, Sydney.

6. Eccles, S. A., and Alexander, P. A. (1974): Macrophage content of tumours in relation to metastatic spread and *Nature,* 250:667.
7. Eccles, S. A., and Alexander, P. (1975): Immunologically-mediated restraint of latent tumour metastases. *Nature,* 257:52.
8. Suit, H. D., Sedlacek, R., Wagner, M., Orsi, L., Silobrcic, V., and Rothman, K. J. (1976): Effect of *Corynebacterium parvum* on the response to irradiation of a C3H fibrosarcoma. *Cancer Res.,* 36:1305.
9. Delorme, E. J., and Alexander, P. (1964): Treatment of primary fibrosarcoma in the rat with immune lymphocytes. *Lancet,* 2:117.
10. Haddow, A., and Alexander, P. (1964): An immunological method of increasing the sensitivity of primary sarcomas to local irradiation with X-rays. *Lancet,* 1:452.
11. Delorme, E. J., Hall, J. G., Hodgett, J., and Alexander, P. (1969): The cellular immune response to primary sarcomata in rats. I. The significance of large basophilic cells in the thoracic duct lymph following antigenic challenge. *Proc. R. Soc. Lond. [Biol.],* 174:237.
12. Sloan, B., Yocum, C., and Clem, L. W. (1975): Recognition of self from non-self in crustaceans. *Nature,* 258:521.
13. Alexander, P. (1976): Surveillance against neoplastic cells—is it mediated by macrophages? *Br. J. Cancer,* 33:344.
14. Riley, V. (1968): Lactate dehydrogenase in the normal and malignant state in mice and the influence of a benign enzyme-elevating virus. Lactate dehydrogenase in the normal and malignant state. In: *Methods of Cancer Research,* edited by H. Busch. Academic Press, New York.
15. Kay, M. B. (1975): Mechanism of removal of senescent cells by human macrophages *in situ. Proc. Natl. Acad. Sci. U.S.A.,* 72:3521.
16. Alexander, P., and Evans, R. (1971): Endotoxin and double stranded RNA render macrophages cytotoxic. *Nature [New Biol.],* 232:76.
17. Bona, C., Damais, C., Dimitriu, A., Chedid, L., Giorbaru, R., Adam, A., Petit, J. F., Lederer, E., and Rosselet, J. P. (1974): Mitogenic effect of a water-soluble extract of *Nocardia opaca:* A comparative study with some bacterial adjuvants on spleen and peripheral lymphocytes of four mammalian species. *J. Immunol.,* 112:2028.
18. Olivotto, M., and Bomford, R. (1974): *In vitro* inhibition of tumor cell growth and DNA synthesis by peritoneal and lung macrophages from mice injected with *Corynebacterium parvum. Int. J. Cancer,* 13:478.
19. Hibbs, J. B. (1973): Macrophage nonimmunological recognition: Target cell factors related to contact inhibition. *Science,* 180:868.
20. Evans, R., and Alexander, P. (1972): Mechanism of immunologically specific killing of tumour cells by macrophages. *Nature,* 236:168.
21. Piessens, W. F., Hallowell Churchill, W., Jr., and David, J. R. (1975): Macrophages activated *in vitro* with lymphocyte mediators kill neoplastic but not normal cells. *J. Immunol.,* 114:293.
22. Hibbs, J. B., Jr., Lambert, L. H., Jr., and Remington, J. S. (1972): Control of carcinogenesis: A possible role for the activated macrophage. *Science,* 177:998.
23. Evans, R., and Alexander, P. (1970): Co-operation of immune lymphoid cells with macrophages in tumour immunity. *Nature,* 228:620.
24. Currie, G. A., and Basham, C. (1975): Activated macrophages release a factor which lyses malignant but not normal cells. *J. Exp. Med.,* 142:1600.
25. Inbar, M., and Shinitzky, M. (1974): Cholesterol as a bioregulator in the development and inhibition of leukemia. *Proc. Natl. Acad. Sci. U.S.A.,* 71:4229.
26. Edelman, G. M., and Yahara, I. (1976): Temperature-sensitive changes in surface modulating assemblies of fibroblasts transformed by mutants of Rous sarcoma virus. *Proc. Natl. Acad. Sci. U.S.A.,* 73(6):2047.
27. O'Neill, F. J. (1974): Control of nuclear division in normal but not in neoplastic mouse cells. *Cancer Res.,* 34:1070.
28. Springer, G. F., Parimal, R. D., and Scanlon, E. F. (1976): Blood group MN precursors as human breast carcinoma-associated antigens and "naturally" occurring human cytotoxins against them. *Cancer,* 37:169.
29. Alexander, P. (1974): Escape from immune destruction by the host through shedding of surface antigens: Is this a characteristic shared by malignant and embryonic cells? *Cancer Res.,* 34:2077.

30. Morell, A. G., Gregoriadis, G., and Scheinberg, I. H. (1971): The role of sialic acid in determining the survival of glycoproteins in the circulation. *J. Biol. Chem.,* 246:1461.
31. Davey, G. C., Currie, G. A., and Alexander, P. (1976): Spontaneous shedding and antibody induced modulation of histocompatibility antigens on murine lymphomata: Correlation with metastatic capacity. *Br. J. Cancer,* 33:9.
32. Scott, M. T. (1972): Biological effects of the adjuvant *Corynebacterium parvum.* II. Evidence for macrophage–T-cell interaction. *Cell. Immunol.,* 5:469–479.
33. Parr, I. B., Wheeler, L. E., and Alexander, P. (1975): Rejection of sarcoma cells at the site of an inflammatory reaction: Macrophages are not the only effector cells. *Cancer Lett.,* 1:49.
34. Parr, I., Wheeler, E., and Alexander, P. (1973): Similarities of the anti-tumour actions of endotoxin, lipid A and double-stranded RNA. *Br. J. Cancer,* 27:370.
35. Holm, G., and Perlmann, P. (1967): Cytotoxic potential of stimulated human lymphocytes. *J. Exp. Med.,* 125:721.
36. Lurie, M. B. (Ed.) (1964): Common denominators in resistance to tuberculosis and to other diseases. In: *Resistance to Tuberculosis. Experimental Studies in Native and Acquired Defence Mechanisms,* pp. 330–336. Harvard University Press, Cambridge.
37. Argyris, B. F. (1968): Role of macrophages in immunological maturation. *J. Exp. Med.,* 129:459.
38. Klein, E., and Holtermann, O. A. (1972): Immunotherapeutic approaches to the management of neoplasms. *Natl. Cancer Inst. Monogr.,* 35:379.
39. Alexander, P. (1973): Activated macrophages and the antitumor action of B.C.G. *Natl. Cancer Inst. Monogr.,* 39:127.
40. Selecki, E. E. (1959): A study of the metastatic distribution of Ehrlich ascites tumour cells in mice. *Aust. J. Exp. Biol. Med.,* 37:489.
41. Hofer, K. G., Prensky, W., and Hughes, W. L. (1969): Death and metastatic distribution of tumour cells in mice monitored with ^{125}I-iododeoxyuridine. *J. Natl. Cancer Inst.,* 43:763.
42. Weiss, L., Glaves, D., and Waite, D. A. (1974): The influence of host immunity on the arrest of circulating cancer cells and its modification by neuraminidase. *Int. J. Cancer,* 13:850.
43. Van den Brenk, H. A. S., Burch, W. M., Kelly, H., and Orton, C. (1975): Venous diversion trapping and growth of blood-borne cancer cells en route to the lungs. *Br. J. Cancer,* 31:46.
44. Sadler, T. E., and Alexander, P. (1976): Trapping and destruction of blood-borne syngeneic leukaemia cells in lung, liver and spleen of normal and leukaemic rats. *Br. J. Cancer,* 33:512.
45. Alexander, P., Eccles, S. A., and Gauci, C. L. L. (1976): The significance of macrophages in human and experimental tumors. *Ann. N. Y. Acad. Sci.,* 276:124.
46. Eccles, S. A., Bandlow, G., and Alexander, P. (1976): Monocytosis associated with the growth of transplanted syngeneic rat sarcomata differing in immunogenicity. *Br. J. Cancer,* 34:20.
47. Normann, S. J., and Sorkin, E. (1976): Cell specific defect in monocyte function during tumor growth. *J. Natl. Cancer Inst.,* 57:135.
48. Moldow, R. E. (1971): *Ann. Intern. Med.,* 74:449.
49. Barrett, J. O. (1970): Monocytosis in malignant disease. *Ann. Intern. Med.,* 73:991–992.
50. Currie, G. A., and Basham, C. (1972): Serum mediated inhibition of the immunological reactions of the patient to his own tumour: A possible role for circulating antigen. *Br. J. Cancer,* 26:427.
51. Currie, G. A., and Alexander, P. (1974): Spontaneous shedding of TSTA by viable sarcoma cells; its possible role in facilitating metastatic spread. *Br. J. Cancer,* 29:72.
52. Bystryn, J.-C. (1976): Release of tumor-associated antigens by murine melanoma cells. *J. Immunol.,* 116(5):1302.

Cancer Invasion and Metastasis: Biologic Mechanisms and Therapy, edited by S. B. Day et al. Raven Press, New York © 1977.

Quantitative Analysis of Tumor:Host Interaction and the Outcome of Experimental Metastasis

*Isaiah J. Fidler, *Douglas M. Gersten, and **Charles W. Riggs

*Basic Research Program and **Information Systems Department, NCI Frederick Cancer Research Center, Frederick, Maryland 21701

The development of tumor metastasis involves five major steps: (a) dislodgment of cells from the primary tumor, invasion into surrounding tissue, and penetration of blood and/or lymph vessels; (b) release of tumor cell emboli into the circulation; (c) arrest of the emboli in small vascular channels of distant organs; (d) tumor cell invasion of the wall of the arresting vessel, infiltration into adjacent tissue, and multiplication; and (e) growth of vascularized stroma into the new tumor (36). The process of invasion, embolization, arrest, and development of emboli can then recommence (8). We are concerned here only with blood-borne metastasis.

It is becoming increasingly clear that the mere presence of tumor emboli in the circulation does not constitute metastasis. Whether metastasis will occur is determined by the ability of tumor emboli to survive the turbulence of the circulation, evade possible host defense mechanisms, and successfully complete the above steps. Thus, when malignant cells are released at the site of a primary tumor or experimentally administered into the circulation, a variety of host and tumor cell factors determines their distribution and fate. Tumor cells can enter the circulation in clumps or as single cells, and then interact with one another (5,35), or with platelets (16,17), lymphocytes (9), soluble blood components (26), and noncirculating host cells (21,22). These cellular interactions may modify the extent and location of subsequent metastases. Most tumor cells die rapidly in the blood (4,27), but many are nonspecifically trapped or specifically arrested in the first capillary bed encountered (8,36). Circulating tumor cells trapped in a given location can then recirculate and arrest at other locations (18,23,37).

The determinant, then, for the outcome of experimental metastasis appears to be an interplay between properties of the host and properties of the tumor cells. In order to sort out the relative contributions of the host immune system, the tumor cells, and the host properties not associated with immunity, we will deal with each separately.

The relationship of the host immune response to the growth and metastasis of malignant tumors is not well understood. Studies of the relationship of lymphocyte-tumor cell interactions to the ultimate outcome of experimental metastasis in animals yielded contradictory results, which, in turn, led to the proposition that two competing tumor cell-lymphocyte interactions might be involved (24). The cell-mediated response in the early development of cancer or when tumors are weakly antigenic might directly stimulate rather than inhibit tumor growth. On the other hand, tumor inhibition could occur with a strongly active immune response or when the neoplasm is highly antigenic (25). It is entirely possible that different tumor cell-immune cell interactions could occur during the pathogenesis of metastasis. One approach to the problem has been to demonstrate the stimulation or inhibition of tumor growth in an experimental metastasis system by varying the ratio of lymphocytes:tumor cells (7). In that study, it was shown that mixtures of both lymphocytes and tumor cells injected intravenously (i.v.) simultaneously into syngeneic mice altered the outcome of experimental metastasis. Injections of tumor cells mixed in low ratios with syngeneic lymphocytes yielded significantly more pulmonary tumor colonies than tumor cells injected alone. In contrast, tumor cells mixed in high ratios with the same lymphocytes yielded significantly fewer lung tumors (7). Earlier studies in that same system showed that injections of homotypic clumps of four to five tumor cells resulted in a markedly greater number of lung tumors than identical numbers injected as single cells (5). All of these observations suggest that tumor-lymphocyte embolus formation could affect the initial arrest in the lungs, thereby explaining the apparent increase in tumor incidence. The inhibition of such tumor colonies could have occurred after arrest or at a different stage in the sequence of metastasis development (5). From studies of experimental metastasis in platelet-depleted (16) and immune-manipulated (31) animals as well as from studies in this laboratory regarding the effect of immune manipulation on the final number of gross metastases, it is apparent that there is no clear-cut relationship between the initial arrest and tumor cells in the lungs and the ultimate number of pulmonary tumor colonies. There is also no simple correlation between the outcome of experimental metastasis and the immune status of the recipient animal as far as the specific tumor is concerned. We will present data to show that holding the tumor cells constant and varying the immune status of the host drastically change the number of pulmonary metastases.

The properties of tumor cells themselves are also important in metastasis. B16 melanoma variant cell lines with enhanced pulmonary implantation and survival potential were selected by repeated i.v. injection of the tumor cells into syngeneic mice and recovery of the resulting pulmonary tumor colonies. From each *in vivo* selective cycle, tumor cell lines were recovered that produced increasing numbers of experimental pulmonary metastases when readministered i.v. into syngeneic recipients (6). In addition, selection of B16 tumor cells *in vivo* for enhanced pulmonary arrest and subsequent growth resulted in concomitant loss of extrapulmonary tumor formation (12,20).

The effects of immune manipulation on the arrest, distribution, and survival of low and high metastatic variants of B16 melanoma were examined after i.v. injection into immune-competent and -incompetent syngeneic and allogeneic hosts. The results indicate that the biological properties and ability of highly metastatic B16-F10 variants to form more experimental tumors than the weakly metastatic B16-F1 variants were maintained regardless of the immune status of the host. That is, although the absolute numbers of tumor colonies could be affected by immune manipulation, the relative differences between tumor formation by B16-F1 and B16-F10 could not be abolished.

Finally, the interaction of tumor cells with circulatory host blood cells was examined. It will be shown that introduction of tumor cells into the circulation of normal, syngeneic animals leads to a leukopenia associated with an accumulation of white blood cells (WBCs) in the lung capillary bed.

MATERIALS AND METHODS

Animals

Inbred mouse strains, C57BL/6 and athymic NIH Swiss nude (nu/nu) and their immune-competent heterozygous littermates (nu/+), were obtained from the Experimental Animal Breeding Facility, Frederick Cancer Research Center. Inbred A mice were purchased from the Jackson Laboratory, Bar Harbor, Maine.

Tumor Cell Lines

The B16 melanoma cell lines were developed as described previously (6). Briefly, C57BL/6 mice were given i.v. injections of 50,000 viable B16 melanoma cells and killed 3 weeks later. Their pulmonary melanoma nodules (colonies) were removed aseptically, pressed through 80-mesh stainless steel sieves (E-C Apparatus, St. Petersburg, Fla.), filtered through gauze, and cultivated *in vitro* on plastic in Eagle's minimum essential medium supplemented with 10% fetal calf serum and a solution containing nonessential amino acids, sodium pyruvate, L-glutamine, and vitamins (CMEM) obtained from Flow Laboratories (Rockville, Md.). Cells were harvested from confluent cultures by overlaying a thin layer of 0.25% trypsin:EDTA for 1 min. The flask was tapped to facilitate removal of cells from the plastic. The process was then repeated 10 times. With each successive *in vivo* cycle the yield of pulmonary colonies increased (6,9). Cell lines from the first and tenth cycles *in vivo* have been designated B16-F1 and B16-F10 for low and high lung implantability and survival, respectively. These tumor cell lines have maintained their metastatic properties whether grown subcutaneously (s.c.), or i.v., or *in vitro* (9).

Embryo Cultures

Embryo cultures were established from 14- to 16-day C57BL/6 fetuses as described previously (11). In general, all studies were conducted with tertiary subcultures of embryo cells in their exponential growth phase.

Procedure for Quantitative Analysis of Tumor Cell Arrest, Distribution, and Survival

B16-F1 or B16-F10 cells prelabeled *in vitro* with ^{125}I-5-iodo-2'-deoxy-uridine ([^{125}I]IUdR) were injected i.v. into mice. This labeling technique has been described in detail elsewhere (4). [^{125}I]IUdR is an analogue of thymidine that is incorporated into the DNA of proliferating cells and remains there until cell death, when it is released and subsequently degraded in the liver. The free radioiodine is then excreted in the urine. Reutilization of the isotope was minimal, and thyroidal accumulation was prevented by supplementing the drinking water with 0.1% NaI. Tumor cell labeling was accomplished by adding [^{125}I]IUdR at 0.3 μCi/ml medium (specific activity, 200 mCi/mM; New England Nuclear, Boston, Mass.) to actively dividing cells for 24 hr. Labeling with [^{125}I]IUdR did not alter the biological behavior of the tumor cells, and practically all cells were labeled as determined by autoradiography (4).

[^{125}I]IUdR-labeled cells were harvested as above. The cells were then washed and resuspended in Hanks' balanced salt solution (HBSS) for injection. Tumor cell viability was about 95% as determined by the trypan blue dye exclusion test. The suspension was diluted to yield 100,000 single, viable, [^{125}I]IUdR-labeled cells per 0.2 ml, the inoculum dose per mouse. Triplicate inocula were placed into vials and monitored for radioactivity in a well-type NaI crystal scintillation counter to determine the activity per cell. Each mouse was given an i.v. injection into the tail vein of 100,000 [^{125}I]IUdR-labeled B16 cells, and five mice from each group were killed at intervals ranging from 2 min to 14 days post-injection. Lung, liver, spleen, and 0.5 ml of blood were collected from each mouse, and the organs were placed into vials containing 70% ethanol. The ethanol was replaced once a day for 3 days to remove practically all the ethanol-soluble ^{125}I. The remaining radioactivity was associated with DNA of tumor cells (4,6). Thus, the number of originally injected tumor cells, which were viable in organs at time of death, was calculated from the activity per cell ratio in the representative inocula samples and corrected for isotope decay. Each sample was counted four times for 2 min each. The number of pulmonary tumor colonies on day 14 after i.v. injection was determined with the aid of a dissecting microscope by two independent observers.

Immune Manipulation Procedures

C57BL/6 mice were injected s.c. with 100,000 viable B16 melanoma cells. Then 10 or 21 days later these tumor-bearing mice were injected i.v. with 100,000 viable [^{125}I]IUdR-labeled cells and processed as described above.

C57BL/6 mice, 4 weeks old, were thymectomized or sham-thymectomized 5 weeks before the experiment. These mice were also X-irradiated (450 R, whole body) 1 week following surgery (4 weeks before the experiments). These adult thymectomized, X-irradiated (ATX) mice and their counterparts, control sham-thymectomized, X-irradiated (STX) mice were injected i.v. with 100,000 viable [^{125}I]IUdR-labeled cells, as described above.

In subsequent experiments, ATX and STX C57BL/6 mice were injected i.v. with a reconstituting dose of 1×10^7 non-glass-adherent syngeneic lymphocytes 24 hr prior to labeled tumor cell injection. The method for obtaining homogeneous non-glass-adherent mononuclear cells (lymphocytes) from spleens and lymph nodes of syngeneic C57BL/6 mice bearing B16 melanoma s.c. has been detailed previously (7).

Immunization of C57BL/6 Mice Against B16 Melanoma

C57BL/6 mice were given injections of 1×10^6 melanoma tumor cells s.c. that had been exposed to 15 kR X-irradiation and mixed with complete Freund's adjuvant. Mice were given injections three times at 2-week intervals and then challenged s.c. with 100,000 viable, unirradiated B16 cells. The viable tumor inoculum dose was calculated to yield 100% takes. Only the mice that rejected the above normally lethal tumor inoculum were designated as "successfully immunized" animals. The mice that failed to reject the s.c. challenge dose were classified as "unsuccessfully immunized." Immune cells from successfully and unsuccessfully immunized mice were previously demonstrated to differ significantly in their *in vitro* cytotoxicity against the B16 melanoma (7,8). Both these groups of mice were injected i.v. with 100,000 viable [^{125}I]IUdR-labeled cells and processed as described above.

Immunization of A Mice Against AC 15091

Adenocarcinoma 15091 (AC 15091) cells syngeneic to A mice were grown intraperitoneally (i.p.) and harvested into cold HBSS containing 2 units/ml heparin. Tumor cells were then frozen and thawed three times as described previously (19). Mice were given s.c. injections of 1×10^6 frozen-thawed cells three times at 2-week intervals and then challenged s.c. with 100,000 viable AC 15091 cells. Again, only mice rejecting this ordinarily lethal tumor inoculum were designated as tumor-immune animals and used in the distribution experiments. Each mouse received an i.v. inoculum of 100,000 viable [^{125}I]IUdR-labeled B16 melanoma cells and processed as described above.

Statistical Methods

At each of the seven sacrifice times, beginning at 2 min and continuing through 14 days, the percentage of originally injected tumor cells still present and viable in the lungs was calculated. These percentages were transformed to probability units (probits) and plotted against the logarithm of time to show the relative rates of disappearance of the labeled cells from the lungs for the several treatments. The covariance analysis on the probit versus log time transformation was performed using a prepackaged program (BMDX82) and was based on the mean values of five mice per treatment group (above).

Preliminary examination of the data suggested that the rate of decrease was frequently shallow for 2 min to 1 hr, fairly steep from 1 hr through 1 day, and then shallow again from 1 day through 14 days. Comparisons of decrease rates and recovery percentages (percent of originally injected cells recovered from the lungs at a given time) were therefore made during the time intervals when the decrease slopes were relatively linear. Accordingly, these comparisons were made over the 1 hr through 1 day interval and from 1 day through 14 days. The period from 2 min to 1 hr was not examined statistically. Duncan's Multiple Range test (3) was applied to identify percent recovery differences among the various treatments. The program used was SAS (North Carolina State University). Mean percent recoveries at 14 days were calculated from the data of individual animals and were compared by a one-way analysis of variance.

Studies of Peripheral Blood Cells

Either 0.145 M NaCl (0.2 ml) or varying numbers of tumor cells were injected into the tail vein of five mice per group. Blood was collected from each mouse by tail bleeding (through a small incision at the proximal part) at 5, 30, 60, and 120 min post-injection. In some experiments these sequential bleedings were performed on normal mice that received no injection. In all mice, the total WBC count and differential determinations were performed.

In a separate experiment, mice were injected i.v. with tumor cells but were tail bled only once, either at 5, 30, 60, or 120 min after injection.

RESULTS

Host Immune Status

The first section deals with arrest and distribution of 100,000 viable B16-F1 cells in hosts that differ in their immune status. The results for lung distribution only, which are shown in Figs. 1 through 3 as probit versus log time transformations, will be analyzed statistically.

Pattern of Tumor Cell Distribution and Fate: Syngeneic C57BL/6 Mice

As can be seen in Fig. 1, 62% of the injected tumor cells were recovered in the lungs at 2 min post-injection. Thus, the majority of circulating B16-F1 cells were indeed arrested in the capillary bed of the first organ they encountered. By 3 hr post-injection, only 30% of the injected cells were found in the lung. This immediate decline in lung counts could have been due in part to recirculation of some tumor cells but primarily was a measure of cell death and not merely escape (4). A significant increase in tumor cell counts was observed in the liver, spleen, and blood during the interval from 2 min to 3 hr post-injection. This increase, however, represents only about 10% of the cells that cleared the lungs over that same interval and is there-

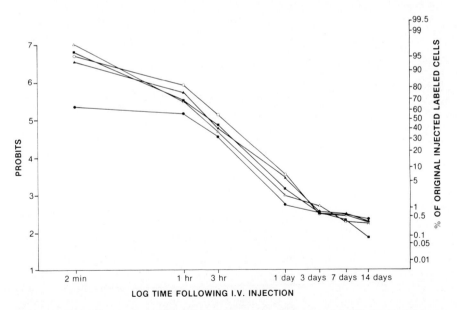

FIG. 1. Probits vs log time transformation of the percentage of originally i.v. injected tumor cells still present in the lungs. (●) Normal C57BL/6 mice; (▲) C57BL/6 mice bearing s.c. tumor for 10 days; (○) C57BL/6 mice bearing s.c. tumor for 21 days; (■) successfully immunized C57BL/6 mice; (△) unsuccessfully immunized C57BL/6 mice.

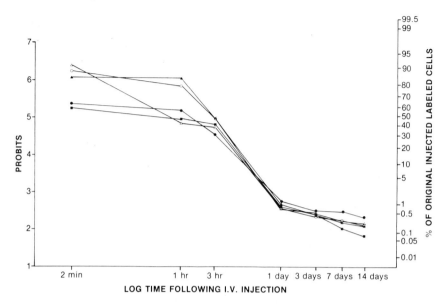

FIG. 2. Probits vs log time transformation of the percentage of originally i.v. injected tumor cells still present in the lungs. (●) Normal C57BL/6 mice; (▲) sham-thymectomized, X-irradiated C57BL/6 mice; (○) sham-thymectomized, X-irradiated, lymphocyte-reconstituted C57BL/6 mice; (■) thymectomized, X-irradiated C57BL/6 mice; (△) thymectomized, X-irradiated, lymphocyte-reconstituted C57BL/6 mice.

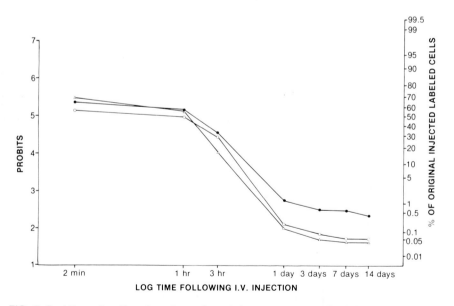

FIG. 3. Probits vs log time transformation of the percentages of originally i.v. injected tumor cells still present in the lungs. The points represent the mean determination of at least 5 mice as detailed in Materials and Methods. (●) Normal C57BL/6 mice; (△) normal A mice; (○) A mice immunized against AC15091.

fore indicative of cell death, not recirculation. At 1 day post-injection, 99% of the originally injected cells died, leaving 1% in the lungs. The liver, spleen, and blood were unremarkable at that time. Tumor cell death began shortly after initial arrest with only 1% of the cells surviving in the lungs 24 hr later; whereas by day 14 after injection, 50 ± 10 gross tumor colonies were observed.

"Tumor-bearing" C57BL/6 mice are those that had been injected s.c. with the B16 melanoma either 10 days or 21 days before the i.v. injection of [^{125}I]IUdR-labeled B16-F1 cells. There was no significant difference between these two groups of animals; therefore, the data were considered together. At 2 min after i.v. injection, 94 to 96% of the tumor cells were arrested in the lungs (Fig. 2). This percentage was significantly greater than the normal counterparts ($p < 0.001$). By 3 hr after injection, the rate of tumor cell clearance from the lungs of tumor-bearing mice was practically identical to the rate in normal recipients at that time. Tumor cell death occurring between 1 and 14 days after i.v. injection was more pronounced in tumor-bearing than in normal mice. At 14 days, there were also fewer tumor cells remaining in the lung, thus yielding a smaller number of visible tumor colonies. The average number of pulmonary nodules was 24 ± 2 for mice bearing s.c. tumor for 10 days, and 19 ± 4 nodules for mice bearing s.c. tumor for 21 days.

Immune manipulated syngeneic animals consisted of four groups: ATX mice, control STX mice, and ATX and control STX mice receiving an i.v. reconstitution of 1×10^7 non-glass-adherent trypan blue excluding syngeneic lymphocytes 24 hr prior to i.v. tumor cell administration. The data suggest that the pattern of initial tumor arrest in ATX mice differed from that in ATX mice reconstituted with syngeneic lymphocytes or both groups of STX mice. The injection of syngeneic lymphocytes into ATX mice 24 hr prior to tumor cell injection significantly increased the initial lung arrest (60 to 92%, $p < 0.001$). Nevertheless, by 3 hr post-injection and continuing until 3 days post-injection, the number of tumor cells in lungs was practically identical in both ATX and ATX-lymphocyte-reconstituted mice. The number of tumor cells in lungs of lymphocyte-reconstituted ATX mice stabilized by day 7, but tumor cell death continued in ATX mice until the termination of the experiment. This tumor cell death was reminiscent of that of mice successfully immunized against the B16 melanoma (below).

The pattern of tumor cell arrest, distribution, and survival observed in STX and lymphocyte-reconstituted STX mice was strikingly similar to the one described for lymphocyte-reconstituted ATX mice. The patterns for these three groups of mice were also clearly related to those found in normal syngeneic animals. By day 14 the number of pulmonary nodules in the four groups of mice in this study differed significantly. ATX mice averaged 6 ± 2 pulmonary nodules, ATX lymphocyte-reconstituted mice averaged 14 ± 2 colonies, STX mice averaged 18 ± 4 colonies, and STX lymphocyte-reconstituted mice averaged 17 ± 6 pulmonary nodules ($p < 0.01$).

The pattern of cell arrest in either successfully or unsuccessfully immunized mice was similar to that observed with tumor-bearing mice, but different from the pattern in normal mice. The decline in lung counts in both groups from 2 min to 1 day post-injection was similar. By day 1, 3.3% of originally injected cells were found in lungs of successfully immunized mice as compared to 2.2% in lungs of unsuccessfully immunized mice. It was interesting to note that the decline in number of cells observed in lungs of unsuccessfully immunized mice from day 1 to day 14 paralleled that seen in both normal and tumor-bearing mice. In contrast, tumor cell death in mice successfully immunized against the B16 melanoma continued steadily until day 14. Indeed, the number of gross pulmonary nodules observed in successfully immunized mice (10 ± 5) was significantly smaller than the corresponding number observed in either unsuccessfully immunized (55 ± 7) or normal mice (50 ± 10) ($p < 0.001$).

Allogeneic Animals

There were no significant differences in the pattern of B16-F1 pulmonary arrest between normal A mice and A mice immunized to their syngeneic tumor, AC 15091 (Fig. 3). However, both allogeneic groups differed significantly from all groups of C57BL/6 mice. The rate of initial cell arrest in lungs of A mice was 65 to 68% (similar to that in normal syngeneic C57BL/6 mice). However, by 3 hr post-tumor cell injection, tumor cell death was greater in A mice than in any C57BL/6 mice. Moreover, by day 1 after i.v. injection about 99.8% of injected labeled cells died or cleared the lungs of allogeneic animals, in contrast to the survival rate of at least 1% seen in any syngeneic mice. Tumor cell death continued, but by 3 days post-injection the number of surviving cells stabilized and by day 14 gross pulmonary metastases averaged 12 ± 4 in normal A mice and 13 ± 2 in A mice immune against AC 15091. Allogeneic A mice always rejected the histoincompatible B16 melanoma when injected s.c. The apparent differences between survival and growth of tumor cells injected s.c. or i.v. into A mice were comparable to those seen by immune-competent heterozygous NIH mice (below) and C57BL/6 mice successfully immunized against syngeneic B16 tumor (above).

The growth of s.c. implanted tumors of syngeneic, allogeneic, or xenogeneic origin occurs in athymic (nude) mice; it is interesting to note, however, that transplanted tumors rarely metastasize in nude mice (28). Table 1 shows the pattern of labeled tumor cell initial arrest, organ distribution, survival, and final development of secondary metastases in immune-incompetent nu/nu and their heterozygous immune-competent nu/+ littermates. Most tumor cells were arrested immediately in the capillary bed of the lung. Tumor cell death began shortly thereafter. The difference in the numbers of arrested tumor cells in lungs of the two groups was clearly demonstrable

TABLE 1. Arrest, distribution, and fate of 100,000 viable [^{125}I]IUdR-labeled B16-F1 melanoma cells injected i.v. into allogeneic nu/nu and nu/+mice

Time of death[a]	nu/nu		nu/nu reconstituted		nu/+		nu/+ reconstituted	
	Lung[b]	Blood[c]	Lung[b]	Blood[c]	Lung	Blood	Lung	Blood
2 min	68,000	200	91,000	300	91,000	290	99,000	130
1 hr	40,000	900	46,000	590	74,000	160	68,000	500
3 hr	10,060	260	13,900	540	30,000	300	30,600	490
1 day	160	20	100	20	800	20	1,600	10
3 days	38	0	30	0	180	0	940	0
7 days	20	0	20	0	80	0	250	0
14 days	10	0	10	0	60	0	200	0
Gross metastases on day 14	2 ± 1		0		12 ± 3		30 ± 8	

[a] Five animals/time interval. Variation from the mean did not exceed 10%.
[b] The difference between the number of cells arrested in the lungs of nu/nu mice and that in nu/+ littermates is highly significant ($p < 0.005$).
[c] 0.5 ml of blood/mouse.

by 2 min post-injection, and was statistically significant at any time interval ($p < 0.005$). The percent survival of B16-F1 tumor cells at 3 hr after injection was about 10% in the nu/nu mice and 30% in the nu/+ littermates. By day 14 post-injection, about 0.06% of the original tumor cells survived in the nu/+ mice, as compared to only 0.01% in nu/nu mice. At this time gross lung metastases in nu/nu or nu/+ mice differed significantly. Nu/nu mice averaged 2 ± 1 nodules, whereas nu/+ mice averaged 12 ± 3 nodules ($p < 0.01$).

It has been suggested that thymus-dependent lymphocytes may enhance the metastasis of some syngeneic tumors (8,9). As seen in Table 1, the initial arrest of tumor cells in lungs of nu/nu mice was lower than in nu/+ controls, but the following questions remained unanswered. Was the decreased arrest due to lack of thymus-dependent lymphocytes; and would nu/nu mice develop as many pulmonary metastases as nu/+ mice if they were injected with 1×10^7 lymphocytes from nu/+ mice 24 hr prior to i.v. injection of tumor cells?

The following experiments were carried out in order to answer the above questions. One day prior to tumor cell injection, nu/nu and nu/+ mice were injected i.v. with 1×10^7 nu/+ lymphocytes, a dose that was sufficient to prevent a decrease in metastases in ATX C57BL/6 mice above. This reconstituting dose was judged to render the nu/nu comparable to the nu/+ for the following reason: Both nu/nu and nu/+ mice were injected i.v. with 1×10^7 non-glass-adherent nu/+ lymphocytes. Twenty-four hours later groups of 10 lymphocyte-treated and non-lymphocyte-treated nu/nu and nu/+ mice were injected s.c. with 100,000 viable B16 melanoma tumor cells. The appearance of a measurable s.c. tumor was monitored in all four test groups. None of the nu/+ mice had visible tumors 16 days after implantation. Of 10 non-lymphocyte-treated nu/nu mice, 8 had palpable tumors averaging 4 × 6 mm, whereas only 1 of 9 lymphocyte-treated nu/nu mice had palpable tumors. Administration of 1 × 10⁷ nu/+ lymphocytes to nu/nu mice 24 hr before s.c. allogeneic tumor challenge therefore protected the mice for at least 16 days after s.c. tumor cell injection. When nu/nu mice were preinjected with nu/+ lymphocytes, then 1 day later given i.v. injection of 100,000 B16-F1 cells, the outcome was not comparable to that of the nu/+ counterparts as for s.c. challenges above. The initial arrest of tumor cells, survival, and outcome of pulmonary metastases differed between lymphocyte-treated and nontreated nu/+ mice (Table 1). Most significantly, gross pulmonary metastases in treated nu/+ mice averaged 30 ± 8, whereas in nontreated nu/+ mice, they averaged 12 ± 3 ($p < 0.005$). Apparently, the preinjection of lymphocytes enhanced metastasis. The arrest and distribution of B16-F1 melanoma cells differed significantly between lymphocyte-treated and nontreated nu/nu mice. The initial arrest of the B16 melanoma in lungs of lymphocyte-treated nu/nu mice was significantly greater than that in non-lymphocyte-treated nu/nu mice ($p < 0.01$). Preinjected nu/nu mice had a pattern of initial tumor cell arrest similar to that of nu/+ mice (Table 1). Nevertheless, by 3 hr post-injection, tumor cell survival in lymphocyte-reconstituted nu/nu was low and close to that in nontreated mice. By day 14 post-i.v. tumor cell injection, the reconstituted nu/nu mice had no gross pulmonary metastases, but their nu/+ littermates averaged 30 ± 8 nodules ($p < 0.001$). Apparently, the increased initial arrest of tumor cells in the pulmonary capillary bed was not reflected in the subsequent development of tumor nodules.

Statistical Analysis

The relationship of the percentage of originally injected cells recovered to time following i.v. injection was expressed by converting the percents to probability units (probits) and time (in hours) to common logarithms. Examination of the resulting curves showed that the rate of decrease of percent recovery could be divided into three fairly distinct phases. First, the rate was usually shallow from 2 min to 1 hr post-injection; second, it was relatively steep from 1 hr to 1 day; and third, the rate was shallow again from 1 day to 14 days post-injection. In view of this nonlinearity, it was felt that the analysis would be more meaningful if the comparisons of decrease rates and recovery percentages were made for those intervals where the slopes were relatively linear.

The 11 different test groups were separated into three categories. In each category, the control group representing the behavior of tumor cells injected into normal, syngeneic, nonmanipulated animals is included. Within each category, the several treatment groups were tested by covariance analysis for parallelism of labeled cell decrease rates and for equality of average percent recovery. Separate analyses were performed for the 1 hr to 1 day and the 1 day to 14 day intervals. The decrease rates over the 1 hr to 1 day interval were essentially parallel within each category. The 2 min to 1 hr interval was not analyzed in this manner.

The first category includes all groups in which mice were exposed to the tumor in some manner before the injection of $[^{125}I]IUdR$-labeled cells and the normal C57BL/6 control group (Fig. 1). The exposed groups are tumor-bearing animals (both 10-day and 21-day) as well as successfully immunized and unsuccessfully immunized animals. Their decrease rates in the final interval (days 1 to 14) were $-0.973, -0.071, -1.084, -0.701,$ and -0.314 (controls), respectively, and the probability that these rate differences may be due to chance alone is 0.12. The mean percent recoveries in the day 1 to day 14 interval were 1.00, 1.04, 0.57, 0.74, and 0.66 (controls), respectively, and the probability of chance variation is 0.54. This category is characterized by moderate departure from parallelism of decrease rates and no statistical differences in the mean percent recoveries of tumor cells in the final interval.

The second category covers the four immune-manipulated groups: sham-thymectomized X-irradiated; sham-thymectomized X-irradiated lymphocyte-reconstituted; thymectomized X-irradiated; thymectomized X-irradiated lymphocyte-reconstituted; and the normal C57BL/6 control group (Fig. 2). These groups are characterized by significant departure from parallelism of their decay rates over the final interval ($-0.485, -0.412,$ $-0.704, -0.411, -0.314; p = 0.012$) and a small but very significant reduction from the normal in the mean percent recoveries (0.41, 0.39, 0.27, 0.39, 0.66; $p = 0.002$).

The third category, shown in Fig. 3, includes normal A, A immunized against AC 15091, and normal C57BL/6 mice as controls. In the day 1 to day 14 interval, the labeled cell decrease rates (in probits/$\log_{10}$ hr) were $-0.317, -0.364,$ and $-0.314,$ respectively. The probability that the rate differences are attributable to chance alone is 0.90, thus indicating random variation. The mean percent recoveries of viable tumor cells in the day 1 to day 14 interval were 0.06, 0.08, and 0.66, respectively. The differences in the mean percent recoveries for allogeneic compared to normal animals are highly significant ($p < 0.0001$). Category 3, then, is characterized by parallel decrease rates and highly significant differences in the mean percent recoveries in the final time interval. Statistical analysis was not performed for any of the other groups.

Tumor Cell Properties

We turn now to the contribution of tumor cell properties to the ultimate outcome of experimental metastasis. We deal here with the differences between the weakly metastatic B16-F1 and their highly metastatic isolates, B16-F10. The approach is similar to that used above in that the behavior of B16-F1 and B16-F10 cells is compared in syngeneic and allogeneic animals.

This injection procedure was repeated for ATX and STX animals. Lymphocyte-reconstituted animals were not used since they are shown above to resemble STX animals. Both groups had similar initial cell arrest in the lungs and tumor cell survival from day 1 to day 14 post-injection; however, tumor arrest and survival in the STX group were always higher (Table 2). Significantly ($p < 0.01$) more cells from line B16-F10 were initially arrested and ultimately survived in the capillary beds of the lungs than line B16-F1 in either group. The most pronounced difference was seen on the first day after i.v. injection. In the ATX mice, B16-F1 cell survival in the lungs was approximately 0.8%, whereas 5.9% of the B16-F10 cells survived ($p < 0.01$). Similarly, in the STX mice the day 1 survival rate of B16-F1 cells was 1.0% compared to 11% for B16-F10 cells ($p < 0.01$) (Table 2), values very close to those obtained with normal animals (Table 3). Cells from line B16-F10 survived in the lungs at a significantly higher level than B16-F1 cells on days 1, 3, 7, and 14 ($p<0.01$). In ATX mice, cells from line B16-F1 yielded 6 ± 2 nodules, whereas B16-F10 yielded $100 \pm$

TABLE 2. *Arrest and survival of* [^{125}I]*IUdR-labeled B16 melanoma variants injected i.v. into syngeneic thymectomized X-irradiated or sham thymectomized X-irradiated C57BL/6 mice*

Time of death	Thymectomized X-irradiated[a]				Sham thymectomized X-irradiated[a]			
	B16-F1		B16-F10		B16-F1		B16-F10	
	Lung	Blood[b]	Lung	Blood[b]	Lung	Blood[b]	Lung	Blood[b]
2 min	64,000[c]	250	94,000[c]	170	85,500[d]	390	91,000[d]	350
1 hr	48,000	460	64,000	650	65,000	580	72,500	220
3 hr	42,000	230	52,500	500	49,000	510	54,000	240
1 day	830	100	5,900	–	1,000	180	11,000	80
3 days	480	–	1,400	–	500	–	3,380	–
7 days	140	–	1,000	–	250	–	2,900	–
14 days	80	–	700	–	210	–	2,100	–
Gross metas-tases on day 14	6 ± 2		100 ± 30		18 ± 4		420 ± 70	

[a] Mean number of labeled tumor cells after i.v. injection of 100,000 viable [^{125}I]IUdR-labeled B16 melanoma cells. Five animals/time interval. Variation from the mean did not exceed 10%.
[b] 0.5 ml of blood/mouse.
[c] The differences were highly significant ($p<0.01$).
[d] The differences were highly significant ($p<0.01$).

TABLE 3. *Arrest and survival of* [^{125}I]*IUdR-labeled B16 melanoma variants injected i.v. into normal syngeneic C57BL/6 mice*

Time of death	B16-F1[a]		B16-F10[a]	
	Lung	Blood[b]	Lung	Blood[b]
2 min	64,000[c]	170	99,000[c]	90
1 hr	57,000	480	97,000	400
3 hr	32,700	530	88,200	380
1 day	1,190	40	12,450	150
3 days	620	–	3,400	–
7 days	600	–	3,290	–
14 days	400	–	2,600	–
Gross metastases on day 14	60 ± 10		269 ± 37	

[a] Mean number of labeled tumor cells after i.v. injection of 100,000 viable [^{125}I]IUdR-labeled B16 melanoma cells. Five animals/time interval. Variation from the mean did not exceed 10%.
[b] 0.5 ml of blood/mouse.
[c] The differences were highly significant ($p < 0.005$).

30 nodules ($p < 0.01$). Similarly, in STX controls B16-F1 and B16-F10 cells yielded 18 ± 4 and 420 ± 70 pulmonary nodules, respectively ($p < 0.001$).

Allogeneic Animals

Table 2 indicates that upon i.v. injection into allogeneic, immune-competent A/J recipients B16-F1 and B16-F10 cells still form pulmonary tumors, albeit at a lower level than in syngeneic recipients. Neither line B16-F1 nor B16-F10 cells, when transplanted s.c. (100,000 viable cells) into allogeneic strain A mice, will grow to form tumors (data not shown). However, when the same number of B16-F1 cells was injected i.v. into strain A mice, some pulmonary melanoma nodules formed (above). The initial arrest of tumor cells in the lung capillary bed and survival at 1 or 14 days post-injection in strain A mice (Table 4) were less than in syngeneic recipients (Table 4), although differences of arrest and survival between B16-F1 and B16-F10 cells remained significant ($p < 0.01$) (Table 4). Again, there were significantly more B16-F10 cells ($p < 0.001$) in A strain mice (Table 4). Therefore, differences in arrest and survival in lung parenchyma between B16-F1 and B16-F10 cells were not abrogated under these conditions.

Pronounced differences were found between the arrest and survival of a B16 melanoma line injected i.v. in allogeneic nu/nu and nu/+ mice. Cells from lines B16-F1 and B16-F10 arrested at higher initial rates, survived

TABLE 4. *Arrest and survival of* [^{125}I]*IUdR-labeled B16 melanoma variants injected i.v. into normal allogeneic A mice*

Time of death	B16-F1[a]		B16-F10[a]	
	Lung	Blood[b]	Lung	Blood[b]
2 min	68,000[c]	190	88,000[c]	210
1 hr	56,000	400	75,200	510
3 hr	16,500	1,300	20,000	1,450
1 day	140	50	1,500	110
3 days	50	0	260	0
7 days	40	0	240	0
14 days	40	0	220	0
Gross metastases on day 14	12 ± 9		109 ± 30	

[a] Mean number of labeled tumor cells after i.v. injection of 100,000 viable [^{125}I]IUdR-labeled B16 melanoma cells. Five animals/time interval. Variation from the mean did not exceed 10%.
[b] 0.5 ml of blood/mouse.
[c] The differences were highly significant ($p < 0.01$).

longer, and formed more lung nodules in the immune-competent heterozygous littermates (Table 5). Cells from line B16-F10 had significantly higher initial rates of arrest in lungs of both nu/nu ($p < 0.01$) and nu/+ line B16-F1 (Table 5). At day 1 post-injection the survival of B16-F10 cells was significantly higher than their B16-F1 counterparts in nu/nu ($p < 0.01$) and nu/+ ($p < 0.01$), and the differences became more pronounced by day 3. B16-F10 cells survived longer than B16-F1 cells in lungs of both nu/nu and nu/+ mice and yielded significantly more pulmonary metastases. Nu/nu mice injected i.v. with cells from line B16-F1 averaged 1.6 ± 1.5 lung nodules, whereas line B16-F10 averaged 22 ± 12 ($p < 0.001$) on day 14 post-injection. The corresponding averages for nu/+ mice were 10 ± 2 and 79 ± 19 nodules, respectively ($p < 0.01$) (Table 5).

Other Host Factors

In the initial experiment, tumor cells or saline was injected into the tail vein of a mouse, and peripheral blood from the same mouse was obtained at several intervals after the injection. It is seen (Fig. 4) that the mere trauma of tail bleeding resulted in an immediate leukocytosis. The leukocytosis reached a maximum at 30 min post-i.v. injection and gradually declined thereafter. The additional trauma associated with an i.v. (tail vein) injection of 0.2 ml of 0.145 M NaCl increased the leukocytosis more than the incision alone. If, however, either 50,000 or 100,000 F1 cells were injected i.v., a moderate decrease (20%) in total WBC at 5 min, followed by a comparatively reduced, but persistent increase at 30 min post-injection, was ob-

TABLE 5. *Arrest and survival of [^{125}I]IUdR-labeled B16 melanoma variants injected i.v. into nu/nu and nu/+ mice*

| | nu/nu mice[a] | | | | nu/+ mice[a] | | | |
| | B16-F1 | | B16-F10 | | B16-F1 | | B16-F10 | |
Time of death	Lung	Blood[b]	Lung	Blood[b]	Lung	Blood[b]	Lung	Blood[b]
2 min	70,000[c]	210	90,000[c]	260	90,000[d]	190	98,000[d]	200
1 hr	44,000	910	81,000	470	74,000	60	97,000	520
3 hr	11,260	330	24,300	420	36,500	400	47,000	430
1 day	175[d]	25	1,760[d]	20	870[e]	17	1,300[e]	—
3 days	48	—	670	—	160	—	1,200	—
7 days	40	—	300	—	60	—	680	—
14 days	10	—	180	—	50	—	460	—
Gross metastases on day 14	1.6 ± 1.5		22 ± 12		10 ± 2		79 ± 19	

[a] Mean number of viable [^{125}I]-labeled tumor cells after i.v. injection of 100,000 [^{125}I]IUdR-labeled B16 melanoma cells. Five animals/time interval. Variation from the mean did not exceed 10%.
[b] 0.5 ml of blood/mouse.
[c] The differences between line F1 and F10 were highly significant ($p < 0.01$).
[d] The differences between line F1 and F10 were highly significant ($p < 0.001$).
[e] The differences between line F1 and F10 were highly significant ($p < 0.01$).

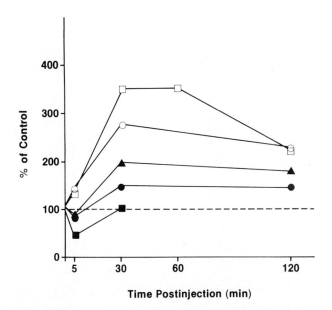

FIG. 4. Circulating leukocyte count as a function of time post-i.v. tumor cell injection. Average of 0 time leukocyte count = 5,300/mm³. (○) No injection, tail bleeding at intervals; (□) saline injection, tail bleeding at intervals; (●) injection of 50,000 B16-F1 cells, tail bleeding at intervals; (▲) injection of 100,000 B16-F1 cells, tail bleeding at intervals; (■) injection of 100,000 B16-F10 cells, tail bleeding of individual animals.

served. The introduction of tumor cells appeared to diminish the effects of the tail bleeding. Sequential tail bleedings led to significant leukocytosis, which might have obscured any leukopenia associated with i.v. tumor cell injection. The lower curve (filled squares) of Fig. 4 represents the second experiment in which individual animals were bled only once at given intervals following tumor cell injection; that is, the same mouse was not bled sequentially. The leukopenia resulting from this experiment was immediate and significant (55% below control, $p<0.01$) but transient. At 30 min post-i.v. injection, no discernible differences in total number of WBCs were noted between normal and injected mice.

Having established that the leukopenia was not due to the trauma of the injection or bleeding procedures, we proceeded to study the effects of i.v. injection of different amounts of either syngeneic tumor or normal cells on the leukopenia. WBC determinations were made 5 min post-i.v. injection. Fig. 5 indicates that i.v. administration of either B16-F1 or B16-F10 in doses from 50,000 to 500,000 per animal resulted in leukopenia. The total WBC count was significantly lower in these mice than in normal mice ($p < 0.01$). The i.v. injection of 200,000 dead B16-F1 cells depressed the WBC count to the same extent as did the administration of viable cells ($p < 0.01$),

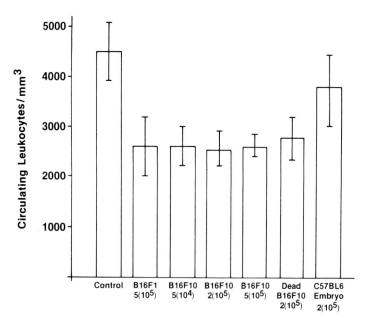

FIG. 5. Circulating leukocyte count in response to i.v. injection of tumor or normal embryo cells. Circulating leukocyte count following all tumor cell injections significantly lower than control ($p<0.01$). Circulating leukocyte count following embryo cell injection not different from control ($0.1 < p < 0.2$).

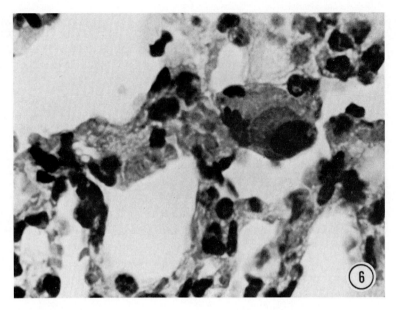

FIG. 6. Lung sections of mice injected i.v. with 500,000 B16 melanoma cells 10 min prior to autopsy. Note accumulation of leukocytes in lung capillary bed; × 600.

whereas administration of normal embryo cells did not significantly change the number of circulating leukocytes ($0.10 < p < 0.20$).

It became necessary, therefore, to account for the disappearance of leukocytes from the circulation. The disappearance of WBCs from the circulation is accompanied by an increase in their number in the lungs (Fig. 6). Other organs were not sectioned since the B16 melanoma rarely yields extrapulmonary colonies when injected in this manner (9).

DISCUSSION

When malignant cells are released at the site of a primary tumor or experimentally administered into the circulation, various host and tumor cell factors determine their distribution and fate. The search for quantitative information regarding the arrest, distribution, and survival of circulating tumor cells has been considerably advanced with the use of radioactive labeling of viable tumor cells. The radiolabel of choice to date has been [^{125}I]IUdR (5). [^{125}I]IUdR is a γ emitter, thus its monitoring is not drastically affected by self-absorption and sample preparation. It has a moderately long half-life (60 days), thereby permitting experiments of a 2- to 3-week duration (5).

Studies of the fate of [^{125}I]IUdR-labeled tumor cells as well as most past studies dealing with tumor cell distribution and fate in experimental animals have employed normal hosts. Even studies dealing with tumor cell modification or host manipulation used non-tumor-sensitized animals. The possibility that such animals may not be a suitable model for studies of the metastatic sequence analogous to that in cancer patients has been recognized by Weiss et al. (31) and by Wexler, Chretien, Ketcham, and Sindelar (33). In order to sort out the relative contributions of different host factors on experimental metastasis, we have analyzed the initial arrest, the death of tumor cells as a function of time post-injection, and the ultimate number of visible tumor colonies at 14 days post-injection in normal, immunized, and immune-manipulated syngeneic and allogeneic recipients.

The various test groups of mice had two major ranges of initial arrest of tumor emboli. Approximately 60% of the i.v. injected B16-F1 cells were arrested at 2 min in the lungs of normal C57BL/6, ATX C57BL/6, both normal A and A immunized to AC15091 and nu/nu mice. All other test groups arrested about 90% of i.v. injected tumor cells. The fact that initial arrest in normal or ATX syngeneic mice was in the 60% range but 90% for the other syngeneic groups confirmed the earlier observation that properties of the host may profoundly enhance the initial arrest of circulating tumor cells (17,31). Lymphocyte depletion (in C57BL/6 ATX and nu/nu mice) appears to abrogate this enhancement. In our system, initial arrest of cells in the lungs never fell below the 60% level in any test group. This raises the speculation that certain inherent tumor cell characteristics establish the base line of their initial arrest in the lungs irrespective of the host status (8). It is entirely possible that, in order to obtain a lower range of initial tumor cell arrest, it is necessary to manipulate the tumor cell surface (12,31).

The initial arrest and kinetics of tumor cell survival by themselves did not correlate with the final number of tumors observed. On one hand, ATX animals exhibited initial arrest patterns similar to those of normal mice, yet they had fewer gross metastases at 2 weeks post-injection; whereas the kinetic pattern of tumor cell survival correlated to that in other animals in immune-manipulated test groups. Animals sensitized to the B16 tumor exhibited a significantly greater initial lung arrest (95%) of labeled tumor cells than normal controls (60%), but the number of gross pulmonary tumor colonies in normal mice was significantly higher than that in most tumor-sensitized animals. In other experiments, the reconstitution of nu/nu mice with lymphocytes from nu/+ increased the initial arrest from 68 to 91% but reduced the number of tumor colonies to 0. The same treatment of nu/+ animals increased the tumor cell arrest from 91 to 99% but increased the number of tumors from 12 to 30.

We thus conclude that initial arrest in the pulmonary bed neither correlates with nor predicts the survival of tumor cells and their subsequent development into visible tumor colonies. It has long been recognized that most i.v. injected tumor cells fail to form metastases (10,37). Our findings have reinforced a widespread opinion that most tumor cell emboli die, and the data seem to rule out the possibility that the emboli remain alive but dormant. In none of the test groups was the appearance of tumor cells in other organs or in the circulation sufficient to account for the loss from the lungs.

Although we did not investigate the detailed mechanisms involved in the survival of the few arrested tumor cells which formed visible tumors, the data suggested that host immune factors might play a major role in this part of the pathogenesis of the disease. Clearly, manipulation of the host immune response affected tumor cell kinetics beyond the stage of initial arrest. As would be expected, tumor cells were destroyed in immunized animals at a faster rate than in all other syngeneic test groups. Successfully immunized mice have been defined as animals capable of rejecting an ordinarily lethal challenge of tumor cells injected s.c. or intramuscularly (i.m.). Nevertheless, in the present studies, such animals did not reject a similar i.v. tumor challenge of 100,000 viable cells. This observation confirmed the previous reports by Wexler, Chretien, and Ketcham (32) regarding lung colonies of so-called immune mice. This paradox also applies to the allogeneic A and nu/+ animals in our studies that ordinarily reject an s.c. tumor allograft of the B16 melanoma. They all permitted the growth of the same tumor following an i.v. challenge, albeit at a lower level than normal syngeneic mice. The nu/nu animals, on the other hand, which ordinarily allow s.c. allografts or even xenografts, had only 2 ± 1 lung tumors and none if they were reconstituted. What i.m. and s.c. tumor injections have in common, but which differs from i.v. administration, might be the existence of a discrete tumor focus. Tumor cells injected i.v. disseminate and arrest in the capillary bed of an organ (lung) in multiple foci. One possible explanation for this discrepancy is that although the host immune response is capable of rejecting tumors in discrete focus, it is ineffective in dealing with tumors that are widely disseminated. Alternatively, the lung might be a more suitable "soil" for growth of melanoma than s.c. sites (8), which may also explain the lack of growth of tumor colonies in the lungs of nu/nu mice.

Data suggesting that tumor cell properties may determine the outcome of metastasis have been reported by several investigators. Tumor cell suspensions from different types of tumors injected into the same organ establish their own unique patterns of metastasis (29). It is well known that tumor cells can traverse different organs at different rates, and that tumor cells from different tumors interact differently within the capillary bed of the same organ (2,14). Moreover, the rate at which tumor cells pass through capillaries was not related to their size but rather was attributed to their plasticity and ability to distort their shape (36). In the B16 system, the mere fact that B16-F1 and B16-F10 could be selected from the original B16 melanoma is sufficient evidence that tumor cell properties participate in this outcome of experimental metastasis.

In the present studies the arrest and survival of melanoma cell lines B16-F1 (low metastasis) and B16-F10 (high metastasis) were compared in normal and immune-manipulated syngeneic and allogeneic animals. We found that initial localization and survival of B16-F10 cells were always significantly greater than in B16-F1 cells in any given group of animals, including nu/nu or nu/+ mice. In every experiment the B16-F10 cell line, which has a higher potential to arrest and survive, formed significantly more lung tumors than B16-F1, *independent of the immune status of the host*, demonstrating that immune status or manipulation did not eliminate the differences in biological properties of these cell lines. However, host properties such as tumor immunity can quantitatively modify tumor cell arrest and survival. The mechanism of immune enhancement to metastasis is not well understood, and it could be due to differing immune properties in each tumor system investigated. In the B16 melanoma variant system, immune enhancement can be attributed, in part, to increased tumor cell-lymphocyte interactions (7) during circulation, leading to formation of large tumor cell-lymphocyte clumps, which should aid in tumor cell arrest and perhaps also in subsequent survival.

Several observations suggest the importance of the interaction between tumor cells and circulating host cells on the final number of experimental metastases. Leukopenia occurred 1 day after tumor cells were introduced i.v. or s.c. into mice and persisted for 3 days (15). Variants of the B16 melanoma with differing capacities to form experimental metastases had different propensities to form tumor cell-lymphocyte heterotypic aggregates *in vitro*. Greater aggregation was observed with the highly metastatic tumor cells (21). Homotypic (tumor cell-tumor cell) clumps of different sizes yielded different numbers of visible tumors when equal cell numbers were injected i.v. (5). *In vitro* mixtures of tumor cells and lymphocytes injected i.v., when compared to injections of an equal number of tumor cells without lymphocytes, gave rise to more tumors when the lymphocyte:tumor cell ratio was low or to fewer tumors when the ratio was high (7). Serum factors may affect tumor embolus size and therefore alter the final outcome of experimental metastasis (34). Thrombocytopenia has also been observed to alter the outcome (16).

When weakly metastatic and highly metastatic B16 derivatives were compared for their ability to aggregate thrombocytes *in vitro,* it was found that the highly metastatic derivative readily aggregated platelets and produced no extrapulmonary metastases. The weakly metastatic tumor cells did not aggregate platelets and produced extrapulmonary metastases in a large percentage of the test group (16). Thrombocytopenia occurring immediately after i.v. tumor cell injection directly correlated to the successful outcome of experimental metastasis. It is reasonable to assume that if circulating emboli bring about aggregation of platelets *in vivo,* release of vasopressive mediators from platelets occurs, and a local pulmonary vasospasm may ensue. Such a vasospasm would begin as a primary mechanical obstruction of vessels and then cause secondary local vasoconstriction and the spread of vasoconstriction to other lobes of the lung. The vasoconstriction brings about a rise in pressure, which in turn leads to the opening of preexisting arteriovenous communications (1).

When B16-F1 and B16-F10 tumor cells are injected into the venous circulation, the majority of cells become lodged in the lungs by 2 min post-injection. Such an injection is associated with a leukopenia, which can be observed 5 min (Fig. 4) post-injection, and which is accompanied by an accumulation of leukocytes in the lungs. Injections of both live and dead tumor cells but not normal cells result in leukopenia (Fig. 5).

The above observations suggest that the formation of an embolus (either homotypic or heterotypic) of some critical size could ensure the arrest of tumor cells in the lung capillary bed. Under the present experimental conditions, it is not clear whether the observed leukopenia is a direct consequence of the tumor cell injection or whether it is merely a measurable indication of vasospasm or other events. A corollary observation, however, is that inflammatory agents such as adrenergic hormones (30) and X-irradiation (13), which would serve to decrease the diameter of the capillary lumen, have been associated with an increase in the number of pulmonary tumor colonies following i.v. injection of tumor cells. The success of the embolus in ultimately forming visible tumors would then depend on both its ability to survive host defenses and its secondary invasion characteristics (8). The results further point out the need to consider that normal host factors, which are seemingly unrelated to the disease, may profoundly alter the outcome of metastatic spread (Figs. 7 through 9).

An alternative to the critical embolus size is that every heterogeneous population of tumor cells may include a small fraction that is destined to home to an organ (lung), implant, and successfully yield clinical tumors after i.v. injection. The actual size of such a fraction would be determined by the relation of the tumor cell properties to the status of the host (8). One prediction which should follow is that the ultimate number of tumor colonies observed in the lungs of animals injected with tumor cells is independent of the first capillary bed tumor cells encounter. This indeed has been observed in our laboratory where B16 melanoma cells injected i.v. into the tail vein or intracardially (arterial circulation) yielded similar numbers of pulmonary B16 colonies (16). A similar result has been reported for fibrosarcoma cells injected i.m. or i.v. into mice (32,33).

In summary, the following conclusions are suggested: (a) Allogeneic animals, as expected, are not appropriate model systems for the study of the metastatic sequence. (b) The initial arrest of tumor cells in organs and tumor cell survival and growth are probably influenced by both tumor cell properties and multiple host factors. (c) Initial tumor cell arrest in organs is not a prediction of nor does it correlate with the ensuing survival kinetics

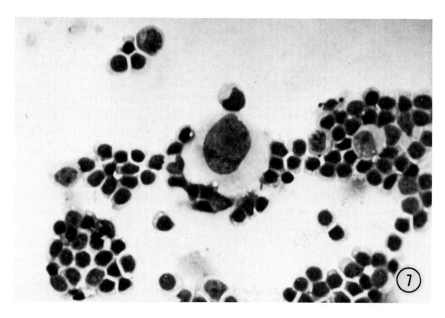

FIG. 7. Heterotypic (tumor cell:lymphocyte) clumping following *in vitro* interaction. Lymphocyte to tumor ratio = 100:1; × 450.

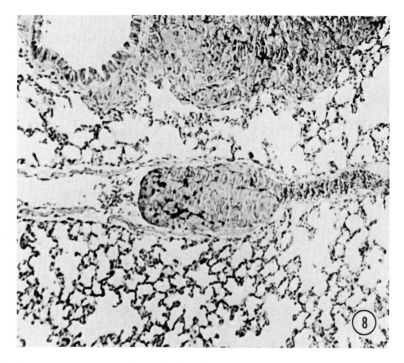

FIG. 8. B16-F10 melanoma colonies in lung. Note one tumor colony growing in the lung parenchyma while another is growing in and obstructing a blood vessel; × 100.

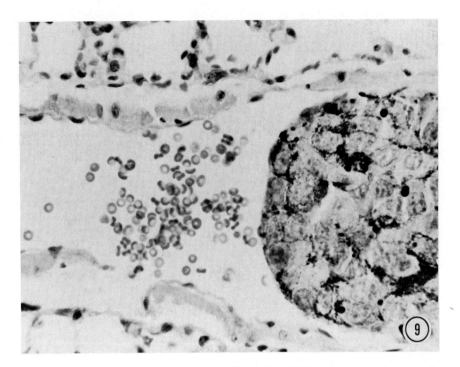

FIG. 9. A higher magnification (× 450) of Fig. 8, i.e., B16 melanoma colony growing inside a blood vessel.

or development into tumor colonies. (d) Mice that rejected an s.c. tumor challenge allowed the same tumor to grow in the lungs after i.v. injection. Therefore, rejection of a s.c. tumor challenge as the sole criterion of host immunity to neoplasms should be questioned. (e) Animals sensitized to a tumor exhibit kinetic patterns of tumor cell arrest and survival that differ from those of normal syngeneic hosts. (f) The patterns of tumor cell arrest and tumor formation in nude mice do not resemble those of their syngeneic or other allogeneic hosts. (g) Tumor cell characteristics are maintained qualitatively regardless of the immune status of the host. (h) Tumor cells interact with seemingly unrelated host factors to an extent not seen for normal cells. (i) The validity of using normal animals in inclusive studies of the pathogenesis of metastasis should be severely questioned according to all the data. Successfully immunized or unsuccessfully immunized (tumor-sensitized) animals might indeed be a more suitable animal model for studies of mechanisms involved in experimental cancer metastasis.

ACKNOWLEDGMENT

This research was sponsored by the National Cancer Institute Contract No. NO1-CO-25423 with Litton Bionetics, Inc.

REFERENCES

1. Avaido, D. M. (1965): *The Lung Circulation, Vol. II*, p. 983. Pergamon Press, London.
2. Barth, R. F., and Singla, O. (1975): Migratory patterns of technetium-99m-labeled lymphoid cells. I. Effects of antilymphocyte serum on the organ distribution of murine thymocytes. *Cell. Immunol.*, 17:83–95.
3. Duncan, D. B. (1955): Multiple range and multiple F tests. *Biometrics*, 11:1–42.
4. Fidler, I. J. (1970): Metastasis: Quantitative analysis of distribution and fate of tumor emboli labeled with ^{125}I-5-iodo-2'-deoxyuridine. *J. Natl. Cancer Inst.*, 45:775–782.
5. Fidler, I. J. (1973): The relationship of embolic homogeneity, number, size and viability to the incidence of experimental metastasis. *Eur. J. Cancer*, 9:223–227.
6. Fidler, I. J. (1973): Selection of successive tumor lines for metastasis. *Nature [New Biol.]*, 242:148–149.
7. Fidler, I. J. (1974): Immune stimulation–inhibition of experimental cancer metastasis. *Cancer Res.*, 34:491–498.
8. Fidler, I. J. (1975): Mechanisms of cancer invasion and metastasis. In: *Biology of Tumors: Surfaces, Immunology, and Comparative Pathology, Vol. 4 of Cancer: A Comprehensive Treatise*, edited by F. F. Becker, pp. 101–131. Plenum Press, New York.
9. Fidler, I. J. (1975): Biological behavior of malignant melanoma cells correlated to their survival *in vivo*. *Cancer Res.*, 35:218–224.
10. Fidler, I. J. (1976): Patterns of tumor cell arrest and development. In: *Fundamental Aspects of Metastasis*, edited by L. Weiss, pp. 275–289. North Holland Publishing Co., Amsterdam.
11. Fidler, I. J., Darnell, J. H., and Budmen, M. B. (1976): Tumoricidal properties of mouse macrophages activated with mediators from rat lymphocytes stimulated with concanavalin-A. *Cancer Res.*, 36:3608–3615.
12. Fidler, I. J., and Nicolson, G. L. (1976): Organ selectivity for implantation, survival and growth of B16 melanoma variant tumor lines. *J. Natl. Cancer Inst.*, 57:1199–1202.
13. Fidler, I. J., and Zeidman, I. (1972): Enhancement of experimental metastasis by X-ray: A possible mechanism. *J. Med. (Basel)*, 3:172–177.
14. Fisher, B., and Fisher, E. R. (1967): The organ distribution of disseminated ^{51}Cr-labeled tumor cells. *Cancer Res.*, 27:412–420.
15. Fisher, B., Saffer, E. A., and Fisher, E. R. (1972): Effect of tumor cell inoculation on circulating lymphocytes. *Proc. Soc. Exp. Biol. Med.*, 139:787–792.
16. Gasic, G. J., Gasic, T. B., Galanti, N., Johnson, T., and Murphy, S. (1973): Platelet-tumor cell interaction in mice. The role of platelets in the spread of malignant disease. *Int. J. Cancer*, 11:704–718.
17. Hagmar, B. (1972): Defibrination and metastasis formation: Effects of arvin on experimental metastases in mice. *Eur. J. Cancer*, 8:17–28.
18. Hagmar, B., and Norrby, K. (1973): Influence of cultivation, trypsinization and aggregation on the transplantability of melanoma B16 cells. *Int. J. Cancer*, 11:663–675.
19. Humphrey, L. J., and Murray, D. R. (1971): Effect of tumor vaccines in immunizing patients with cancer. *Surgery*, 132:437–442.
20. Nicolson, G. L., and Brunson, K. W. (1977): Organ specificity of malignant B16 melanomas: *In vivo* selection for organ preference of blood-borne metastasis. *Gann (in press)*.
21. Nicolson, G. L., and Winkelhake, J. L. (1975): Organ specificity of blood-borne tumour metastasis determined by cell adhesion? *Nature*, 255:230–232.
22. Nicolson, G. L., Winkelhake, J. L., and Nussey, A. C. (1976): An approach to studying cellular properties associated with metastasis: Some *in vitro* properties of tumor variants selected *in vivo* for enhanced metastasis. In: *Fundamental Aspects of Metastasis*, edited by L. Weiss, pp. 307–319. North Holland Publishing Co., Amsterdam.
23. Parks, R. C. (1974): Organ-specific metastasis of a transplantable reticulum cell sarcoma. *J. Natl. Cancer Inst.*, 52:971–973.
24. Prehn, R. T. (1971): Perspectives in oncogenesis: Does immunity stimulate or inhibit neoplasia? *J. Reticuloendothel. Soc.*, 10:1–12.
25. Prehn, R. T., and Lappé, M. A. (1971): An immunostimulation theory of tumor development. *Transplant. Rev.*, 7:26–54.
26. Proctor, J. W., Rudenstam, C. M., and Alexander, P. (1973): A factor preventing the development of lung metastases in rats with sarcomas. *Nature*, 242:29–31.

27. Salsbury, A. J. (1975): The significance of the circulating cancer cell. *Cancer Treatment Rev.,* 2:55–72.
28. Schmidt, M., and Good, R. A. (1975): Transplantation of human cancers to nude mice and effects of thymus grafts. *J. Natl. Cancer Inst.,* 55:81–84.
29. Sugarbaker, E. D. (1952): The organ selectivity of experimentally induced metastases in rats. *Cancer,* 5:606–612.
30. Van den Brenk, H. A. S., Stone, M. G., Kelly, H., and Sharpington, C. (1976): Lowering of innate resistance of the lungs to the growth of blood-borne cancer cells in states of topical and systemic stress. *Br. J. Cancer,* 33:60–78.
31. Weiss, L., Glaves, D., and Waite, D. A. (1974): The influence of host immunity on the arrest of circulating cancer cells and its modification by neuraminidase. *Int. J. Cancer,* 13:850–862.
32. Wexler, H., Chretien, P. B., and Ketcham, A. S. (1972): Effect of tumor immunity on production of lung tumors after intravenous inoculation of antigenically identical tumor cells. *J. Natl. Cancer Inst.,* 48:657–663.
33. Wexler, H., Chretien, P. B., Ketcham, A. S., and Sindelar, W. F. (1975): Induction of pulmonary metastases in both immune and nonimmune mice. Effect of the removal of a transplanted primary tumor. *Cancer,* 36:2042–2047.
34. Wexler, H., Sindelar, W. F., and Ketcham, A. S. (1976): The role of immune factors in the survival of circulating tumor cells. *Cancer,* 37:1701–1706.
35. Winkelhake, J. L., and Nicolson, G. L. (1976): Determination of adhesive properties of variant metastatic melanoma cells to BALB/3T3 cells and their virus-transformed derivatives by a monolayer assay. *J. Natl. Cancer Inst.,* 56:285–298.
36. Zeidman, I. (1957): Metastasis: A review of recent advances. *Cancer Res.,* 17:157–162.
37. Zeidman, I., Gamble, W. J., and Clovis, W. L. (1956): Immediate passage of tumor cell emboli through the liver and kidney. *Cancer Res.,* 16:814–815.

Cancer Invasion and Metastasis: Biologic Mechanisms and Therapy, edited by S. B. Day et al. Raven Press, New York © 1977.

Host Serum Factors Versus Tumor Factors in Immune Resistance to Metastases

Jan Vaage

Department of Cancer Therapy Development, Pondville Hospital, Walpole, Massachusetts 02081

There are, among many other factors, two factors that can influence growth of tumors and the development of metastases: one is free circulating tumor products and tumor components, which may have debilitating effects on the host's general as well as immunospecific resistance and may therefore promote the establishment and growth of metastases. A second factor is the immunoglobulins, which can neutralize free tumor antigens and can also act with complement directly on tumor cells, inhibiting the development of metastases. I have used pathogen-free,[1] 10- to 12-week-old female C3H or C3Hf mice and syngeneic mammary carcinomas, as well as a syngeneic fibrosarcoma, to study the effects of humoral factors on neoplastic growth in different anatomical locations. The experimental conditions of these immunological studies, however, simulated only one aspect of metastasis: tumor cells in the circulation. And the cells were injected, not spontaneously released from a primary tumor. These investigations of immune protection against metastases used passive transfer of serum and lymphocytes to tumor-implanted recipients which had been prepared to simulate conditions of (a) vascular tumor dissemination and (b) tumor antigen overload.

TUMOR-ASSISTED PROTECTION AGAINST VASCULAR SPREAD OF CANCER

Immune serum factors, presumably antibodies, can be shown to participate, in a positive role, in the rejection of implanted tumor cells. The demonstration requires carefully prepared experimental conditions. First, the test animals must be irradiated with sublethal whole-body irradiation before challenge to preclude a primary immune response from developing as a result of the challenge injection of living antigenic tumor cells. A pri-

---

[1] The mice carry only the following nonpathogenic enteric bacteria: Clostridium sp., Peptostreptococcus sp., Bacillus sp., and Bacteroides sp.

mary immune response can easily obscure the kind of protection provided by injected antiserum. Second, the mice must be injected with adequate quantities of antiserum before and after challenge. Third, the mice must be at least partially restored with injections of normal lymph node cells after irradiation. Finally, the protective effect of antiserum is most easily seen if the test animals are challenged intravenously. If the mice are challenged s.c., the protection is not noticeable. Because the lungs are well protected in immune mice (1), the tail vein route of challenge, which gives tumor growth almost entirely in the lungs, was chosen to test for protection by transferred immune cells or immune serum.

In the tests for the effect of passive transferred lymph node cells and serum on tumor growth, actively sensitized control mice had their sensitizing subcutaneous tumor implants surgically removed 4 days before challenge after a growth period of 20 days. The irradiated mice received 400 R whole-body X-radiation 4 days before challenge. On the third day before challenge, the appropriate groups of mice were treated with intraperitoneal injections of lymph node cells and/or serum as indicated in Table 1. The mice injected with lymph node cells each received per inoculum the equivalent of one-half of the quantity of cells obtained from two axillary, two brachial, and two inguinal lymph nodes. Since the suspensions contained pieces of lymph node tissue as well as single cells, it was roughly estimated

TABLE 1. *Effect of transferred lymph node cells and serum on the growth of intravenously transplanted mammary carcinoma cells*

Group	Immune status	Treatment	Challenge[a]	
			No. of mice with tumors	Average tumor growth
1	Irradiated	Immune lymph node cells	4/10	0.88
2	Irradiated	Normal lymph node cells	10/10	2.50
3	Irradiated	Normal cells + immune serum	7/10	1.26
4	Irradiated	Normal cells + normal serum	10/10	2.60
5	Irradiated	Immune serum	10/10	2.60
6	Irradiated	Normal serum	10/10	2.40
7	Irradiated	No treatment	10/10	2.70
8	Sensitized	No treatment	0/10	0
9	Unsensitized	No treatment	6/10	1.26
10	Unsensitized	Immune serum	5/10	1.20

[a] The mice were treated with i.p. injections of normal or immune lymph node cells and/or normal or immune serum 3 days before challenge, again at time of challenge, and 3 days after challenge. The mice were challenged with 3.3×10^4 live tumor cells injected into the tail vein. The differences in mean tumor growth were evaluated by Student's t-test. Group 1 vs each of groups 2, 4, 5, 6, or 7, $p < 0.01$; group 3 vs each of groups 2, 4, 5, 6, or 7, $p > 0.05$; group 1 vs group 3, $p < 0.05$; group 8 differs significantly from all other groups. Values from 0 to 3 express the amount of tumor growth found in the lungs at autopsy. The mean value for each group was derived by dividing the sum of the values by the number of mice. (From *Isr. J. Med. Sci.*, 12:334, 1976.)

that each inoculum contained about 5×10^6 cells. The mice injected with serum received 0.5 ml per inoculum. The mice given both cells and serum received mixed aliquots of cells and serum in a single inoculum. These injections were repeated a few hours before challenge and again 3 days after challenge. All of the mice were challenged with 3.3×10^4 viable tumor cells injected into the tail vein.

Frequent examinations of the mice for signs of dyspnea indicated the termination time for the mice. The test animals were killed by asphyxiation in 100% CO_2 gas 18 days after challenge and their lungs examined for the extent of tumor growth. To describe the amount of tumor growing in the lungs where accurate measurements were not practical, I assigned values from 0 to 3 at blind readings according to the number and size of growths found at autopsy.

The results presented in Table 1 show that the transfer of lymph node cells from mice sensitized against the mammary carcinoma had given a significant degree of resistance to the growth of mammary carcinoma cells (group 1 versus group 7).[2] Similar transfer of normal cells was not effective (group 2 versus group 7). The transfer of normal lymph node cells plus serum from mice immunized against the mammary carcinoma also gave the irradiated recipients significant protection against challenge (group 3 versus group 7), whereas normal lymph node cells plus normal serum or serum alone (groups 4 through 6 versus group 7) gave no protection. Actively sensitized, unirradiated mice were strongly resistant to challenge (group 8). Normal untreated mice and normal serum-treated mice were relatively resistant compared to irradiated untreated mice (groups 9 and 10 versus group 7). Treatment of normal mice with immune serum did not significantly increase their resistance (group 9 versus group 10).

A second experiment reexamined the results seen in the previously described experiment, in which irradiated mice were protected by normal lymph node cells plus immune serum, and examined this effect in the different anatomical locations reached by intravenous and subcutaneous tumor cell implantations. This experiment followed the pretreatment and treatment procedures described for the previous experiment, giving three transfers of normal lymph node cells and/or injections of immune serum. The mice were challenged with 3.3×10^4 living tumor cells injected into the tail vein, or with 1×10^5 cells injected subcutaneously at the left shoulder and at the left hip. The experiment was terminated 18 days after challenge for the animals challenged intravenously, and 28 days after challenge for the animals challenged subcutaneously. The incidence and the amount of tumor growth in the lungs were checked and recorded as in the previously de-

---

[2] In each of the experiments reported here, when immune cells and immune serum were used to passively transfer immunity, immune lymphocytes invariably worked better. However, cellular transfer of immunity is already a well-established phenomenon, and this chapter is considering and emphasizing the role of humoral factors in tumor immunity.

scribed experiment. The incidence of tumors at the subcutaneous injection sites was checked at weekly intervals, and their size was measured with calipers and recorded from the time they became palpable. The experiment was terminated when more than one mouse in any group became cachectic because of progressive s.c. tumor growth. The mean values per group at the last recording of tumor sizes are presented in the results.

The results presented in Table 2 show that the transfer of normal lymph node cells plus serum from mice immunized against the mammary carcinoma gave the irradiated recipients significant protection against intravenous challenge (group 2 versus group 4), whereas normal lymph node cells alone or immune serum alone gave no protection (groups 1 and 3 versus group 4). Protection by normal cells and immune serum was not seen in irradiated recipients challenged subcutaneously (group 8 versus group 10). Actively immunized mice were strongly resistant to challenge (group 5 versus group 6, and group 11 versus group 12). Normal untreated mice were relatively resistant compared to irradiated untreated mice (group 4 versus group 6,

TABLE 2. *Effect of transferred lymph node cells and serum on the growth of intravenously and subcutaneously transplanted mammary carcinoma cells*

				Challenge[a]	
Group	Immune status	Treatment	Injection route	No. of mice with tumors, or No. of tumors	Average tumor growth
1	Irradiated	Normal lymph node cells	Tail vein	10/10	1.90
2	Irradiated	Normal cells + immune serum	Tail vein	8/10	0.96
3	Irradiated	Immune serum	Tail vein	10/10	2.40
4	Irradiated	No treatment	Tail vein	10/10	2.70
5	Sensitized	No treatment	Tail vein	3/10	0.60
6	Unsensitized	No treatment	Tail vein	8/10	1.36
7	Irradiated	Normal cells	Subcutaneous[b]	19/20	8.63 mm
8	Irradiated	Normal cells + immune serum	Subcutaneous	20/20	8.01 mm
9	Irradiated	Immune serum	Subcutaneous	20/20	9.10 mm
10	Irradiated	No treatment	Subcutaneous	20/20	8.84 mm
11	Sensitized	No treatment	Subcutaneous	8/20	3.67 mm
12	Unsensitized	No treatment	Subcutaneous	16/20	8.68 mm

[a] The mice were treated with i.p. injections of normal lymph node cells and/or immune serum 3 days before challenge, again at the time of challenge, and 3 days after challenge. The mice were challenged with 3.3×10^4 live mammary carcinoma cells injected into the tail vein, or were challenged with 1×10^5 live cells injected s.c. both at the left shoulder and at the left hip. The differences in mean tumor growth were evaluated by Student's t-test. Group 2 vs each of groups 1, 3, or 4, $p < 0.05$; group 2 vs group 5, $0.05 < p < 0.1$. Group 5 vs group 6, $p < 0.05$. Group 11 vs each of groups 7, 8, 9, 10, or 12, $p < 0.05$. Values from 0 to 3 express the amount of tumor growth found after i.v. challenge. Subcutaneous growth was measured directly. The mean value for each group was derived by dividing the sum of the values or measurements by the number of mice.

[b] Two subcutaneous challenge implants per mouse. (From *Isr. J. Med. Sci.*, 12:334, 1976.)

and group 10 versus group 12). Irradiated mice challenged s.c. were not protected by passive transfer of normal lymph node cells and/or immune serum.

RELATIVE EFFECTIVENESS OF IMMUNE RESISTANCE AGAINST SECONDARY PULMONARY OR SUBCUTANEOUS TUMOR GROWTH WITH PROGRESSIVE PRIMARY TUMOR GROWTH

As reported in a previous publication (1), the immune resistance against mammary carcinoma cells injected into the circulation appeared to be significantly more effective than the immune resistance facing tumor cells that had been deposited s.c. It was observed that if that number of tumor cells that would give 100% growth s.c. in normal mice was injected into immunized mice, tumor growth would occur in about 50% of the mice. In other words, immune resistance factors available s.c. could reduce growth by about 50%. On the other hand, if that number of cells of the same tumor that would give 100% growth in the lungs after i.v. injection into normal mice was injected i.v. into immunized mice, tumor growth would occur in less than 10% of the animals. Therefore, it seemed that immune resistance was more effective against tumor cells that were in the blood, the lungs, or both, than against tumor cells that had been deposited s.c.

The phenomenon of specific impairment of immune resistance by excess tumor antigen and the recovery of resistance following tumor-curative therapy have been described in previous publications (1-6). Circulating excess tumor antigens have been found to be a cause of declining resistance to tumor growth, although antibodies promote recovery by neutralizing excess free antigen (5). In the experiment described here, I investigated and compared, as the sensitizing tumors grew larger, the ability of mice to resist the growth of tumor cells implanted in the lungs with the ability to resist s.c. tumor growth.

The mice were sensitized with s.c. implants of living pieces of mammary carcinoma tissue, which were excised after various predetermined periods of growth. The levels of resistance in the various groups were tested by i.v. or s.c. challenge implants of living tumor cells in suspension. The challenge implants were always made 3 days before the sensitizing tumors were removed. Each group received 1×10^5 cells injected s.c. at the left shoulder and at the left hip or 3.3×10^4 cells injected i.v.

Table 3 represents the combined data from several similar tests; the figures for groups 1 through 6 and 11 and 12 are the results of three separate tests, the figures for groups 7 through 10 are the results of two separate tests, and the figures for the unsensitized control groups are the combined data from five tests. Figure 1 presents the data from Table 3 in graphic form.

The results show that resistance to challenge was detectable after a sensitization period of 10 days and was fully developed in about 2 weeks. Fully immunized animals challenged i.v. were able to reduce by 96% the amount

TABLE 3. *Effect of growing mammary carcinoma (MC) on the resistance of the host to i.v. and s.c. MC challenge[a]*

Group	Status of host	Challenge route	No. of mice with tumor[b]	Average tumor growth[c]	Rejection response (%)[d]
			Challenge		
1	MC removed day 13, at 3.5 mm	i.v.	14/15	1.80	21
2	MC removed day 13, at 3.5 mm	s.c.	26/30	9.80	11
3	MC removed day 16, at 4 mm	i.v.	5/15	0.47	80
4	MC removed day 16, at 4 mm	s.c.	17/30	6.13	45
5	MC removed day 22, at 6 mm	i.v.	3/15	0.20	91
6	MC removed day 22, at 6 mm	s.c.	13/30	4.93	55
7	MC removed day 28, at 9 mm	i.v.	2/20	0.10	96
8	MC removed day 28, at 9 mm	s.c.	19/40	5.55	50
9	MC removed day 37, at 15 mm	i.v.	5/20	0.30	87
10	MC removed day 37, at 15 mm	s.c.	31/40	8.73	21
11	MC removed day 41, at 18 mm	i.v.	11/15	1.20	48
12	MC removed day 41, at 18 mm	s.c.	23/30	9.00	19
13	Unsensitized	i.v.	35/35	2.29	0
14	Unsensitized	s.c.	64/70	11.06	9

[a] Live sensitizing tumors were implanted s.c. in the right flank and excised, after various periods of growth, 3 days after challenge.
[b] The tumor incidence for mice challenged s.c. means the number of tumors/number of implants (2/mouse).
[c] The average growth values s.c. are expressed in mm. The average tumor growth in the lungs is expressed in values from 0 to 3 (see text). The average values for each group were derived by dividing the sums of values by the number of mice (s.c. by the number of implants).
[d] These values represent the percent difference between the average growth in sensitized mice and the average growth in tumor-positive normal control mice (average for s.c. positive sites, 12.1 mm). The values were used to construct Fig. 1. (From ref. 1.)

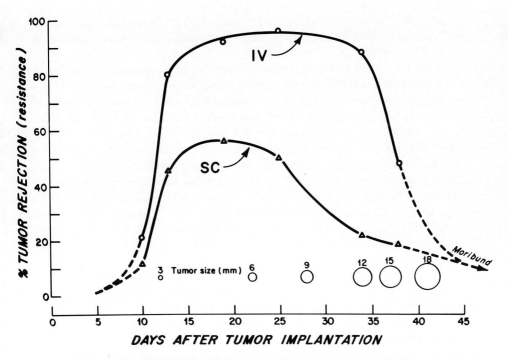

FIG. 1. Development and decline of immune resistance in the lungs (i.v.) and s.c. under the influence of a progressively growing s.c. mammary carcinoma. For detailed data, see Table 3. (From ref. 1.)

of tumor growth found in the lungs of unsensitized control animals compared to a maximum reduction of 55% in sensitized animals challenged s.c. The results also show that the antitumor resistance in the lungs remained effective longer than did the s.c. resistance, before declining with the increasing tumor load.

By tracing the two curves of Fig. 1 on pieces of paper covering an area of the graph from day 5 to day 45 and from 0 to 100%, and then cutting out and weighing the areas under the curves, I obtained an idea of the relative effectiveness of s.c. and pulmonary resistance to challenge for the period from primary tumor onset to terminal disease. The average of several such estimates gave the value for s.c. immune resistance as 31% and the value for pulmonary resistance as 65% of the theoretical total resistance.

FREE TUMOR ANTIGEN VERSUS IMMUNE SERUM FACTORS IN TUMOR IMMUNITY

Possibly the most important negative factor in immune resistance to tumor growth and tumor dissemination is tumor antigen itself, in excess, free in the circulation. It is well recognized in the clinic that a heavy tumor load can be both generally and immunospecifically detrimental. Experimentally, it has been observed that as an antigenic tumor implant grows, a syngeneic host develops the ability to reject additional implants of the same tumor, although it is unable to reject the already established primary tumor implant. This is the well-known phenomenon of concomitant immunity. However, as a primary tumor implant grows larger, the level of concomitant immunity declines, that is, the animal begins to lose the ability to reject additional implants of the same tumor. This phenomenon has been related to a number of immunological concepts—tolerance, energy, and blocking—but is actually poorly understood, except that it seems related to excess tumor antigen. Recovery of immune resistance follows soon after surgical removal of a large antigenic tumor. If a tumor is killed by a single dose of local radiation, immune recovery is delayed for as long as vascular connections between the host and the killed tumor mass persist. If daily injections of killed tumor material are made from the time of surgical removal, immune recovery is also delayed.[3] These situations are described graphically in Fig. 2.

In the following experiment, mice with large s.c. mammary tumor implants, and therefore with depressed immune resistance, had the tumors removed. At this time some of the mice were injected with serum presumed to contain tumor antigen, and some were in addition injected with the antiserum. The purpose of this procedure was to test what effect antigen and antibody present in the blood of the animal at the same time could have on the recovery of immune resistance. Serum presumed to contain soluble tumor antigen came from mice which had first been irradiated to prevent an immune response, then the mice were literally loaded with killed tumor cells: one injection i.p. and one s.c. of 50 mg each, every day for 6 days. A few hours after the last injection the mice were bled. The serum was presumed to contain soluble tumor antigen but no antibody because the animals had been sublethally preirradiated. The antiserum came from mice that had an s.c. sensitizing tumor implant removed, then a week after surgery the mice received a small booster injection of killed tumor cells. A week later the mice were bled. The serum was presumed to contain antibodies but no antigen.

In the tests for the effect of passively transferred antiserum on tumor growth in mice immunodepressed by excess tumor antigen, the experimental mice had been prepared in the following manner: 26 days before the day of challenge, the mice received implants of two 1-cu mm pieces of living mammary carcinoma in the right flank. On the 28th day of growth, when the

---

[3] These observations in a mouse tumor model may mean that a large number of postsurgical clinical attempts at specific immunotherapy with cancer autovaccines may, probably and unfortunately, have been the wrong procedure at the wrong time. Antigenic tumor material may often have been reinjected when a patient would have benefited most from a reduced tumor load.

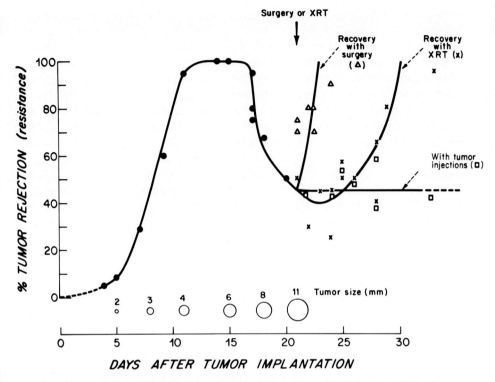

FIG. 2. Recovery of immune resistance following tumor-curative surgery and following injections of radiation-inactivated tumor cells, and recovery following a single local dose of 6,000 R of gamma-radiation (XRT, x). (From *Cancer Res.*, 33:493–503, 1973.)

tumors were on the average 15 × 15 mm, the tumors were removed surgically. Previous studies (2,4,6) have shown that with an antigenic tumor that large the host would be in a state of depressed concomitant immunity, and that immune recovery would follow soon after tumor excision. However, just after the tumor has been removed by surgery, the immune status of the mouse is in balance and can move in either of two directions: immune resistance recovers if the animal is left alone, or resistance remains depressed if tumor antigen is injected.

The surgically cured mice were divided into six groups of five mice each, and their resistance levels were tested on the day following surgery by two simultaneous challenge inocula of 10^5 suspended living mammary carcinoma cells injected s.c. at the left shoulder and at the left hip. Groups of 10 unsensitized, untreated control mice were challenged with cell suspensions containing 3.3×10^5, 1×10^5, or 3.3×10^4 living cells per inoculum to confirm that the challenge dose of 10^5 cells for the experimental animals constituted neither an excessive nor an insufficient dose. All mice in any particular experiment were challenged at the same time with tumor cells from the same suspension. The results of this experiment are presented in Table 4.

The mice in experimental group 1 received no treatment other than surgery. The mice in group 2 were given s.c. injections of 5 mg of radiation-killed mammary carcinoma cells in the right flank on the day of surgery, again on the day of challenge, and for 4 consecutive days thereafter (the same schedule was used to treat the mice of the remaining experimental groups). Previous studies (2,4,6) have shown that this procedure prevents the recovery from specific immune impairment that normally follows the excision of a large antigenic tumor. The mice in group 3 were given i.p. injections of 0.5 ml of serum from irradiated donors treated with killed mammary carcinoma cells. The mice in group 4 were given i.p. injections of 0.5 ml of serum from irradiated donors treated with killed fibrosarcoma cells. The mice in group 5 were given i.p. injections of both 0.5 ml of serum from irradiated donors treated with killed mammary carcinoma cells and 0.5 ml of mammary carcinoma antiserum. The mice in group 6 were treated like the mice in group 5 but were given fibrosarcoma antiserum in place of the mammary carcinoma antiserum. The i.p. injections of antiserum preceded the i.p. injection of serum from irradiated donors each time. The

TABLE 4. *Effect of injecting serum from irradiated, MC-treated mice[a] and serum from immunocompetent, MC-treated mice on resistance to MC challenge*

Group	Treatment[b]	Challenge[c]		
		No. of cells injected	No. of tumors[d]	Average tumor size (mm)[e]
1	Surgery only	1×10^5	9/30	2.70
2	Surgery + killed MC cells	1×10^5	21/30	7.0
3	Surgery + MC serum	1×10^5	17/30	5.57
4	Surgery + FS serum	1×10^5	10/30	2.87
5	Surgery + MC serum + MC antiserum	1×10^5	14/30	3.83
6	Surgery + MC serum + FS antiserum	1×10^5	18/30	5.97
7	Unsensitized	3.3×10^5	60/60	12.30
8	Unsensitized	1×10^5	60/60	10.95
9	Unsensitized	3.3×10^4	47/60	8.67

[a] MC, mammary carcinoma; FS, fibrosarcoma. (From *Isr. J. Med. Sci.,* 12:334, 1976.)

[b] The sensitizing mammary carcinoma implants were removed after 28 days of growth at an average size of about 15×15 mm. For description of treatment procedures, see text.

[c] All the mice were challenged with s.c. injections of tumor cells at the left shoulder and hip. Group 8 differs significantly from each of groups 1 to 6. Group 1 (or group 4 or 5) vs group 2 (or group 3 or 6), $p < 0.05$; group 1 (or group 4 or 5) vs group 2 (or group 3 or 6) vs group 8, $p < 0.001$.

[d] Only the differences in mean tumor size have been evaluated statistically.

[e] The mean value for each group was derived by dividing the sum of the tumor sizes by the total number of s.c. challenge implantations (2/mouse) in each group.

incidence and size of tumors at the s.c. challenge injection sites were checked and recorded as in the previously described experiment.

Table 4 presents the results of three separate but identical experiments. Since the results of the three experiments were similar, the data have been combined. Statistical evaluations of the differences in tumor development show that resistance was strong in the mice treated with tumor excision only (group 1 versus group 8) and that resistance was impaired by the injection of killed mammary carcinoma cells (group 2) or by the injection of serum from irradiated and mammary carcinoma-treated mice (group 3) but not by the injection of serum from irradiated mice treated with the fibrosarcoma (group 4). The impairment produced in the mice of group 3 was partially averted by the additional injection of mammary carcinoma antiserum (group 5), but not by the additional fibrosarcoma antiserum (group 6).

DISCUSSION

On the strength of evidence from mouse experiments, it appears that antitumor immune resistance functions most effectively against tumor cells that have been injected into the circulation and least effectively against tumor cells injected s.c. It is not known whether the i.v. injected tumor cells are destroyed primarily within the blood vessels or after the cells have implanted. Nor is it known why there is a difference in the effectiveness of immune resistance against tumor cells injected i.v. and cells injected s.c. It may simply be that immune resistance factors are more readily and more abundantly available against tumor cells injected into the blood. In any event, it is encouraging to find that tumor immunity is particularly effective in test conditions that simulate metastasis, much more effective than could have been assumed from the mass of information derived from s.c. transplantation studies.

The results of the experiments described in this chapter have shown that immune serum factors, presumed to be antibodies, can act in favor of the tumor host in at least two circumstances: (a) Immune serum plus normal lymph node cells gave protection to irradiated, unsensitized mice against tumor cells injected i.v. in single cell suspension. (b) In passive transfer, immune serum neutralized the specific immune impairment associated with excessive tumor burden.

The demonstration of the protective effect of antibodies (Tables 1 and 2) required carefully selected and prepared conditions: The immune serum recipients had to be preirradiated to preclude that the challenge injection of antigenic tumor cells gave rise to a primary immune response which could obscure the effect of the serum transfer. Furthermore, the irradiated mice had to be partially reconstituted with injected normal lymph node cells.

And, lastly, the serum recipients had to be challenged intravenously and not subcutaneously to display the protection transferred with immune serum. The protective effect of immune serum, much less conspicuous than protection by transferred immune cells, was nevertheless significant in the two tests with intravenous challenge. These observations resemble the *in vitro* observations by Pollack (7) that antitumor serum made normal syngeneic lymph node cells active in the *in vitro* destruction of syngeneic tumor target cells. She has given the effect the descriptive term "arming" of lymphocytes by antibody. This arming mechanism could have provided the protection by lymph node cells and serum against tumor challenge seen most distinctly in irradiated recipients. The resulting protection could have been inadequate in unrestored irradiated mice due to lack of normal lymphocytes, discernible in irradiated mice partially restored with normal lymph node cells, and present in intact mice but obscured by the rapid development of the primary immune response stimulated by the challenge injection of antigenic tumor cells (4).

If an "arming" mechanism functions in antitumor immune resistance, an additional process must be proposed, which can explain how circulating antitumor antibodies may be "arming" and thereby committing to one specificity possibly the entire population of one class of uncommitted lymphocytes without creating a persistent state incompatible with the normal immune responses and functions of an intact animal. The known rapid turnover of a great portion of the small lymphocyte population (8–10) and the relatively short half-life of some immunoglobulins (11) could explain how "arming" of normal lymphocytes by cytophilic antibody could be a very effective, but temporary, immune defense mechanism.

The need to transfer normal lymph node cells along with antiserum to demonstrate protection in irradiated recipient mice suggests another explanation, speculative, but open to testing: in the mixed population of normal lymph node cells, one kind of cell may be both particularly radiosensitive and particularly important in immune resistance actions in which antibodies play a part. If this were the case, the identification of the cell would be of considerable theoretical as well as practical interest. For one, the biological units which function together in the development and execution of the immune responses are currently under intense investigation. Secondly, this information could suggest ways to protect against, or to repair, radiation-induced damage to the immune system.

The results presented in Table 4 constitute evidence that immune serum factors, presumed but not yet proven to be antibodies, may act in immune protection by neutralizing other serum factors presumed to be free tumor antigens. Free tumor antigen in excess has been proposed as the most significant negative factor in antitumor immune resistance by a number of investigators (2–6, 12–14). Therefore, any process that would tend to reduce the amount of free antigen, such as neutralization by antibody and uptake by the liver (15), would favor the protective action of immune resistance factors against living tumor cells.

These results show that immune serum can be effective against tumor cells injected into the bloodstream and can also be effective against excess tumor antigens free in the circulation. Consequently, humoral factors may be of particular importance in preventing metastases directly by cytotoxic effects, as well as indirectly by neutralizing the growth-promoting effects of tumor antigen overload.

SUMMARY

These investigations have studied the role of immune serum factors, presumably antibodies, in resistance to vascular dissemination of tumor growth, and have studied the influence of excess free tumor antigens on antitumor transplantation immunity. The studies used a methylcholanthrene-induced fibrosarcoma and a spontaneous mammary carcinoma, both syngeneic in C3H mice.

In one study the recipient mice were first prepared by being given 400 R whole-body irradiation. This procedure precluded the development of a primary immune response which could obscure the protective effect of passively transferred immune serum. After irradiation, repeated injections of immune serum plus normal lymph node cells protected the mice against pulmonary metastases following injection of fibrosarcoma cells. Injections of immune serum and normal lymphocytes did not protect irradiated mice against s.c. injection of fibrosarcoma cells.

In a second study which compared pulmonary and s.c. immune resistance against implanted mammary carcinoma cells, the following observations were made:

1. During progressive growth of a sensitizing primary tumor implant, concomitant antitumor immunity reached a higher level of effectiveness in the lungs than in s.c. tissues. This was demonstrated by the relatively greater reduction, by immunization, of pulmonary growth following i.v. injection of tumor cells than of the growth of s.c. implanted tumor cells.

2. The concomitant immune resistance declined under the burden of a tumor implant which had grown to a size larger than 10 mm. The immune resistance against tumor cells injected i.v. remained effective longer, however, under the increasing antigenic burden than did resistance against tumor cells injected s.c.

A third study investigated the opposing influences of antigen and antibody, present in the blood of an animal at the same time, on resistance to implanted tumor cells. Immune resistance, depressed by a large tumor, would normally recover soon after excision of the tumor. The recovery could be delayed, however, by several injections of serum from donors that had received

400 R whole-body radiation and then been given six daily injections of 100 mg of radiation-inactivated tumor homogenate. This serum was presumed to contain soluble tumor antigen but no antitumor antibody. The additional injections of serum from immunized donors would neutralize the effect of the serum presumed to contain antigen and assist the recovery of resistance to the growth of implanted tumor cells. This suggests that immune serum factors, presumed but not yet proven to be antibodies, may play a role in tumor resistance by neutralizing factors which are probably free tumor antigens.

ACKNOWLEDGMENTS

This work was supported by U.S.P.H.S. Grants CA13018, CA15960, and CA16039, and by a Cancer Research Scholar Award from the American Cancer Society, Massachusetts Division, Inc.

REFERENCES

1. Vaage, J., and Agarwal, S. (1976): Stimulation or inhibition of immune resistance against metastatic or local growth of a C3H mammary carcinoma. *Cancer Res.,* 36:1831–1836.
2. Vaage, J. (1971): Concomitant immunity and specific depression of immunity by residual and reinjected syngeneic tumor tissue. *Cancer Res.,* 31:1655–1662.
3. Vaage, J. (1972): Specific desensitization of resistance against a syngeneic methycholanthrene-induced sarcoma in C3Hf mice. *Cancer Res.,* 32:193–199.
4. Vaage, J. (1973): Influence of tumor antigen on maintenance versus depression of tumor specific immunity. *Cancer Res.,* 34:493–503.
5. Vaage, J. (1974): Circulating tumor antigens versus immune serum factors in depressed concomitant immunity. *Cancer Res.,* 34:297–298.
6. Vaage, J. (1973): Concomitant immunity and specific desensitization in murine tumor hosts. *Isr. J. Med. Sci.,* 9:332–343.
7. Pollack, S. (1973): Specific "arming" of normal lymph node cells by sera from tumor-bearing mice. *Int. J. Cancer,* 11:138–142.
8. Caffrey, R. W., Rieke, W. O., and Everett, N. B. (1962): Radiographic studies of small lymphocytes in the thoracic duct of the rat. *Acta Haematol. (Basel),* 28:145–154.
9. Metcalf, W. K., and Osmond, D. G. (1966): A radio-autographic investigation of the identity of phytohaemagglutinin responsive cells in the lymphoid tissues of the rat. *Exp. Cell Res.,* 41:669–672.
10. Robinson, S. H., Brecher, G., Lourie, I. S., and Haley, J. S. (1965): Leukocyte labeling in rats during and after continuous infusion of tritiated thymidine: Implications for lymphocyte longevity and DNA revitalization. *Blood,* 26:281–295.
11. Waldman, T. A., and Strober, W. (1969): Metabolism of immunoglobulins. *Prog. Allergy,* 13:1–110.
12. Alexander, P. (1974): Escape from immune destruction by the host through shedding of surface antigens: Is this a characteristic shared by malignant and embryonic cells? *Cancer Res.,* 34:2077–2082.
13. Currie, G. A., and Gage, J. O. (1973): Influence of tumor growth on the evolution of cytotoxic lymphoid cells in rat bearing a spontaneously metastasising syngeneic fibrosarcoma. *Br. J. Cancer,* 28:136–146.
14. Thomson, D. M. P., Eccles, S., and Alexander, P. (1973): Antibodies and soluble tumor-specific antigens in blood and lymph of rats with chemically induced sarcomata. *Br. J. Cancer,* 28:6–15.
15. Vaage, J. (1972): The immunogenic activity of tumor antigen retained by the reticuloendothelial cells of tumor-bearing mice. *Cancer Res.,* 32:898–903.

Cancer Invasion and Metastasis: Biologic Mechanisms and Therapy, edited by S. B. Day et al. Raven Press, New York © 1977.

Immunosuppression and Metastasis

Jan Stjernswärd and Pelham Douglas

Ludwig Institute for Cancer Research, Lausanne Branch, and Department of Radiotherapy, Cantonal University Hospital, Lausanne, Switzerland

Immunosuppression may be one of many mechanisms important for metastasis, and it has been shown by experiment to facilitate the take and outgrowth of metastases. Experimental animal data clearly demonstrate that immunosuppression by irradiation of the host or thoracic duct drainage accelerates the appearance of occult metastases (11), that large-volume irradiation of the host outside the true tumor area facilitates metastases (48), that chemical-induced immunosuppression facilitates the take of antigeneic tumor transplant (41,51), and that there exists a correlation between changes in host immunity with age and ability of take and outgrowth of antigeneic tumor cells (41). Immunosuppression may thus be one of the many complex mechanisms important in metastases. Radiation of the tumors may also enhance distant metastases, although the mechanism here still is unclear (12,13).

The question arises as to whether the observed mechanisms of facilitation of metastasis by immunosuppression found in a clear-cut experimental animal model system are relevant phenomena occurring in the human cancer setting. The first part of our chapter will investigate this question. In two clinical situations routine therapy is applied to treat the previous site of the tumor "prophylactically" after it has been removed so as to prevent local recurrence, although later mortality data show that at the time of operation there existed widespread occult disease outside the treated area. This routine treatment is radiotherapy. It induces a unique and long-lasting lymphopenia (42,44,45). Irradiation, as opposed to chemotherapy, has only a local-regional tumor-neutralizing effect; although both induce lympho-penia, chemotherapy also may effect systemic disease. Operable breast cancer in stage II, e.g., with tumor less than 5 cm and positive axillary lymph nodes, and ovarian cancer in stage I have, up to now, mostly received postoperative irradiation locally as the only adjuvant therapy to surgery, although the statistics show that many die from distant metastases.

Does irradiation in such a situation accelerate the appearance or increase the total number of distant metastases, parallel with results from experimental animal model systems? When routine postoperative irradiation is used in the two tumors above in the disease stages mentioned, it offers a unique opportunity to investigate whether changes of one immune parameter such as lymphopenia will correlate with changes in frequency of distant metastases. The lymphopenia may not have an adverse effect on the immune response. However, *a priori*, it is not unreasonable to suppose a decrease in immunocompetence. The lymphopenia caused by postoperative irradiation is much more long-lasting and gives a much more dramatic change in lymphocyte count than any nonspecific immunostimulants currently used for boostering the immune response. The irradiation-induced lymphopenia may be considered as an "inverted" study of the possible role of immunotherapy. Although there are many preliminary and encouraging data from controlled studies using "immunotherapy," up to today, in spite of numerous studies, not one single trial has produced convincing statistical evidence that nonspecific immunostimulants work in the clinical routine as therapy for micrometastases. All studies await confirmation (27).

Enhancement of metastatic spread into apparently normal tissue after its irradiation (usually skin or lung) has been observed both in man—in well-documented examples (7,9,38,39)—and in experimental animal tumor systems (4,14,15,17,21,30,33,49,52). This phenomenon does not involve immune depression according to most investigators. The second part of our chapter will document results showing that nidation and/or local outgrowth of tumor cells may be facilitated in irradiated tissues. The existence of important mechanisms may sometimes be indicated by rare occurrences.

IRRADIATION AND SECONDARY SPREAD IN HUMAN CANCER

Breast Cancer

More than 4,000 patients have been investigated over the last 20 years in clinically controlled trials in which the main comparison has been between different forms of surgery plus or minus irradiation. Formally, the various trials considered are not comparable because varying surgical and radiotherapeutic elements have been used. Biologically, however, the differences in surgery have been shown to be of no importance for changing survival or distant metastases. Therefore, biologically the main difference in the trials is whether or not the patient has received postoperative radiotherapy. Prophylactic postoperative adjuvant radiotherapy has a general systemic effect inducing a long-lasting severe lymphopenia (42,45), with various changes in the white blood cell subpopulations, as yet not fully understood. This in a situation in which occult disseminated disease is outside the irradiated area in more than 50% of the patients with positive axillary lymph nodes, as confirmed by later mortality. Immunological tumor-host relationships in which the tumor-antagonistic immune defense reactions of the host have been documented as cellular changes in the lymphoreticular system exist, and they have been shown to correlate with disease and survival characteristics (44).

Table 1 gives survival data from all available controlled clinical trials, without any selection. The major difference between the two treatment groups compared in each study is the use or non-use of radiotherapy. The surgical procedures vary but have been shown to be of minor importance

TABLE 1. *Increased mortality after adding irradiation postoperatively to operable breast cancer patients: analysis of all available randomized trials for survival*

Study/Reference	Year postop	Increased mortality in irradiated groups (%)	Remarks
Manchester Q	5	+1.5	Includes $N_{(-)}$ pat.[a]
(10,32)	7	+2.6	
	10	+1.3	
Manchester P	5	+4.5	Includes $N_{(-)}$ pat.
(10,31,32)	7	+2	
	10	+3.3	
Copenhagen (22)	5	+1	Includes $N_{(-)}$ pat.
Edinburgh	5	+2.9	Includes $N_{(-)}$ pat.; premenopausal women castrated by irradiation too
(5,19)			
N.S.A.B.P.	1		Includes $N_{(-)}$ pat.
(16)	3	+7	
	4	+8	
	5	+6	
CRC Trial	1	+9.4	Only known $N_{(+)}$ cases
(26)	2	+9.9	included
	3	+8.1	
	4	+9.2	
St. Mary-Cardiff	1	No difference in	All $N_{(+)}$
(M. Roberts and A. M. P. Forrest,	2	mortality but	
personal communication)	3	+20% in dissemi-	
	4	nated disease in	
	5	"radical" radiation therapy group	
Oslo I (20)	5	+0.3	$N_{(+)}$ pat.
Oslo II	5	-13	All $N_{(+)}$; pre-
(H. Höst, *personal communication*)			menopausal castrated
Stockholm (37)	1	0.0	
Malmo (3)	1	-2	Palpatory lymph node
	2	+1	status only, and $N_{(-)}$
	3	+3	for all patients in-
	4	0	cluded; no difference
	5	+8	in mortality but +11%
	6	+2	of disseminated disease after 6 years in the group where irradiation was added

[a] $N_{(-)}$ pat., lymph node = negative patients; $N_{(+)}$ pat., lymph node = positive patients.

for survival. The table shows a consistent trend of an increased mortality among the radiotherapy treated groups. Out of the 9 randomized studies, 9 allow the estimation of survival at 4 or 5 years. Moreover, 7 of these 9 trials show an increased mortality rate in the group that is irradiated. This in itself is significant. Node-negative patients were included in 6 of the 9 trials, and in 2 adjuvant castration was carried out in all premenopausal women, thereby possibly eliminating a group at high risk for increased distant metastases after irradiation, as is shown in Table 2. The observed decreased survival after adding postoperative radiotherapy is revealed even though in most trials 5 years postoperatively has been arbitrarily used as the time of assessment of survival, most of the trials include lymph node-negative patients, and certain high-risk groups may have been eliminated by castration. If one looks only at survival at 5 years, an accelerated appearance of metastases without total increase may be missed. Two trials in which data are available to judge this question indicate that this is the case. The Oslo I trial shows no increased mortality at 5 years, although at 1 year 9 out of 109 patients had distant disease in the irradiated group as compared to none of 92 in the group of patients treated by surgery only (20). In the CRC trial (26), 173 patients could be identified with positive lymph nodes and were randomized into either simple mastectomy or simple mastectomy plus postoperative radiotherapy. During the first year there were 13 deaths in the group in which radiotherapy was added, as compared to only 5 in the group with surgery, which in itself was claimed as a statistically significant difference (26). Within the same study there were 18 patients with distant metastases in the irradiated group as compared to 6 in the surgery only group during the first year.

Patients with negative axillary lymph nodes are a group with low risk of microdissemination. If such patients are included in a study, it will be unlikely to find an increase of distant metastases after irradiation-induced immunosuppression as compared to that in a group of lymph node-positive

TABLE 2. *Increased earlier mortality after postoperative irradiation compared with operation only in premenopausal noncastrated women with breast cancer*

Study	Nodal status	Years postop	Increased mortality in irradiated group (%)
Manchester	Q technique	5	+7
Manchester	P technique	5	+19
N.S.A.B.P.	+ and −	3	+14
		4	+22
		5	+9
N.S.A.B.P.	+ only	3	+16
N.S.A.B.P.	+ 1–3 nodes	3	+25
	+ 4 nodes	3	+13

patients. Seven of the ten studies in Table 1 include lymph node-negative patients. In spite of this, an increased mortality is found.

Certain subgroups, such as premenopausal women with positive axillary lymph nodes, may have a high risk of accelerated mortality after irradiation (45), as indicated in Table 2. In two of the studies this subgroup is identifiable. Table 2 shows that they seem to carry a higher risk of mortality if postoperative irradiation is added to surgery. In two of the studies listed in Table 1, Edinburgh and Oslo II, this high-risk group was eliminated by irradiation-castration of all premenopausal women (5; H. Höst, *personal communication*).

In conclusion, there seems to be concordance between the results in the experimental animal systems (11–13,15,17,21,23,25,40,46,48) and human cancer data, showing increased disseminated disease after irradiation. Irradiation-induced immunosuppression is one very likely mechanism suggested to be of relevance from the experimental animal data to explain the above observation.

Ovarian Cancer, Stage I

The role of postoperative therapy as a useful adjuvant to surgery in stage I ovarian cancer is, within the clinical community, an unsettled question (1,18,35). Stage I disease calls for the use of postoperative routine radiotherapy, a biological situation very similar to that of operable breast cancer, stage II. In both, irradiation is given "prophylactically" to target tissue where the primary tumor has been removed but where there will be distant micrometastases outside the irradiated target tissue as confirmed by later mortality. Such a situation offers the possibility for insight into the biological mechanism documented in animal models which will reveal whether the confirmed increase of metastases after irradiation-induced immunosuppression in animal systems is also relevant in humans. The irradiation confined to a small target volume leads to a "geographic miss" of the tumor invasion outside the irradiated volume. However, when remaining tumor clearly is left or a large tumor is within the irradiated target volume, as in more advanced stages of disease, it is logical to suspect, as has been confirmed, a beneficial effect of irradiation. This holds true for stage III, e.g., as well as for breast cancer and ovarian cancers.

Table 3 summarizes the survival in stage I ovarian cancer in patients treated with surgery only and with surgery plus postoperative irradiation. All studies are retrospective. A high degree of patient selection thus cannot be excluded. It cannot, then, be ruled out completely that clinical intuition for disease prognosis within the same stage of disease has been better and given a larger survival difference than that which exists between different stages of disease after pathological staging. It is open to question whether

TABLE 3. *Survival in ovarian cancer, stage I, with and without postoperative irradiation*

Study/Reference	Survival at 5 years (%)		Increased mortality in irradiated groups (%)	No. of patients at start of study		Comments
	Surgery only	Surgery + radiotherapy		Surgery	Surgery + radiotherapy	
Decreased survival						
Rubin et al. (35)	91	62	+29	11	12	
Maus et al. (28)	66.7	57.9	+8.8	33	28	
Munnell (29)	78	53	+24	98	81	Stage I A
Munnell (29)	80	54	+26	20	35	Stage I B
Dalley (8)	88	67	+21	8	12	
Barr et al. (2)	72	65	+7	40	17	
Bagley et al. (1)	63	66	−3			Stage I A
Bagley et al. (1)	70	50	+20			Stage I B
Webb et al. (50)	89.3	73.4	+15.9	105	98	Complete surgery compared to complete surgery + radiation; groups biologically not balanced
Webb et al. (50)	88.2	52	+36.2	43	25	Complete surgery compared to complete surgery + radiation; groups biologically balanced
Clark et al. (6a)	60	53	+7	46	101	
Increased survival						
Kent et al. (24)	46.4	71.1	−24	69	45	Stage I

the allocation of patients to surgery only or to postoperative radiotherapy has been the factor that can explain the differences. However, it cannot be excluded that the observed mortality after adding postoperative radiotherapy may be due to the treatment modality itself. It is to be noted that most irradiation has been done with orthovoltage therapy to relatively limited pelvic target volumes and with limited doses. Modern radiotherapy with megavoltage irradiation and with large and shaped treatment fields carried to relatively high irradiation doses and including irradiation of the whole abdomen by, for instance, the moving strip technique, and thereafter adding pelvic boosted doses of irradiation may neutralize micrometastases outside the conventional irradiation fields of the orthovoltage irradiation plotted in Table 3. This newer form of radiotherapy should not be compared biologically in its mechanism with the above data. Irradiation by the larger volumes and doses currently used, especially in stage II, seems to result in increased survival after irradiation (18).

As can be seen from Table 3, eight out of the nine studies indicate an increased mortality when postoperative radiotherapy has been added after surgery. The reason for this remains unclear. However, besides the more conventional explanation that it may be due to patient selection within the same stage of disease, it cannot be excluded that the data may reflect an interesting biological mechanism of importance in explaining increased metastases after irradiation, parallel with mechanisms found in experimental animal systems (13).

CLINICAL SUPPORT FOR THE RELEVANCE OF THE "SOIL THEORY"

At the end stage of the many mechanisms important for metastases are factors that influence the nidation and the fixation of circulating cells, and consequently their possibility to grow out locally. The factors that determine the localization of metastases are largely unknown (6,36), but some of these mechanisms may be revealed by rare occurrences.

Figures 1, 2, and 3 show a fortunately rare phenomenon in the clinic in which outgrowth of tumor cells has been limited exactly to the field of irradiation. In the patient in Fig. 2, the tumor recurrence started with multiple small nodules that were histologically confirmed, and approximately 2 months later the picture given in Fig. 1 was seen with confluent tumor growth limited strictly to the irradiated area. Notice that tumors grow also on the medial side of the remaining breast, which by the technique of irradiation with two tangential fields was also irradiated.

Twelve similar cases were documented in a larger oncological center during the routine follow-up of breast cancer patients during a year. Tissue damage, whether caused by irradiation or surgery, is probably the underlying cause of the phenomenon, which may not be related to immunology,

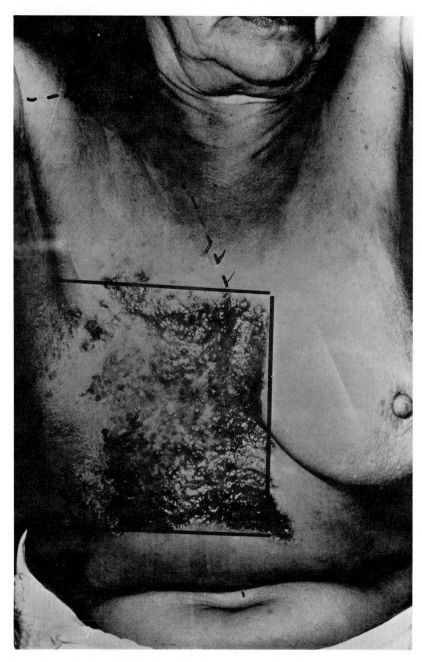

FIG. 1. Chest wall field irradiated with 15 mev electrons as outlined in black, as well as irradiated axillary field with ⁶⁰Co. Tumor growth limited strictly to the chest wall field. Visible tumor growth occurred 7 months after irradiation.

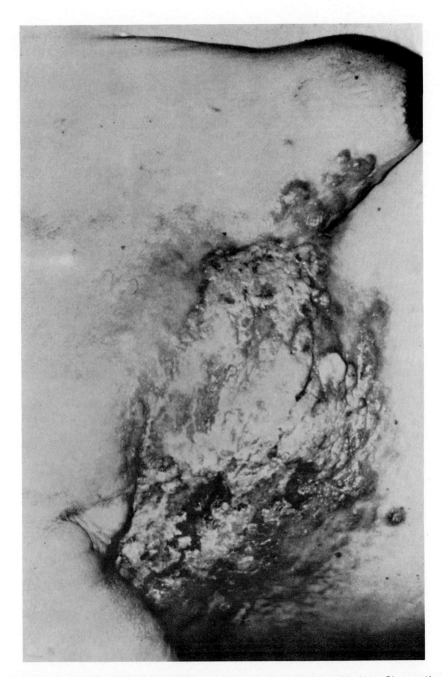

FIG. 2. Patient irradiated with 2 tangential fields, ^{60}Co, 4,400 rads/30 days. Six months later tumor growth appeared, strictly limited to irradiated area. Notice growth of tumor on the medial side of the remaining breast. Growth occurs here in skin which was included in the target area when using two tangential fields.

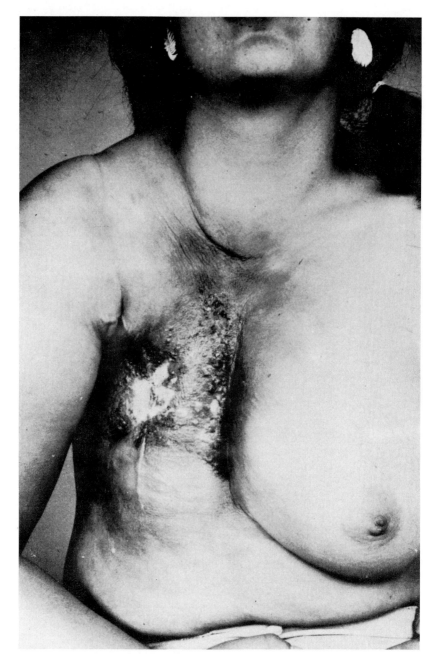

FIG. 3. Tumor growth limited to the irradiated skin area 9 months after postoperative irradiation, ^{60}Co, 2 tangential fields.

although a decreased ability to raise a delayed hypersensitivity reaction within the irradiated area could be documented, as compared to the opposite nonirradiated breast in two of the above three patients. The decreased ability to mount a delayed hypersensitivity reaction is probably an epiphenomenon to the tissue damage. More likely explanations are morphological changes such as microthrombi in blood vessels, endothelial damage, or fibrosis. A review of suggested mechanisms explaining observed increased metastases after irradiation, including irradiation of the primary tumor, irradiation of normal tissue, and irradiation of the host, has been summarized elsewhere (13). Earlier clinical observations (7,9,38,39) have been confirmed in experimental animal models (4,15,30,33,47,49,52) showing that tissue damage as such may facilitate nidation of tumor cells.

CONCLUSION

Sufficient data exist to support the concept that irradiation-induced immunosuppression may be one of many mechanisms important to metastases. Prophylactic irradiation of the tumor bed after complete removal of the primary tumor may be harmful when there is a high frequency of occult disseminated disease outside the irradiated area. This is indicated by the given data from human breast cancer and ovarian cancer. These data are in concordance with experimental animal data. It remains to be shown whether the accelerated appearance of distant metastases after irradiation could be explored positively and therapeutically by adequate chemotherapy, as more rapidly dividing micrometastases ought to be more sensitive to cell-specific cytotoxic agents. In rare circumstances, not yet understood, tissue damage after irradiation may facilitate nidation and/or local outgrowth of metastases.

REFERENCES

1. Bagley, C. M., Jr., Young, R. C., Canellos, G. P., and Devita, T. (1972): Treatment of ovarian cancer: Possibilities for progress. *N. Engl. J. Med.,* 287:856–861.
2. Barr, W., Cowell, M., and Chatfield, W. R. (1970): The management of ovarian carcinoma: A review of 420 cases. *Scott. Med. J.,* 15:250–256.
3. Borgström, S., Wenckert, A., Gynning, I., Langeland, P., and Linell, F. (1976): Är Körtelutrymning Och Röntgenbehandling Indicerad På Cancer Mammae Patienter Utan Lymfkörtelmetastaser? *Swed. Soc. Med. Oncol.,* 5:40.
4. Brown, J. M. (1973): The effect of lung irradiation on the incidence of pulmonary metastasis in mice. *Br. J. Cancer,* 46:613–618.
5. Bruce, J. (1971): Operable cancer of the breast: A controlled clinical trial. *Cancer,* 28:1443–1452.
6. Carter, R. L. (1976): Metastasis. In: *Scientific Foundation of Oncology,* edited by T. Symington and R. L. Carter, pp. 172–180. William Heineman Medical Books Ltd., London.
6a. Clark, D., Hilaris, B., Roussis, C., and Burnschwig, A. (1973): The role of radiation therapy (including isotopes) in the treatment of cancer of the ovary. (Results of 614 patients treated at Memorial Hospital, New York, N.Y.) *Prog. Clin. Cancer,* 5:227–235.
7. Cole, H., and Halnan, K. E. (1971): Facilitation of tumour spread in irradiated tissue after

prophylactic post-operative x-ray therapy for breast cancer. *Clin. Radiol.,* 22:133–135.

8. Dalley, V. M. (1969): Radiotherapy in malignant disease of the ovary. *Proc. R. Soc. Med.,* 62:359–361.

9. Dao, T. L., and Kovaric, J. (1962): Incidence of pulmonary and skin metastasis in women with breast cancer who received post-operative irradiation. *Surgery,* 52:203–212.

10. Easson, E. C. (1968): Post-operative radiotherapy in breast cancer. In: *Prognostic Factors in Breast Cancer,* edited by A. P. M. Forrest and P. B. Kunkler, pp. 118–127. E. S. Livingstone Ltd., Edinburgh.

11. Eccles, S. A., and Alexander, P. (1975): Immunologically-mediated restraint of latent tumour metastases. *Nature,* 257:52–54.

12. von Essen, C. F., and Kaplan, H. S. (1952): Further studies on metastasis of a transplantable mouse mammary carcinoma after roentgen irradiation. *J. Natl. Cancer Inst.,* 12:883–892.

13. von Essen, C. F., and Stjernswärd, J. (1977): Radiation and metastasis. In: *Secondary Spread of Cancer,* edited by R. Baldwin. Academic Press, New York.

14. Fidler, I. J. (1975): Immunologic factors in experimental metastases formation: Current concepts in cancer. *Radiat. Oncol. Biol. Phys.,* 1(1/2):93–96.

15. Fidler, I. J., and Zeidman, I. (1972): Enhancement of experimental metastasis by x-ray: A possible mechanism. *J. Med. (Basel),* 3:172–177.

16. Fisher, B., Slack, N. H., Cavanaugh, P. J., Gardner, B., and Ravdin, R. G. (1970): Postoperative radiotherapy in the treatment of breast cancer: Results of the NSABP clinical trial. *Ann. Surg.,* 172:711–732.

17. Fisher, E. R., and Fisher, B. (1969): Effects of X-irradiation on parameters of tumor growth, histology and ultrastructure. *Cancer,* 24:39–55.

18. Fuks, Z. (1975): External radiotherapy of ovarian cancer: Standard approaches and new frontiers. *Semin. Oncol.,* 2:253–266.

19. Hamilton, T., Langlands, A. O., and Prescott, R. J. (1974): The treatment of operable cancer of the breast: A clinical study in the south-east region of Scotland. *Br. J. Surg.,* 61:758–761.

20. Höst, H., and Brennhovd, I. O. (1975): Combined surgery and radiation therapy versus surgery alone in primary mammary carcinoma. I. The effect of ortho-voltage radiation. *Acta Radiol. Scand.,* 14:25–32.

21. Kaae, S. (1953): Metastatic frequency of spontaneous mammary carcinomas in mice following biopsy and following local roentgen irradiation. *Cancer Res.,* 13:744–750.

22. Kaae, S., and Johansen, H. (1968): Simple versus radical mastectomy in primary breast cancer. In: *Prognostic Factors in Breast Cancer,* edited by A. P. M. Forrest and P. B. Kunkler, E. S. Livingstone Ltd., Edinburgh.

23. Kaplan, H. S., and Murphy, E. D. (1949): The effect of local roentgen irradiation on the biological behavior of a transplantable mouse carcinoma. I. Increased frequency of pulmonary metastasis. *J. Natl. Cancer Inst.,* 9:407–413.

24. Kent, S. W., and McKay, D. G. (1960): Primary cancer of the ovary. An analysis of 349 cases. *Am. J. Obstet. Gynecol.,* 80:430–438.

25. Krebs, C. (1929): Effect of roentgen irradiation on the interrelation between malignant tumors and their hosts. *Acta Radiol. [Suppl.] (Stockh.),* 8:1–133.

26. McDonald, A. M., Simpson, J. S., and MacIntyre, J. (1976): Treatment of early cancer of the breast. Histological staging and role of radiotherapy. *Lancet,* 1:1098–1100.

27. Mastrangelo, M. J., Berd, D., and Bellet, R. E. (1976): Critical review of previously reported clinical trials of immunotherapy with non-specific immunostimulants. *Ann. N.Y. Acad. Sci.,* 277:94–122.

28. Maus, J. H., Mackay, E. N., and Sellers, A. H. (1968): Cancer of the ovary: A 21 year study of 1722 patients treated in the Ontario cancer clinics, 1938–1958 inclusive. *Am. J. Roentgenol. Radium Ther. Nucl. Med.,* 102:603–607.

29. Munnell, E. W. (1968): The changing prognosis and treatment in cancer of the ovary. *Am. J. Obstet. Gynecol.,* 100:790–805.

30. Owen, L. (1975): Influence of radiotherapy. *Eur. J. Cancer,* 11:35–36.

31. Paterson, R. (1962): Breast cancer. A report of two clinical trials. *J. R. Coll. Surg. Edinb.,* 7:243–254.

32. Paterson, R., and Russell, M. H. (1959): Clinical trials in malignant disease. Part III. Breast cancer: Evaluation of postoperative radiotherapy. *J. Fac. Radiol.,* 10:175–180.

33. Peters, L. J. (1974): The potentiating effect of prior local irradiation of the lungs on the development of pulmonary metastases. *Br. J. Cancer,* 47:827–829.
34. Report of an International Multicentre Trial (1976): Management of early cancer of the breast. Cancer Research Campaign. *Br. Med. J.,* 1:1035–1038.
35. Rubin, P., Grise, J. W., and Roger, T. (1962): Has postoperative irradiation proved itself? *Am. J. Roentgenol. Radium Ther. Nucl. Med.,* 88:849–866.
36. Salsbury, A. J. (1975): The significance of the circulating cancer cells. *Cancer Treatment Rev.,* 2:55–72.
37. de Schryver, A. (1976): The Stockholm breast cancer trial: Preliminary report of a randomized study concerning the value of pre-operative radiotherapy in operable disease. *Int. J. Oncol. Biol. Phys.,* 1:601–609.
38. Schürch, O. (1935): Ueber Hautmetastasen in Bestrahlungsfeld bei Phyloruscarcom. *Z. Krebsforsch.,* 41:47–50.
39. Schwarz, G. (1935): Ueber die Nachbestralung bei operiertem Mammaskarzinom. *Strahlentherapie,* 53:674–681.
40. Sheldon, P. W., and Fowler, J. F. (1973): The effect of irradiating a transplanted murine lymphosarcoma on the subsequent development of metastases. *Br. J. Cancer,* 28:508–514.
41. Stjernswärd, J. (1966): Age-dependent tumor-host barriers and effect of carcoiogen-induced immunodepression on rejection of isografted methylcholanthrene-induced sarcoma cells. *J. Natl. Cancer Inst.,* 37:505–512.
42. Stjernswärd, J. (1972): Immunological changes after radiotherapy for mammary carcinoma. *Ann. Inst. Pasteur Lille,* 122:883–894.
43. Stjernswärd, J. (1974): Decreased survival correlated to local irradiation in "early" operable breast cancer. *Lancet,* 2:1285–1287.
44. Stjernswärd, J. (1977): Radiotherapy, host immunity and cancer spread. In: *Secondary Spread in Breast Cancer, Vol. III, New Aspects of Breast Cancer,* edited by B. Stoll, pp. 139–167. Heinemann Medical Books Ltd., London.
45. Stjernswärd, J., Jondal, M., Vanky, F., Wigzell, H., and Sealy, R. (1972): Lymphopenia and change in distribution of human B and T lymphocytes in peripheral blood induced by irradiation for mammary carcinoma. *Lancet,* 1:1352–1356.
46. Suit, H. D., and Kastelan, A. (1970): Immunologic status of host and response of a methyl-cholanthrene-induced sarcoma to local x-irradiation. *Cancer,* 26:232–238.
47. Thompson, S. C. (1974): Tumour colony growth in the irradiated mouse lung. *Br. J. Cancer,* 30:337–341.
48. Vaage, J., Doroshow, J. H., and DuBois, T. T. (1974): Radiation-induced changes in established tumor immunity. *Cancer Res.,* 34:129–137.
49. Van den Brenk, H. A. S., and Kelly, H. (1974): Stimulation of growth of metastases by local x-irradiation in kidney and liver. *Br. J. Cancer,* 23:349–353.
50. Webb, M. J., Decker, D. G., Mussey, E., and Williams, T. J. (1973): Factors influencing survival in Stage I ovarian cancer. *Am. J. Obstet. Gynecol.,* 116:222–228.
51. Wigzell, H., and Stjernswärd, J. (1966): Age dependent rise and fall of immunological reactivity in the CBA mouse. *J. Natl. Cancer Inst.,* 37:573–577.
52. Wither, H. R., and Milas, L. (1973): Influence of pre-irradiation of lung on development of artificial pulmonary metastases of fibrosarcoma in mice. *Cancer Res.,* 33:1931–1936.

Cancer Invasion and Metastasis: Biologic
Mechanisms and Therapy, edited by S. B. Day
et al. Raven Press, New York © 1977.

Patterns of Metastases in Hemopoietic Neoplasms: Immunologic Correlations

Harry L. Ioachim, Antonia Pearse,
and Steven E. Keller

*Departments of Pathology, Lenox Hill Hospital and College of Physicians and
Surgeons of Columbia University, New York, New York 10032*

The spread of malignant tumors in the human body appears to be erratic and unpredictable. Yet the prognosis, treatment, and final outcome of most neoplasms are largely dependent on their metastasizing capacity for which reliable criteria of evaluation are not presently available. Clinical staging and histologic grading of primary tumors provide two useful parameters for this assessment; however, they are insufficient for the establishment of consistent criteria of prognosis.

In the presence of a malignant tumor we would like to know (a) if it has a potential for dissemination, (b) at what time it will metastasize, and (c) where secondary tumors would localize. Considering these questions, one first has the impression that total inconsistency characterizes the timing and distribution of metastases. Not infrequently, against expectations, well-differentiated tumors metastasize early whereas poorly differentiated tumors remain localized for long periods of time. Sometimes primary tumors are cured by surgical treatment only to recur many years later at various secondary sites. And yet, at closer examination, some events seem to repeat themselves in the evolution of metastases and some patterns seem to emerge from the study of their distribution. Lymphocytic lymphomas are known to metastasize earlier and wider than histiocytic lymphomas (1,2); clear cell carcinomas of the kidneys consistently invade the veins (3), whereas carcinomas of prostate and pancreas frequently infiltrate perineural spaces (4); follicular carcinomas of the thyroid metastasize preferentially to bones in contrast to papillary carcinomas of the thyroid that spread to the lymph nodes (5). Similar selectivity for secondary sites is displayed by carcinomas of the lung for the adrenals, by carcinomas of the prostate for the bones, and by carcinomas of the lung for the cerebrum. These of course are only empirical observations; however, their consistency indicates the existence of certain correlations based on mechanisms that unfortunately are still obscure. Needless to say, the understanding of such mechanisms would represent an essential contribution to the treatment of cancer.

To investigate such mechanisms, it seems that two approaches are available: the study of various types of human tumors from the point of view of their metastatic capacity and the reproduction in animal systems of experimental models of metastasizing tumors, similar to those observed in human oncology.

In the present chapter we examine problems of metastasis in the area of hemopoietic tumors and report on our attempts to investigate such problems in an experimental system.

Hemopoietic tumors are unique among all other neoplasms in that their tissue of origin is not restricted to one organ but is part of an integrated ubiquitous system. The concept of the reticuloendothelial system (RES) introduced by Aschoff and Kiyono in 1913 (6) has successfully withstood the challenge of time and was confirmed by the discoveries made in the fields of hematopoiesis and immunobiology.

According to this concept, organs and tissues apparently as dissimilar as the bone marrow, thymus, lymph nodes, spleen, tonsils, bronchial and gastrointestinal lymphoid follicles, interstitial hepatic tissue, and others belong to an integrated system and include stem cells endowed with the capacity of multipotential differentiation. A consequence of this concept was the idea that tumors of hemopoietic or lymphopoietic origin are always multicentric, developing from the beginning in different areas of the RES. This belief was strengthened by the consistent finding that lymphomas, myelomas, and leukemias at the time of clinical onset had already involved multiple tissues and organs. For this reason the concept of tumor dissemination by metastasis was thought not to be applicable to hemopoietic tumors, an idea that influenced for a long time the treatment of these neoplasms. However, in recent years, diagnosis of early lesions and their successful treatment by megavoltage radiotherapy showed that complete cure, free of recurrences, can be achieved (7,8), implicitly demonstrating the existence of unifocal lymphopoietic proliferative and hemopoietic tumors. With the present opportunities to examine very early lesions, it is not infrequent to find focal involvement by lymphoma of a lymph node that is otherwise histologically unchanged.

A new perspective on the problem of dissemination of RES tumors was obtained with the introduction of staging procedures in Hodgkin's and non-Hodgkin's lymphomas (9) which revealed the existence of a large number of unsuspected abdominal lesions at the time of initial diagnosis when only one group of cervical lymph nodes appeared to be involved. Before the introduction of lymphangiography (10) and particularly of exploratory laparotomy (11), the involvement of abdominal lymph nodes and spleen was grossly underestimated, which is not surprising since we have seen that lesions are often found in spleens of normal weight.

Methodical studies of Kaplan and his group at Stanford (12,13) established that Hodgkin's disease may arise in a single lymph node and then spread in an orderly fashion along the lymphatic channels, progressively involving subsequent lymph nodes. Segmental involvement of lymph nodes by Hodgkin's and non-Hodgkin's lymphomas in the course of dissemination is occasionally seen, not dissimilar to that of metastatic carcinoma in lymph nodes. To a certain extent the involvement of certain groups of lymph nodes occurs predictably, and several studies have shown the consistency of such a relationship (12,13). Thus, according to Dorfman (14), abdominal involvement in Hodgkin's disease occurred in 54% of his 171 cases in association with that of the left cervical lymph nodes and only in 17% with that of the right cervical lymph nodes. Mediastinal disease in Kaplan's experience occurs in relation to the involvement of the lower cervical lymph nodes.

Kaplan (13), based on a large number of cases, has reported that in Hodgkin's disease the liver is hardly ever involved in the absence of spleen involvement, which clearly indicates a direct metastatic spread from spleen to liver. Therefore, the latter must be hematogenous, just as the extranodal lesions, particularly the bone marrow involvement, cannot be explained on the basis of lymphatic spread alone (Fig. 1).

The hematogenous dissemination in Hodgkin's disease has been well

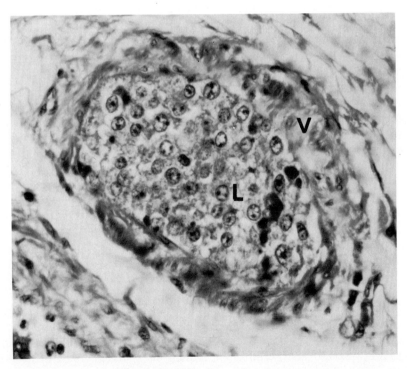

FIG. 1. Vascular invasion in lymphoblastic lymphoma. Vein (V) plugged by large embolus of neoplastic lymphoid cells (L) in patient with retroperitoneal lymphoma (×400).

documented by the studies of Rappaport and his associates (15). They have shown that in 6 to 14% of patients with lymph node involvement and in 20% of those with spleen and lymph node involvement, extranodal lesions are also present. They found vascular invasion in 83% of patients with visceral involvement and in 56% of patients presenting with lesions in nonadjacent areas. Only a minority among these cases did not show vascular invasion. The survival data clearly indicate the importance of vascular involvement as a prognostic criterion in Hodgkin's disease.

There are a few more arguments supporting the existence of hematogenous spread in Hodgkin's disease. One of these is the constancy of histologic patterns in different locations, a fact confirmed by several authors (1,14). It means that if a cervical lymph node exhibits the pattern of nodular sclerosis or mixed cellularity, the splenic lesions will probably be similar. This also means that histologic patterns generally associated with a better prognosis do not necessarily imply limited disease.

Almost all data on hematogenous dissemination in hemopoietic neoplasia available in the literature refer to Hodgkin's disease; however, it is fair to assume that the mechanisms of metastasis are more or less similar in non-Hodgkin's lymphomas. Consequently, it could be concluded that the dissemination of hemopoietic tumors by lymphatic and hematogenous spread is apparently not unlike the spread of any other tumors. And yet when lymphopoietic or hemopoietic tumors spread, it is primarily to other lymphoid or myeloid tissues, always within the confines of the reticuloendothelial system.

The spleen, which is only exceptionally the site of metastatic carcinoma, is invariably and precociously involved in Hodgkin's and non-Hodgkin's lymphomas (11,16). It is thus apparent that the simple mechanics of circulation cannot account for this selectivity of metastases. If the locations of metastases were the result of random spread of tumor emboli, there would be no difference between the frequency of splenic involvement in carcinomas and lymphomas. It appears that the localization of secondary involvement in lymphomas, and probably in other types of tumors as well, is the result of both circulatory mechanisms and cellular selectivity, which is the predilection of tumor cells for a favorable microenvironment. The consistent location of secondary tumors in particular organs may be the result of either a special tropism or attraction of the circulating tumor cells to those tissues or the survival of only those tumor cells that have fortuitously landed in compatible organs.

To gain insight into some of these problems, we attempted their study in an experimental system using several lines of hemopoietic tumors of rats. The role of immunity in the occurrence, amount, and distribution of metastases was studied in experiments in which the immune status of the host and the antigenic expression of the tumor cells were separately investigated (17–20). In other experiments we explored the selectivity of metastasis by

TABLE 1. *Metastases in W/Fu rats transplanted with GLV-induced leukemic cells[a]*

Recipient	Leukemic cell	Local tumor[b]	Metastasis[b]
Normal adults	MuLV$^+$	2/68	0/68
" "	A-B/MuLV^{-c}	36/36	0/36
" "	C-E/MuLV^{-d}	11/11	11/11
Normal infants	MuLV$^+$	17/35	35/35
" "	MuLV$^-$	14/14	13/14
X-irradiated adults	MuLV$^+$	12/12	9/12
" "	MuLV$^-$	9/9	8/9
Tolerant adults	MuLV$^+$	9/10	8/9
" "	MuLV$^-$	7/7	7/7

[a] Figures represent total of rats transplanted s.c. and i.p.
[b] Results are given as number of rats with tumors over number of rats transplanted.
[c] A, B—serially transplantable lines of MuLV$^-$ leukemic cells that grow at site of transplant and do not metastasize.
[d] C, D, E—serially transplantable lines of MuLV$^-$ leukemic cells that grow at site of transplant and metastasize widely.

using two lines of hemopoietic tumor cells expressing different patterns of dissemination (21,22).

In all cases, tumor cells in similar amounts were inoculated subcutaneously or intraperitoneally (Table 1).

The recipients were W/Fu rats of the following kinds:

1. Normal adults (2 to 4 months old)—immunologically competent
2. Normal infants (2 to 8 days old)—immunologically incompetent
3. X-irradiated adults (400 R, total body)—immunologically incompetent
4. Tolerant adults (injected at birth with Gross leukemia virus soluble antigen)—immunologically tolerant

The transplanted cells were of the following kinds:

1. Gross leukemia virus (GLV)-induced, syngeneic rat leukemic cells expressing murine leukemia virus-associated membrane antigens—MuLV$^+$ cells.[1]
2. GLV-induced, syngeneic rat leukemic cells lacking the expression of murine leukemia virus-associated membrane antigens as a result of antigenic modulation. There were several transplantable lines (A, B, C, D, E) of leukemic cells—MuLV$^-$ cells.[1]

---

[1] As detected in indirect immunofluorescence (IIF) after being reacted with anti-MuLV rat antiserum and stained with fluorscein isothiocyanate (FITC)-labeled goat antirat serum according to a method previously described (19,20).

The results were similar in the rats transplanted s.c. and i.p. and are given as total figures in Table 1. Normal adult rats, being immunologically competent, in close to 100% rejected the leukemic cells expressing viral antigens (MuLV[+]) and as a result did not develop metastases (19–24). In contrast, infant rats and X-irradiated rats, being immunologically incompetent, accepted the tumors which grew at the transplantation site and metastasized to distant locations, always within the confines of the reticuloendothelial system (20,22,23). In newborns due to the short survival time, some recipients died of metastases without forming local tumors (22). The rats conditioned at birth with soluble antigen, although immunologically competent, displayed specific unresponsiveness to MuLV antigens and therefore behaved like incompetent recipients and presented with tumors both locally and metastatic (18,19). Leukemic cells that had lost the expression of MuLV antigens by passage through X-irradiated recipients as previously described (17,19,24) resulted in several lines of serially transplanted tumors, designated A to E. All these lines were entirely MuLV[−] as assayed by IIF and consistently grew at the site of transplantation in normal, immunologically competent recipients resulting in huge local tumors that eventually killed the host. However, although some lines (A and B) did not metastasize, others (C, D, E) produced numerous large metastases in distant organs (24). Serial transplantation increased the propensity of such tumors for wide metastases, which in later generations affected not only lymphoid organs but also the kidneys (Fig. 2) and occasionally the liver, lungs, and brain.

The distribution of metastases was investigated in a different set of experiments in which two different types of leukemic cells were compared in regard to their patterns of dissemination (Table 2) (21,22).

The recipients were, as before, W/Fu rats—adults, infants, and X-irradiated. The leukemic cells were of two types: (a) GLV-induced W/Fu rat leukemic cells expressing surface MuLV[+] antigens (25); and (b) dimethylbenz(a)anthracene (DMBA)-induced W/Fu rat leukemic cells, as previously described (25).

Although the two lines were morphologically similar, it was determined by histochemical and ultramicroscopic studies (25) that the cells were of different origins: the virus-induced leukemic cells were lymphoid and the chemically induced leukemic cells were myeloid. They also differed substantially in their localization, the former in the thymus and lymph nodes, the latter in the liver and spleen.

To determine their respective patterns of metastasis, we injected similar numbers of the two kinds of leukemic cells in young W/Fu littermate rats (22). Intraperitoneal and subcutaneous administration of leukemic cells were used in parallel experiments. The results were remarkable, as the cells of lymphoid leukemia produced in all cases tumors in the thymus and lymph nodes, whereas the cells of myeloid leukemia produced tumors in the spleen and liver without any involvement of the thymus (Figs. 3 and 4).

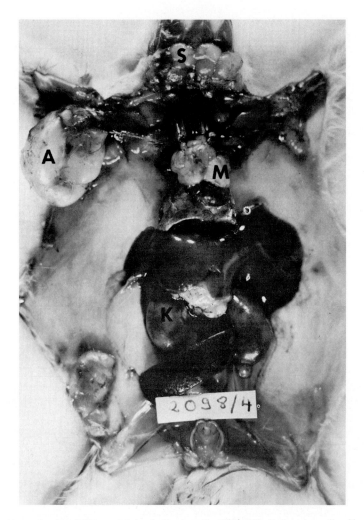

FIG. 2. Normal adult W/Fu rat injected s.c. with C/MuLV⁻ leukemic cells. Numerous metastases in axillary (A), submaxillary (S), and mediastinal (M) lymph nodes, kidneys (K), and spleen, larger than the transplanted tumor.

When the two types of cells were injected s.c., the same selective patterns of localization were obtained.

To examine the possible role of anatomic circulation in this selective localization, we labeled both types of cells with ^{51}Cr and injected them i.v. in similar numbers (22). Animals were sacrificed at regular intervals from 30 min to 20 days, and the amount of radioactivity in various organs was estimated with a scintillation counter. The results showed that in the first 24 to 48 hr the spread of cells to different organs was rather uniform with

TABLE 2. *Metastases in W/Fu rats transplanted with GLV-induced and DMBA-induced leukemic cells[a]*

Recipient	Leukemic cell	Local tumor (T/L[b])	Metastasis T/L[b]	Metastasis Site[c]
Normal adults	GLV[d]	2/68	0/6	— —
" "	DMBA[e]	0/19	10/19	Liv. Spl.
Normal infants	GLV	17/35	35/35	Thy.LN
" "	DMBA	9/25	19/25	Liv. Spl.
X-irradiated adults	GLV	12/12	9/12	Thy.LN
" "	DMBA	0/4	4/4	Liv. Spl.

[a] Figures represent total of rats transplanted s.c and i.p.
[b] Results (T/L) are given as number of rats with tumors over number of rats transplanted.
[c] Liv., liver; Spl., spleen; Thy., thymus; LN, lymph nodes.
[d] GLV-induced.
[e] DMBA-induced.

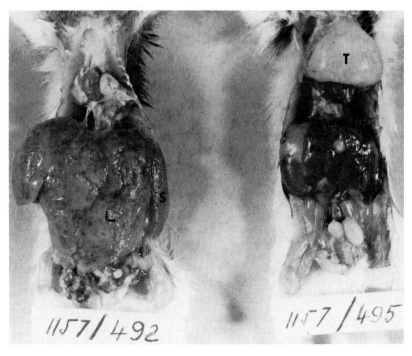

FIG. 3. Two W/Fu rat littermates injected i.p. at 3 weeks of age with 500,000 DMBA-induced leukemic cells (1157/492) and 500,000 GLV-induced leukemic cells (1157/495). The rat at left (1157/492) shows massive tumor invasion of liver (L) and spleen (S) without thymus involvement. The rat at right (1157/495) shows massive involvement of thymus (T) without spleen and liver involvement.

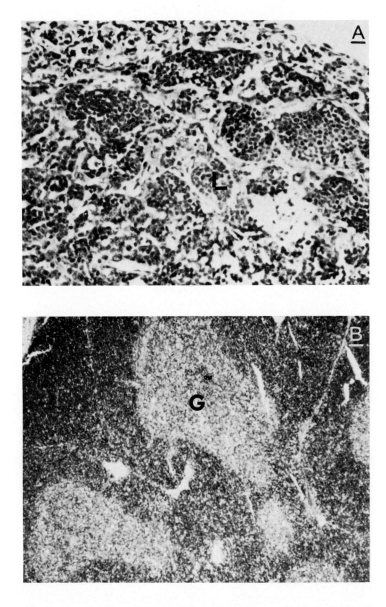

FIG. 4. A: W/Fu rat thymus massively invaded by large aggregates of GLV-induced leukemic cells (L). Liver and spleen were not involved (×120). **B:** W/Fu rat thymus uninvolved by DMBA-induced leukemic cells that produced tumors in liver and spleen. Normal thymus structure showing intact germinal centers (G) (×120).

no significant differences between the two types of cells. Only later, specific organ patterns began to emerge, indicating that tumor emboli circulate uniformly through different organs and that the eventual location of metastases does not depend solely on circulatory mechanics.

It was thought that perhaps the localization of circulating tumor cells is determined by recognition of specific cellular markers and that this process is under the control of immune-like mechanisms, particularly since one of the lines of leukemic cells expressed strong specific antigenicity. To investigate the possible role of immunity in the localization of metastases (Table 2), we gave an immunosuppressive dose of 400 R total-body X-irradiation to all recipients and subsequently injected the two types of leukemic cells as before. Immunosuppression did not alter the pattern of tumor distribution. Similarly, when lymphoma cells were injected in newborn animals (Table 2) which are obviously immunodeficient hosts, the same metastatic localization was consistently reproduced.

COMMENTS

The role of immunity in the occurrence, timing, and distribution of metastases of several lines of hemopoietic tumors was explored in the present experiments and the results are summarized in Table 3. Some of these observations seem to provide a sufficient basis for drawing general conclusions; others indicate only that complex mechanisms are operative in the process of metastasis and that additional investigation is needed for their elucidation.

It appears from this table that tumor cells that express strong membrane antigenicity are recognized and destroyed by the immune system of competent hosts. Conversely, despite their antigenicity, such tumor cells can proliferate and metastasize unrestrictedly in immunologically deficient hosts such as infants and immunosuppressed (X-irradiated) adults. The favorable effect of immunodeficiency on tumor growth has also been observed in animals treated with thymectomy (26,27), X-irradiation (28,29), steroids (30,31), and antilymphocytic serum (ALS) (32).

These various agents affect the immune system in different ways, not al-

TABLE 3. *Metastases in immune competent and immune-deficient hosts*

Host W/Fu rats	Tumor cells	Local tumor	Distant selective	Distant nonselective
Immune competent	MuLV+	−	−	−
"	A-B/MuLV−	+	−	−
"	DMBA	+	+	−
"	C-E/MuLV−	+	+	+
Immune incompetent (infants; irradiated adults)	All	+	+	+

ways producing global suppression, as originally thought, but rather creating imbalances between the various arms of the system (33–36).

The disturbance of immune homeostasis with predominance of the B- or T-cell populations results in defective immune reactions which may considerably affect tumor growth and dissemination. Recent work from our laboratory (24) shows that by passage through X-irradiated rats, leukemic cells undergo antigenic changes that endow them with the capacity to grow progressively and metastasize widely when transplanted in normal, immune-competent hosts. These experiments indicate that under the pressure of host immune reactions, new, less antigenic and more invasive clones of tumor cells may emerge.

The natural selection of tumor cells that are less likely to be recognized and destroyed yet better equipped to invade and proliferate in unfavorable environments appears to be the paradoxical result of some of the host's defensive efforts. And, at least in some human tumors, the selection of more invasive populations of tumor cells may be the result of our own therapeutic efforts that have inadvertently upset immunological homeostasis.

Further examination of Table 3 shows that in contrast to the tumor lines designated C-E/MuLV$^-$, which as a result of their antigenic deletion have become increasingly malignant and metastatic, the tumor lines designated A-B/MuLV$^-$ have remained incapable of metastasis in spite of years of serial transplantation in normal recipients. This striking difference in the metastatic capacity of two lines of cells that have the same origin and are morphologically and immunologically similar has no readily available explanation and will be the subject of future investigations.

Finally, the aspect of tissue selectivity in the distribution of tumor metastasis is revealed by the results of our comparative experiments with viral- and chemically induced leukemic cells. Invariably, when transplanted, GLV-induced leukemic cells metastasized to the thymus and lymph nodes, whereas DMBA-induced leukemic cells formed tumors in the liver and spleen. These characteristic patterns of dissemination that remained consistent regardless of the route of injection were also similarly reproduced in infant and X-irradiated recipients. These findings were rather surprising since it was expected that immunoincompetent hosts, offering no resistance to the spread of tumors, would present with a picture of generalized, randomly distributed metastases. In fact, ^{51}Cr-labeled leukemic cells of both kinds did show random organ distribution at short intervals after intravenous injection in all recipients (22). However, the tumors that eventually developed were not localized according to anatomic circulatory pathways but in organs consistent with their respective metastatic patterns. The persistence of this specific distribution in immunosuppressed animals indicates that the localization of circulating tumor cells is dependent not on immune mechanisms but rather on intrinsic cellular properties that determine their preferential growth in certain tissues and organs.

We concluded therefore that although the local growth and metastatic potential of a tumor may be dependent on immune surveillance, the site of metastasis is conditioned by genetic cellular qualities that determine the compatibility between tumor cell and microenvironment.

And in a sense this brings us back to the original hypothesis of the "congenial soil" formulated in the *Lancet* of March, 1889 (37), by Stephen Paget of London, an earlier observer bewildered by the illogical behavior of metastases.

ACKNOWLEDGMENT

This work was supported by Research Grant CA 16997–03 from the National Cancer Institute.

REFERENCES

1. Lukes, R. J. (1968): The pathologic picture of the malignant lymphomas. In: *Proceedings of the International Conference on Leukemia-Lymphoma,* edited by C. J. D. Zarafonetis, pp. 333–356. Lea & Febiger, Philadelphia.
2. Dorfman, R. F. (1975): The non-Hodgkin's lymphoma. In: *The Reticulo Endothelial System,* edited by J. W. Rebuck et al., pp. 262–281. William & Wilkins Co., Baltimore.
3. Anderson, W. A. D., and Jones, D. B. (1971): Carcinomas of the kidneys. In: *Pathology, Vol. 2,* edited by W. A. D. Anderson, p. 822. C. V. Mosby Co., St. Louis.
4. Lacy, P. E., and Kissane, J. M. (1971): Carcinoma of pancreas. In: *Pathology, Vol. 2,* edited by W. A. D. Anderson, p. 1285. C. V. Mosby Co., St. Louis.
5. Sommers, S. C. (1971): Thyroid carcinoma. In: *Pathology, Vol. 2,* edited by W. A. D. Anderson, pp. 1445–1446. C. V. Mosby Co., St. Louis.
6. Aschoff, L., and Kiyono (1913): Zur Frage der grossen Mononukleären. *Folia Haematol.,* 15:383–390.
7. Kaplan, H. S. (1962): The radical radiotherapy of regionally localized Hodgkin's disease. *Radiology,* 78:553–561.
8. Easson, E. C., and Russell, M. (1963): The cure of Hodgkin's disease. *Br. Med. J.,* 1:1704–1707.
9. Rosenberg, S. A. (1966): Report of the committee on the staging of Hodgkin's disease. *Cancer Res.,* 26:1310.
10. Lee, B. J., Nelson, J. H., and Schwarz, G. (1964): Evaluation of lymphangiography, inferior venacavography and intravenous pyelography in the clinical staging and management of Hodgkin's disease and lymphosarcoma. *N. Engl. J. Med.,* 271:327–337.
11. Glatstein, E., Guernsey, J. M., Rosenberg, S. A., and Kaplan, H. S. (1969): The value of laparotomy and splenectomy in the staging of Hodgkin's disease. *Cancer,* 24:709–718.
12. Rosenberg, S., and Kaplan, H. S. (1966): Evidence for an orderly progression in the spread of Hodgkin's disease. *Cancer Res.,* 26:1225–1231.
13. Kaplan, H. S. (1972): *Hodgkin's Disease.* Harvard University Press, Cambridge.
14. Dorfman, R. F. (1971): Relationship of histology to site in Hodgkin's disease. *Cancer Res.,* 31:1786–1793.
15. Rappaport, H., Strum, S. B., Hutchison, G., and Allen, L. W. (1971): Clinical and biological significance of vascular invasion in Hodgkin's disease. *Cancer Res.,* 31:1794–1798.
16. Lowenbraun, S., Ramsey, H., Sutherland, J., and Serpick, A. A. (1970): Diagnostic laparotomy and splenectomy for staging Hodgkin's disease. *Ann. Intern. Med.,* 72:655–663.
17. Ioachim, H. L., Dorsett, B., Sabbath, M., and Keller, S. (1972): Loss and recovery of phenotypic expression of gross leukemia virus. *Nature [New Biol.],* 237:215–218.
18. Ioachim, H. L., Keller, S., and Dorsett, B. (1975): Transplantability, immunological unresponsiveness and loss of cellular antigenicity in gross virus lymphoma. In: *Comparative*

Leukemia Research, 1973, Leukemogenesis, edited by Y. Ito and R. M. Dutcher, pp. 301–310. S. Karger, Basel.

19. Ioachim, H. L., Keller, S., Dorsett, B., and Pearse, A. (1971): Induction of partial immunologic tolerance in rats and progressive loss of cellular antigenicity in gross virus lymphoma. *J. Exp. Med.,* 139:1382–1394.

20. Ioachim, H. L., Keller, S., Sabbath, M., and Dorsett, B. (1974): Antigenic expression as a determining factor of tumor growth in gross virus lymphoma. Immunology of cancer. *Prog. Exp. Tumor Res.,* 19:284–296.

21. Ioachim, H. L. (1971): Homing to original organs of syngeneic transplanted cells. *Fed. Proc.,* 30:1210.

22. Ioachim, H. L., Pearse, A., and Keller, S. (1976): Role of immune mechanisms in metastatic patterns of hemopoietic tumors in rats. *Cancer Res.,* 36:2854–2862.

23. Ioachim, H. L., Cali, A., and Sinha, D. (1965): Age-dependent transplantability in rats of virus-induced thymic lymphoma cultures in vitro. *Cancer Res.,* 25:132–139.

24. Ioachim, H. L., Pearse, A., and Keller, S. (1977): Antigenic deletion and malignant enhancement induced in lymphoma cells by passage through X-irradiated hosts. *Nature* 265:55–57.

25. Ioachim, H. L., Sabbath, M., Andersson, B., and Keller, S. (1971): Viral and chemical leukemia in the rat: Comparative study. *J. Natl. Cancer Inst.,* 47:161–177.

26. Miller, J. F. A. P., Grant, G. A., and Roe, F. J. C. (1963): Effect of thymectomy on the induction of skin tumours by 3,4,benzopyrene. *Nature,* 199:920–922.

27. Ting, R. C., and Law, L. W. (1965): The role of thymus in transplantation resistance induced by polyoma virus. *J. Natl. Cancer Inst.,* 34:521–527.

28. Dao, T. L., and Yogo, H. (1967): Enhancement of pulmonary metastasis by X-irradiation in rats bearing mammary cancer. *Cancer,* 20:2020–2025.

29. Fidler, I. J., and Zeidman, I. (1972): Enhancement of experimental metastasis by x-ray: A possible mechanism. *J. Med. (Basel),* 3:172–177.

30. Pomeroy, T. C. (1954): Studies on the mechanism of cortisone-induced metastases of transplantable mouse tumors. *Cancer Res.,* 14:201–204.

31. Baserga, R., and Shubik, P. (1954): The action of cortisone on transplanted and induced tumors in mice. *Cancer Res.,* 14:12–16.

32. Gershon, R. K., and Carter, R. L. (1970): Facilitation of metastatic growth by antilymphocyte serum. *Nature,* 226:368–370.

33. Stjernswärd, J., Jondal, M., Vanky, F., Wigzel, H., and Sealy, R. (1972): Lymphopenia and change in distribution of human B and T lymphocytes in peripheral blood induced by irradiation for mammary carcinoma. *Lancet,* 1:1352–1356.

34. Cosimi, A. B., Brunstetter, F. H., Kemmerer, W. T., and Miller, B. N. (1973): Cellular immune competence of breast cancer patients receiving radiotherapy. *Arch. Surg.,* 107: 531–535.

35. Raben, M., Walach, N., Galili, U., and Schlesinger, M. (1976): The effect of radiation therapy on lymphocyte subpopulations in cancer patients. *Cancer,* 37:1417–1421.

36. Fink, M. P., Parker, C. W., and Shearer, W. T. (1975): Antibody stimulation of tumor growth in T-cell depleted mice. *Nature,* 255:404–405.

37. Paget, S. (1889): The distribution of secondary growths in cancer of the breast. *Lancet,* 1:571–573.

Cancer Invasion and Metastasis: Biologic
Mechanisms and Therapy, edited by S. B. Day
et al. Raven Press, New York © 1977.

Role of T and B Lymphocytes in the Development and Growth of Experimental Metastases

John M. Yuhas

Cancer Research and Treatment Center and Department of Radiology, University of New Mexico, Albuquerque, New Mexico 87131

Although the appearance and growth of neoplastic disease may or may not reflect failure of the immune system to recognize and control aberrant cells, it is clear that the elements required for such reactions (tumor-specific antigens, specific immune reactivity, etc.) do exist. Even if it should eventually be shown that failure of some component of the immune process is not the basis of disease appearance, it remains possible that appropriate stimulation of the immune system, i.e., immunotherapy, might result in effective anti-tumor effects.

It is unlikely, however, that immunotherapy will be able to address large tumor burdens, but rather it will be restricted to the therapy of metastases or residual tumor following primary tumor treatment. Even within this limited area, a full knowledge of the mechanisms involved is required, including the role of each effector arm, in order to avoid the application of ineffective therapy in certain patients or actual tumor enhancement.

Since the eventual aim of immunotherapy studies is clinical application, then it follows that the systems used and the method of analysis parallel, as closely as possible, the clinical condition. We have pointed out elsewhere (1) that strongly immunogenic tumors growing in young adult mice bear little in common with the clinical cancer situation, and demonstrated that simulation of metastasis by the intravenous injection of large numbers of tumor cells (artificial metastasis) differs at least quantitatively and possibly qualitatively from spontaneous metastatic spread.

We have extended these studies to include a comparison of the role of T and B lymphocytes in spontaneous and artificial metastasis, and report below the results of these experiments.

MATERIALS AND METHODS

Mice

The mice used throughout these studies were 4-month-old BALB/c females, which were housed eight per cage with food and chlorinated water provided *ad libitum*.

Assay of Metastases

A full description of the methods involved in the study of spontaneous and artificial metastases has been provided elsewhere (2,3). In brief, spontaneous metastases were quantitated by counting the number of metastatic foci in the lungs of mice which had received an s.c. transplant of 5×10^7 line 1 carcinoma cells. It should be noted that this highly malignant alveolar cell carcinoma metastasizes to all organs but is most easily quantitated in the lungs. Artificial metastases were determined by counting similar lung tumor foci 21 days after the i.v. injection of tumor cells.

X-Irradiation

Mice were exposed to 300 kVp X-rays at a dose rate of 110 rads/min (total dose = 500 rads). In all experiments, the interval between exposure and transplant was 2 hr.

Cell Preparation

Spleen cells were harvested from normal and immunized (three weekly injections of 5×10^7 heavily irradiated line 1 cells) mice and partially purified by passage through prewetted sterile cotton. At least 90% of the cells in these suspensions were indistinguishable from lymphocytes (stained smears and phase contrast). For selective killing of T lymphocytes or B lymphocytes, we incubated the lymphocytes for 30 min with either antithymocyte sera (ATS) or antimouse globulin (AMG) at 5°C. Complement was then added and a further 45-min incubation at 37°C was performed. Routinely, ATS killed 25 to 35% of the spleen lymphocytes and AMG killed 60 to 75%. We refer, for the sake of convenience, to cells which survive ATS treatment as B lymphocytes and those which survive AMG treatment as T lymphocytes.

RESULTS

Table 1 summarizes the data for spontaneous and artificial metastasis in control and irradiated BALB/c mice. Exposure of the mice to 500 rads of X-rays 2 hr prior to s.c. transplant of the line 1 carcinoma accelerates the appearance of spontaneous metastases by approximately 1 week in both the bioassay and gross observation systems. In the artificial metastasis system, the same exposure increases the yield of countable lung tumor colonies by factors of 5 (Table 1) to 20, depending on the specific experiment. Local radiation effects within the lung are not responsible for these increases, since such exposures have no effect on the development of spontaneous metastases and induce only a transient 20% increase in the yield of artificial metastases (3).

TABLE 1. *Spontaneous and artificial metastatic patterns of the line 1 lung carcinoma*

Metastases	Control	500 rads
Spontaneous		
A. Bioassay (lungs)		
First detectable	Day 6	Day 4
100% incidence	Day 18	Day 11
B. Grossly observable		
First detectable	Day 25	Day 18
100% incidence	Day 35	Day 28
Day 35 mean	4.8 ± 1.7	40.6 ± 3.4
Artificial[a]		
Lung colonies/10⁴ cells	20.3 ± 3.1	108.4 ± 10.1
Survival time	38.1 ± 3.2 days	24.6 ± 1.4 days

[a] Other organs affected: brain, heart, kidney, liver, lymph nodes, and spleen.

Since local effects could not account for the increases, and forms of immunosuppression other than irradiation (hydrocortisone, senescence, etc.) were also associated with an increase in the yield of both types of metastasis (3), we considered it likely that the increase was a result of immunosuppression. To test this more directly, we transplanted spleen lymphocytes from immunized mice into the irradiated recipients just prior to s.c. (spontaneous metastasis) or i.v. (artificial metastasis) tumor transplant. Table 2 summarizes the results of these studies, and demonstrates quite clearly that spleen lymphocytes from immunized mice are able to reverse the radiation-induced enhancement of metastasis in both systems. The fact that normal spleen lymphocytes (Table 2) and spleen lymphocytes from mice immunized against other tumors (data not shown) are less effective in reversing this enhancement suggests that the reversal is dependent on specific immunologic reactions directed against line 1 tumor cell antigens.

In order to determine which cells in the spleen lymphocyte inocula were responsible for the reversal, we exposed the inocula to ATS or AMG prior to injection, yielding "B-lymphocyte" and "T-lymphocyte" preparations,

TABLE 2. *Spontaneous and artificial metastases in irradiated mice which received spleen cells from normal and immunized mice following exposure but before tumor transplant*

Experimental group (N = 16–24)	Spontaneous metastases[a]	Artificial metastases[b]
Unirradiated	4.0 ± 1.1	11.5 ± 3.1
500 rads	31.6 ± 2.2	97.0 ± 8.6
500 rads + 5 × 10⁷ immunized spleen cells	5.6 ± 1.0	15.0 ± 3.2
500 rads + 5 × 10⁷ normal spleen cells	21.0 ± 3.6	37.8 ± 7.6

[a] Measured 35 days after s.c. transplant of 5 × 10⁷ line 1 carcinoma cells.
[b] Measured 21 days after i.v. transplant of 2 × 10⁴ line 1 carcinoma cells.

respectively. Table 3 summarizes the results of these studies in which the total spleen lymphocyte inocula was compared to these two subpopulations for the ability to reverse radiation-induced enhancement of both types of metastasis. In the spontaneous metastasis system, the B-lymphocyte inocula was as effective in reversing the radiation effect as was the total inocula, but the T lymphocytes had no detectable effects. Quite the reverse in the artificial metastasis system: T lymphocytes were effective, although B lymphocytes were not. In these experiments, both s.c. and i.v. inocula were prepared from s.c. tumors harvested 10 days after transplant. Similar patterns are observed when the source of the tumor tissue is from spontaneous lung metastases or from tissue culture-maintained line 1 carcinoma cells. We conclude, therefore, that the primary immunologic effector involved in the control of spontaneous metastases is the B lymphocyte, whereas the T lymphocyte is the major effector involved in control of artificial metastases.

Additional data presently accumulating in our laboratory suggest that the qualitative difference in the involved effector arm in the two systems is actually a reflection of quantitatively different antigen burdens. In the artificial metastasis system, 20,000 cells are injected and only 20 form lung tumor colonies, leaving the remainder to trigger immunologic recognition. Although not subject to quantitation, the antigen exposure in the spontaneous metastasis system is obviously far lower and more gradual. To test the possibility that a greater antigen exposure would allow triggering of the T-lymphocyte compartment, even in the spontaneous metastasis system, we compared the effects of T-lymphocyte reconstitution on the development of spontaneous metastases, with and without the addition of extrinsic tumor antigen. Table 4 summarizes the results of this study. Three injections of heavily irradiated tumor cells had no effect on the development of spontaneous metastases, nor did the injection of T lymphocytes from immunized mice. However, when the two procedures were used together, the reduction in the incidence of spontaneous metastases (Table 4) equalled that observed with B-lymphocyte preparations (Table 3). We interpret these data as demonstrating that triggering of the T-lymphocyte compartment requires large amounts of antigen, whereas the B-lymphocyte compartment is

TABLE 3. *Effects of selective T- or B-lymphocyte killing on the ability of immunized spleen cell inocula to reverse the radiation enhancement of spontaneous and artificial metastasis*

Immunized spleen lymphocyte inocula	Metastases	
	Spontaneous	Artificial
None	51.3 ± 7.1	115.3 ± 10.9
Total lymphocytes	17.3 ± 3.4	21.8 ± 2.4
B lymphocytes	18.4 ± 4.3	126.5 ± 11.4
T lymphocytes	45.4 ± 3.5	11.7 ± 2.0

TABLE 4. *Effects of injection of dead tumor cells during the first week post-transplant on the ability of various spleen lymphocyte inocula to reverse radiation enhancement of metastasis*

Spleen lymphocyte inocula[a]	Dead line 1 cells[b]	Metastases	
		Spontaneous	Artificial
None	No	47.1 ± 0.9	87.4 ± 3.2
	Yes	56.7 ± 2.3	98.3 ± 4.3
Total lymphocytes	No	5.0 ± 1.6	21.0 ± 3.6
	Yes	4.0 ± 0.7	25.4 ± 4.9
5×10^7 B lymphocytes	No	7.0 ± 1.7	79.8 ± 5.4
	Yes	8.3 ± 3.0	67.3 ± 3.6
10^7 B lymphocytes	No	28.7 ± 4.6	101.4 ± 7.8
	Yes	21.6 ± 1.9	83.4 ± 9.1
5×10^7 T lymphocytes	No	39.5 ± 2.1	19.8 ± 5.1
	Yes	1.8 ± 0.3	25.4 ± 7.3
10^7 T lymphocytes	No	45.7 ± 6.3	31.0 ± 4.5
	Yes	10.1 ± 3.2	15.0 ± 3.0

[a] Numbers refer to number of lymphocytes prior to ATS or AMG treatment.
[b] 5×10^7 heavily irradiated line 1 carcinoma cells injected 1, 3, and 7 days after transplant.

effectively triggered by the small amounts of antigen which are released spontaneously.

DISCUSSION

The results presented above demonstrate quite clearly that spontaneous and artificial metastasis are not quantitatively the same process, and that they place qualitatively different stresses on the immune system. The gradually developing spontaneous metastases appear insufficient to trigger an effective T-lymphocyte response, and therefore are affected only by the B-lymphocyte compartment. Artificial metastases, on the other hand, are produced in the presence of large amounts of antigen and therefore effective T-lymphocyte responses are induced. Experiments presently in progress indicate that the B lymphocyte can be the major effector when the cell dose used in the artificial metastasis system is below 100.

In summary, the B lymphocyte is the major effector involved in the control of spontaneous metastasis in the line 1 lung carcinoma system, and studies conducted in the artificial metastasis system yield misleading information regarding the relative importance of B- versus T-lymphocyte control.

REFERENCES

1. Yuhas, J. M., and Ullrich, R. L. (1976): Responsiveness of senescent mice to the antitumor properties of Corynebacterium parvum. *Cancer Res.,* 36:161–166.

2. Yuhas, J. M., Pazmino, N. H., and Wagner, E. (1975): Development of concomitant immunity in mice bearing the weakly immunogenic line 1 lung carcinoma. *Cancer Res.*, 35: 237–241.
3. Yuhas, J. M., and Pazmino, N. H. (1974): Inhibition of subcutaneously growing line 1 lung carcinomas due to metastatic spread. *Cancer Res.*, 34:2005–2010.

Cancer Invasion and Metastasis: Biologic
Mechanisms and Therapy, edited by S. B. Day
et al. Raven Press, New York © 1977.

Discussion Summary: Immunologic Aspects and Tumor Immunity

Martin G. Lewis

Cancer Unit, McGill University, Montreal, Quebec, Canada

The first few chapters were devoted to various aspects of immunological control of metastasis. Lewis pointed out the importance of recognizing antibodies which were protective against blood-borne metastases, but also the presence of antibodies against the internal components of the tumor cell which produced no protective value but in fact invoked the production of immune complexes. These were seen in relative proportions both in the peripheral blood and in the draining lymph nodes. The presence of these immune complexes and various types of antiimmunoglobulin was taken in conjunction to indicate a state of immune derangement in the production of metastatic spread of tumors.

Alexander pointed out the importance of recognizing an innate form of host-tumor interaction at the earliest stages of malignancy, which was not specific immunologically, but mediated through monocytes, macrophages, and possibly polymorphonuclear leukocytes. He emphasized the importance of the granulocyte series and the monocyte macrophage series in combatting disease in general, and the relative importance of this system, and then pointed out that this was the most important aspect of the early control of malignancy, whereas other more specific immune factors may be operative later in the secondary line of defense against metastatic spread. It was pointed out during the discussion, however, that the earliest aspects of malignancy that one recognizes in human pathological material, namely, *in situ* malignancy of the cervix and other sites and early malignant melanoma, were not particularly marked by the presence of monocyte macrophages, but clearly by the presence of small lymphocytes, so that these reactions were not necessarily universal in their pattern or type.

Fidler then reviewed experiments with artificial metastases using labeled tumor cells and their distribution in immunized and nonimmune animals. During this he answered questions which were raised several times on the problems of labeled cells, and pointed out that if the tissues were washed for 3 or 4 days in ethanol to remove the detached label, then this would obviate these problems considerably. He pointed out the problems in using thymectomized irradiated animals for these types of experiments and also the problem of allogeneic animals not being appropriate.

The use of co-cultivation of lymphocytes and tumor cells with surviving cells which were no longer able to be killed by the lymphocytes was interpreted as selectivity for a particular type of metastatic cell, and this was argued as to its relative importance. Several times in the discussion the problem of the various selective pressures on *in vitro* production of cells was again raised.

Fidler stated that man was the best model for metastases, but failing this, the dog had many features which would enable it to be a close laboratory counterpart.

Stjernswaard presented data which show that lymphocyte-mediated immunity was markedly depressed for up to 4 to 5 years after radiotherapy and that in experimental animals local irradiation of the tumor increased lung metastases. He also reviewed a series of trials throughout the world of radiotherapy in the treatment of breast carcinoma, pointing out that it offered little and, if anything, produced detrimental effects. This was to some extent countered by other suggestions during the discussion which pointed out the complexity of irradiated tissue, particularly the effect that the primary irradiated tissue may have on the immune system and other parameters. Also, the preirradiation of lung sometimes does not increase metastases but may in fact be effective against micrometastases. It became clear from these discussions that the problem had to be considered in detail rather than as a generalization.

Some argument occurred about whether this was a particular specific immune suppression; why did generalized suppression fail to occur with the increased risk of infection? It was, however, stated by several individuals that the immune suppression due to radiotherapy may under certain circumstances be very specific, depending on the relative balance of T and B cells and tumor-directed immune cells present at the time, and therefore a rather tumor-selective immune suppression may occur.

Ioachim then discussed the patterns of metastatic spread in hemopoietic neoplasms with particular emphasis on the way metastatic spread via the lymphatics may occur in some lymphomas, pointing out that these may be true lymphatic metastases rather than multifocal disease. He also emphasized the difference in the ability of tumors to spread via the hematogenous rather than the lymphatic route.

Ioachim then described the differences in two experimental systems using a viral-induced leukemia and a chemical-induced lymphoma showing the differences in metastatic spread and the ability to present different metastatic patterns. Yuhas presented data concerning lung metastases in spontaneous and artificial circumstances, pointing out the effect that the spleen cells have in the prevention of both of these procedures. He concluded that macrophages were not responsible, that T cells were partly responsible in artificial metastases, whereas B lymphocytes may have importance in spontaneous metastases. The key to the issue is balance of antigen — too much antigen, or too little, is detrimental to the immune response. This raised the issue of the importance of immunogenicity of tumor cells under varying circumstances, which was pointed out by Vaage and others. Immunogenicity is of considerable importance in the host-tumor interaction and therefore in the subsequent distribution and survival of metastases, yet it is difficult at times to establish with certainty.

McCullough presented work entitled "Leukemia — the ultimate metastasis," pointing out that in leukemia the malignant cells circulate continuously, or at least very frequently. He then proposed examples to support the clonal origin for hemopoietic malignancies, namely, chronic and acute myeloid leukemia, polycythemia, and myelofibrosis syndrome. He pointed out that colony-forming units vary in different patterns and that the regulation of these clones determines in a leukemic patient the state of the disease.

The question was raised during the discussion as to the evidence for the clonal origin of acute myeloid leukemia in humans and several detailed arguments occurred, but as McCullough pointed out, this was a strongly suggestive series of arguments.

Further consideration was given to the problem of the macrophage and its role in the recognition of tumors, both early and late. It seems clear that the macrophage can act in a nonspecific way, and this was again emphasized by Alexander and Vaage. The importance, however, of its role in early recognition was questioned on several grounds, although clearly it remains a theoretical possibility. The question of the entire regulation of the immune system was raised, namely, the interactions among antigen, macrophage, T suppressor and helper cells, and various other subfractions of the immune system. What was clearly needed was a model of complete congenital absence of macrophages which would allow the animal to live long enough for the importance of tumor interaction to be demonstrated. Such a model is not at present available. The use of the nude mouse as a means of seeing the importance of total T-cell absence was used as an analogy.

Finally, the role of the macrophage in dealing with liberated internal components of normal cells and thus preventing autoimmune reactions against cellular antigens was pointed out, and the phenomenon of apoptosis described by Kerr et al. was mentioned as a possible normal mechanism to prevent this, so that if tissue destruction occurred beyond the normal ability to be dealt with, the macrophage might well be of extra importance in preventing immune reaction against self-antigens. This may also be involved in the early problems in tumor-host interaction.

Cancer Invasion and Metastasis: Biologic Mechanisms and Therapy, edited by S. B. Day et al. Raven Press, New York © 1977.

Factors that Modify the Rate and Extent of Spontaneous Metastases of Prostate Tumors in Rats

Morris Pollard, Gary R. Burleson, and Phyllis H. Luckert

Lobund Laboratory, University of Notre Dame, Notre Dame, Indiana

Three lines of transplantable adenocarcinomas (designated tumors I, II, and III) were derived from prostate tumors that appeared spontaneously in aged germfree Lobund Wistar rats (1,2). The tumor cells spread from the subcutaneous inoculation site through lymphatic channels to the lungs, and from the lungs to visceral organs (liver, kidney) and less frequently to bones. The lung lesions produced by prostate tumors I and III are precise and localized; however, those produced in the lungs by prostate tumor II are diffuse, and thus are difficult to quantitate. Since the pattern of metastasis is spontaneous and predictable in all Lobund Wistar rats (males and females), especially in those inoculated subcutaneously (s.c.) with prostate tumors I and III, we have attempted to analyze the phenomenon through treatments which either accelerate or interfere with the pattern of metastasis. We wish to determine if rats with either of these prostate tumor lines will show the same responses to modifying agents; i.e., is there a common denominator in the phenomenon of tumor metastasis? The effects of the following agents on metastasis were assessed: *Corynebacterium parvum*, aspirin, inhaled anesthetic agents (chloroform, halothane, ether), and sodium barbiturate.

METHODS

Male and female conventional weanling Wistar rats of the Lobund line were inoculated s.c. with minced tumor or with tissue culture-propagated (3) tumor cells. The two tumor lines (designated I and III), have the following similarities and differences: both are scirrhous in appearance and texture and consist of epithelial cells arranged as glands and sheets in a prominent matrix of connective tissue. Both tumor cell lines are being propagated *in vitro* as similar-appearing cell monolayers (3). Rats show a leukemoid reaction to the growth of prostate tumor I, which is not manifested by rats with prostate tumor III. The latter tumor line grows and metastasizes faster than tumor I. Both tumors grow at the s.c. inoculation site and invariably ulcerate to the surface. In spreading, they cause swollen, hard ipsilateral lymph nodes (filled with tumor cells) and distinct round foci of tumor cells in and on the lungs. The transit time from the s.c. site to the lungs ranges from 10 to 20 days. The tumors can be transplanted by the intravenous (i.v.), intramuscular, intradermal, and s.c. routes. Through the latter route, tumors develop on the dorsolumbar area, in the footpad, and in the tail. Actually, metastasizing tumors will develop wherever adequate numbers of cells are deposited: at least 10 cells of prostate tumor III and 10^4 cells of prostate tumor I have initiated such tumors. Tumor II is softer, more cellular, and consists of tight packets of prominent epithelial cells in a sparse matrix of connective tissue. Tumor II develops into very large s.c. masses, the tumor cells enlarge the lymph nodes to 10 to 50 times normal size and produce diffuse lesions in the lungs which are less precise, and thus more difficult to count. No immunogenicity could be demonstrated with the three tumor lines, nor could a microbial flora be detected in them.

Assays of metastases by tumors I and III were based on numbers of visible tumor foci that developed on the lungs. Rats were inoculated s.c. either in the dorsolumbar area or in the right hind footpad. At intervals thereafter, each rat was subjected to one of the treatment regimes noted below. At 30 to 50 days after inoculation of tumor cells, all rats, including untreated tumor-bearing controls, were killed by ether anesthesia, exsanguinated from the heart, and subjected to gross and microscopic examinations to determine the rate and extent of tumor spread from the s.c. inoculation site. Each rat was weighed, gross observations of tissues were recorded, and the s.c. tumor, lymph nodes, spleen, and liver were excised and weighed. Weights of tumors in the amputated feet were determined by subtracting the weight of the left foot from that of the right foot. The lungs were inflated with Bouin's solution through the trachea, and 24 hr later they were stored in 70% ethanol. The white tumor foci were then counted with the aid of a duoloupe. Tumor-related tissues were fixed in Bouin's solution, embedded in paraffin, sectioned, and processed for histological examinations.

At intervals after s.c. inoculation of tumor I or III cells, groups of male and female Lobund Wistar rats were subjected to the treatment regimes noted below, and then examined for resultant changes in the pattern of tumor growth and metastasis compared with the untreated control rats.

A. Coincident with s.c. inoculation of tumor cells, rats were each inoculated i.v. with 1.4 mg killed. *C. parvum*.[1] In addition, some groups of rats were inoculated i.v. with *C. parvum* at 3 weekly intervals thereafter. Control rats were inoculated i.v. with the same volume of sterile physiological saline.

B. Rats were fed *ad libitum* acetylsalicylic acid (aspirin) in the drinking water for the entire period of each experiment starting at 1 week prior to s.c. inoculation of the tumor cells. The aspirin was diluted (620 mg/liter

---

[1] Burroughs Welcome Laboratories *C. parvum:* CN6134, Batch PX398, 7 mg dry weight/ml.

deionized water) and provided fresh each day. The control rats were fed deionized water.

C. At intervals after s.c. inoculation of tumor cells, groups of rats were each administered an anesthetic agent by inhalation. Each rat was placed in a jar with a drug-soaked sponge, maintained anesthetized for 3 min, and then returned to the animal cage for further observations and examinations. The effects of chloroform, halothane, and ether were examined.

D. Groups of rats were fed *ad libitum* 0.1% sodium diethylbarbiturate (sodium barbital N.F.) in the drinking water for 1 week. Each rat was then inoculated with tumor cells and continued on the drug-supplemented drinking water until the termination of the experiment. Control tumor-bearing rats were fed water without the drug. At a specified time after inoculation of tumor cells, all of the rats were anesthetized, exsanguinated from the exposed heart, and subjected to autopsy examinations.

The experimental rats were of the random-bred conventional Lobund Wistar strain which had been propagated for over 30 generations in this laboratory. Other strains of Wistar rats were not susceptible to the tumor cells. The rats were propagated and maintained in an isolated animal facility, fed sterilized diet L-485 (4) and tap water *ad libitum*. They were free of demonstrable pathogenic agents, and up to age 1 year they were free of spontaneous diseases (5).

RESULTS

As indicated in previous reports (1,2), the cells of prostate tumors I and III were disseminated from the s.c. inoculation site through draining lymph nodes in which they produced distinct round solid foci of adenocarcinomas which could be counted. The lung tumors appeared light colored and distinct on a yellow background. The rate and extent of tumor spread were assessed on the basis of s.c. tumor weight, on comparative weights of individual contralateral lymph nodes, and on numbers of tumor foci on the lungs. A peripheral lymph node from a disease-free rat weighed about 0.05 g.

A. Rats which were inoculated simultaneously with *C. parvum* i.v. and with prostate tumor III cells s.c. developed reduced numbers of tumor foci in the lungs compared to those tumor-bearing rats which had been inoculated i.v. with saline (Table 1). Four i.v. inoculations of *C. parvum,* each at weekly intervals, resulted in further reductions of tumor foci on the lungs: average 4 per lung compared with average 58 per lung in a single saline-treated control male rat. The numbers of tumor foci on the lungs were lower in untreated female rats than in male rats; however, i.v. inoculated *C. parvum* (four doses, each at weekly intervals) also caused a further reduction of tumors on their lungs: average 1.2 per lung compared to average 20 per lung in the saline-treated controls. Spleens and livers in all of the *C. parvum*-treated rats were significantly enlarged, and the latter organs showed peri-

TABLE 1. *Effects of* C. parvum *inoculations on metastatic spread of prostate tumor III*[a]

No. of rats	Sex	C. parvum[b]	Avg. weights/g (range)			Avg. metastatic foci/lung (range)
			Tumor	Popliteal lymph node	Liver	
1	M	0	1.5	0.17	7.5	58
7	F	0	0.42 (0.23–0.55)	0.23	6.4 (4.3–7.4)	20 (5–44)
2	M	1X	0.57 (0.47–0.67)	0.15	9.6 (8.6–10.6)	26.5 (21–32)
5	F	1X	0.55 (0.40–0.60)	0.19	8.78 (7.3–10.6)	6 (0–9)
2	M	4X	0.74 (0.57–0.91)	0.24	9.65 (8–11)	4 (3–5)
5	F	4X	0.33 (0.29–0.39)	0.126	7.5 (4–7.9)	1.2 (0–6)

[a] Weanling Lobund Wistar rats were inoculated into the right hind footpad with 10^5 *in vitro* propagated tumor cells, and killed for examinations after 34 days.

[b] Killed *C. parvum* (strain CN6134, Wellcome Research Laboratories) inoculated i.v. (1.4 mg dry weight) on day 0; and, where indicated, at 4 weekly intervals thereafter. Control rats received 0.2 ml physiological saline i.v.

vascular aggregations of mononuclear cells. The primary tumors and the lymph nodes were not markedly reduced in size by the *C. parvum* treatment, except in those female rats which received four i.v. doses of the organism.

In rats with prostate tumor I cells, four i.v. doses of *C. parvum* (each at weekly intervals) also caused a marked reduction in numbers of lung tumors at 41 days, compared to that in the saline-treated control rats (Table 2). There was no consistent reduction in size or character of the primary (s.c.) tumor in the *C. parvum*-treated rats. In a second experiment, rats that re-

TABLE 2. *Effect of* C. parvum *on metastatic spread of prostate tumor I*[a]

Experiment	No. of rats	Treatment	Avg. weights/g (range)		Avg. tumors/lung (range)
			Tumor	Spleen	
I	5	Saline 4X	0.63 (0.25–1.1)	0.61 (0.43–0.78)	13.6 (8–25)
	6	C. parvum 4X	0.78 (0.49–1.9)	1.12 (0.88–1.3)	1.3 (0–2)
II	2	Saline 1X	1.13 (0.84–1.4)	0.57 (0.56–0.58)	126 (15–240)
	4	C. parvum 1X	2.38	0.79 (0.71–0.88)	22 (0–58)
III	4	Saline 4X	6.4 (3.5–9.8)	0.925 (0.7–1.1)	123.5 (36–240)
	5	C. parvum 4X	4.6 (1.8–6.9)	1.18 (1.0–1.4)	12.4 (3–21)

[a] Wistar rats were inoculated s.c. with prostate tumor I cells into the right hind footpad (I) or in the dorsolumbar area (II and III) simultaneously with 1.4 mg *C. parvum* i.v. Where indicated, the latter inoculum was repeated 3× at weekly intervals. Experiments I, II, and III were terminated after 41, 30, and 50 days, respectively. Tumor weights were calculated from weights of right foot minus left foot.

ceived one i.v. dose of *C. parvum* had fewer lung tumors than the saline-inoculated control rats.

B. Groups of rats were fed aspirin in deionized water (620 mg/liter water) *ad libitum,* and 2 days later each was inoculated s.c. with prostate I tumor cells. Fresh aspirin was provided in the drinking water at daily intervals for the duration of the experiment; and control rats were given deionized water. Female and male rats each consumed approximately 45 and 80 mg aspirin/kg body weight/day, respectively. After treatment for 48 days, the aspirin-fed male rats had fewer metastatic tumors on their lungs than the untreated control rats (Table 3): males—0.3 tumors per lung and 8.3 tumors per lung in one trial; and in a second trial 13.8 tumors per lung and 138.8 tumors per lung, respectively. The results in female rats were less significant (Table 3). The rats in the two groups showed no significant differences in weights of bodies, tumors, and livers, nor in microscopic appearances of their tumors.

The effects of aspirin in rats with prostate tumor III were similar to those noted above with prostate tumor I; male rats that were fed aspirin developed fewer focal tumors per lung than those without aspirin. The trend was the same in female rats (Table 4).

C. Rats with prostate tumor I developed increased numbers of metastatic tumors on their lungs following inhalation of chloroform or halothane (Table 5). The increase was more marked in the male than in the female

TABLE 3. *Effect of aspirin on metastasis of prostate tumor I in Wistar rats[a]*

	No.	Sex	Aspirin	Weights/g (range)			Avg. metastases/lung (range)
				Body	Tumor	Liver	
I.	3	M	−	271 (251–300)	6.2 (4.8–7.6)	10.4 (9.5–11.9)	8.3 (1–15)
	6	M	+	271 (250–309)	6.4 (1.5–10)	11.4 (9.8–12)	0.33 (0–1)
	3	F	−	175 (170–180)	5.7 (5.2–6.4)	7.5 (7.1–7.7)	10.3 (2–23)
	4	F	+	170 (165–173)	6.5 (5.1–7.8)	7.3 (7–7.7)	7 (0–16)
II.	4	M	−	282 (261–303)	4.53 (2.2–7.3)	10.82 (10.2–11.3)	138.8 (69–178)
	5	M	+	303 (294–307)	5.7 (4.1–8.5)	10.16 (9.3–10.9)	13.8 (0–47)

[a] Lobund Wistar rats were inoculated s.c. in the dorsolumbar area with prostate I tumor. One group was given deionized water. The second group was given deionized water with aspirin (620 mg/liter water) starting 2 days before tumor inoculation and continuing with daily changes for subsequent 48 (I) and 43 (II) days when all of the rats were killed for examinations.

TABLE 4. *Effects of aspirin on metastatic spread of prostate tumor III*

No. of rats	Sex	Aspirin[a]	Avg. weights/g (range)					Avg. metastatic foci/lung (range)
			Body	Tumor	Popliteal lymph node	Liver	Spleen	
5	M	−	278	0.52 (0.23–0.64)	0.38 (0.2–0.9)	10.7 (9.4–12.2)	0.69 (0.59–0.8)	47.5 (19–111)
3	M	+	251	0.48 (0.3–0.66)	0.28 (0.19–0.42)	10.38 (9.2–11.8)	0.71 (0.64–0.82)	10.6 (8–16)
5	F	−	181	0.34 (0.09–0.58)	0.31 (0.1–0.58)	7.5 (6.4–8.5)	0.49 (0.4–0.52)	59.4 (1–71)
4	F	+	179	0.37 (0.3–0.57)	0.28 (0.3–0.57)	8.8 (8–9.5)	0.64 (0.54–0.7)	24.5 (8–68)

[a] Male and female Wistar rats were inoculated with tumor cells (10^4) into the right hind footpad. One group was given deionized water; the other group was given aspirin in deionized water (620 mg/liter water) starting 2 days before tumor inoculation and continuing with daily change of aspirin for 42 days when all rats were killed for examinations.

TABLE 5. *Effect of inhaled anesthetic agents on metastatic spread of prostate tumor I*[a]

	Drug	Sex	No.	Avg. tumors/lung (range)	
I.	Controls	M	3	19.3 (15–35)	
		F	3		21 (14–26)
II.	Halothane	M	5	43.8 (35–58)	
		F	5		27.5 (9–40)
III.	Ether	M	4	41.25 (13–65)	
		F	4		23 (9–40)
IV.	CHCl$_3$	M	4	48.5 (37–60)	
		F	3		42.3 (41–43)

[a] Male and female Wistar rats were inoculated with tumor cells into the right hind footpad. Seven days later each rat was placed in a jar with anesthetic agent and maintained anesthetized for 3 min. The rats were examined for lesions at day 39 after inoculation of tumor cells.

rats. Among groups of rats bearing tumor III and exposed at weekly intervals to one, two, or three treatments with chloroform, all had developed more lung tumors than the untreated control rats (Table 6). There were no significant differences between treated and untreated rats in size or in character of their s.c. tumors, nor in extent of involvement of their lymph nodes.

D. Rats that consumed sodium diethylbarbiturate in drinking water (about 100 mg/kg/day/rat) while carrying prostate tumors I or III developed larger s.c. tumors and metastatic popliteal lymph nodes and more lung tumors than the rats on drug-free water (Tables 7 and 8). The drug-consuming rats appeared active and alert during the experimental period. Body weights were essentially the same in both groups of rats, but livers were

TABLE 6. *Effect of inhaled chloroform on metastatic spread of prostate tumor III*[a]

			Avg. weights/g (range)			
				Right lymph nodes		
	No.	Day of anesthesia	Tumor[b]	Popliteal	Inguinal	Metastases/lung (range)
Controls	8		1.05 (0.23–3.23)	0.19	0.11	48 (3–212)
CHCl$_3$	8	7	0.81 (0.2–1.35)	0.19	0.15	108 (18–220)
CHCl$_3$	8	7,14	1.49 (0.35–3.51)	0.21	0.11	109 (46–225)
CHCl$_3$	8	7,14,21	1.06 (0.1–3.1)	0.30	0.13	97 (13–297)

[a] Prostate adenocarcinoma cells inoculated s.c. in right hind footpad. Each rat was maintained anesthetized for 3 min. At 35 days after inoculation, the rats were killed by ether anesthesia and exsanguination from the exposed heart.
[b] Right foot minus left foot.

TABLE 7. *Effect of sodium barbiturate on metastatic spread of prostate tumor III*[a]

Sex and No. of rats	Drug	Avg. weights/g (range)				Avg. tumors/lung (range)
		Body	Tumor	Lymph node	Liver	
Male—6	Control	201 (194–219)	0.29 (0.14–0.39)	0.16 (0.07–0.23)	7.9 (7–8.8)	75.1 (34–130)
Female—6	Control	145 (132–154)	0.34 (0.2–0.54)	0.20 (0.11–0.34)	6.7 (5.7–8)	75.5 (12–149)
Male—6	Sodium barbiturate	232 (211–266)	0.6 (0.19–1.03)	0.27 (0.15–0.43)	11.7 (9.2–12.4)	260 (56–554)
Female—6	Sodium barbiturate	147 (139–154)	0.6 (0.28–1.9)	0.20 (0.14–0.35)	7.8 (7.0–8.6)	101 (33–197)

[a] Wistar rats were inoculated with *in vitro* propagated tumor cells (5×10^5) into the right hind footpad. Na barbiturate (0.1%) was fed *ad libitum* in deionized water from day 11 to the end of the experimental period 28 days after inoculation of tumor cells. The rats were then killed and examined for lesions.

TABLE 8. *Effect of sodium barbiturate on metastasis of rat prostate tumor I*[a]

No.	Sodium barbiturate	Avg. weights/g (range)				
		Body weight		Ratio right foot/left foot	Right popliteal lymph node	Metastases/lung (range)
		Male	Female			
11	+[a]	259.7	168	1.45	0.41 (0.18–0.87)	9.9 (1–21)
10	−	246.6	171.4	1.2	0.27 (0.13–0.46)	4.6 (1–19)

[a] Sodium barbiturate (0.1% in drinking water) fed to rats *ad libitum* beginning 1 week before inoculation of tumor cells s.c. into right footpad. Rats were killed and examined 1 month after inoculation of tumor cells.

heavier in the drug-treated rats. In a separate trial, rats were fed the drug for only 1 week prior to inoculation of tumor III cells. A second group was fed the drug from 1 week prior to inoculation of tumor cells until the termination of the experiment 28 days later. The control rats had average 74.37 tumors per lung, a level similar to that of the rats which received the drug for only 1 week (79.6/lung). The third group of rats that received the drug continuously had 141.4 tumors per lung.

DISCUSSION

The rate and extent of experimental tumor metastases have been modified by a wide variety of drugs and manipulations (6–8). Some of the experimental tumor systems in those reports were not optimal: some of them were lymphomas, with some tumors the patterns of spread were sporadic, and with others the tumor cells spread only if inoculated intravenously. The rat prostate tumors I and III are solid carcinomas that show a predictable and spontaneous pattern of spread through regional lymph nodes to the lungs.

The phenomenon of metastasis needs clarification: Is it regulated by characteristics unique to the tumor cells, or by mechanisms in the host which regulate rates and organ locations, or by interactions by both host and tumor cell?

An immunosuppressive and oncolytic drug, cyclophosphamide (CPA) destroyed subcutaneous prostate tumors in rats and interfered with the rate and extent of metastases (9). As indicated in the present chapter, i.v. inoculated *C. parvum,* an immunopotentiating agent, interrupted the spread of tumor cells to the lungs without significant change in the size and character of the primary s.c. tumor. This may be related to a barrier effect of macrophages in the stimulated reticuloendothelial system (10). Orally administered aspirin also interfered with the rate of metastasis, possibly through its thrombocytopenic effect (11) or by inhibition of prostaglandin synthetase (12). The three agents noted above are associated with a suppression of metastasis, but their physiologic effects differ: one is immunosuppressive (CPA), one is immunopotentiating (*C. parvum*), and the third (aspirin) has no known effect on immunity. These actions may have no direct relationship to metastasis, which means that other, as yet unidentified, factor(s) may be involved in this phenomenon.

The deep inhalation of chloroform, halothane, or ether enhanced the rate and extent of metastatic spread of tumor cells to the lungs. Chloroform and halothane are purported to be hepatotoxic in animals, including man. Oral administration of sodium barbiturate stimulates hepatic functions through activation of a mixed-function oxidase system (13). Rats fed sodium barbital developed enlarged livers and larger tumors and manifested accelerated rates of tumor metastases to the lungs compared to untreated control rats. Does this suggest that the liver has a metastasis-regulating function?

We have described the effects of four groups of unrelated agents on the process of metastasis in rats by two adenocarcinomas of prostate origin. The spread patterns of prostate tumors I and III were enhanced by inhalations of halothane and chloroform and by ingestion of sodium barbital, but the effects of these drugs on observable liver functions differed. In contrast, the metastatic spread patterns of both tumors were retarded by regimes involving *C. parvum* and aspirin—two agents that differ in their effects on the host. For significance, we must determine if these effects are manifested by other tumors in rats and in other species. From the results recorded here, however, either metastasis involves a complexity of mechanisms, or the agents noted above share some physiological effects on the tumor cells which have not yet been revealed.

ACKNOWLEDGMENTS

This investigation was supported in part by Public Health Service Research Grants No. RR00294 from the Animal Resources Branch, No.

CA17559 from the National Cancer Institute, and The Elsa U. Pardee Foundation.

REFERENCES

1. Pollard, M. (1973): Spontaneous prostate adenocarcinomas in aged germfree Wistar rats. *J. Natl. Cancer Inst.*, 51:1235–1241.
2. Pollard, M., and Luckert, P. (1975): Transplantable metastasizing adenocarcinomas in rats. *J. Natl. Cancer Inst.*, 54:643–649.
3. Chang, C. F., and Pollard, M. (1977): In vitro propagation of prostate adenocarcinoma cells from rats. *Invest. Urol.*, 14:331–334.
4. Kellogg, T. F., and Wostmann, B. S. (1969): Stock diet for colony production of germfree rats and mice. *Lab. Anim. Care*, 19:812–814.
5. Pollard, M. (1971): The germfree rat. *Pathobiol. Annu.*, 1:83–94.
6. Fisher, B., and Fisher, E. R. (1968): Studies of metastatic mechanisms employing labeled tumor cells. In: *The Proliferation and Spread of Neoplastic Cells*, pp. 555–582. Williams & Wilkins Co., Baltimore.
7. Wood, S., Jr., and Strauli, P. (1973): Tumor invasion and metastasis. In: *Cancer Medicine*, edited by J. F. Holland and E. Frei, III, pp. 140–151. Lea & Febiger, Philadelphia.
8. Hoover, H. C., Jr., and Ketcham, A. S. (1975): Techniques for inhibiting tumor metastases. *Cancer*, 35:5–14.
9. Pollard, M., and Luckert, P. H. (1976): Chemotherapy of metastatic prostate adenocarcinomas in germfree rats. *Cancer Treatment Rep.*, 60:619–621.
10. Halpern, B. N., Prevot, A. R., Biozzi, G., Stiffel, C., Mouton, D., Morard, J. C., Bouthillier, Y., and Decreusefond, C. (1964): Stimulation of the phagocytic activity of the reticuloendothelial system provoked by *Corynebacterium parvum*. *J. Reticuloendothel. Soc.*, 1:77–96.
11. Gasic, G. J., Gasic, T. B., Galanti, N., Johnson, T., and Murphy, S. (1973): Platelet-tumor-cell interactions in mice. The role of platelets in the spread of malignant disease. *Int. J. Cancer*, 11:704–718.
12. Vane, J. R. (1971): Inhibition of prostaglandin synthetase. *Nature [New Biol.]*, 231:232.
13. Orrenius, S., Ericsson, J. E., and Ernster, L. (1965): Phenobarbital induced synthesis of the microsomal drug-metabolizing enzyme system and its relationship to the proliferation of endoplasmic membranes. A morphological and biochemical study. *J. Cell Biol.*, 25:627.

Cancer Invasion and Metastasis: Biologic Mechanisms and Therapy, edited by S. B. Day et al. Raven Press, New York © 1977.

An Inhibitory Mechanism of Blood-Borne Metastasis by Sulfated Polysaccharides

Eiro Tsubura, Takashi Yamashita, and Yuhji Higuchi

Third Department of Internal Medicine, School of Medicine, Tokushima University, Tokushima, Japan

The inhibition of cancer metastasis is a major research effort in the control of malignancy. Vascular spread of cancer occurs mainly through the lymphatic or hematogenous route. Hematogenous metastasis consists of four stages: (a) release of tumor cells from the primary site, (b) their migratory transport in blood vessels, (c) their lodgment in capillary beds far from the primary site, and (d) extravascular growth of these cells. The inhibition of lodgment of tumor cells in the capillary is important in preventing blood-borne metastasis. What factors concern tumor cell lodgment? We must consider them from the standpoint of both the tumor cell and host. Much information has been accumulated on the lodgment of tumor cells and on the intravascular events, such as hemodynamics, blood coagulation, fibrinolysis, platelets, and biological characteristics of tumor cells.

We attempted to find reliable antimetastatic agents against blood-borne metastasis in rats. Xylan sulfate, a sulfated polysaccharide, was found to inhibit metastasis markedly. Its effect on the blood coagulation system was studied in relation to its mechanism of action.

INTRAVASCULAR COAGULATION AND TUMOR CELL LODGMENT

Some interest has focused on tumor cell emboli and their attachment to the vascular endothelium. Baserga and Saffiotti (3) suggested that these tumor cell emboli became lodged in the capillary vessels either by adhering to the vascular endothelium or by plugging the lumen of capillaries. Wood (62) demonstrated the intravascular behavior associated with metastasis formation in a rabbit ear chamber by intravital microcinematography. He showed that the most important feature of the intravascular behavior of tumor cells was their selective, firm adhesion to the vascular endothelium of small postcapillary venules; such cells initiated the formation of a blood clot composed predominantly of fibrin, platelets, and leukocytes. Subsequently, the tumor cells moved through the endothelial defects into the perivascular connective tissue within which the cells proliferated, thereby producing a metastasis. Sato (53) observed by microcinematography of the mesenteric arterioles of rats that changes in microcirculatory hemodynamics occurred after intravasation of tumor cells, and that the cells then became attached to the injured endothelium forming an extravascular tumor growth. Using histological and immunofluorescent techniques, Jones et al. (36) reported that tumor cells became lodged singly or in small groups in capillaries and arterioles, surrounded by a meshwork resembling monomeric fibrin. Tanaka et al. (58) and Chew and Wallace (11) observed similar phenomena by electron microscopy; tumor cells accompanied by a platelet mass were seen in arterioles; fibrin occurred very early in small amounts in association with tumor cell emboli, but had largely disappeared while the cells were still intravascular.

On the other hand, malignant cells contain and secrete a thromboplastin-like substance (34,41,46,59). O'Meara (46) called it the "cancer coagulative factor" (CCF). The chemical properties of these substances were reported (7,33,45). Folkman et al. (18,19) reported a different biological substance from tumor cells, the so-called tumor angiogenesis factor (TAF).

SUBSTANCES INHIBITING AND ENHANCING METASTASIS

Anticoagulants and fibrinolytic agents inhibit whereas antiplasmins enhance blood-borne metastasis. Anticoagulants such as heparin (1,4,6,16, 29,40,56,65) and coumarins (2,10,28,47,51), and fibrinolytic agents such as plasmin (13,16,23,30,48,63), urokinase (38), and antifibrinogen(Arvin®) (27,64) reduce metastasis. Conversely, ϵ-aminocaproic acid (EACA) (4, 6,12), *trans*-4-aminomethyl cyclohexyl-1-carboxylic acid (*trans*-AMCHA) (38,48), and aprotinin (Trasylol®) (6) increase metastasis. However, results with these compounds were not consistent under different experimental conditions.

INHIBITION OF PULMONARY METASTASIS BY SULFATED POLYSACCHARIDES IN RATS

The sulfated polysaccharides tested were xylan sulfate (XS), dextran sulfate (DS), chondroitin polysulfate (CPS), chondroitin sulfate (CSN), glucose polysulfate (GPS), sulfated alginic acid (Alg-S), agar sulfate (Aga-S), laminaran sulfate (LS), and mannan sulfate (MS). The molecular weight, sulfur contents, and chemical structures of these compounds are shown in Table 1 and Fig. 1. We screened the antimetastatic effect of these compounds on intravenously induced pulmonary metastasis in rats. The animals used were 8- to 10-week-old female Donryu strain rats, weighing approximately 100 g; tumor used was rat ascites hepatoma AH-109A.

When ^{125}I-labeled AH-109A cells were inoculated into rats via the tail vein, they passed through the lung but remained for a short time. On the

TABLE 1. *Sulfated polysaccharides tested*

Sulfated polysaccharides	Molecular weight	Sulfur content (%)
Xylan sulfate (XS)	$3 \sim 4 \times 10^3$	ca 18.0
Dextran sulfate (DS)	$6 \sim 7 \times 10^3$	" 18.0
Chondroitin polysulfate (CPS)	$6 \sim 7 \times 10^3$	" 15.0
Chondroitin sulfate (CSN)	$30 \sim 40 \times 10^3$	" 6.0
Glucose polysulfate (GPS)	ca 360	" 18.0
Sulfated alginic acid	Undetermined	" 13.4
Agar sulfate (Aga-S)	"	" 10.8
Laminaran sulfate (LS)	"	" 18.0
Mannan sulfate (MS)	"	" 18.0

other hand, the anticoagulative and fibrinolytic activities of sulfated polysaccharides reached a maximum in the plasma 1 hr after intraperitoneal injection. Therefore, these compounds were routinely injected intraperitoneally 1 hr before tumor inoculation (60).

The inhibitory effects of these compounds were examined 2 weeks after tumor inoculation by comparing the number of metastatic nodules on the pulmonary surface of control rats and those injected with these compounds. The results are summarized in Tables 2 and 3. A dose of 100 mg/kg of XS and DS strongly inhibited the development of pulmonary metastases ($p < 0.001$); CPS was less inhibitory, and CSN and GPS were not inhibitory. Sulfated alginic acid, agar sulfate, and mannan sulfate were moderately

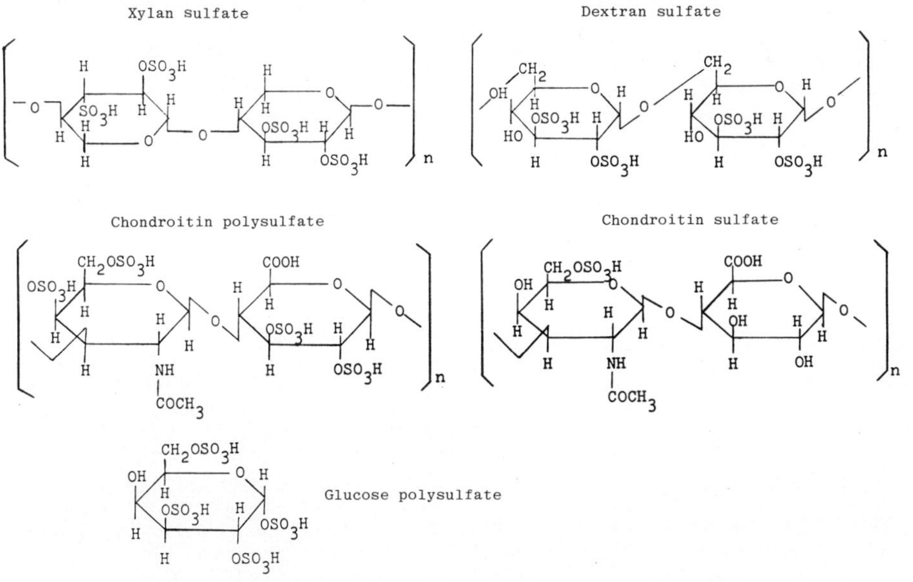

FIG. 1. Chemical structures of sulfated polysaccharides tested.

TABLE 2. *Effect of sulfated polysaccharides on blood-borne pulmonary metastases*

Dose (mg/kg)	Saline (control)	XS	DS	CPS	CSN	GPS
		No. of metastatic nodules on the surface of the lungs				
10	39.0 ± 5.2 (12/12)	16.4 ± 3.6[b] (9/10)	NT	26.4 ± 6.1[c] (12/12)	NT	NT
25	53.2 ± 6.8 (15/15)	10.5 ± 2.4[a] (13/15)	14.1 ± 4.0[a] (11/12)	15.0 ± 3.1[a] (15/15)	NT	NT
50	53.2 ± 6.8 (15/15)	4.3 ± 1.4[a] (13/15)	2.3 ± 1.3[a] (4/11)	9.4 ± 2.3[a] (15/15)	NT	NT
100	62.3 ± 6.3 (10/10)	0.7 ± 0.4[a] (4/10)	1.4 ± 0.6[a] (5/9)	1.9 ± 0.5[a] (8/10)	50.6 ± 6.2[c] (10/10)	65.1 ± 9.0[c] (10/10)

Each rat was inoculated intravenously with 5×10^6 cells of AH-109A. A dose of 10, 25, 50, or 100 mg of sulfated polysaccharides was injected i.p. 1 hr before tumor inoculation. Values are mean ± SE. The incidences of pulmonary metastases are shown in parentheses (number of rats with pulmonary metastases/number of rats tested). Significance of differences of values from that of control by the Student's t-test.
[a] $p < 0.001$.
[b] $p < 0.005$.
[c] Not significant.
NT, not tested.

inhibitory at a dose of 50 mg/kg ($p < 0.001$). Thus, XS caused the strongest inhibition of pulmonary metastasis. The inhibition of pulmonary metastasis by sulfated polysaccharides depends on dose and time of administration (Table 4); these compounds seemed to act at a very early stage of blood-borne pulmonary metastasis.

TABLE 3. *Effect of other sulfated polysaccharides on blood-borne pulmonary metastases*

	Saline (control)	XS	Alg-S	Aga-S	LS	MS High MW	MS Low MW
		No. of metastatic nodules on the surface of the lungs					
Exp. 1	229.5 ± 18.6 (10/10)	36.3 ± 9.0[a] (10/10)	49.8 ± 9.5[a] (10/10)	90.3 ± 12.2[a] (10/10)			
Exp. 2	183.2 ± 8.7 (10/10)				60.7 ± 13.8[a] (10/10)	91.1 ± 8.7[a] (10/10)	67.3 ± 9.6[a] (10/10)

Each rat was inoculated intravenously with 10^7 cells of AH-109A in each experiment. A dose of 50 mg/kg of sulfated polysaccharides was injected i.p. 1 hr before tumor inoculation. Values are mean ± SE. The incidences of pulmonary metastases are shown in parentheses (number of rats with pulmonary metastases/number of rats tested). Significance of differences of values from that of the control by the Student's t-test.
[a] $p < 0.001$.

TABLE 4. *Time dependency of inhibition of pulmonary metastases by sulfated poly-saccharides*

		No. of metastatic nodules on the surface of the lungs			
Treatment schedule		Saline (control)	XS	CPS	CSN
Exp. 1	Four injections of 10 mg/kg, at 6-hr intervals from 7 hr before tumor inoculation	99.0 ± 21.0 (12/12)	4.7 ± 0.9[a] (11/12)	28.0 ± 9.0[b] (12/12)	NT
Exp. 2	Five injections of 50 mg/kg, once daily from day 3–7 after tumor in-oculation	17.3 ± 2.8 (15/15)	17.5 ± 3.4[c] (12/12)	14.9 ± 2.0[c] (13/13)	12.4 ± 2.3[c] (13/13)

Rats were inoculated intravenously with 7×10^6 or 3×10^6 cells of AH-109A in Exp. 1 and 2, respectively. Values are mean ± SE. The incidences of pulmonary metastases are shown in parentheses (number of rats with pulmonary metastases/number of rats tested). Significance of differences of values from that of the control by the Student's *t*-test.

[a] $p < 0.001$.
[b] $p < 0.01$.
[c] Not significant.

RELATIONSHIP BETWEEN ANTIMETASTATIC AND ANTICOAGULATIVE ACTIVITY OF SULFATED POLYSACCHARIDES

The coagulative activity of blood was measured by determining whole-blood clotting time (43), partial thromboplastin time (42), prothrombin time (50), and thrombin time. We examined the anticoagulative activities of three sulfated polysaccharides, XS, CPS, and CSN, which have strong, weak, and no inhibitory effect on metastasis, respectively (Fig. 2). The anticoagulative activity of XS was strongly dose dependent. The anticoagulative activity of CPS was less than that of XS; the former had no detectable effect on prothrombin or thrombin time. These results indicate that the antimetastatic activity of sulfated polysaccharides correlated well with their anticoagulative activity.

We then investigated the effect of these compounds on blood coagulation factors. Coagulation factor activity was determined by the correction required to restore control activity to factor-deficient substrate plasma. The degree of correction was determined by the Quick prothrombin time (50). Control plasma was considered to give 100% correction. As shown in Fig. 3, the surface contact factors, factor XII (Hageman factor) and factor XI (plasma thromboplastin antecedent) in the plasma obtained from rats injected with 100 mg/kg of XS were markedly inactivated. Moderate inactivation of factors II, V, VII, VIII, IX and X were noted in the plasma (Fig. 4).

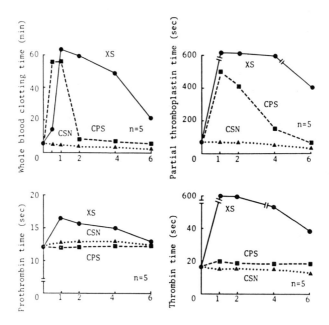

FIG. 2. Change in coagulative activities of blood after i.p. injection of sulfated polysaccharides into rats. Single dose of 100 mg/kg of xylan sulfate (XS), chondroitin polysulfate (CPS), or chondroitin sulfate (CSN) was injected into rats. Each point is expressed as the average of 5 rats.

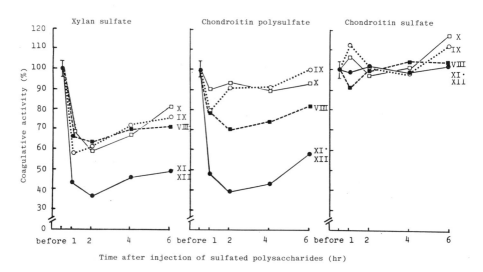

FIG. 3. Change in intrinsic coagulative factors of blood after i.p. injection of sulfated polysaccharides into rats. 100 mg/kg of XS, CPS, or CSN was injected into rats. Each point is expressed as average of 3 rats.

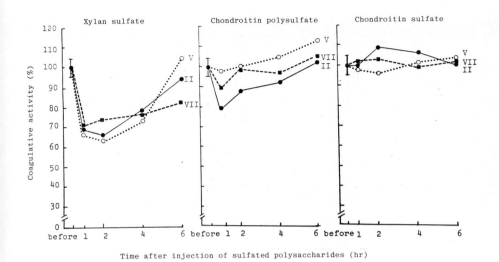

FIG. 4. Change in other coagulative factors of blood after i.p. injection of sulfated poly-saccharides into rats. 100 mg/kg of XS, CPS, or CSN was injected into rats. Each point is expressed as average of 3 rats.

Marked inactivation of factors XI and XII and moderate inactivation of factor VIII were noted in the plasma of rats injected with CPS. CSN did not cause any inactivation of blood coagulation factors. These results indicate that the inactivation of the surface contact factor was also closely related to the inhibitory effects on blood-borne metastasis.

EFFECT OF SULFATED POLYSACCHARIDES ON PLATELETS

Platelets play an important role on the circulation and arrest of tumor cells (61). Gasic et al. (21) reported that thrombocytopenia and altered platelet function decreased metastasis formation. Suzuki and Sato (57) and Gastpar (22) reported that dipyridamole reduced tumor cell stickiness by blocking platelet aggregation. Hilgard and Gordon-Smith (32) found that injection of tumor cells caused thrombocytopenia in animals and that reduction in the number of platelets was proportional to the number of tumor cells injected. Studies of ^{51}Cr-labeled platelets and ^{125}I-labeled fibrinogen suggested that the disappearance of platelets from the circulation was due to thrombus formation around tumor cell emboli in target organ.

We determined platelets in the blood of rats after injecting 100 mg/kg of three sulfated polysaccharides; platelets were counted by the method of Brecher and Cronkite (9). The platelet counts, however, did not change after injection of these compounds (Fig. 5). To examine platelet functions, we measured retention and aggregation in the blood of rats injected with the three compounds by the method of Salzman (52) and Born (8), respectively.

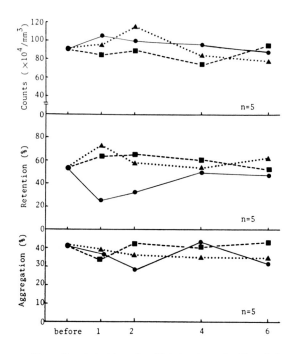

FIG. 5. Change in platelet counts and function on blood after i.p. injection of sulfated polysaccharides into rats. 100 mg/kg of XS, CPS, or CSN was injected into rats. Each point is expressed as average of 5 rats. ●——● XS; ■----■ CPS; ▲....▲ CSN.

There was reduced retention of platelets in blood for 2 hr after injection of XS. No significant change in platelet aggregation was noted in any of the rats. According to Jaques (35), heparin inhibits platelet adhesion to intercellular cement. Silver (55) found small doses of heparin had no effect on platelet adhesiveness, but with larger doses the antiaggregating effects increased in proportion to the dose. Furthermore, Gröttum (24) reported that increasing the concentration of heparin increased their electrophoretic mobility but did not aggregate platelets. Eika (14) found that heparin inhibited thrombin-induced platelet aggregation and release of adenine nucleotides.

EFFECT OF XYLAN SULFATE ON THE DISAPPEARANCE OF TUMOR CELLS FROM THE LUNG

The effect of XS on the disappearance of tumor cells from the lung after intravenous inoculation of tumor cells was examined. AH-109A tumor cells were labeled with ^{125}I-5-iodo-2-deoxyuridine (^{125}IUDR), and the total radioactivity in the lung was estimated after injection 10^7 ^{125}IUDR-labeled

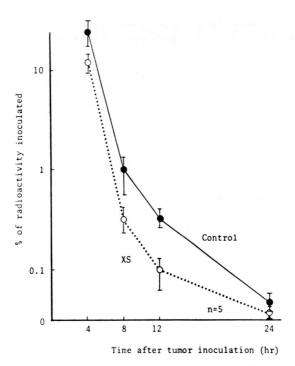

FIG. 6. Effect of xylan sulfate on the disappearance of [125]IUDR-labeled tumor cells inoculated intravenously from the lung of rats. Each rat was inoculated intravenously with 10^7 cells of [125]IUDR-labeled AH-109A. 100 mg/kg of XS was injected i.p. 1 hr before tumor inoculation into rats.

tumor cells intravenously. The radioactivity in the lungs of rats treated with XS decreased faster than that in controls (Fig. 6). XS may increase the rate of disappearance of tumor cells from the lung by impairing attachment to the endothelium of pulmonary capillary vessels. Suemasu and Ishikawa (56) reported similar effects of heparin and dextran sulfate on ^{51}Cr-labeled Sato lung cancer cells. Brown (10) also observed increased clearance of ^{125}I-labeled KHT sarcoma cells from the lung when mice were treated with warfarin. However, Fisher and Fisher (15) could not find any difference between heparin-treated and control animals using ^{51}Cr-labeled Walker 256 carcinosarcoma cells or V_2 carcinoma cells.

EFFECT OF XYLAN SULFATE ON PULMONARY METASTASES AND SURVIVAL OF RATS BEARING DIFFERENT TUMOR STRAINS

Biological characteristics of tumor strains, such as plasticity, deformability, cell surface charge, thromboplastic or fibrinolytic activity, and enzymes play an important role in determining metastasis (37,39).

The effect of xylan sulfate on the pulmonary metastasis 2 weeks after tumor inoculation as well as effect on survival of the rats inoculated with three types of ascites hepatomas (AH-109A, AH-130, and AH-100B) having different biological properties was studied. In particular, AH-109A cells are highly deformable, AH-100B are slightly deformable, and AH-130 are moderately deformable (54).

In order to study the effect of XS on these tumors, we inoculated a number of cells of each intravenously so as to obtain appropriate rate of death in the controls of each strain: 5×10^6 cells of AH-109A, 10^7 of AH-130, and 10^4 of AH-100B were inoculated into the rats. XS was administered intraperitoneally 100 mg/kg 1 hr before tumor inoculation.

The inhibition of pulmonary metastatic nodules by XS was significant and approximately similar in each tumor strain at 2 weeks after the tumor cells were injected (Table 5).

However, survival rates between XS-treated and control groups of rats were quite different, as shown in Fig. 7. With AH-109A, survival rates between the treated and control groups were similar. In AH-130 and AH-100B, marked prolongation of survival was observed in the XS-treated rats.

To explain these diverse results, we note first that XS has no direct cytotoxic action.

We assume at the present time that the major point here may depend on cell deformability. AH-100B is characterized by low deformability but AH-109A is highly deformable. Therefore, AH-100B tumor cells are easily

TABLE 5. *Effect of xylan sulfate on blood-borne pulmonary metastases with different tumor strains*

	No. of metastatic nodules on the surface of the lungs	
Tumor	Saline (control)	Xylan sulfate
AH-109A	62.3 ± 6.3	0.7 ± 0.4^a
AH-130	348.4 ± 36.4	26.5 ± 11.5^a
AH-100B	127.6 ± 15.9	35.8 ± 9.1^a

Each rat was inoculated intravenously with 5×10^6 cells of AH-109A, 10^7 cells of AH-130, or 10^4 cells of AH-100B. A dose of 100 mg/kg of xylan sulfate was injected i.p. 1 hr before tumor inoculation. Pulmonary surface nodules were assayed 14, 16, or 20 days after intravenous inoculation of AH-109A, AH-130, or AH-100B, respectively. Values are mean $\pm$ SE. Significance of differences of values from that of control by the Student's t-test.
$^a p < 0.001$.

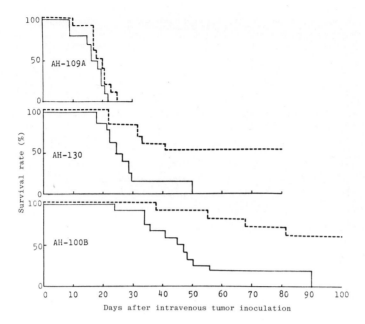

FIG. 7. Effect of xylan sulfate on the survival rates of rats bearing different tumors. Each group consisting of 10, 14, or 12 rats was inoculated with 10^6 cells of AH-109A, 10^7 cells of AH-130, or 10^4 cells of AH-100B, respectively. A dose of 100 mg/kg of xylan sulfate was injected i.p. into rats 1 hr before tumor inoculation. ——— Control; ------ XS treated.

trapped in the capillaries in the lung after intravenous inoculation. The escaped cells from the lung tend to die in postpulmonary circulation. In other words, postpulmonary metastasis is rare in AH-100B. This allows longer survival than in the controls. On the other hand, AH-109A cells, being highly deformable, survive better in the postpulmonary circulation, and thus induce death. But this is our tentative speculation; these points will have to be studied in more detail in the future.

There are other reasons for considering the influence of extrapulmonary metastasis on the survival results. For instance, Fisher and Fisher (17) have pointed out an interrelation between hematogeneous and lymphatic vessels. Anticoagulants such as heparin may act on transmigration of tumor cell in both vessels on some occasions (26,29,31). Indeed, enhancement of extrapulmonary metastasis by heparin has been observed (26,29).

DISCUSSION

The first important step in the establishment of hematogenous metastasis is the firm attachment of transported tumor cells to the endothelium of capillaries. Intravascular coagulation occurs chiefly at this point, and this mechanism was thought responsible for (a) obstruction of blood flow by

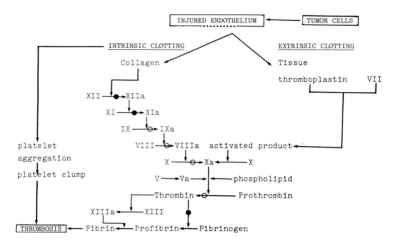

FIG. 8. Inhibiting points of xylan sulfate on blood coagulation mechanism. ●: major inhibition; ○: minor inhibition.

tumor cell emboli, (b) release of the tissue thromboplastin from the injured endothelium, (c) activation of contact factors by tumor cells, and (d) activation of the extrinsic coagulation factors by tumor cells. It is necessary to know the exact intravascular events by which antimetastatic substances such as heparin or other sulfated polysaccharides exert their activity.

Heparin is a well-known, typical anticoagulant as well as antimetastatic agent. It interferes directly with the formation of thrombin and thromboplastin (55a) and also interferes mostly with intrinsic coagulation factors *in vitro* and *in vivo* (20,25,44,49). Sulfated polysaccharides are chemically similar to heparin, and have *o*-sulfate groups and polyanionic properties. But the precise mode of action of anticoagulative and other biological properties of sulfated polysaccharides has not been fully clarified. The anticoagulative mechanism of sulfated polysaccharides became clear in our studies. XS showed the most potent antimetastatic activity among tested sulfated polysaccharides, and the parallelism between the antimetastatic and anticoagulative activity was evident. Our results lead to a tentative conclusion of the inhibitory mechanism of intravascular coagulation by XS and are schematically illustrated in Fig. 8. Major or minor inhibiting sites are pointed out in this figure. At any rate, intrinsic anticoagulability apparently plays a major role on the inhibitory mechanism of blood-borne metastasis by xylan sulfate.

ACKNOWLEDGMENT

This work was supported by a Grant-in-Aid for Scientific Research from the Ministry of Education, Science and Culture of Japan.

REFERENCES

1. Agostino, D., and Cliffton, E. E. (1962): Anticoagulants and the development of pulmonary metastases. *Arch. Surg.,* 84:449–453.
2. Agostino, D., Cliffton, E. E., and Girolami, A. (1966): Effect of prolonged coumadin treatment on the production of pulmonary metastases in the rat. *Cancer,* 19:284–288.
3. Baserga, R., and Saffiotti, U. (1955): Experimental studies on histogenesis of blood-borne metastases. *A. M. A. Arch. Pathol.,* 59:26–34.
4. Boeryd, B. (1965): Action of heparin and plasminogen inhibitor (EACA) on metastatic tumor spread in an isologous system. *Acta Pathol. Microbiol. Scand.,* 65:395–404.
5. Boeryd, B. (1966): Effect of heparin and plasminogen inhibitor (EACA) in brief and prolonged treatment on intravenously injected ascites tumor cells. *Acta Pathol. Microbiol. Scand.,* 68:347–354.
6. Boeryd, B. (1966): Effect of heparin and plasminogen inhibitor (EACA) on intravenously injected ascites tumor cells. *Acta Pathol. Microbiol. Scand.,* 68:547–552.
7. Boggust, W. A., O'Meara, R. A., and Fullerton, W. W. (1968): Diffusible thromboplastins of human cancer and chorion tissue. *Eur. J. Cancer,* 3:467–473.
8. Born, G. V. R. (1962): Aggregation of blood platelets by adenosine diphosphate and its reversal. *Nature,* 194:927–929.
9. Brecher, G., and Cronkite, E. P. (1950): Morphology and enumeration of human blood platelets. *J. Appl. Physiol.,* 3:365–377.
10. Brown, J. M. (1973): A study of the mechanism by which anticoagulation with warfarin inhibits blood-borne metastases. *Cancer Res.,* 33:1217–1224.
11. Chew, E. C., and Wallace, A. C. (1976): Demonstration of fibrin in early stages of experimental metastases. *Cancer Res.,* 36:1904–1909.
12. Cliffton, E. E., and Agostino, D. (1964): Effect of inhibitors of fibrinolytic enzymes on development of pulmonary metastases. *J. Natl. Cancer Inst.,* 33:753–763.
13. Cliffton, E. E., and Grossi, C. E. (1956): Effect of human plasmin on the toxic effects and growth of blood-borne metastasis of the Brown-Pearce carcinoma and the V_2 carcinoma rabbit. *Cancer,* 9:1147–1152.
14. Eika, C. (1971): Inhibition of thrombin induced aggregation of human platelets by heparin. *Scand. J. Haematol.,* 8:216–222.
15. Fisher, B., and Fisher, E. R. (1961): Anticoagulants and tumor cell lodgement. *Cancer Res.,* 27:421–425.
16. Fisher, B., and Fisher, E. R. (1961): Experimental studies of factors which influence hepatic metastases. VIII. Effect of anticoagulants. *Surgery,* 50:240–247.
17. Fisher, B., and Fisher, E. R. (1966): The interrelationship of hematogenous and lymphatic tumor cell dissemination. *Surg. Gynecol. Obstet.,* 122:791–798.
18. Folkman, J. (1972): Anti-angionesis. New concept for therapy of solid tumors. *Ann. Surg.,* 175:409–416.
19. Folkman, J., Merler, E., Abernathy, C., and Williams. G. (1971): Isolation of a tumor factor responsible for angiogenesis. *J. Exp. Med.,* 133:275–288.
20. Fremont, R. E. (1964): Pharmacodynamics of parenteral and oral anticoagulants. *Angiology,* 15:152–162.
21. Gasic, G. J., Gasic, T. B., Galanti, N., Johnson, T., and Murphy, S. (1973): Platelet-tumor-cell interactions in mice. The role of platelets in the spread of malignant disease. *Int. J. Cancer,* 11:704–718.
22. Gastpar, H. (1974): Inhibition of cancer cell stickiness by the blocking of platelet aggregation. *S. Afr. Med. J.,* 48:621–627.
23. Grossi, C. E., Agostino, D., and Cliffton, E. E. (1960): The effect of human fibrinolysin on pulmonary metastases of Walker 256 carcinosarcoma. *Cancer Res.,* 20:605–608.
24. Gröttum, K. A. (1969): Platelet surface charge and aggregation. Effects of polyelectrolytes. *Thromb. Diath. Haemorrh.,* 21:450–462.
25. Haas-Weston, C. F. (1971): Anticoagulants and their site of action. *Southwest Med.,* 52:119–126.
26. Hagmar, B. (1970): Experimental tumor metastases and blood coagulability. *Acta Pathol. Microbiol. Scand.* [*Suppl.*], 211:5.

27. Hagmar, B. (1972): Defibrination and metastasis formation: Effects of Arvin on experimental metastases in mice. *Eur. J. Cancer,* 8:17–28.
28. Hagmar, B., and Boeryd, B. (1969): Distribution of intravenously induced metastases in heparin and coumarin-treated mice. *Pathol. Eur.,* 4:103–111.
29. Hagmar, B., and Boeryd, B. (1969): Disseminating effect of heparin on experimental tumor metastases. *Pathol. Eur.,* 4:274–282.
30. Hiemeyer, V., and Merkle, P. (1968): Über den Einfluss von Plasmin auf die Metastasierung von Impfttumoren der Ratte. *Z. Krebsforsch.,* 70:325–330.
31. Hilgard, P., Beyerle, L., Hohage, R., Hiemeyer, V., and Kübler, M. (1972): The effect of heparin on the initial phase of metastasis formation. *Eur. J. Cancer,* 8:347–352.
32. Hilgard, P., and Gordon-Smith, E. C. (1974): Microangiopathic hemolytic anemia and experimental tumor-cell emboli. *Br. J. Haematol.,* 26:651–659.
33. Holyoke, E. D., and Ichihashi, H. (1966): The C3H/St/Ha mammary tumor. 1. Thromboplastin content. *J. Natl. Cancer Inst.,* 36:1049–1056.
34. Holyoke, E. D., Frank, A. L., and Weiss, L. (1972): Tumor thromboplastin activity in vitro. *Int. J. Cancer,* 9:258–263.
35. Jaques, L. B. (1963): The chemistry, pharmacology and assay of heparin. *Thromb. Diath. Haemorrh.* [*Suppl.*], 11:27–36.
36. Jones, D. S., Wallace, A. C., and Fraser, E. E. (1971): Sequence of events in experimental metastases of Walker 256 tumor: light, immunofluorescent, and electron microscopic observations. *J. Natl. Cancer Inst.,* 46:493–504.
37. Khato, J., Suzuki, M., and Sato, H. (1974): Quantitative study on thromboplastin in various strains of Yoshida asictes hepatoma cells of rat. *Gann,* 65:289–294.
38. Kodama, Y. (1974): Experimental studies on significance of coagulation-fibrinolysis system in growth and metastasis formation of rabbit V_2 and V_7 carcinomas. *Fukuoka Med. J.,* 65:941–966.
39. Kodama, Y., Kohga, S., and Tanaka, K. (1972): Coagulative and fibrinolytic activities of ascites tumor cells of rat. *Igaku-no-Ayumi,* 83:530–531.
40. Koike, A. (1964): Mechanism of blood-borne metastases. 1. Some factors affecting lodgement and growth of tumor cells in the lungs. *Cancer,* 17:450–460.
41. Laki, K., Tyler, H. M., and Yancey, S. T. (1966): Clot forming and clot stabilizing enzymes from the mouse tumor YPC-1. *Biochem. Biophys. Res. Commun.,* 24:776–781.
42. Langdell, R. D., Wagner, R. H., and Brinkhous, K. M. (1953): Effect of antihemophilic factor on one stage clotting tests. *J. Lab. Clin. Med.,* 41:637–647.
43. Lee, R. I., and White, P. D. (1913): A clinical study of the coagulation time of blood. *Am. J. Med. Sci.,* 145:495–503.
44. Niewiarowski, S., and Wegrzynwicz, Z. (1960): Studies on the mechanism of the anticoagulant action of heparin. *Symposium on Thrombosis and Anticoagulant Therapy.* Dundee.
45. Ogura, T., Tatsuta, M., Tsubura, E., and Yamamura, Y. (1967): Localization of fibrinogen in the tumor tissue. *Gann,* 58:403–413.
46. O'Meara, R. A. Q. (1958): Coagulative properties of cancer. *Ir. J. Med. Sci.,* 394:474–479.
47. Orme, S. K., and Ketcham, A. S. (1967): Effect of prolonged anticoagulation on spontaneous metastases. *Surg. Forum,* 18:84–85.
48. Peterson, H. I. (1968): Experimental studies on fibrinolysis in growth and spread of tumor. *Acta Chir. Scand.* [*Suppl.*], 394:42.
49. Pitlick, F. A., Lundblad, R. L., and Davie, E. W. (1969): The role of heparin in intrinsic blood coagulation. *J. Biomed. Mater. Res.,* 3:95–106.
50. Quick, A. J., Stanly, B. M., and Bancroft, F. W. (1935): A study of the coagulation defect in hemophilia and in jaundice. *Am. J. Med. Sci.,* 190:501–511.
51. Ryan, J., Ketcham, A. S., and Wexler, H. (1968): Warfarin treatment of mice bearing autochthonous tumors: Effect on spontaneous metastases. *Science,* 162:1493–1494.
52. Salzman, E. W. (1960): Measurement of platelet adhesiveness: a simple in vitro technique demonstrating an abnormality in von Willebrand's disease. *J. Lab. Clin. Med.,* 62:724–735.
53. Sato, H. (1967): Cancer metastasis, from pathological studies on ascites tumors. *Trans. Soc. Pathol. Jpn.,* 56:9–36.
54. Sato, H., and Suzuki, M. (1976): Deformability and viability of tumor cells by transcapillary passage, with reference to organ affinity of metastasis in cancer. In: *Fundamental Aspects of Metastasis,* edited by L. Weiss, pp. 311–317. North-Holland, Amsterdam.

55. Silver, M. J. (1970): Platelet aggregation and plug formation: Studies on mechanism of action. *Am. J. Physiol.,* 218:389–395.
55a. Soulier, J. P. (1963): Action of heparin in the blood coagulation system. *Thromb. Diath. Haemorrh.* [*Suppl.*], 9:37–44.
56. Suemasu, K., and Ishikawa, S. (1970): Inhibitive effect of heparin and dextran sulfate on experimental pulmonary metastasis. *Gann,* 61:125–130.
57. Suzuki, M., and Sato, H. (1972): Mechanism in intravascular attachment of cancer cell: Lodgement on blood-borne metastasis. *Blood Vessels,* 3:501–509.
58. Tanaka, K., Kodama, Y., and Kohga, S. (1972): Cancer and blood coagulation, fibrinolysis. *Blood Vessels,* 3:1025–1040.
59. Thornes, R. D. (1974): Oral anticoagulant therapy of human cancer. *J. Med.* (*Basel*), 5:83–91.
60. Tsubura, E., Yamashita, T., Kobayashi, M., and Higuchi, Y. (1976): Effect of sulfated polysaccharides on blood-borne pulmonary metastasis in rats. *Gann,* 67:849–856.
61. Warren, B. A. (1970): The ultrastructure of platelet pseudopodia and adhesion of homologous platelets to tumor cells. *Br. J. Exp. Pathol.,* 51:570–580.
62. Wood, S., Jr. (1958): Pathogenesis of metastasis formation observed in vivo in the rabbit ear chamber. *Arch. Pathol.,* 66:550–568.
63. Wood, S., Jr. (1964): Experimental studies of the intravascular dissemination of ascitic V₂ carcinoma cells in the rabbit, with special reference to fibrinogen and fibrinolytic agents. *Bull. Schweiz. Akad. Med. Wiss.,* 20:92–121.
64. Wood, S., Jr., and Hilgard, P. (1973): ARVIN-induced hypofibrinogenemia and metastasis formation from blood-borne cancer cells. *Johns Hopkins Med. J.,* 133:207–213.
65. Wood, S., Jr., Holyoke, E. D., and Yardley, J. H. (1961): Mechanisms of metastasis production by blood-borne cancer cells. *Can. Cancer Conf.,* 4:167–223.

Cancer Invasion and Metastasis: Biologic
Mechanisms and Therapy, edited by S. B. Day
et al. Raven Press, New York © 1977.

Hereditary Adenomatosis of the Colon and Rectum: A Model of Tumor Progression

L. Kopelovich

Cornell University Graduate School of Medical Sciences, Memorial Sloan-Kettering Cancer Center, New York, New York 10021

Heritable forms of neoplasia in man provide a model for analysis of the differential genetic susceptibility to cancer, the specific biochemical events leading to the acquisition of oncogenic potential *in vivo,* and the physiologic manisfestations of tumor progression (10,12,13,18–22,24,29).

Several cellular parameters associated with the growth pattern of normal and transformed cells in culture have been resolved. The ability of mammalian cells to grow in culture is dependent on the presence of serum and nutrients and is affected by cell density and anchorage to solid substratum (7,14–16,31,39). Normal cells become quiescent in either the G1 or G0 phase of the cell cycle at a density proportionate to the concentration of serum and nutrients present in the growth medium (5,16). In contrast, transformed cells do not become quiescent under usual monolayer conditions; they require lower amounts of serum factors for growth and are anchorage independent (7,8,14–16,28,31,33,40,41,44–46). The acquisition of oncogenic potential *in vivo* was best correlated with loss of anchorage (11,42). Two additional biochemical correlates of *in vivo* malignancy are increased production of plasminogen activator and deformed actin matrices (34–37).

This chapter summarizes experiments on the growth characteristics of human skin fibroblasts (SF) obtained from individuals with hereditary adenomatosis of the colon and rectum (ACR). It concerns serum requirement, contact inhibition, levels of plasminogen activator, intracellular distribution of actin matrices, and differential genetic susceptibility to transformation by an RNA oncogenic virus. The acquisition by the virally transformed cells of growth in the absence of anchorage and ability to form tumors in athymic mice is reviewed. These may possibly be related to the presence of early and previously undetected biochemical lesions in SF from ACR genotypes.

METHODS

Parts of these studies, including all methods used here, have been published elsewhere (11,23,29,30,33,48).

RESULTS

Serum Requirements and Growth Pattern of Human SF

The serum requirement and growth pattern of primary SF cultures derived from ACR phenotypes were examined. SF from ACR subjects and a portion of their clinically asymptomatic progeny (first filial generation, abbreviated as F_1), but not from individuals with nonhereditary colon carcinomas or normals, grew in 1% fetal calf serum (FCS) (Table 1) and showed lack of contact inhibition (Fig. 1). The final saturation density of these cells in 15% FCS was about 95% higher than that of normal SF. Cell cultures from ACR individuals exhibited extensive regions of crisscrossed arrays and multilayered pattern, whereas normal cell cultures grew in well-organized monolayers resembling the highly structured whorls of a fingerprint (Fig. 1).

SF from several children of ACR individuals did not grow in 1% FCS (Table 1). This bimodal response of the clinically asymptomatic F_1 ACR progeny (Table 1) reflects the expected distribution of an inherited trait in a human population in which involvement of an autosomal dominant gene and possibly modifier genes have been implicated (2,25,26).

Plasminogen Activator and Intracellular Actin Matrices in Human SF

The levels of plasminogen activator and intracellular organization of actin matrices in primary SF cultures representing ACR phenotypes and controls were determined. The activity level of plasminogen activator in Triton X-100-treated whole cells from ACR individuals and a number of

TABLE 1. *Serum requirements of SF from ACR individuals*

Group	No. of subjects	1% FCS		15% FCS	
		Mean	p	Mean	p
I. Symptomatic ACR	13	2.68 ± 0.28	<0.001	6.57 ± 1.53	ns
II. Asymptomatic progeny					
a. Low serum positive	10	2.28 ± 0.13	<0.001	4.78 ± 0.84	ns
b. Low serum negative	4	0.95 ± 0.05	ns	4.64 ± 1.56	ns
III. Normals					
a. Spouses	5	0.96 ± 0.03	–	6.30 ± 1.54	–
b. Healthy volunteers	5	0.96 ± 0.02	–	3.73 ± 0.87	–
IV. Nonhereditary colon carcinoma	4	0.92 ± 0.06	ns	3.51 ± 0.27	ns
V. Normals (ATCC)	13	0.95 ± 0.02	–	2.98 ± 0.13	–

Results are taken from ref. 30. ± denotes SEM. The p values represent group analyses and express the probability of obtaining a difference with respect to the average value of groups III and V. ns, Not significant.

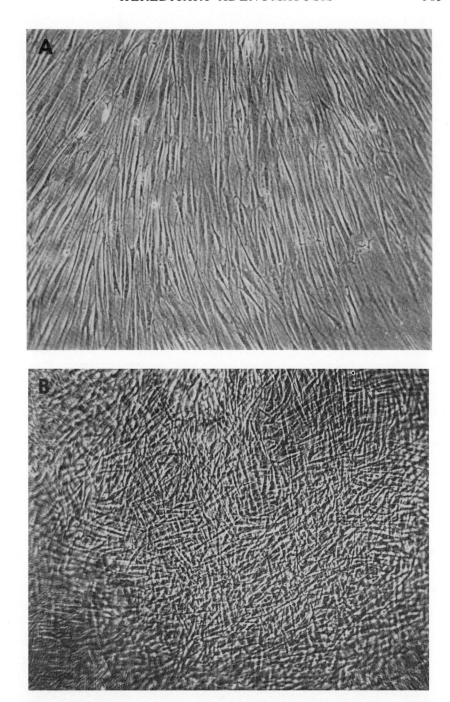

FIG. 1. Morphologic demonstration of confluent human SF. **(A):** Normal subject. **(B):** ACR subject (30).

TABLE 2. *Levels of plasminogen activator in SF from ACR individuals*

Group	No. of experiments	Plasminogen activator (%)[a]	p
I. Symptomatic ACR	15	46.7 ± 6.5	<0.001
II. Asymptomatic progeny			
a. Low serum positive; virus susceptible	2	38.8 ± 11.2	<0.001
b. Low serum negative; virus resistant		ND	
III. Normals	10	7.3 ± 2.3	—

[a] Activity is expressed as percent of control containing plasminogen plus trypsin.

± denotes SEM. The *p* values represent group analyses and express the probability of obtaining a difference with respect to the average value of group III. ND, not done due to lack of experimental material.

the F_1 ACR progeny was significantly higher than that found in normal SF (Table 2). It is of interest that SF cultures from ACR phenotypes showed a decreased expression of actin-containing sheaths as determined by immunofluorescence (Fig. 2; 21). Thus, SF from ACR phenotypes appear to have lost about two-thirds of their actin matrices as compared with control SF (Table 3; 21). This result is presumably due to a redistribution, rather than to a lower amount of actin in cells derived from ACR phenotypes (34). A comparison of the levels of plasminogen activator and intracellular actin matrices in individuals representing all genotypes within the F_1 ACR progeny was not possible due to lack of experimental material. Those used were the low serum-positive and virus-susceptible SF (Tables 1 and 4; 29,30).

Differential Susceptibility of Human SF to Transformation by an RNA Oncogenic Virus

Virally induced cell transformation has been used to study variations in susceptibility of human cell lines with genetic abnormalities or neoplasia

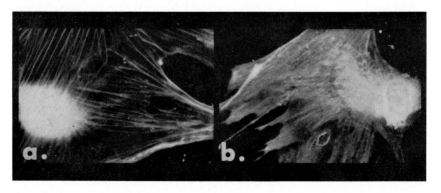

FIG. 2. Visualization of intracellular actin sheaths by specific immunofluorescence staining of human SF. **(a):** Normal individual. **(b):** ACR subject (21).

TABLE 3. *Distribution of actin cables in SF from ACR individuals*

Group	No. of experiments	Presence of actin cables (%)[a]	p
I. Symptomatic ACR	46	31.6 ± 2.99	<0.001
II. Asymptomatic progeny			
a. Low serum positive; virus susceptible	17	31.2 ± 3.7	<0.001
b. Low serum negative; virus resistant	3	74.7 ± 4.3	ns
III. Normals	27	77.8 ± 2.96	—

[a] Results are expressed as percent of total cells counted (21).

± denotes SEM. The p values represent group analyses and express the probability of obtaining a difference with respect to the average value of group III.

(1,17,47). In the present chapter the differential genetic susceptibility of the various human SF cultures to transformation by Kirsten murine sarcoma virus (KiMSV) was determined. Transformed foci were observed in 34 of the 36 cultures tested, albeit to varying degrees (Table 4). The most resistant cultures [log 10 focus-forming units per milliliter (FFU/ml) <1.0] were derived from normal volunteers chosen at random, normal cultures obtained from the American Type Culture Collection (ATCC), and a portion of the clinically asymptomatic F_1 ACR progeny. In contrast, cultures susceptible to transformation by KiMSV (log 10 FFU/ml > 2.0) included all ACR individuals and a number of their asymptomatic F_1 ACR progeny (Table 4). Thus, SF cultures taken from ACR phenotypes and a fraction of the clinically asymptomatic F_1 ACR progeny were 100 to 1,000-fold more susceptible to transformation than were all other human cell cultures tested. The morphological alterations of the transformed foci were characterized by refractile spindle-shaped and round cells which grew on top of the monolayers, exhibiting large cytoplasmic vacuoles (Fig. 3).

It is of considerable interest that SF cultures from several clinically asymptomatic ACR progeny were resistant to transformation (Table 4; 29),

TABLE 4. *Transformation of human SF from ACR individuals by Kirsten murine sarcoma virus*

Group	No. of subjects	Mean log titer (FFU/ml)	p
I. Symptomatic ACR	11	3.00 ± 0.09	<0.001
II. Asymptomatic progeny			
a. High susceptibility	6	2.96 ± 0.09	<0.001
b. Low susceptibility	3	0.46 ± 0.09	ns
III. Normals			
a. Spouses	5	0.61 ± 0.05	—
b. Volunteers	5	0.55 ± 0.07	—
c. ATCC	6	0.51 ± 0.13	—

Human SF cultures were infected with virus as described in ref. 29. ± denotes SEM. The p values represent group analyses and express the probability of obtaining a difference with respect to the average value of group III.

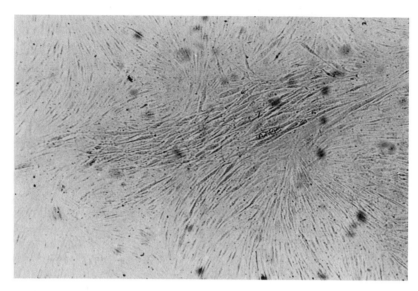

FIG. 3. Morphologic demonstration of human SF transformed by KiMSV (29).

since we have previously shown a similar dichotomy within individuals of asymptomatic F_1 ACR progeny with regard to growth properties (Table 1; Fig. 1; 30). Specifically, SF from asymptomatic progeny of ACR individuals were classified as (a) those which were not contact inhibited and grew in low serum, and (b) those which were contact inhibited and did not grow in low serum. SF from individuals in the first category were susceptible to viral transformation, whereas SF from the second category were resistant to transformation by KiMSV (Table 4; 29).

Growth of Virus-Transformed Human SF in Methylcellulose (Methocel ®) Suspension and Ability to Form Tumors in Athymic Mice

Alterations in cellular growth properties following viral transformation were determined. Several susceptible SF cultures infected with KiMSV (log 10 FFU > 2.0) have been plated in a semisolid medium (38,42). The cells formed spherical colonies at an efficiency greater than 2% of the initial cell number plated. Cell cultures from normal subjects which did transform also grew in methylcellulose, but at a lower efficiency. The latter result may possibly be due to the lower number of foci present in these cultures. Mock-infected cultures derived from ACR individuals, their progeny, and normals showed a plating efficiency of less than 0.001%.

KiMSV-transformed cultures capable of growth in methylcellulose were injected into congenitally athymic BALB/c, *nu/nu* mice. These virally transformed cultures induced the formation of palpable tumor masses at the site of injection within 8 to 10 weeks. Cultures of mock-infected SF were non-tumorigenic in athymic mice. The results indicate that selection for anchorage-independent cells effected the simultaneous selection of tumorigenic cells within the virally transformed human SF.

DISCUSSION

This chapter shows that phenotypic expressions that have previously been attributed to chemical or viral transformation of mammalian cells *in vitro* occur in cultured SF genetically predisposed to cancer, presumably a result of a germinal mutation (22,29,30). This mutation effected the expression of several growth abnormalities within normal-appearing SF obtained from ACR genotypes. These consisted of loss of contact inhibition, low serum requirement, elevated levels of plasminogen activator, redistribution of actin matrices, and increased susceptibility to transformation by an RNA oncogenic virus, but not loss of anchorage or ability to form tumors in athymic mice. Anchorage independence was not present in ACR cells prior to transformation by KiMSV, indicating that loss of anchorage in these cells is a consequence but not a cause of transformation by an oncogenic agent.

The results suggest that transformation of ACR cells by KiMSV had presumably been facilitated to a large degree by a germinal mutation. Whether induction of abnormal growth properties and susceptibility to viral transformation occur concurrently, and whether susceptibility to an RNA oncogenic virus may effect neoplastic transformation of ACR cells *in situ* and/or represent a generally increased sensitivity to other carcinogens is, at present, a matter of conjecture. In this respect, growth abnormalities associated with increased propensity for malignant transformation have been recently reported for cultured fibroblasts derived from individuals with bronchial carcinomata and osteogenic sarcoma (3,4,43).

Evidence from revertants of transformation and correlative studies indicates that malignancy may occur in the absence of one or more phenotypic expressions generally found in cells undergoing malignant transformation (38; Proceedings of the 1st International Congress of Cell Biology, Boston, 1976). However, the appearance of these growth abnormalities in ACR cells supports the notion that oncogenesis *in vivo* might indeed be an all-inclusive temporal multistage process. The ability of transformed cells, in some instances, to form tumors in the absence of certain abnormal expressions may point to a complex interaction of epigenetic mechanisms during the post-mutational period. Isolation of revertants among cultured ACR cells that had not been transformed by KiMSV would be of considerable importance.

Table 5 delineates our perception of events in the malignant transformation of ACR cells. The preneoplastic phase could be defined as those steps preceding the ability of cells to grow in the absence of anchorage, whereas

TABLE 5. *Possible relationship of phenotypic expressions in human SF derived from ACR individuals to metastasis*

Stages in metastasis	Phenotypic expressions in SF						
	Growth in low serum →	Loss of contact inhibition →	Elevated levels of plasminogen activator →	Deformed actin cables →	Susceptibility to viral transformation →	Anchorage independence →	Ability to form tumors
	Preneoplastic transformation				Neoplastic transformation		
Transformation at site A	+	+	+	+			
Angiogenesis at site A	ACR phenotypes may provide an abundant source of angiogenic factor?				+	+	+
Detachment from site A	+	+	+	+			
Penetration[a]			+	+			
Travel[a]			?				
Thrombosis[a]			?				
Trapping[a]			?				
Penetration into site B		+	+				
Growth at site B	+				+		
Angiogenesis at site B	ACR phenotypes may provide an abundant source of angiogenic factor?				+		+

Horizontal arrows suggest a possible sequence of events in ACR genotypes during cell transformation *in situ*. Vertical arrow indicates the transforming event. In our system the transforming agent was Kirsten murine sarcoma virus.

[a] Events taking place in the hemopoietic and lymphatic systems.

the malignant phase also included the ability of cells to grow without anchorage and form tumors *in vivo*. The possibility exists, however, that cell transformation in other model systems does not conform to a two-hit mutation indicated for ACR cell transformation.

The heritable nature of ACR suggests that individuals carrying this trait might be susceptible to tumors at more than one organ site. Indeed, ACR is regarded as a disease in which colonic and extracolonic malignancies occur (2,12,26,27). Although multiple primaries would appear to account for the production of tumors at several organs of an ACR genotype (2,12,26), metastasis may well be a significant contributor. Further, the role of host cells other than those which form a tumor should be considered. For example, defective vascular endothelial and lymphatic systems, and biochemically altered cells passing through them, may enhance metastasis to a considerable extent.

Based on our results, Table 5 provides a partial account of the possible interrelationships between the phenotypic abnormalities found in ACR cells and certain steps involved in metastasis. Thus, malignant transformation in and detachment of tumor cells from tissue A could be explained by those expressions associated with cells undergoing neoplastic transformation (Table 5). Similarly, growth of tumor cells in tissue B as a result of metastasis would appear to depend on these factors. Angiogenesis of tumors may be greatly enhanced by the secretion of large amounts of angiogenic factor (9) from ACR cells, SF, and possibly other host cell types as well. The occurrence of elevated plasminogen activator may in part account for the ability of malignant cells to spread. It can facilitate movement of tumor cells across basal membranes (6,37,48) and unmask cell surface components in a manner analogous to the action of other proteolytic enzymes. The latter mechanism may increase cell recognition and aggregation of self and nonself target cells which participate in the processes of travel, thrombosis, and trapping of malignant cells during metastasis (49). The possible application of *in vitro* culture methods for the analysis of metastasis has been reviewed (32) and is currently under consideration in our laboratory.

The experimental results suggest that growth in low serum, loss of contact inhibition, elevated levels of plasminogen activator, intracellular distribution patterns of actin sheaths, and susceptibility to viral transformation might be used as diagnostic indices for individuals with latent ACR or those who are at high risk of other forms of cancer (19,21,29,30).

CONCLUSION

Hereditary adenomatosis of the colon and rectum indicates a propensity to develop colonic and extracolonic malignancies. At present it is believed that this trait is carried by an autosomal dominant gene, although it seems probable that additional genes may pleiotropically modify its expression. Assuming that phenotypic expressions which appear in primary cell cultures closely reflect biologic abnormalities occurring *in situ*, the study of SF derived from ACR genotypes provided a unique system for analysis of the oncogenic process. It was shown that SF taken from ACR subjects manifest growth abnormalities heretofore seen only in chemically or virally transformed cells. The results further suggest that growth in low serum, loss of contact inhibition, augmented levels of plasminogen activator, and deformed actin matrices are not in themselves sufficient to confer oncogenic potential *in vivo*. Rather, an RNA oncogenic virus was essential for malignant transformation to occur, evidenced by loss of anchorage and ability to form tumors in athymic mice. These growth abnormalities represent steps in the changing phenotypic expression of cells undergoing neoplastic transformation. Although no causal relationship could be clearly established, it is conceivable that cell transformation *in situ* is a temporal multistage process presumably similar to that found in cell cultures transformed *in vitro*. The possible involvement of phenotypic abnormalities occurring in SF and other host cells in metastasis was indicated. Identification of the phenotypic expressions associated with oncogenesis may facilitate their use as diagnostic indices for the detection of latent forms of colon cancer in man.

ACKNOWLEDGMENTS

I wish to thank Mr. J. O'Malley and Miss L. Stern for technical assistance, Mr. L. Pfeffer for his considerable contribution to these studies, and Dr. M. Lipkin for his advice and support. This work was supported by NCI contract NO1 CP 43366 and Grant CA 08748.

REFERENCES

1. Aaronson, S., and Todaro, G. (1975): Transformation and virus growth by murine sarcoma viruses in human cells. *Nature*, 225:458–459.
2. Alm, T., and Licznerski, G. (1973): The intestinal polyposes. In: *Clinics in Gastroenterology*, Vol. 2, edited by R. McConnell, pp. 577–602. Saunders, Philadelphia.
3. Azzarone, B., and Pedulla, D. (1976): Spontaneous transformation of human fibroblast cultures derived from bronchial carcinomata. *Eur. J. Cancer*, 12:557–561.
4. Azzarone, B., Pedulla, D., and Romanzi, C. A. (1976): Spontaneous transformation of human skin fibroblasts derived from neoplastic patients. *Nature*, 262:74–75.
5. Baserga, R. (1968): Biochemistry of the cell cycle: A review. *Cell Tissue Kinet.*, 1:167–191.
6. Beers, W. H., Strickland, S., and Reich, E. (1975): Ovarian plasminogen activator: Relationship to ovulation and hormonal regulation. *Cell*, 6:387–394.
7. Clarke, G., Stoker, M., Ludlow, A., and Thornton, M. (1970): Requirement of serum for DNA synthesis in BHK 21 cells: Effects of density, suspension and virus transformation. *Nature*, 227:798–801.
8. DiPaolo, J., Donovan, P., and Nelson, R. (1969): Quantitative studies of in vitro transformation by chemical carcinogens. *J. Natl. Cancer Inst.*, 42:867–876.

9. Folkman, J. (1975): Tumor angiogenesis: A possible control point in tumor growth. *Ann. Intern. Med.*, 82:96-100.
10. Fraumeni, J., Jr. (1973): Genetic factors. In: *Cancer Medicine*, edited by J. Holland and E. Frei, III, pp. 7-15. Lea & Febiger, Philadelphia.
11. Freedman, V., and Shin, S. (1974): Cellular tumorigenicity in nude mice: Correlation with cell growth in semi-solid medium. *Cell*, 3:355-359.
12. Gardner, E., and Richards, R. (1953): Multiple cutaneous and subcutaneous lesions occuring simultaneously with hereditary polyposis and osteomatosis. *Am. J. Hum. Genet.*, 5:139-148.
13. Hirschhorn, K., and Block-Shtacher, N. (1970): Transformation of genetically abnormal cells. In: *The University of Texas M.D. Anderson Hospital and Tumor Institute at Houston, 23rd Annual Symposium on Fundamental Cancer Research*, pp. 191-202. Williams & Wilkins, Baltimore.
14. Holley, R. (1972): A unifying hypothesis concerning the nature of malignant growth. *Proc. Natl. Acad. Sci. U.S.A.*, 69:2840-2841.
15. Holley, R. (1974): Serum factors and growth control. In: *Control of Proliferation in Animal Cells*, edited by B. Clarkson and R. Baserga, pp. 13-18. Cold Spring Harbor Laboratory, Cold Spring Harbor, New York.
16. Holley, R., and Kiernan, J. (1968): "Contact inhibition" of cell division in 3T3 cells. *Proc. Natl. Acad. Sci. U.S.A.*, 60:300-304.
17. Klement, V., Friedman, M., McAllister, R., Nelson-Rees, W., and Huebner, R. (1971): Differences in susceptibility of human cells to mouse sarcoma virus. *J. Natl. Cancer Inst.*, 47:65-73.
18. Knudson, A., Jr., Strong, L., and Anderson, D. (1973): Heredity and cancer in man. *Prog. Med. Genet.*, 9:113-158.
19. Kopelovich, L. (1977): Phenotypic markers in human skin fibroblasts as possible diagnostic indices of hereditary adenomatosis of the colon. *Cancer (in press).*
20. Kopelovich, L. (1977): Levels of plasminogen activator in skin fibroblasts derived from individuals with hereditary adenomatosis of the colon and rectum. *(Preliminary observations).*
21. Kopelovich, L., Conlon, S., and Pollack, R. (1977): Intracellular organization of actin matrices in cultured skin fibroblasts derived from individuals with hereditary adenomatosis of the colon and rectum. *Proc. Natl. Acad. Sci. U.S.A. (in press).*
22. Kopelovich, L., Pfeffer, L., and Lipkin, M. (1976): Recent studies on the identification of proliferative abnormalities and of oncogenic potential of cutaneous cells in individuals at increased risk of colon cancer. *Semin. Oncol.*, 3:369-372.
23. Lazarides, E., and Weber, K. (1974): Actin antibody: The specific visualization of actin filaments in non-muscle cells. *Proc. Natl. Acad. Sci.*, 71:2268-2272.
24. Lynch, H. T. (1976): *Cancer Genetics.* Charles C Thomas, Springfield, Ill.
25. McConnell, R. (1966): *The Genetics of Gastrointestinal Disorders.* Oxford University Press, London.
26. Morson, B., and Bussey, H. (1970): Predisposing causes on intestinal cancer. In: *Current Problems in Surgery*, pp. 1-50. Year Book Medical Publishers, Chicago.
27. Morson, B., and Dawson, I. (1972): Benign epithelial neoplasma. In: *Gastrointestinal Pathology*, pp. 522-538. Blackwell, Oxford.
28. Paul, D., Henahan, M., and Walter, S. (1974): Changes in growth control and growth requirements associated with neoplastic transformation in vitro. *J. Natl. Cancer Inst.*, 53:1499-1503.
29. Pfeffer, L., and Kopelovich, L. (1977): Differential genetic susceptibility of cultured human skin fibroblasts to transformation by Kirsten murine sarcoma virus. *Cell*, 10:313-320.
30. Pfeffer, L., Lipkin, M., Stutman, O., and Kopelovich, L. (1976): Growth abnormalities of cultured human skin fibroblasts derived from individuals with hereditary adenomatosis of the colon and rectum. *J. Cell Physiol.*, 89:29-38.
31. Pollack, R. (Ed.) (1975): *Readings in Mammalian Cell Culture.* Cold Spring Harbor Laboratory, Cold Spring Harbor, New York.
32. Pollack, R. (1976): A strategy for the in vitro analysis of the metastatic process. *Gann (in press).*
33. Pollack, R., Green, H., and Todaro, G. (1968): Growth control in cultured cells: Selection

of sublines with increased sensitivity to contact inhibition and decreased tumor producing ability. *Proc. Natl. Acad. Sci.*, 60:126–133.

34. Pollack, R., Osborn, M., and Weber, K. (1975): Patterns of organization of actin and myosin in normal and transformed cultured cells. *Proc. Natl. Acad. Sci. U.S.A.*, 72:994–998.

35. Pollack, R., Risser, R., Conlon, S., and Rifkin, D. (1974): Plasminogen activator production accompanies loss of anchorage regulation in transformation of primary rat embryo cells by SV40. *Proc. Natl. Acad. Sci. U.S.A.*, 71:4792–4796.

36. Pollack, R., Risser, R., Conlon, S., Freedman, V., Shin, S., and Rifkin, D. (1975): Production of plasminogen activator and colonial growth in semi-solid medium are in vitro correlates of tumorigenicity in the immune deficient nude mouse. In: *Proteins and Biological Control*, edited by E. Reich, D. Rifkin, and E. Show, pp. 885–900. Cold Spring Harbor Laboratory, Cold Spring Harbor, New York.

37. Rifkin, D. B., Gilula, N. B., Quigley, J. P., Loskutoff, D., Ossowski, L. Unkeless, J. C., Dan, K., and Piperno, A. (1974): Proteases associated with malignant transformation. In: *Mechanisms of Virus Disease*, edited by W. Robinson and C. F. Fox, pp. 315–325. Benjamin, New York.

38. Risser, R., and Pollack, R. (1974): A nonselective analysis of SV40 transformation of mouse 3T3 cells. *Virology*, 59:477–489.

39. Rubin, H. (1970): Growth regulation in cultures of chick embryo fibroblasts. In: *Symposium on Growth Control in Cell Cultures*, edited by G. Wolstenholme and J. Knight, pp. 127–145. Churchill Livingstone, London.

40. Sanford, K. (1974): Biologic manifestation of oncogenesis in vitro: A critique. *J. Natl. Cancer Inst.*, 53:1481–1485.

41. Scher, C., and Todaro, G. (1971): Selective growth of human neoplastic cells in medium lacking serum growth factor. *Exp. Cell Res.*, 68:479–481.

42. Shin, S. I. L., Freedman, V. H., Risser, R., and Pollack, R. (1975): Tumorigenicity of virus-transformed cells in nude mice is correlated specifically with anchorage independent growth in vitro. *Proc. Natl. Acad. Sci. U.S.A.*, 72:4435–4439.

43. Smith, H. S., Owens, R. B., Hiller, A. J., Nelson-Rees, W. A., and Johnston, J. O. (1976): The biology of human cells in tissue culture. I. Characterization of cell derived from osteogenic sarcomas. *Int. J. Cancer*, 17:219–237.

44. Stenners, C., Till, J., and Siminovitch, L. (1963): Studies on the transformation of hamster embryo cells in culture by polyoma virus. *Virology*, 21:448–463.

45. Todaro, G., Green, H., and Goldberg, B. D. (1964): Transformation of properties of an established cell line by SV40 and polyoma virus. *Proc. Natl. Acad. Sci. U.S.A.*, 51:66–73.

46. Todaro, G., Lazar, G., and Green, H. (1965): The initiation of cell division in a contact-inhibited mammalian cell line. *J. Cell. Physiol.*, 66:325–333.

47. Todaro, G., and Martin, G. (1967): Increased susceptibility of Down syndrome fibroblasts to transformation by SV40. *Proc. Soc. Exp. Biol. Med.*, 124:1232–1236.

48. Unkeless, J. C., Tobia, A., Ossowski, L., Quigley, J. P., Rifkin, D. B., and Reich, E. (1972): An enzymatic function associated with transformation of fibroblasts by oncogenic viruses. *J. Exp. Med.*, 137:85–93.

49. Weiss, L. (Ed.) (1976): *Fundamental Aspects of Metastasis*. North Holland, Amsterdam.

Discussion

S. B. Day: Dr. Kopelovich, would you comment on the potential of the model you have described for the elucidation of biologic mechanisms related to cancer invasion and metastasis.

L. Kopelovich: The first point I would like to make is related to our ability to effectively diagnose a primary tumor and metastatic forms of neoplasia. Have our recent efforts indicated progress toward cancer detection? Dr. Bodansky has noted (*this volume*) that biochemical correlates of *in vivo* malignancy presumably measure a state of advanced metastatic growth and the clinical status of the patient. But to date no biochemical parameter has been found which identifies an *incipient* primary, latent forms of neoplasia in particular. Cytology of pap smears, sputum, and lavage has been effectively used in some instances in the detection of carcinoma *in situ*. For example, following the introduction of smear cytology as a tool for early diagnosis of cervical carcinoma, a large number of cases of carcinoma *in situ* were reported. However, organ topology limits the extent to which this approach can be applied.

Our recent work on hereditary forms of cancer suggests that host cells at a site removed from a primary can be tapped directly, possibly even before a tumor appears, for information concerning cancer causation and cancer progression. This information need not be restricted to *bona fide* forms of genetic predisposition to neoplasia. Systemic disorders occurring within stromal cells of high-risk individuals may be considerably more extensive than has been thus far suspected (Kopelovich, *this volume*). I submit that identification of abnormal phenotypic expressions occurring systemically within stromal cells, in conjunction with biochemical correlates and smear cytology, will provide comprehensive diagnostic measures for cancer detection, and possibly effective prophylactic measures as well.

The second point concerns our concept of tumor dormancy. Tumor dormancy has been defined by Wheelock et al. (*this volume*) as "a state in which tumor cells persist in the host without metastasis or outgrowth to overt disease." Hereditary adenomatosis of the colon and rectum is characterized by a period from birth (germinal mutation) through puberty which we now define as premalignant, but during which no clinical manifestations are apparent (*this volume*). I choose to describe this period as tumor latency rather than tumor dormancy and propose to reserve the latter term to mean the clinically quiescent state effected by successful treatment and host regulatory mechanisms (Wheelock et al., *this volume*). The distinction between tumor latency and tumor dormancy is conceptually important to our understanding of prospective measures. I further suggest that the premalignant state is intrinsically linked to cancer. However, whether tumor latency and a state of premalignancy are physiologically synonymous remains to be established.

Cancer Invasion and Metastasis: Biologic Mechanisms and Therapy, edited by S. B. Day et al. Raven Press, New York © 1977.

Enhancement of Artificial Lung Metastases by Cyclophosphamide: Pharmacological and Mechanistic Considerations

Lester J. Peters and Kathryn Mason

Section of Experimental Radiotherapy, The University of Texas System Cancer Center, M.D. Anderson Hospital and Tumor Institute, Houston, Texas 77030

In contrast to the extensive literature concerning the effects of irradiation on the transplantability of experimental tumors, relatively little attention has been directed at cytotoxic chemotherapeutic agents in this regard. In 1975 van Putten et al. (1) published data showing the effect of pretreatment of mice with some 30 different cytotoxic agents on the subsequent development of lung colonies from intravenously injected tumor cells. Although most of the agents they tested promoted lung colony-forming efficiency (CFE) to a greater or lesser extent, cyclophosphamide stood out as being singularly effective, increasing CFE by up to 1,000 times. This uniqueness of cyclophosphamide was emphasized by the relative inefficiency of the closely related drugs isophosphamide and trophosphamide.

In this chapter we report studies of the pharmacodynamics of the cyclophosphamide effect, and we compare and contrast the actions of the drug and irradiation.

MATERIALS AND METHODS

Mice and Tumor

C3Hf/Bu mice were bred in the specific pathogen-free colony maintained at the M.D. Anderson Hospital, Section of Experimental Radiotherapy. Within each experiment mice of the same sex, aged 10 to 12 weeks, were used. Animals were housed five to a cage and were maintained on a sterilized diet with a 12-hr light-dark cycle.

The tumor used in these experiments is a methylcholanthrene-induced fibrosarcoma (FSa) showing moderately strong immunogenicity for its syngeneic hosts (2). Source material for the experiments described in this chapter was derived from injection of fourth generation isotransplants. The method used for preparing single-cell suspensions from this tumor has been described previously (3).

Lung Colony Assay

Single-cell suspensions of FSa in medium 199 supplemented with 5% fetal calf serum were prepared. The required number of viable tumor cells was injected in a volume of 0.25 ml. For the scoring of lung colony formation, we killed mice 14 days after tumor cell injection, after which their lungs were removed and fixed in Bouin's solution, and the number of macroscopic tumor colonies was counted.

Cyclophosphamide

Cyclophosphamide (Cytoxan ®) was obtained commercially in 100-mg vials. After initial reconstitution with sterile distilled water, the solution was further diluted as required with physiological saline to give the required dose in a volume of 0.01 ml/g body weight. Except where *in vitro* premetabolism was undertaken (see below), the drug was administered immediately after dissolution.

In vitro *Metabolism*

The method used was adapted from that of Dolfini et al. (4). The microsomal fraction obtained from the livers of 20 female donor mice was used. The livers were removed under sterile conditions, cooled to 0°C, and homogenized in 4 volumes of cold Dulbecco's PBS (pH 7.4). This homogenate was centrifuged at 9,000 g for 20 min, following which the supernatant containing the microsomal fraction was centrifuged in a Beckman model L5-50 ultracentrifuge at 105,000 g for 1 hr. The microsomal pellet was washed by resuspending in PBS and was recentrifuged at 105,000 g for 1 hr. The final microsomal fraction was resuspended in 5 ml PBS from which two 2-ml aliquots were taken. To one aliquot were added the cofactors required for an NADPH-generating system: 200 mg glucose-6-phosphate (G-6-P); 10 units G-6-P dehydrogenase; 10 mg NADP and 40 mg $MgCl_2 \cdot 6 H_2O$ all suspended in 2 ml sterile water; and 20 mg cyclophosphamide in a volume of 2 ml. The other aliquot of microsomes was made up to 6 ml with saline. These two preparations plus a control solution of 20 mg cyclophosphamide in 6 ml were agitated at 37°C for 18 hr prior to injection into mice of 0.02 ml/g of each (s.c.) corresponding to 67 μg/g cyclophosphamide.

Irradiations

Mice received whole-body irradiation (WBI) in a ^{137}Cs γ-irradiator at a dose rate of 260 rads/min calculated at the midplane of each mouse. Dose variation across the thickness of the mouse amounted to $\pm 10\%$.

Local thoracic irradiation (LTI) was administered to anesthetized mice using a double-headed ^{137}Cs unit delivering 1,060 rads/min through a 3-cm diameter circular portal (5). Dose variability with this set-up was $\pm 3\%$.

Radiolabeling of Tumor Cells

Short-term cell cultures were established from tumors growing *in vivo* by plating 2.5×10^7 FSa cells into 32-oz glass flasks containing 50 ml of Hsu's medium plus 20% fetal calf serum. After 24 hr in culture, the medium was replaced with fresh medium containing ^{125}IUdR at a concentration of 0.4 μCi/ml. After a further 24 hr in culture the medium was poured off, and after rinsing of the flasks with solution A the cells were trypsinized and then washed repeatedly in fresh medium until the activity of the supernatant was less than 0.2% of that of the cell suspension. Counts of viable cells were then made on phase-contrast appearance. Autoradiography showed the labeling index of tumor cells to be >90%. No evidence of radiotoxicity was observed with this technique as measured by the cloning efficiency of cultured labeled cells.

Measurement of Lung Radioactivity

At the appropriate times after injection of the radioactive cell suspension, groups of three to six mice were killed. Their lungs were removed, washed in water, and placed in plastic tubes for counting in a Nuclear Chicago Automatic Gamma Sample Counter. Concurrently, samples of the cellular inoculum and of the supernatant fluid from the inoculum were counted also. The net residual cellular activity in the lungs was calculated as

$$\frac{\text{cpm (lungs)} - \text{background}}{\text{cpm (inoculum)} - \text{cpm (supernatant)}}.$$

RESULTS

Dose-Response Relationship

In Fig. 1 we have plotted the lung colony-forming efficiency of 10^4 intravenously injected FSa tumor cells as a function of cyclophosphamide (Cy) dose over a range of 10 to 300 μg/g. The drug was given as a single dose subcutaneously 2 days prior to tumor cell injection. The CFE of FSa cells increased progressively with dose of Cy, showing a peak enhancement factor of 18 at 300 μg/g. This is the maximum dose permitting survival of mice for the 14-day duration of the lung colony assay (Table 1), and is in fact above the $LD_{50/30}$ for hemopoietic death.

Also in Fig. 1 are plotted data from van Putten et al. (1). The slope of the dose response they obtained for a C3H mammary carcinoma is very similar

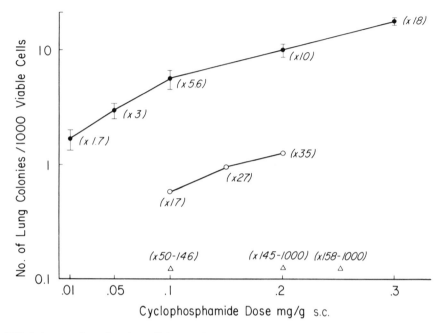

FIG. 1. Lung colony-forming efficiency (CFE) as a function of dose of cyclophosphamide given s.c. 2 days before tumor cell injection. Numbers in parentheses indicate the enhancement factor relative to the CFE in untreated mice. (●), C_3Hf/Bu fibrosarcoma (FSa) used in the current experiments; (○) and (△), data from van Putten et al. (1) referring to a C_3H mammary carcinoma and the C22LR osteosarcoma, respectively. Absolute values of CFE for the latter tumor were not quoted.

to that observed in our system, although the enhancement factors were somewhat greater. Absolute values of CFE for their osteosarcoma were not given, but the enhancement factors for 100, 200, and 250 $\mu g/g$ Cy are an order of magnitude greater than we observed.

Effect of Timing and Route of Administration

Cy was administered at a dose of 150 $\mu g/g$ either s.c. or i.v. from 7 days before through 1 day after tumor cell injection. It can be seen in Fig. 2 that

TABLE 1. *Cyclophosphamide toxicity*

Single dose ($\mu g/g$)	Proportion dying	Survival (days)
100	0/4	—
200	0/4	—
300	4/4	16, 21, 30, 30
400	4/4	6, 6, 8, 9
500	6/6	<1, <1, 6, 6, 6, 6 (acute pulmonary edema in 2 mice)

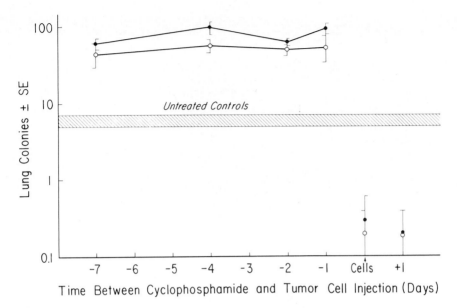

FIG. 2. Effect of timing and route of administration of cyclophosphamide on the number of lung colonies from 10^4 FSa cells injected intravenously. Cy was given as a single dose of 150 μg/g. (●) and (○), s.c. and i.v. administration of Cy, respectively. Pretreatment with Cy by the s.c. route was consistently slightly more efficient in promoting lung CFE. When given 10 min prior to tumor cell injection or 1 day thereafter, Cy dramatically reduced lung colony formation.

the promotion of lung CFE was essentially constant when Cy was given from 7 days to 1 day before tumor cells. The s.c. route gave a consistently higher yield of lung colonies, although the difference was individually significant at only one time point (−4 days). When Cy was administered on the same day as (10 min before) or 1 day after tumor cell injection, its cytotoxic action on the tumor cells far outweighed its conditioning effect on the lung.

Effect of Split Doses of Cy

The effect of two doses of 100 μg/g s.c. separated by 1 to 96 hr was compared with a single dose of 200 μg/g. The single dose, or the second half of each split dose, was given 2 days before tumor cell challenge. The results, plotted in Fig. 3, show a split dose to be less effective: the yield of lung colonies from the single dose was significantly higher than that from 2 doses separated by 3 hr or more. However, not until the dose was split by 96 hr was the effect consistent with that of the second dose of 100 μg/g alone.

Additivity of Effects of Cy and Irradiation

The lung CFE of FSa cells can be promoted by irradiation of the lungs of mice prior to tumor cell injection (5). Irradiation may be localized to the

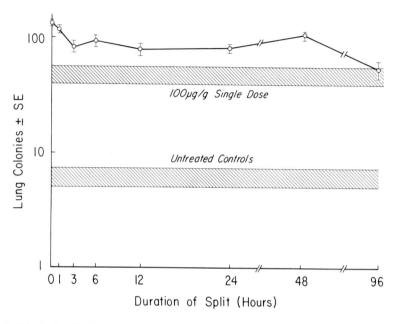

FIG. 3. Effect of split-dose administration of cyclophosphamide. Cy was given as a single dose of 200 μg/g s.c. or as two equal doses of 100 μg/g separated by from 1 to 96 hr. The second dose in each case was given 2 days before tumor cell injection. Split doses were significantly less effective when separated by 3 hr or more, but some cumulative effect was apparent for dose intervals up to 48–96 hr. By 96 hr the effect could be accounted for by either 100-μg/g dose independently.

thorax (LTI) or may include the whole body (WBI), but, curiously, irradiation of the whole body *except* thorax does not increase lung CFE even for an immunogenic tumor such as FSa (6). Evidence that the effect of Cy is not based on its immunosuppressive action is provided by our finding that the effect of a modest 150 μg/g dose of Cy is additive to that of both LTI and WBI at doses of 1,000 rads (Table 2). A dose of 1,000 rads WBI is profoundly immunosuppressive, and is lethal unless bone marrow reconstitution

TABLE 2. *Additivity of effects of cyclophosphamide and irradiation*

No irradiation	Lung colonies ± SE 14 days after 10^4 FSa i.v. 6 mice/group	
	No Cy	Cy 150 μg/g s.c. day-2
	6.2 ± 1.1	57.5 ± 13.4
LTI 1,000 rads day-1	34.7 ± 7.3	103.8 ± 29.8
WBI 1,000 rads day-1[a]	113.8 ± 10.9	Confluent >250 (mean lung weight 246% of controls)

[a] Rescued with 4 × 10^6 bone marrow cells day + 4.

is undertaken. In these experiments, 4×10^6 bone marrow cells were given 4 days after tumor cell injection, i.e., 6 days after Cy—long after its cyto-toxic activity had ceased.

Dynamics of Tumor Cell Retention in Lungs and Lung CFE After Irradiation or Cy

After intravenous injection of ^{125}IUdR-labeled tumor cells, almost all the injected activity is initially trapped in the lungs. The rate of loss of tumor cells from the lungs depends on the total number of tumor cells injected (7): for example, untreated mice retained only 0.5% of 10^4 tumor cells 24 hr after their injection, compared with 16% retention of 10^7 tumor cells. The rate of loss of tumor cells from the lungs is further modified by conditioning influences such as irradiation or Cy. In Fig. 4, the percentage retention of labeled cells in the lungs is plotted for control (C), LTI, WBI, and Cy-treated mice over a range of inoculum sizes from 10^4 to 10^7 cells. It can be seen that in terms of 24-hr retention of cells in the lungs, Cy (150 μg/g s.c.) is significantly more efficient than either LTI or WBI (1,000 rads).

When, however, the colony-forming efficiency of injected cells in irradi-

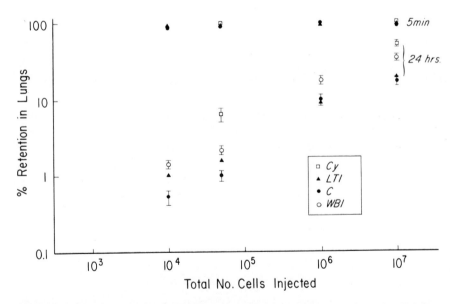

FIG. 4. Percentage retention of ^{125}IUdR-labeled FSa tumor cells in the lungs as a function of the total number of cells injected 5 min and 24 hr after i.v. tumor cell injection. (●), control, untreated mice; LTI mice (▲) received 1,000 rads local thoracic irradiation on day −1; WBI mice (○) received 1,000 rads whole-body irradiation on day −1; and Cy mice (□) received 150 μg/g cyclophosphamide s.c. on day −2. Tumor cells were injected on day 0. Errors are SEM of 3–6 mice/point. For clarity, error bars were omitted from the 5-min points and the 24-hr points for LTI mice. Differences in residual radioactivity at 24 hr between WBI and Cy mice are highly significant.

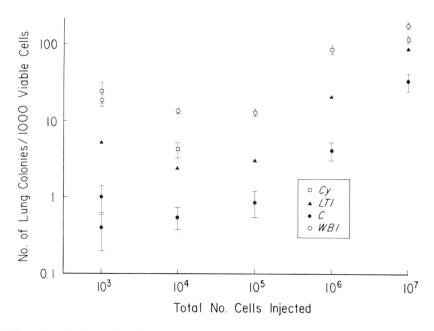

FIG. 5. Lung CFE as a function of the total number of tumor cells injected. Symbols are as for Fig. 4. For these experiments, WBI mice were reconstituted with 4×10^6 syngeneic bone marrow cells 4 days after tumor cell injection to prevent hemopoietic death. Errors are SEM of 6–8 mice/point. The CFE following injection of 10^4 and 10^7 FSa cells was significantly lower in Cy than in WBI mice.

ated or Cy-treated animals was compared (Fig. 5), Cy was significantly less efficacious than 1,000 rads WBI for inoculum sizes of 10^4 and 10^7 tumor cells. (There was no significant difference in the CFE of 10^3 injected tumor cells in Cy-treated or WBI mice.) From these observations, we deduce that the effect of Cy is exerted earlier after tumor cell injection than that of WBI, and is perhaps explicable in terms of increased efficiency of vascular transmigration and interstitial lodgment of tumor cells in the lungs. This temporal difference in the manifestation of the effects of Cy and WBI and our demonstration that the two effects are additive strongly suggest that their mechanisms differ in at least some important respects.

Effect of Modifications of Cy Metabolism

The basic pathway of Cy metabolism is indicated in the following schema:

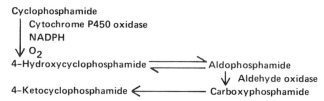

TABLE 3. *Effects of modifiers of cyclophosphamide metabolism—phenobarbital and chloramphenicol*

			Lung colonies $\pm$ SE 14 days after 10^4 FSa i.v. 8 mice/group	
Control	4.0 ± 0.6	Control	9.6 ± 1.1
Cy[a]	62.6 ± 7.3	Cy[a]	55.4 ± 6.0
Cy[a] + Phenobarbital[b]	21.4 ± 3.7	Cy[a] + Chloramphenicol[c]	75.9 ± 6.3
Phenobarbital[b]	2.0 ± 0.6	Chloramphenicol	10.0 ± 2.2

[a] Cy dose 150 μg/g s.c. 2 days before FSa.
[b] Phenobarbital dose 40 μg/g i.p. b.d. for 5 days before Cy.
[c] Chloramphenicol dose 600 μg/g s.c. 30 min before Cy.

TABLE 4. *Effect of* in vitro *premetabolism of cyclophosphamide (dose equivalent 67 μg/g)*

	Lung colonies $\pm$ SE 14 days after 10^4 FSa i.v. 8 mice/group
Control	3.1 ± 0.8
Cy incubated with buffer	9.1 ± 1.7
Microsomes and cofactors only	12.9 ± 3.3
Cy incubated with liver microsomes and cofactors	26.9 ± 5.7

To exert its alkylating action, cyclophosphamide requires biotransformation which is mediated predominantly by liver microsomal mixed-function oxidases (8). Many drugs act to modify the activity of these enzymes and so alter the rate of Cy biotransformation. The effects of phenobarbital, which accelerates Cy metabolism, and of chloramphenicol, which inhibits it, are shown in Table 3. A significant decrease in lung CFE resulted from phenobarbital pretreatment, whereas the administration of chloramphenicol before Cy further increased the lung colony yield. These findings suggested the possibility that the promotion of CFE by cyclophosphamide might be due to some action of the parent molecule rather than to the alkylating activity of its metabolites. We therefore tested the effect of premetabolism of cyclophosphamide *in vitro* by incubating the drug with hepatic microsomes and NADPH-generating cofactors at 37°C for 18 hr prior to administration. In this experiment, injection of microsomes and cofactors alone stimulated lung CFE; however, the additional effect of Cy metabolites was very similar to that of unmetabolized Cy on untreated control mice (Table 4). It is therefore unlikely that Cy itself acts directly to increase lung colony formation (see Discussion).

DISCUSSION

The stimulation of lung CFE we observed with single doses of Cy is in general agreement with the report of van Putten et al. (1), although the magnitude of the stimulation in our system was much less (Fig. 1). This was rather surprising since Cy is immunosuppressive and the tumor used in the present experiments is moderately strongly immunogenic (2), whereas no immune response could be demonstrated against the C22LR osteosarcoma of van Putten et al. The scope for enhancement of lung CFE of course depends to a certain extent on the base-line CFE of the tumor in intact animals, and this in turn varies with the number of tumor cells injected. From Fig. 5 it can be seen that the CFE for our tumor in untreated mice varies from 0.05 to 0.1% with inocula of 10^3 to 10^5 cells to 3% with an injection of 10^7 cells. Thus, to achieve an enhancement factor of 1,000 would be essentially impossible in our system.

The effect of Cy appears to be largely the result of increased early cell retention in the lungs. DeRuiter et al. (9) reported that mice pretreated with 250 μg/g Cy retained 48.2% of 2.5 to 5×10^6 osteosarcoma cells in their lungs 24 hr after tumor cell injection. These data are very similar to our observation (Fig. 4) that 50% of 10^7 FSa cells were retained for 24 hr in mice receiving 150 μg/g Cy. When the effects of Cy and WBI are compared, it is seen that although Cy is more efficient in securing the lodgment of FSa cells in the lungs, the yield of lung colonies is greater in WBI mice, implying a higher mortality rate of the cells initially lodging in the lungs of Cy-treated mice. According to Turk et al. (10), Cy is relatively sparing to T lymphocytes, whereas the immune response to our FSa tumor is T-cell dependent (11). Winkelstein (12) reported that although the expression of a delayed hypersensitivity response to tuberculin was inhibited in guinea pigs undergoing Cy treatment, no inhibition of the intradermal reaction was observed when Cy was administered for 5 days prior to immunization. Thus, it is conceivable that the effect of Cy in promoting CFE in our system was partly offset by a T lymphocyte-mediated immune response which was abrogated by WBI. However, we have reported elsewhere (6) that T cell reconstitution fails to restore the resistance of WBI mice to i.v. FSa tumor cell injection. Hence the precise reason(s) for the increased rate of delayed cell death in the lungs of Cy mice must remain *subjudice*. We may confidently conclude, however, that the stimulation of FSa lung colony formation by Cy is not predominantly due to the drug's immunosuppressive function (even though the tumor is immunogenic) since its effect is additive to and temporally distinct from that of a massive 1,000-rad dose of WBI. A mechanism divorced from specific immunological reactions is also indicated by the dramatic effect of Cy observed by van Putten et al. (1) in a nonimmunogenic tumor system. Winkelstein (12) showed that macrophage/monocyte precursors in the bone marrow of guinea pigs were highly sensitive to fractionated doses of Cy. However, there is no evidence to suggest that resident lung macrophages are acutely depleted by the drug. We have found (*unpublished data*) that a single 150-μg/g dose of Cy given 5 days after stimulation of macrophages by *Corynebacterium parvum* does not abrogate the protection against FSa afforded by *C. parvum*. If, however, Cy is given 1 to 2 days after *C. parvum,* when a proliferative response is occurring in reticuloendothelial precursor cells, then the effect of *C. parvum* is significantly reduced. Finally, inhibition of macrophage lysosomal enzymes with trypan blue, which reduces macrophage cytotoxicity, does not simulate the effect of Cy (7). Thus it seems unlikely that impairment of nonspecific macrophage-mediated host defenses can explain the action of Cy.

The reason for the increased efficiency of cell lodgment in the lungs of Cy-treated mice is unclear. Cy in very high doses produces acute pulmonary edema (13), and in our toxicity studies (Table 1) two of six mice given 500 μg/g died soon after injection with acute pulmonary edema. However, the much lower doses which caused dramatic enhancement of lung CFE produced no discernible morphologic changes in the lungs as assessed by light microscopy. We are presently undertaking EM studies. Possible Cy-induced alterations in endothelial stickiness and/or permeability are as yet unassessed.

Pharmacological considerations indicate that the lesion(s) induced by Cy is produced rapidly and is relatively long-lasting. Recently Carmel and Brown (14) reported an enhanced CFE of intravenously injected KHT sarcoma cells when Cy was given up to 8 weeks previously. In our system, the effect was essentially constant when Cy was given 1 to 7 days before tumor cells. Two doses of 100 μg/g Cy separated by 3 hr or more were significantly less effective than a single 200-μg/g dose, and with a dose interval of 96 hr, the effect on CFE was accountable by one 100-μg/g dose alone. Thus, although the effect of a given dose of Cy is long-lasting, repeated doses of the same size appear not to be additive in effect. The route of administration of Cy appears to be of little consequence (Fig. 2), although the s.c. route was slightly more effective than the i.v. Acceleration of the biotransformation of Cy to its alkylating metabolites by phenobarbital-induced stimulation of liver microsomal enzymes resulted in a reduced effect on CFE. Conversely, inhibition of the biotransforming enzyme system with chloramphenicol increased the effect of Cy. Taken together with the uniqueness of the Cy action compared with that of other alkylating agents, these findings suggested that the Cy molecule itself might be acting (possibly idiosyncratically in the mouse) on the lung. This possibility was rejected, however, when we found a comparable effect of *in vitro* premetabolized Cy compared with the parent drug (Table 4), and we conclude that just as some of the toxic effects of Cy metabolites observed clinically (e.g., hemorrhagic cystitis) are unique to the agent, so is probably its effect on the mouse lung. The reduced enhancement of CFE by Cy that we observed in phenobarbital pretreated mice and the increased effect following chloramphenicol contrast with the reported effects of these drugs on Cy-induced hemopoietic toxicity. Hart and Adamson (15), Cohen and Jao (16), and

Sladek (17) all reported increased hemopoietic toxicity from Cy after phenobarbital pretreatment, whereas Dixon (18) observed a protective effect of chloramphenicol. Pharmacokinetic studies by Field et al. (19), Alberts and van Daalen Wetters (20), and Donelli et al. (21) all show that although the biotransformation of Cy is accelerated by phenobarbital treatment, the rate of detoxification of its alkylating metabolites is also increased. Thus, the serum alkylating activity shows an initially higher peak, but a more rapid decay, and the integrated total alkylating activity is reduced. By contrast, inhibitors of Cy biotransformation such as chloramphenicol or 2-diethylaminoethyl-2,2-diphenylvalerate (SKF525A) cause a prolonged low level of alkylating activity with an increase in the integrated total (19). From this, we might conclude that a prolonged exposure to lower concentrations of Cy metabolites produces a greater effect on the lungs than a short exposure to higher concentrations. This would be consistent with our finding that s.c. administration of Cy is a little more effective than i.v.

The intriguing question as to whether Cy-induced enhancement of lung CFE is of clinical importance remains unanswered. In the therapeutic setting, the cytotoxic effect of Cy on FSa tumor cells far outweighed its conditioning effect on the lung. Nevertheless, it is conceivable that the metastatic potential of a tumor type resistant to Cy would be enhanced. To date, the enhancement of lung CFE by Cy has been studied only in mice, and it is possible that the marked difference in effect between Cy and other cytotoxic drugs could be an idiosyncrasy of that species. Clearly, more studies are necessary to delineate the potential hazards of chemotherapy quite apart from considerations of immunosuppression. However, irrespective of their possible clinical relevance, studies of the mechanisms involved in the modulation of tumor transplantability by agents such as Cy are important for their contribution to our understanding of the pathogenesis of metastasis.

SUMMARY

Pretreatment of mice with cyclophosphamide increases the lung colony-forming efficiency of intravenously injected tumor cells in a dose-dependent fashion. The effect is slightly greater when Cy is given subcutaneously compared with intravenously. By both routes, the effect is constant from 1 to at least 7 days prior to tumor cell injection. Two equally divided doses of Cy are less effective than a single dose, but some cumulative effect is present with a dose interval of up to 48 to 96 hr. Increasing the rate of biotransformation of Cy decreases its effect on CFE, whereas inhibition of Cy metabolism further increases CFE. Premetabolism of Cy *in vitro* does not abolish its action. These observations suggest that the integrated total exposure to Cy metabolites determines the drug's effectiveness. The increase in CFE caused by a moderate 150-μg/g dose of Cy is additive to that of a massive 1,000-rad dose of whole-body irradiation. When these treatments are separately examined, retention of tumor cells in the lungs 24 hr after injection is much greater in Cy-treated than in WBI mice, but the ultimate number of lung colonies formed is less. We conclude that the major effect of Cy is to condition the lungs in such a way as to promote lodgment and survival of cells soon after i.v. dissemination, when they are most vulnerable. Its immunosuppressive action appears not to be important in this regard. An idiosyncratic reaction to one of its metabolites may explain the marked effect of Cy on CFE compared with other alkylating agents.

ACKNOWLEDGMENTS

We are grateful to Nehama Dubravsky for the autoradiography of ^{125}IUdR-labeled tumor cells; to Dr. H. Rodney Withers for his interest and helpful advice; and to Ellen Hilton and her staff for the supply and care of the mice used in these experiments. This investigation was supported in part by N.I.H. Research Grants CA-06294 and CA-17769 from the National Cancer Institute.

REFERENCES

1. van Putten, L. M., Kram, L. K. J., van Dierendonck, H. H. C., Smink, T., and Fuzy, M. (1975): Enhancement by drugs of metastatic lung nodule formation after intravenous tumour cell injection. *Int. J. Cancer*, 15:588–595.
2. Suit, H. D., and Kastelan, A. (1970): Immunologic status of host and response of a methylcholanthrene induced sarcoma to local x-irradiation. *Cancer*, 26:232–238.
3. Milas, L., Hunter, N., Mason, K., and Withers, H. R. (1971): Immunological resistance to pulmonary metastases in C$_3$Hf/Bu mice bearing syngeneic fibrosarcoma of different sizes. *Cancer Res.*, 34:61–71.
4. Dolfini, E., Martini, A., Donelli, M. G., Morasca, L., and Garattini, S. (1973): Method for tissue culture evaluation of the cytoxic activity of drugs active through the formation of metabolites. *Eur. J. Cancer*, 9:375–378.
5. Withers, H. R., and Milas, L. (1973): Influence of preirradiation of lung on development of artificial pulmonary metastases of fibrosarcoma in mice. *Cancer Res.*, 33:1931–1936.
6. Peters, L. J., McBride, W. H., and Mason, K. A. (1976): T cell depletion and tumor metastasis. *Int. J. Radiat. Biol. [Supp.]*, 1:106.
7. Peters, L. J., Mason, K., and McBride, W. H. (1977): Enhancement of lung colony forming efficiency by local thoracic irradiation—interpretation of labelled cell studies. *Radiology* (*in press*).
8. Brock, N., and Hohorst, H. J. (1967): Metabolism of cyclophosphamide. *Cancer*, 20:900–904.
9. DeRuiter, J., Smirk, T., and van Putten, L. M. (1976): Studies on the enhancement by cyclophosphamide (NSC 26271) of artificial lung metastasis after labeled cell inoculation. *Cancer Treatment Rep.*, 60:465–470.
10. Turk, J. L., Parker, D., and Poulter, L. W. (1972): Functional aspects of the selective depletion of lymphoid tissue by cyclophosphamide. *Immunology*, 23:493–501.
11. Milas, L., Kogelnik, H. D., Basic, I., Mason, K., Hunter, N., and Withers, H. R. (1976): Combination of *C. parvum* and specific immunization against artificial pulmonary metastases in mice. *Int. J. Cancer*, 16:738–746.
12. Winkelstein, A. (1973): Mechanisms of immunosuppression: Effects of cyclophosphamide on cellular immunity. *Blood*, 41:273–284.

13. O'Connell, T. X., and Berenbaum, M. C. (1974): Cardiac and pulmonary effects of high dose cyclophosphamide and isophosphamide. *Cancer Res.,* 34:1586–1591.

14. Carmel, R. J., and Brown, J. M. (1977): The effect of cyclophosphamide and other drugs on the incidence of pulmonary metastases in mice. Abstract Ih1, Proceedings of 24th Annual Meeting of the Radiation Research Society. *Cancer Res.,* 37:145–151.

15. Hart, L. G., and Adamson, R. H. (1969): Effect of microsomal enzyme modifiers on toxicity and therapeutic activity of cyclophosphamide in mice. *Arch. Int. Pharmacodyn. Ther.,* 180:391–401.

16. Cohen, J. L., and Jao, J. Y. (1970): Enzymatic basis of cyclophosphamide activation by hepatic microsomes of the rat. *J. Pharmacol. Exp. Ther.,* 174:206–210.

17. Sladek, N. E. (1972): Therapeutic efficacy of cyclophosphamide as a function of its metabolism. *Cancer Res.,* 32:535–542.

18. Dixon, R. L. (1967): Effect of chloramphenicol on the metabolism and lethality of cyclophosphamide in rats. *Proc. Soc. Exp. Biol. Med.,* 127:1151–1155.

19. Field, R. B., Gang, M., Kline, I., Venditti, J. M., and Waraodekar, V. S. (1972): The effect of phenobarbital or 2-diethylaminoethyl 2, 2-diphenylvalerate on the activation of cyclophosphamide *in vivo. J. Pharmacol. Exp. Ther.,* 180:475–483.

20. Alberts, D. S., and van Daalen Wetters, T. (1976): The effect of phenobarbital on cyclophosphamide antitumor activity. *Cancer Res.,* 36:2785–2789.

21. Donelli, M. G., Bartosek, I., Guaitani, A., Martini, A., Colombo, T., Pacciarini, M. A., and Modica, R. (1976): Importance of pharmacokinetic studies of cyclophosphamide (NSC 26271) in understanding its cytotoxic effect. *Cancer Treatment Rep.,* 60:395–401.

Cancer Invasion and Metastasis: Biologic Mechanisms and Therapy, edited by S. B. Day et al. Raven Press, New York © 1977.

Effect of Cyclophosphamide and Other Drugs on Artificial Pulmonary Metastases in Mice

J. M. Brown

Department of Radiology, Stanford University Medical Center, Stanford, California 94305

With a similar experimental model, we have obtained results that closely resemble those described in the previous chapter of Peters and Mason (1,2).

We have used the KHT sarcoma, a tumor that arose spontaneously and has been maintained by serial subcutaneous passage in C3H mice. No immunogenicity of this tumor in this host can be demonstrated using either the number of lung colonies following an i.v. injection or the TD_{50} assay, in mice that have been subjected to repeated "immunizations" with heavily irradiated tumor cells or have had a cured primary tumor. In most of our experiments single-cell suspensions of KHT tumor cells were prepared from solid tumors, and a known number of cells were injected via the tail vein in a volume of 0.2 ml. The mice were sacrificed 17 or 18 days later and the colonies were counted.

Various drugs in common use as chemotherapeutic agents were injected i.p. into recipient mice (at a dose of roughly two-thirds LD_{50}) and 24 hr later KHT cells were injected. There was a slight enhancement of pulmonary metastases (lung colony formation) by actinomycin D and mithramycin, but a far greater enhancement (by a factor of roughly 100) with cyclophosphamide. Figure 1 shows a dose-response curve for the number of lung colonies in mice treated 1 day prior to tumor cell injection with various doses of cyclophosphamide. Unlike the dose-response curve for local thoracic irradiation (1), the dose-response curve is highly sigmoidal.

The kinetics of development and decay of the colony enhancement effect are shown in Fig. 2. As soon as 2 hr after cyclophosphamide injection, much of the enhancement had developed. In other experiments we have found that the colony-enhancing effect is much reduced between 1 and 4 weeks after cyclophosphamide injection, but a significant enhancement is still present 8 weeks after injection. We have also found that, although the enhancing effect of a dose of 100 mg/kg remains virtually undiminished for up to 1 week after injection, a second dose of 100 mg/kg does not interact with the first dose to give an effect comparable to that produced by a single

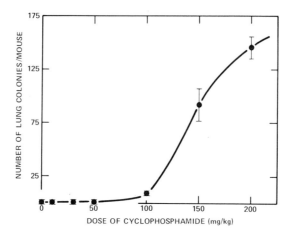

FIG. 1. The number of lung colonies per mouse as a function of the dose of cyclophosphamide injected 1 day prior to the injection of 10^4 KHT tumor cells (from ref. 2).

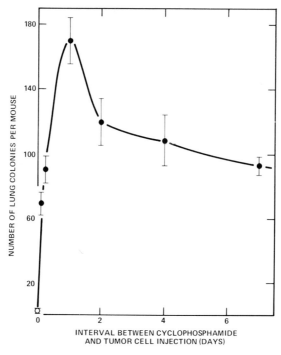

FIG. 2. The number of lung colonies per mouse as a function of the time interval between cyclophosphamide treatment (200 mg/kg) and cell injection (from ref. 2).

dose of 200 mg/kg unless less than 24 hr separates the two doses. This is consistent with the data presented by Peters and Mason (*this volume*).

We have performed various experiments designed to ascertain the mechanism of the effect. We agree with Peters and Mason (*this volume*) that colony enhancement by cyclophosphamide is not by suppression of any specific immune response. However, we have not yet ruled out the possibility that nonspecific host defenses involving macrophages, lymphocytes, or both are involved. We have evidence that increased clot formation around the trapped tumor cells is not involved (2). On the basis of preliminary light and electron microscope studies, it appears that a more rapid migration of tumor cells from the capillaries to alveoli may be involved.

REFERENCES

1. Brown, J. M. (1977): Effects of radiation and chemotherapeutic agents on the incidence and treatment of blood-borne metastases. *Gann* (*in press*).
2. Carmel, R. J. and Brown, J. M. (1977): The effect of cyclophosphamide and other drugs on the incidence of pulmonary metastases in mice. *Cancer Res.*, 37:145–151.

Cancer Invasion and Metastasis: Biologic Mechanisms and Therapy, edited by S. B. Day et al. Raven Press, New York © 1977.

Discussion Summary: Current Experimental Approaches to Metastasis Control

Stacey B. Day

Sloan-Kettering Institute for Cancer Research, New York, New York 10021

Not unremarkably, chapters in this section dealt with widely different aspects of metastasis, although the emphasis throughout was from the viewpoint of the experimentalist rather than from that of the clinician. For that reason the chapters were predictably satisfying and unsatisfying, for as Hellman said elsewhere in this volume, the human is one of the worst models possible, and this applies no less to animal models too: there are heterogenous factors in tumors, patients, and animal models. Among such variables must be nature and site of the primary tumor, time, the approach studied, as well as the nature of the challenge used to evaluate the experiment.

This section brought to the fore some of the difficulties inherent in experimental studies seeking to evaluate the nature of metastasis, and presented a variety of models and strategies aimed at accomplishing this task.

Pollard presented an interesting discussion of germ-free prostate adenocarcinomas with metastasis to the lungs. He noted this finding in three lines of spontaneous tumors of this type with cells migrating via the lymphatics. Pollard's studies showed that cyclophosphamide, *Corynebacterium parvum,* and aspirin, although not curative, could retard metastases. He noted that treatment with ICRF 159 reduced the rate and extent of tumor metastases to the lungs.

To the present observer, his report that chloroform, halothane, ether, and sodium barbiturate anesthesia all appeared to accelerate metastases was of great interest. In most model systems involving animals, as well as in clinical studies in man, *the role of anesthesia is seldom, if ever, evaluated.* That anesthesia increased the average number of tumors in Pollard's studies might suggest possibilities for pathophysiologic (enzyme) changes in the liver, which both in man and in animals may be a susceptible site for tumor metastasis. The physiologic importance of the liver is often overlooked in both clinical studies in man and experimental "variables" in the laboratory. Some years ago, while working with a rather enthusiastic burn team given to advocating frequent debridement (every 2 to 3 days) in patients with burns over 30% total body surface, I noted a surprisingly high incidence of bleeding from the gastrointestinal tract. Burns of severe magnitude were

415

debrided under anesthesia, and it was my view then (and still is) that the postdebridement GI bleeding was a result more of the anesthesia provoking metabolic problems than of the mechanical action of the procedure.

I thought Pollard's point most worthwhile.

Tsubura presented elegant work studying mechanisms of inhibition of blood-borne tumors by sulfated polysaccharides, and disclosed that such inhibition was closely related to their anticoagulative activities. His results suggest that anticoagulative therapy may be helpful in preventing blood-borne metastases in cancer patients. He qualified this view by remarking that before we use these compounds clinically further studies are needed. But there is the point; without being ungenerous of spirit, and acknowledging the interest of the studies, one must take the issue to task. How long are we to hear the phrase "more studies needed"? We seem, year after year, always back to "more studies." Fisher took the bull by the horn and asked the assembled faculty how many had actually used anticoagulative therapy over the years in patients? There were no respondents. The truth is that few do use this approach, and one presumes this sort of therapy is still unlikely to come in clinical cases of human cancer.

Kopelovich moved to an approach quite different from that taken in the preceding chapters. He argued a case for biologic parameters in hereditable forms of neoplasia as a model for analysis of differential genetic susceptibility to cancer. This strategy for the analysis of the metastatic process was well received and elicited favorable comment.

In this same section Dr. Philip Levine presented remarks on anti-A or anti-P as neoantigens in prevention of metastasis.

Dr. Schabel has presented an authoritative discussion on micrometastasis. (One tends to review the chapters of Schabel, Fisher, and Krakoff as falling within the same domain. There is a measure of authority and experience in their work, and an understanding of the cancer problem that, when presented, becomes a fascinating learning experience in the biology of cancer.) Schabel related the size of the primary to the surgical cure rate. The larger the primary, the larger the body burden. Cure rate parallels tumor size. If the primary is removed, surgery and synergistic chemotherapy aid the surgical cure rate, and although time is a factor, the metastatic kill rate is alleviated. In Schabel's view aggressive chemotherapy (adjuvant combination therapy) raises the life span of "dying" animals.

Drugs ineffective against advanced disease do show results against small tumor body burden—thus cyclophosphamide may increase life span if given early enough. Schabel's views might be reasonably summarized as (a) remove the primary, (b) reduce the total body burden, and (c) treat aggressively and make use of adjuvant chemotherapy. He noted that a small body burden may be effectively treated with drugs that fail in advanced cases of cancer. His emphasis throughout was to lower the burden as much as possible.

Cancer Invasion and Metastasis: Biologic
Mechanisms and Therapy, edited by S. B. Day
et al. Raven Press, New York © 1977.

The Lewis Lung Carcinoma as a Model for Carcinoma of the Bronchus and Pulmonary Metastases: Effect of ICRF 159, Radiotherapy, and Oxytetracycline

K. Hellmann, S. E. James, H. A. Atherton, and *A. J. Salsbury

*Chemotherapy Department, Imperial Cancer Research Fund, Lincoln's Inn Fields,
London; and *Cardio-Thoracic Institute, Brompton Hospital,
London SW3, England*

In a controlled, randomized trial of radiotherapy with ICRF 159 [(±)1,2-bis(3,5-dioxopiperazin-1-yl) propane; NSC 129, 943] compared to radiotherapy alone in patients with carcinoma of the bronchus, survival times of those who had the combination seemed at first to be shorter than those of the controls. This was especially so among patients who also developed severe esophagitis (M. F. Spittle and K. Hellmann, *unpublished observations*). A paucity of information concerning terminal episodes led to the conjecture that pulmonary infections might have played an important part in the apparently shortened survival times.

It therefore seemed of some interest to determine the effect of ICRF 159 in combination with radiation on an animal model of carcinoma of the bronchus, but since no suitable model was available, studies on the development of experimental lung metastases appeared to be a possible compromise. The tumor system chosen was the Lewis lung carcinoma (3LL). This tumor when implanted s.c. into the flank of $C_{57}BL$ female mice metastasizes spontaneously and regularly to the lungs within 21 days of tumor implantation (1). Serial daily excision of the primary 3LL tumor has shown that by 9 days post-implantation, tumor cells which subsequently form pulmonary metastases have already been disseminated (3). Thus 3LL tumor-bearing mice were subjected to primary tumor removal 10 days post-implantation and treatment was given days 14 to 18 inclusive. The preliminary results of the experiments were similar to the clinical trial in that there were a considerable number of early deaths, but they were not attributable to tumor in the lung.

In the clinical trial there were a large number of cases with (a) postirradiation esophagitis and (b) leukopenia, and this raised the possibility that increased morbidity could have resulted from decreased food intake and/or decreased resistance to lung infections. Consequently, the experimental

417

esophagii and lungs were kept for histological examination, and total white cell counts were carried out during and after treatment. To clarify the possibility that infection might have played a part in the results, we performed further experiments in which mice were given a broad-spectrum antibiotic alone and in addition to treatment.

MATERIALS AND METHODS

Drugs

Mice received 30 mg/kg ICRF 159 suspended in 0.2 ml of 0.5% carboxymethyl cellulose (CMC) i.p., and controls received 0.2 ml CMC i.p. only on days 14 to 18 inclusive. ICRF 159 or CMC was given 1 hr before irradiation. Oxytetracycline hydrochloride (Terramycin®) was given at a concentration of 1% *ad libitum* in the drinking water. Each mouse took a mean dose of 15 mg/day.

Excision of Primary Subcutaneous Implant

C57/B1 SPF female mice were given s.c. implants in the flank of 0.1 g finely minced 3LL tumor on day 0. On day 10 primary implants were excised surgically under tribromoethanol (Avertin®) anesthesia (250 mg/kg body weight i.p.). A wide margin of skin surrounding the tumor and the underlying part of the peritoneal wall was excised with the implant to minimize the possibility of tumor regrowth. Those mice surviving operation (95%) were randomly allocated into treatment groups.

Radiotherapy

A total dose of 1,500 R was delivered to the whole lung in five consecutive daily doses of 300 R from days 14 to 18 inclusive. Mice were anesthetized with tribromoethanol (as above) and placed in the supine position under a lead shield with the thorax exposed through a triangular aperture. A 250-kv Pantak machine was the X-ray source: the half-value layer (HVL) was 0.5 mm Cu, and with a 13-mA setting at 240 kv, the dose rate was 250 rads/min at a distance of 15 inches from the source. The nonirradiated control mice were also anesthetized with tribromoethanol during treatment days 14 to 18.

Prophylactic Antibiotic Treatment

In a preliminary experiment, mice subjected to tumor excision on day 10 were given either radiotherapy in combination with ICRF 159, radiotherapy alone, or no treatment. In a subsequent experiment, mice subjected to tumor excision were treated in the same way but an additional group received a combination of radiotherapy, ICRF 159, and a 1% solution of oxytetracycline *ad libitum* in their drinking water from day 14 until termination of the experiment. Subsequently, further studies included a group of mice receiving only oxytetracycline in the drinking water.

Blood Leukocyte Counts

Blood samples for total white cell counts were taken from the tail veins of each of six marked mice per treatment group on days 14 to 18 and on days 21 and 23. Blood was taken within 10 min of the induction of anesthesia in all groups.

Survival of Mice

Deaths were recorded after daily observation of the mice, and routine postmortem examinations were carried out. Lungs and esophagii were fixed in 10% neutral buffered formalin, sectioned (5 μm thickness), stained with hematoxylin and eosin, coded, and examined blind for evidence of pathological changes. Those mice with evidence of tumor regrowth at the excision site were discarded (approximately 2%).

Oxytetracycline Effect on Primary 3LL Tumor *in situ*

C57/B1 SPF female mice received 0.1 ml of 3LL tumor mash subcutaneously in the flank on day 0. Treatment with oxytetracycline was started immediately and continued until day 21 when the animals were sacrificed, the tumors were excised and weighed, and the lungs examined for the presence of metastases using Indian ink (1).

RESULTS

Effect of Treatment on Survival Time after Primary Excision

The median survival times (MSTs) of mice in the first experiment are shown in Table 1. Although the survival time for mice receiving the combination therapy was increased, early deaths which were not attributable to tumor growth in the lungs occurred in this and the other two groups from the first day of treatment (day 14 post-implantation).

Deaths directly attributable to the presence of tumor in the lung were not noted in any treatment group until at least day 25 post-implantation. After this time deaths of control mice and those treated with radiotherapy (RTX) alone were due to almost complete replacement of pulmonary tissue by tumor. However, postmortem examination of those animals receiving a

TABLE 1. *Comparison of the effects of radiation plus ICRF 159 on survival*

Treatment (day 14–18)	No. per group	MST of nonsurvivors (days)	No. deaths not attributable to lung secondaries	No. indefinite survivors
1,500 R + 30 mg/kg ICRF 159	14	53.0	10	8 (d 308)
1,500 R	13	32.2	3	1 (d 308)
CMC only	10	29.1	3	0

combination of ICRF 159 and radiotherapy at no time revealed the presence of pulmonary tumor growth. Detailed histological examination of these lungs receiving combination therapy at 25 days after implantation showed signs of inflammation including lymphocytic cuffing, dilated blood vessels, and lining of the vessels with polymorphs. Very few, probably non-viable tumor cells were visible. In contrast, those lungs that had received RTX alone were only slightly inflamed, and large deposits of 3LL cells were actively growing. Control lungs were not inflamed, and very large metastases had displaced much of the lung tissue.

The survival of mice in a further experiment, in which an additional group of mice received oxytetracycline and combination therapy (RTX + ICRF 159) is shown in Table 2.

Again, early deaths (Table 2) not attributable to tumor growth in the lungs occurred in those mice receiving no treatment, radiotherapy alone, and radiotherapy + ICRF 159. However, the addition of oxytetracycline to the drinking water appeared to prevent such deaths. The survival times of the mice in the four groups are shown in Table 2.

When a group of mice receiving oxytetracycline alone was included in a subsequent experiment (Fig. 1), the number of survivors in this group was less than in a group receiving combination therapy and oxytetracycline, and the MST of nonsurvivors was also less (Table 3). Further experiments comparing oxytetracycline treatment alone directly to a control receiving only tap drinking water showed that the MST of nonsurvivors at 50 days in the oxytetracycline-treated group (35.7 days + 10 survivors) was greater than that of the control group (27.6 days + 3 survivors). In another experiment there were no significant differences between the two groups.

Blood Counts

The mean total white cell counts (±SE) of those mice receiving radiotherapy, radiotherapy + ICRF 159, or no treatment are shown in Fig. 2. Although leukopenia occurred during treatment with both radiotherapy

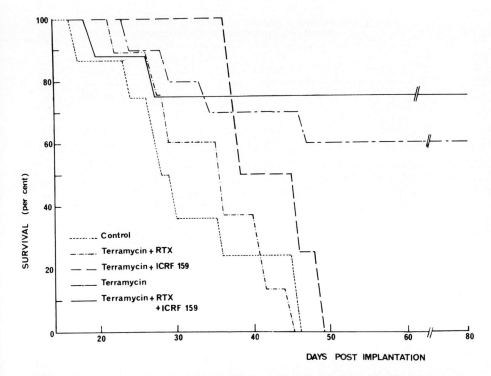

FIG. 1. Survival curve of mice inoculated with Lewis lung carcinoma in the flank (removed 10 days later) and treated with CMC only, radiotherapy alone, ICRF 159 and radiotherapy, or ICRF 159 and radiotherapy but given oxytetracycline (Terramycin®) in the drinking water during the period of treatment. For details of experiments, see text.

TABLE 2. *Comparison of radiation plus ICRF 159 in mice with and without prophylactic antibiotic treatment*

Treatment (day 14–18)	No. per group	MST (days) nonsurvivors	No. deaths not attributable to lung secondaries	No. deaths attributable to secondaries	No. indefinite survivors
1,500 R + 30 mg/kg ICRF 159 + oxytetracycline	16	69.0	2	0	14 (d 133)
1,500 R + 30 mg/kg ICRF 159	13	33.3	4	2	7 (d 133)
1,500 R	14	33.2	6	6	2 (d 133)
CMC	15	33.7	1	12	2 (d 133)

TABLE 3. *Comparison of radiation plus ICRF 159 in mice with and without prophylactic antibiotic treatment*

Treatment (day 14–18)	No. per group	MST (days) nonsurvivors	No. indefinite survivors
1,500 R + 30 mg/kg ICRF 159 + oxytetracycline	10	44.7	2 (day 80)
Oxytetracycline	10	33.5	6 (day 80)
Oxytetracycline + 1,500 R	9	33.8	0 (day 80)
Oxytetracycline + 30 mg/kg ICRF 159	9	34.4	0 (day 80)
CMC	11	31.3	0 (day 80)

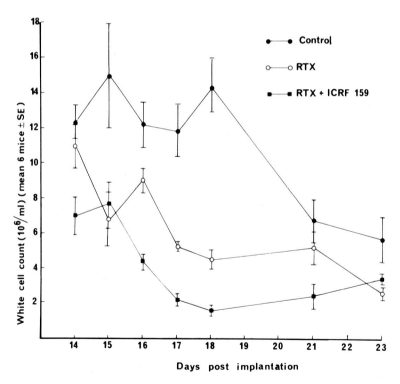

FIG. 2. Total white cell count of mice after implantation of the Lewis lung carcinoma (removed surgically after 10 days) and then treatment with either CMC or radiotherapy alone, or radiotherapy and ICRF 159. For details of experiments, see text.

alone and ICRF 159 and radiotherapy combined, this was more pronounced in the latter group.

Effect of Oxytetracycline on the Growth of 3LL Tumor Left *in situ*

The effects of continuous oxytetracycline treatment on tumor weights and the number of lung metastases at 21 days when the primary 3LL implant was allowed to remain *in situ* are shown in Table 4. No effect on 3LL primary size was seen at any time, but in two of four experiments oxytetracycline significantly decreased the number of lung secondaries.

TABLE 4. *Effect of oxytetracycline on the primary weight and number of lung metastases from 3LL tumor growing in C57 female mice at day 21 post-implantation*[a]

	Control (tap water *ad lib.*)		Oxytetracycline 1% (in tap water *ad lib.*)	
	Primary tumor weight (g)	No. lung metastases	Primary tumor weight (g)	No. lung metastases
Exp. 1	6.94 ± 1.02	51.83 ± 6.1	5.59 ± 0.71	15.5 ± 3.5 ($p < 0.05$)
Exp. 2	4.99 ± 0.57	27.1 ± 2.03	5.53 ± 0.82	14.3 ± 3.42 ($p < 0.05$)
Exp. 3	7.5 ± 0.9	53.1 ± 7.40	8.23 ± 1.04	41.25 ± 5.67
Exp. 4	5.64 ± 0.91	25.8 ± 4.8	6.01 ± 0.67	41.14 ± 2.46

[a] All values are mean ±SEM; *p*, probability value Student's *t*-test.

DISCUSSION

Although the metastatic Lewis lung carcinoma may have its limitations as a model for carcinoma of the bronchus, treatment of it highlights the complexities encountered when combined modality treatments are used on such critical and sensitive tissues as the lung and mediastinum.

ICRF 159 in combination with radiotherapy to the lungs for only 5 days clearly resulted in a greatly increased survival time as well as more long-term survivors, i.e., a much greater antitumor effect than in comparable animals receiving radiation alone or in those receiving chemotherapy alone. ICRF 159 at 30 mg/kg given to mice with primary 3LL tumors excised on day 10, although increasing the survival time, does not result in any long-term survivors (2).

Combination therapy was very successful in preventing tumor growth in the lung, but early deaths, although not due to 3LL metastatic growth in the lungs, occurred. It was distinctly possible that these deaths were due to pneumonitis and infection, and these would have been further aggravated by the leukopenia observed in mice receiving the combination therapy. The fact that oxytetracycline given to mice receiving combination therapy prevented the early deaths suggested, among other possibilities, that ICRF 159 and radiation together caused a life-threatening lung infection that was sensitive to this antibiotic.

However, the ability of oxytetracycline given alone to increase survival time in two of three experiments was unexpected. If the action of oxytetracycline was through its antibiotic effect, then it must be supposed that infection may actually help tumor growth, and this may be the case if lung congestion consequent to the infection helps to establish the small foci of pulmonary metastases by more effective trapping and support.

Another possibility is that oxytetracycline has a cytotoxic effect of its own, and this has been confirmed in tissue culture experiments with 3LL cells, but doses between 10 and 100 μg/ml were required before activity became evident (T. Cawte, *unpublished observations*). It is not excluded that both activities are involved in producing the unexpectedly long survival times sometimes seen in mice with 3LL on oxytetracycline alone.

In conclusion, these studies have shown that compared to each modality used alone, ICRF 159 used in combination with radiotherapy prolongs the survival time and increases the number of survivors in mice with 3LL carcinoma in the lung. Deaths occurring during treatment — but not due to tumor growth — could be largely prevented by the use of oxytetracycline in the drinking water. The effect of oxytetracycline used alone on this tumor system was variable, and may have reflected differences in the bacterial population and inflammatory state of the lungs.

REFERENCES

1. Hellmann, K., and Burrage, K. (1969): Control of malignent metastases by ICRF 159. *Nature*, 224:273–275.
2. James, S. E. (1975): Factors influencing dissemination of tumor cells. Ph.D. thesis. London University, London.
3. James, S. E., and Salsbury, A. J. (1974): Effect of (±)-1,2-*bis*(3,5-dioxopiperayin-1-yl)-propane on tumor blood vessels and its relationship to the antimetastatic effect in the Lewis lung carcinoma. *Cancer Res.*, 34:839.

Cancer Invasion and Metastasis: Biologic
Mechanisms and Therapy, edited by S. B. Day
et al. Raven Press, New York © 1977.

Factors Influencing Development
of Bone Metastases

Trevor J. Powles, G. C. Easty, D. M. Easty, M. Dowsett, and
A. M. Neville

Department of Medicine, Royal Marsden Hospital, Surrey, England

One curious feature of cancer is the distinctive distribution of metastases which occurs with various tumors. For example, patients with melanoma have a high risk of developing liver metastases, those with testicular tumors, lung metastases, and those with breast tumors, bone metastases. It is equally curious how gross metastatic disease can develop in one site presumably from blood-borne metastasees, with little or no development at other sites. One possible explanation for this is that some tumor cells produce substances locally which allow preferential development and tumor growth in a particular site. For example, tumor cells may release substances that break down bone, thereby allowing the cells trapped in the marrow to develop into osteolytic deposits. Tumors that possess this property and whose cells can pass into the circulation may find the bones a preferred site for development, an advantage that would not necessarily apply to other sites.

We have found that most breast tumors when cultured *in vitro* possess a marked ability to break down bone in organ culture (1). These tumors are able to synthesize prostaglandins as well as other osteolytic factors (2), and this *in vitro* osteolysis can, in part, be inhibited by prostaglandin synthesis inhibitors such as aspirin or indomethacin (1). Production of nonprostaglandin osteolytic agents, as well as prostaglandins, by the tumor cells is inhibited by these drugs.

We have found that only patients whose tumors possess *in vitro* osteolytic activity have or develop bone metastases and hypercalcemia (3), suggesting that development of tumor metastases in bone may depend on the ability of tumors to release substances to break down bone. Bennett et al. (4) have described how some breast tumors, particularly those from patients with bone metastases, are able to synthesize materials with prostaglandin-like biological activity.

The types of prostaglandins produced by osteolytic tumors *in vitro* have not so far been identified. The nonprostaglandin osteolytic agents, although they have been shown to be nondialyzable and are probably not protein-bound prostaglandins or parathyroid hormone, have also not been identified (2). The possibility that osteolytic enzymes are involved in the process is at present under investigation. Collagenase and trypsin have been found to possess marked osteolytic activity *in vitro* (1). These enzymes may be produced by tumor cells and depend for their production and release on prostaglandin synthesis. We have shown that fibrinolysins are released from osteolytic tumors *in vitro* (5). The role of collagenolytic enzymes in tumor invasion of bone and perhaps other collagen-supported structures needs to be investigated.

The significance of prostaglandin synthesis and osteolysis in the mechanisms for development of metastases *in vivo* has been studied in several animal tumor models. Prostaglandin synthesis has been shown to be involved in nonmetastatic osteolysis by the H.S.D.M. mouse tumor, which gives rise to hypercalcemia (6). We have used the Walker tumor, which possesses marked *in vitro* osteolytic p operties, in the rat to study the mechanisms for development of bone metastases. We found that using prostaglandin synthesis inhibitors such as aspirin we could prevent development of osteolytic bone deposits and hypercalcemia in rats with this tumor (7). Galasko (8,9) has shown that indomethacin can prevent the early development of the osteolytic VX2 tumor in the femur of the rabbit. He notes that early osteolytic development depends on osteoclast activity presumably stimulated by something released from the tumor cells. Established osteolytic deposits appear to have a direct osteolytic effect on the bone, independent of osteoclasts, and are not influenced by prostaglandin synthesis inhibitory drugs. We have shown that prostaglandin synthesis might be involved in osteoclast activity (10,11), and it is therefore possible that prostaglandin synthesis by the bone cells, and not the tumor cells, is the more important factor in the initial development of bone deposits. This is supported by our observation that prostaglandin synthesis inhibitory agents such as aspirin and indomethacin fail to normalize hypercalcemia or increased hydroxyproline excretion seen with patients who have obvious bone metastases from breast cancer (12).

The part played by macrophages, which may be present in the metastases, is not known. Inflammatory cells are able to synthesize prostaglandins and release osteolytic enzymes. The staphylococcus, which is not osteolytic, is able to stimulate inflammatory cells to cause osteolysis in osteomyelitis, and a similar process could occur with metastases in bone.

Prostaglandin synthesis by host inflammatory cells may be an important factor in the host defense against metastatic development. Therefore, use of prostaglandin synthesis inhibitory agents such as aspirin might enhance metastatic growth in tissues where the antiosteolytic effect is not important. For example, in three out of a series of nine experiments with rats injected intra-aortically with Walker tumor cells, use of aspirin, although inhibitory to development of bone deposits, significantly increased the development of soft tissue tumor (1). In this allogeneic system the host defense may be very important in soft tissue tumor development, particularly when only a small amount of tumor is present, and it is therefore of interest that this apparent enhancement occurred in those experiments where there was relatively little soft tissue tumor.

In conclusion, it seems possible that the ability of tumors to metastasize to bone may not entirely depend on chance, and the subsequent development of metastases in bone may not depend purely on a physical process. Rather, the spread and behavior of tumors in bone may depend on biochemical and biological properties of the tumor cells, particularly the production of biologically active agents such as prostaglandins. A study of these properties may help us to develop methods to control tumor metastases.

REFERENCES

1. Powles, T. J. (1975): A study of in vivo and in vitro osteolysis by human and experimental mammary tumour. Ph.D. Thesis, London University, London.
2. Dowsett, M., Easty, G. C., Powles, T. J., Easty, D. M., and Neville, A. M. (1976): Human breast tumour induced osteolysis and prostaglandins. *Prostaglandins*, 2:447.
3. Powles, T. J., Dowsett, M., Easty, D. M., Easty, G. C., and Neville, A. M. (1976): Breast cancer osteolysis, bone metastases and anti-osteolytic effect of aspirin. *Lancet*, 1:608.
4. Bennett, A., Macdonald, A. M., Simpson, J. S., and Stanford, I. F. (1976): Breast cancer, prostaglandins and bone metastases. *Lancet*, 1:1218.
5. Dowsett, M., Gazet, J. C., Powles, T. J., Easty, G. C., and Neville, A. M. (1976): Benign breast lesions and osteolysis. *Lancet*, 1:970.
6. Tashjian, A. H., Voelkel, E. F., Levine, L., and Goldhaber, P. (1972): Evidence that the bone resorption stimulating factor produced by mouse fibro-sarcoma cells is Prostaglandin E_2. A new model for the hypocalcaemie of cancer. *J. Exp. Med.*, 136:1329.
7. Powles, T. J., Easty, D. M., Easty, G. C., and Neville, A. M. (1973): Inhibition by aspirin and indomethacin of osteolytic tumour deposits and hypercalcaemia in rats with Walker tumour and its possible application to human breast cancer. *Br. J. Cancer*, 28:316.
8. Galasko, C. S. B. (1976): Mechanisms of bone destruction in the development of skeletal metastases. *Nature*, 263:507.
9. Galasko, C. S. B., and Bennett, A. (1976): Relationship of bone destruction in skeletal metastases to osteoclast activation and prostaglandins. *Nature*, 263:508.
10. Powles, T. J., Easty, G. C., Easty, D. M., Bondy, P. K., and Neville, A. M. (1973): Aspirin inhibition of in vitro osteolysis stimulated by PTH and PGE. *Nature [New Biol.]*, 245:83.
11. Dowsett, M., Eastman, A. R., Easty, D. M., Easty, G. C., Powles, T. J., and Neville, A. M. (1976): Prostaglandin mediation of collagen-induced bone resorption. *Nature*, 263:72.
12. Coombes, R. C., Neville, A. M., Bondy, P. K., and Powles, T. J. (1977): Failure of indomethacin to lower the serum calcium in hypercalcaemia complicating breast cancer. *Prostaglandins (in press)*.

Discussion

P. M. Gullino: Two points are not clear. The first concerns the osteotropism of mammary metastases. In human lesions the metastatic localization is mostly in the spongy bone where bone marrow is often present. What evidence do we have that the metastatic localization is bone oriented and not bone marrow oriented? I am asking this question because in the rat model of primary mammary carcinomas induced by methylnitrosourea (1), metastatic spread occurs in the bone marrow first and hypercalcemia occurs later, without signs of bone erosion, and it is eliminated by feeding aspirin (P. M. Gullino, *unpublished*).

The second point concerns the facilitation of metastatic growth allegedly related to prostaglandin production by epithelial cells of mammary carcinomas. What evidence do we have to sustain this supposition? In the methylnitrosourea-induced mammary carcinomas we tried to influence the accumulation of metastatic cells by continuous infusion of prostaglandin E_1 into the bone marrow cavity of the femur. Thus far we have had no success; we have not yet tried infusion of aspirin. I do not know of other experiments aimed at assessing whether products of mammary carcinoma cells favor their capacity for metastatic growth, do you?

T. Powles: It seems to me that there are at least two possible mechanisms for the predominant development of bone metastases in some patients with cancer. One hypothesis is that tumors produce osteolytic substances that are able to circulate throughout the body. This may cause generalized osteolysis and make the bones more susceptible to development of metastases from circulating malignant cells.

An alternative hypothesis is that tumors produce osteolytic substances which can break down bone but which may not be of great importance as circulating factors — for example, the substances may be rapidly inactivated in the circulation or when passing through the lungs. Although a systemic effect is not important, if these tumor cells are able to reach the bones, then production of osteolytic substances locally, causing breakdown of bone, may facilitate the development of tumor deposits at these sites. This advantage would not necessarily apply at other sites. We have shown some evidence that breast tumors are able to produce osteolytic substances, particularly prostaglandins, and that this may in fact predispose to development of bone metastases. The role of circulating prostaglandins in initiation of metabolic bone disease and hypercalcemia is in considerable doubt.

Various experimental models have demonstrated the ability of tumors to produce substances that can circulate and cause metabolic bone disease and hypercalcemia. None of these models has shown a predisposition to development of bone metastases, and to my knowledge, no experiments have been done to show that administration of osteolytic substances enhances development of bone metastases. I therefore think that the local effect in breast cancer is a more attractive hypothesis.

P. M. Gullino: What is the significance of prostaglandin production by tumor cells in sites other than bone?

T. Powles: I think there is a real possibility that production of prostaglandins by tumor or host cells may stimulate the inflammatory host cell response, which could inhibit development of the metastases. It is therefore of some concern that anti-inflammatory agents could enhance metastatic development. Recently it has been shown that prostaglandins can have a direct antitumor effect *in vitro* in soft tissue transplants (2). It is therefore of some concern that inhibition of prostaglandin synthesis could inhibit development of bone deposits by an antiosteolytic effect but enhance development of soft tissue tumor by an anti-inflammatory or direct tumor-stimulating effect.

DISCUSSION REFERENCES

1. Gullino, P. M., Pettigrew, H. M., and Grantham, F. H. (1975): N-Nitrosomethylurea as mammary gland carcinogen in rats. *J. Natl. Cancer Inst.,* 54:401.
2. Santoro, M. G., Philpott, G. W., and Jaffe, B. M. (1976): Inhibition of tumour growth in vivo and in vitro by prostaglandin E. *Nature,* 263:777.

Cancer Invasion and Metastasis: Biologic Mechanisms and Therapy, edited by S. B. Day et al. Raven Press, New York © 1977.

Osteotropism of Human Breast Cancer

Richard S. Bockman and W. P. Laird Myers

Laboratory of Calcium Metabolism, Memorial Sloan-Kettering Cancer Center, New York, New York 10021

Cancer of the breast was the most frequent malignancy and the leading cause of cancer-related deaths in American women from 15 to 74 years of age in 1974 (USPHS, 1974). It was estimated by the American Cancer Society that 88,000 new cases of breast cancer were diagnosed in 1975, and some 32,600 women died of the disease in that same year.

It has long been known that breast cancer preferentially metastasizes to bone. In one autopsy study 75% of the patients demonstrated skeletal involvement (1). More significantly, in a series of patients post-mastectomy, 26% had skeletal involvement as their first sign of recurrence, second only to recurrence in the integument (11). Serial bone scans of a similar group of patients revealed a 23% incidence of bony recurrence within 3 to 24 months after mastectomy (13). In a 10-year follow-up study the incidence of bone metastasis in patients with lymph node involvement in the lower one-third of the axilla (level I), beneath the pectoralis minor muscle (level II), or cephalad to the pectoralis minor muscle at the apex of the axilla (level III) was 18, 34, and 41%, respectively (J. A. Urban, *unpublished observations*). Furthermore, it has been shown that with primary lesions less than 2 cm in diameter 15.6% of the patients developed disease metastatic to bone, whereas in patients with primary lesions from 2 to 4 cm in diameter, 29.2% subsequently manifested disease metastatic to bone during a 10-year follow-up (38). As an additional complication of their disease, up to 40% of patients have been reported to develop hypercalcemia at some time in the course of their disease, the greater percentage of such patients having skeletal involvement (14,20,29).

Although these clinical features of breast carcinoma are well described, the basic mechanism by which the tumor cells show preference to implant themselves, survive, and grow in bone are unclear. The factors which may lead to the implantation and growth of bone metastasis and some of the metabolic disturbances associated with such lesions fall into several groups.

FACTORS LEADING TO IMPLANTATION AND TUMOR GROWTH IN BONE

Biological Activity of Tumors

Evidence for the production by tumors of chemically active substances that may act directly on bone tissue causing osteolysis has increased sharply in recent years. Tumor cell implantation in bone with or without hypercalcemia has been suggested as the result of the elaboration of these substances. On the other hand, a significant number of patients with a variety of cancers may manifest hypercalcemia and/or hypercalciuria in the absence of demonstrable bone metastases (24), and such findings suggest that humoral mediators of bone dissolution could be involved in osteolysis without subsequent tumor cell implantation in bone. Examples of such humoral factors include prostaglandins, and parathyroid hormone.

Prostaglandins

Prostaglandins are 20-carbon fatty acids produced by virtually every tissue in the body. PG content and synthesis has been measured in a variety of animal and human tumors (43,45,49). It has been shown in a chemically induced rat mammary carcinoma that tumor content of PGE_2 and the tumor's synthetic capacity to convert precursor ^{14}C-arachidonic acid to PGE_2 were much greater than those of the adjacent "unstimulated" normal breast tissue (44). In 23 patients with breast cancer, PGE and PGF content and synthesis in the tumor tissues were significantly greater than those of adjacent normal breast tissue or of benign adenomas (3). It should be noted that there are inherent difficulties in comparing PG levels in normal and cancerous breast tissues. In the rat mammary carcinomas the authors do not elaborate on what was histologically identified as normal "unstimulated" breast. Furthermore, the amount of normal glandular breast tissue available for assay in the unstimulated rat is virtually insignificant. In postmenopausal women, tissue adjacent to tumors is essentially adipose tissue; thus, it is not apparent that such comparisons are valid. Nevertheless, in experimental animals as well as in human breast cancer, PG production, particularly of the E class, seems well established but the synthesizing cell has yet to be identified.

In two remarkable animal model experiments tumor growth in bone has been shown to be associated with PG activity. Powles and colleagues (33) have injected Walker carcinoma tumor cells into the abdominal aorta of rats. All rats so injected developed tumors in the soft tissue and bones of their lower extremities. On the average each animal had four tumor deposits in the bones of the lower extremities, and all the animals became hypercalcemic. If these animals were pretreated with aspirin or indomethacin, inhibitors of PG synthetase, growth with bone breakdown was prevented as was the development of hypercalcemia. However, soft-tissue tumor weights were unchanged compared to those of untreated animals (33). Of interest was that histological examination of the lower extremities of the treated animals demonstrated Walker carcinosarcoma cells in the bone marrow but there was no evidence of osteolysis (T. J. Powles, *personal communication*). It would appear that tumor-induced lysis of bone but not tumor localization in bone was specifically inhibited either directly or indirectly. Generalized tumor growth inhibition, i.e., in terms of decreased DNA, RNA, protein synthesis, and metabolic functioning, was unlikely since the tumors grew unimpeded in adjacent soft tissues. This experiment is so provocative that studies directed to understanding the mechanism of aspirin and indomethacin inhibition of tumor growth in bone are in order.

More recently, Strausser and Hume (42) have shown decreased bone invasion to result from pretreatment with indomethacin of mice injected with Maloney sarcoma virus (MSV). In these studies BALB/c mice with MSV-induced leg tumors were shown on histological examination to have tumor invasion of adjacent bone with osteolytic changes seen in the involved bones. Treatment with indomethacin begun at the time of tumor induction reduced tumor growth, and no bone invasion or osteolysis was seen (42). This effect of PG-related tumor invasiveness and growth in bone seems to depend in part on physiological mechanisms which are separate and distinct from that of immune suppression. Nevertheless, immune suppression in the tumor-bearing host clearly plays an important part in promoting the malignant process, and recent experiments have suggested that this may be an indirect mechanism by which PG may facilitate tumor growth.

Parathyroid Hormone

In spite of the current attention focused on PG, all the osteolytic activity found in tissues and sera of breast cancer patients may not be attributable to PG. In 103 of 108 unselected, hypercalcemic cancer patients, inappropriately elevated levels of circulating immunoreactive parathyroid hormone (iPTH) have been reported (4). Fourteen of these patients had breast cancer; four of these had iPTH levels significantly beyond the normal range (4). Although these authors refer to the inappropriate iPTH levels as "ectopic," they failed to demonstrate this. Specifically, (a) tumor tissues were not tested for iPTH, (b) iPTH levels before and after surgical removal of the tumor were not measured, (c) iPTH levels on the afferent and efferent sides of the tumor were not measured, and, lastly, (d) the chemical nature of the "ectopic" iPTH was not studied in the majority of their patients. This last point is particularly telling since the same authors suggested that chemical differences existed between PTH and its tumors immunologues (5,37).

In sharp contrast to the Benson studies are recent reports of hypercalcemic cancer patients with nonmeasurable iPTH levels in their sera (32,39). To confuse matters further, there appears to be a significant occurrence of primary hyperparathyroidism in the breast cancer patient population. In a series of 100 patients with documented primary hyperparathyroidism sequentially observed at Memorial Hospital, 34 had a history of cancer occurring before, coincident with, or following discovery of hyperparathyroidism, and 10 of these patients had breast carcinoma (9,47). Two patients with breast cancer and probable (nonsurgically documented) primary hyperparathyroidism recently followed at Memorial Hospital highlight the possible role of PTH in facilitating metastasis to bone. A 54-year-old woman presented with a breast mass in 4/75 for which she underwent a modified radical mastectomy for infiltrating duct cancer. At the time of surgery she was noted to be hypercalcemic and her iPTH level was found to be 83 μlEq/ml, far exceeding the upper range of normal (40 μlEq/ml). Within 6 months of her surgery a skeletal survey (which initially showed no evidence of bone disease) revealed widespread lytic bone metastases. A similarly rapid course was more recently observed in a 39-year-old patient whose iPTH level at the time of mastectomy was 190 μlEq/ml. She developed lytic bone disease within 18 months of tumor detection.

Impairment of Local Immune Response

Certain factors impair local immune response, which is necessary for impeding tumor growth in bone tissue. Immune deficiency in cancer patients and tumor-bearing animals has previously been described (15,21,23). Circulating tumor antigens, antigen-antibody complexes (8,40), and serum blocking factors (16,17) have been postulated to be mechanisms of blocking host immunity. More recently, spleen-derived suppressor cells have been demonstrated in tumor-bearing mice. Such animals with suppressed T-cell response to mitogenic stimulation could have this reactivity restored by the removal of an adherent macrophage cell population (22,23). Interestingly, unstimulated human monocytes have been demonstrated to produce significant amounts of PGE, 1.0 ng/10⁶ cells. PGE has been shown to inhibit the production of macrophage inhibitor factor (MIF) by T lymphocytes and to inhibit antibody production by B lymphocytes (7,27,36,41). Furthermore, aspirin and indomethacin could reverse the tumor immunosuppression (mimicked by PGE_2 in vitro) in mice bearing experimental cancers (30,31, 42). The retardation of tumor growth seen in the latter PG synthesis-inhibited animals presumably was due to the restoration of the host's immune responsiveness.

Activation of Other Biological Systems

Factors related to the activation of other biological systems of the body by the tumor result in local or generalized skeletal and metabolic disturbances. Specifically, circulating mononuclear cells are known to produce a host of biologically active substances when stimulated. Recently, an osteolytic substance known as osteoclast-activating factor (OAF) has been described (19). Initially, OAF was demonstrated in the supernatant media of phytohemagglutinin (PHA)-stimulated peripheral blood leukocytes (19,46). OAF was noted to be released within 6 hr of PHA stimulation, and its peak production coincided with the peak of amino acid incorporation into protein, i.e., before the peak of DNA synthesis. OAF was found to be released by stimulated lymphocytes, but in order to initiate release the presence of an adherent macrophage population was required (18). However, OAF-like activity has been demonstrated by fetal rat bone assay following PHA stimulation of human T cells cultured in the absence of adherent cells. OAF was subsequently demonstrated to be produced by unstimulated lymphoid cell lines from patients with myeloma and Burkitts' and malignant lymphomas (28). Partially characterized, OAF appears to be a protein with a molecular weight of 18,000 with differing heat and enzymatic degradation susceptibilities when compared to PTH (25). Smaller molecular forms of OAF have been described (G. R. Mundy, *personal communication*).

It should be noted that stimulated lymphocytes have been demonstrated to facilitate tumor growth and metastasis to soft tissues *in vitro* (8,35). As suggested previously, osteolysis could initiate or facilitate breast carcinoma metastasis to bone, possibly via OAF. Such metastases could then be nurtured by lymphocytes stimulated by passage through breast cancer tissues. In this sense the tumor could be subverting normal host defenses. The circulating mononuclear cells are prime candidates for being recruited by tumors as they travel freely throughout the body and notably in bone.

Invaded Bone Tissue

Factors inherent in the invaded bone tissue may render it more or less vulnerable to tumor invasion and more or less reactive locally or generally to such an invasion. Such factors may include the state of mineralization, collagen turnover, and the ground substance. At the present time there is no evidence in the literature that such factors play any role in the osteotropism of breast cancer.

EXPERIMENTAL DATA

In a recently published study, the osteolytic activity of breast cancer tissue from 38 patients was analyzed. Tumors from 23 patients were found to have osteolytic activity when the tumor tissues were co-cultured with fetal rat calvaria *in vitro,* whereas those from the 15 other patients did not. Follow-up of the patients over a 3-year period revealed seven patients to have developed bone metastases, and four of these became hypercalcemic. All seven of the latter patients came from the tumor group with osteolytic activity (34). The osteolytic activity found in these tumors has not been characterized chemically or by dose dependency curves in bone cultures.

It would seem that in order to establish which if any of the previously mentioned factors determine the osteotropism of breast cancer, the following sequence of experimental steps needs to be carried out. A population of breast cancer patients in whom the risk of metastatic disease is high should be followed prospectively in order to study: (a) the presence or appearance of circulating osteolytic factors and the chemical identification of these factors; and (b) the immune status of these patients with regard to mitogen responsiveness and OAF (lymphokine) production. Initial results of such a study which are presented in this volume are considered preliminary and base-line values from which correlations with subsequent clinical course will be drawn.

METHODS

Patient Selection

Patients with breast cancer were selected for study at the time of their primary surgery. Study patients were chosen on the basis of having an operable infiltrating carcinoma where the primary lesion was 2 cm or greater with or without nodal disease. Such patients, as previously noted, have a significant incidence of developing metastatic disease to bone. None of the patients had received prior radiation or chemotherapy. Initial serum samples and circulating cells were obtained prior to surgery and/or medical treatment. Tissue samples were obtained at the time of mastectomy.

Circulating Osteolytic Factors

Parathyroid Hormone

Fasting serum samples were assayed for immunoreactive PTH by the method of Arnaud et al. (2). The upper limit of normal by this method is about 40 μlEq/ml.

Prostaglandin E

Serum- or tissue-conditioned media samples were immediately extracted with acidified ethylacetate, then fractionated on a silicic acid column to isolate prostaglandin E (PGE). The PGE was measured by radioimmuno-assay using a double antibody method, which proved capable of measuring as little as 10 pg of PGE. The antibody was highly specific for the parent

PGE compounds cross-reacting only 1/60th to 1/400th as well with the major blood metabolites 15-keto PGE_2 and 13,14-dihydro PGE_2, respectively.

Immune Cells

Isolation and Culture

Mononuclear cells comprising approximately 80 to 90% lymphocytes and 10 to 20% monocytes were isolated from heparinized blood by differential sedimentation in ficoll hypaque (6). The cells washed free of the ficoll hypaque were suspended in McCoy's media (26) with 10% heat-inactivated fetal calf serum (FCS), and incubated at 37° in a 5% CO_2 atmosphere for 72 hr without and with purified phytohemagglutinin (Burroughs Wellcome). Tritiated thymidine incorporation was measured between the 72nd and 90th hr of culture. Cell-free medium harvested at 72 hr was subsequently assayed by radioimmunoassay for prostaglandin E as well as tested for osteolytic activity in a fetal rat bone assay system.

Tumor Tissues

Tumor tissues freshly obtained from frozen biopsy specimens were cut into 1-mm cubes and either co-cultured with fetal rat bones or cultured alone in the McCoy's. The latter tumor-conditioned medium (TCM) was subsequently tested in the fetal rat bone assay. Radioimmunoassay for PGE was carried out on the TCM.

Fetal Rat Bone Culture System

Some 16-day pregnant Sprague-Dawley rats were injected (s.c.) with 400 to 500 μCi $^{45}CaCl_2$ to deep label the fetal rat bones. The embryos were collected on the 19th day and the ^{45}Ca-labeled fetal rat ulnae and radii were dissected free of surrounding tissues. Intact paired bones were used as control (C) and experimental (E) bones, respectively. The individual bones were cultured separately on stainless steel rafts according to a modification of the technique described by Fell and Mellanby (10) in Biggers media (5a) with 5% heat-inactivated fetal calf serum; the experimental media also contained an aliquot of a test substance (TCM, lymphocyte condition media, PTH, or PG). After a 72-hr incubation at 37°C in a 5% CO_2 atmosphere, the media were counted in a liquid scintillation counter to measure ^{45}Ca released into the media. Each paired sample served as its own control with the data expressed as the ratio (E/C) of ^{45}Ca as counts per minute released by the experimental bones divided by the ^{45}Ca counts per minute of the control. The mean ratio of 45 control/control bones was found to be

0.97 ± 0.02 ($\bar{X}_{45}$ ± SEM); therefore, any E/C exceeding 1.01 ($\bar{X}$ ± 2 SEM) can be assumed to be significant with *p* less than 0.05. Dose-dependent bone resorption in this *in vitro* system can be used to identify the osteolytic agent. PTH has a very steep dose dependency where E/C can vary from 1.0 to 2.0 over the molar range of 2×10^{-8} to 10^{-7}, whereas PGE_2 and its active metabolite 13,14-dihydro PGE_2 have a shallow dose dependency where E/C varies from 1.0 to 1.5 over the molar range of 10^{-9} to 10^{-5}M. Histological sections of the cultured fetal rat bones were analyzed.

RESULTS

Patient Population

Of the 24 patients initially studied, 11 fulfilled the requirements for entry into the prospective study (Table 1). All 11 patients had infiltrating duct carcinoma and all underwent radical mastectomy. Five of eleven had nodal involvement on pathological examination. The age range of these patients was 32 to 69 years with a median of 57 years. One of the eleven patients was found by bone scan and skeletal survey to have X-ray evidence of a single metastatic lesion at the head of the humerus at the beginning of this study. The initial serum calcium was elevated in one patient (11.8 mg%), and the serum phosphorus was low in one other patient (2.4 mg%). Alkaline phosphatase determinations were elevated in 4 of 11 patients studied, and all 4 of these patients had nodal involvement but normal serum calciums and negative bone X-rays or scans. None of these patients had abnormal renal or liver function tests. The patients have been entered into the study for more than 6 months with 9 months being the longest follow-up. No recurrent disease has yet been reported. Only two of these patients have received postoperative chemotherapy.

Circulating Osteolytic Factors

Parathyroid Hormone

In the six patients in whom it was measured, immunoreactive PTH was found to be elevated in two patients, range 45 to 47 μlEq/ml. In one of

TABLE 1. *Summary of clinical findings*

Patient (No.)	Age range	Nodal disease			Highest level				Size of primary (cm)		
		0	1–3	>4	0	I	II	III	1–1.9	2–2.9	≥3
11	32–69	6	2	3	6	1	0	4	0	3	8

these patients the serum calcium was at the upper limit of normal, 10.8 mg%. In both of these patients the serum phosphorus was within normal limits, whereas the serum alkaline phosphatase activity was elevated in one patient.

Prostaglandin E

The average serum value of PGE for the seven patients with measurable values was 2.47 ± 0.88 ng/ml (± SEM); the range for all patients was less than 0.01 to 5.53 ng/ml. This average is significantly elevated when compared to the mean of six normals (0.56 ± 0.19 ng/ml (± SEM).

Immune Cells

Cell Counts and Thymidine Incorporation

No significant differences in the absolute or relative mononuclear cell counts were noted when the normals were compared to breast cancer patients. Nor was there a significant difference in the response to the mitogen PHA measured either as tritiated thymidine incorporation or by cytological methods between the normal and the breast cancer patients. Mononuclear cells from normals when incubated with PHA and tritiated thymidine showed incorporation of 33,590 ± 4,560 dpm/100,000 cells (± SEM) compared to breast cancer patients of 30,980 ± 3,792 dpm/100,000 cells (± SEM).

Prostaglandin E

PGE levels measured in the cell-free media from the lymphocyte cultures of the 11 breast cancer patients averaged 0.22 ng/ml (± SEM) for plain cultures and 0.19 ± 0.07 ng/ml (± SEM) in the PHA-stimulated cultures at the end of 72 hr of incubation. In no case was the level of PGE measured sufficient to account totally for the resorption caused by that conditioned medium in the bone culture assay system (Table 2).

TABLE 2. PGE production

Lymphocyte-conditioned media[a]		Tumor-conditioned media[b]
Plain	+PHA	
0.22 ± 0.08	0.19 ± 0.7	0.60 ± 0.25

[a] ng PGE/ml produced by 10^6 mononuclear cells after 72 hr in McCoy's and fetal calf serum—heat inactivated, isolated from peripheral blood of breast cancer patients.

[b] ng PGE/ml produced by 1-mm^3 breast cancer slice (wet weight $\bar{X}_7 = 0.028 \pm 0.004$ mg) in 2 ml of McCoy's media.

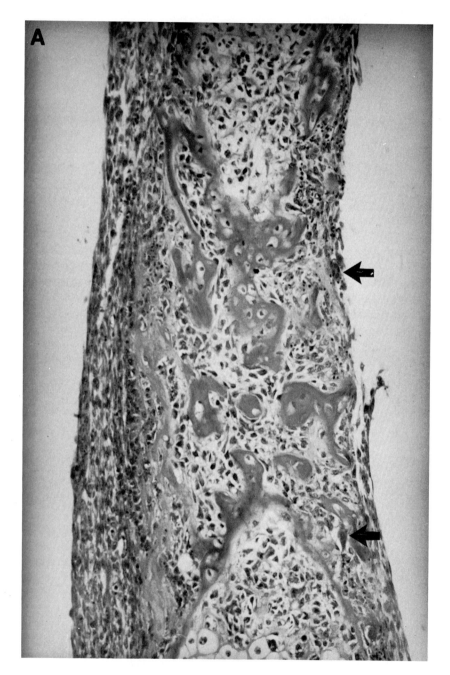

FIG. 1. Shaft portion of fetal rat ulnae, explanted on day 19 and cultured for 72 hr (×10). **(A):** Control bone. **(B):** Experimental bone co-cultured with 1-mm slice of breast cancer, E/C of ^{45}Ca release after 72 hr in culture was 1.5 ± 0.15 (± SEM). Marked diminution in bone matrix and an increase in the number of multinucleated osteoclasts (*arrows*) are evident.

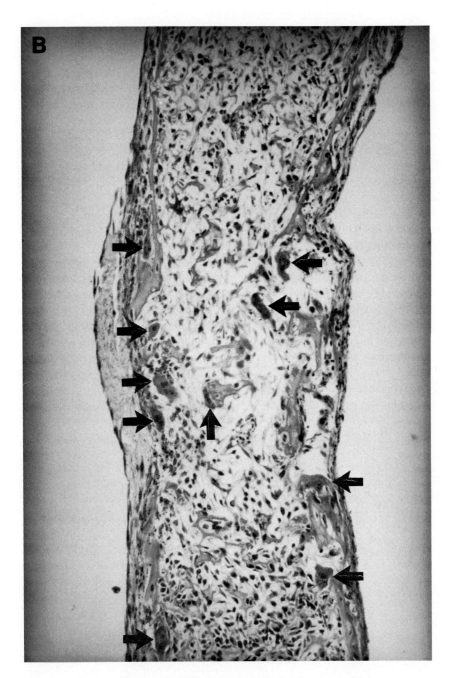

FIG. 1. (*continued*).

Tumor Tissues

The amount of PGE released into the media from a 1-mm³ slice of tumor tissues from 8 of 11 patients was measured by radioimmunoassay. The average PGE level per milliliter of media was 0.60 ± 0.25 ng ($\pm$ SEM) (Table 2).

Media conditioned by 1-mm³ slices of tumor tissue were tested in the bone culture assay. Only one of these tumor-conditioned media of the eight tested demonstrated significant bone resorbing activity, E/C = 1.1. The PGE concentration for this TCM was 2.22 ng/culture. The average E/C of ^{45}Ca release for the TCM was 0.81 ± 0.06 ($\pm$ SEM) from 1 ml of conditioned medium.

Tumor tissue slices from four patients with breast cancer were co-cultured with fetal rat bones in the bone assay system. Tumor tissues from two patients demonstrated significant bone resorption—E/C ^{45}Ca release equal to 1.5 ± 0.15 and 1.14 ± 0.3 ($\overline{X}_4 \pm$ SEM) for each test sample compared to control cultures 0.97 ± 0.02 ($\overline{X}_{45} \pm$ SEM); $p < 0.001$ and < 0.05, respectively, in the two-tailed Student's t-test.

Histological review of the fetal rat bones co-cultured with the human breast tumor slices that caused ^{45}Ca release confirmed marked loss of bone matrix. An increase in osteoclastic activity was evidenced by an increase in the number of multinucleated and vacuolated osteoclasts seen compared to those in sections from control bones. The normal marrow elements appeared diminished in number (Fig. 1).

Lymphocyte-Derived Osteoclast-Activating Factor

The lymphocyte-derived OAF was studied in 11 patients by measuring the ability of lymphocyte-conditioned media (LCM) to release ^{45}Ca from labeled fetal rat bones. Compared to control cultures where no LCM had been added, the LCM of all 11 patients were active in causing significant resorption. The latter occurred with and without the mitogen PHA being present in the lymphocyte culture. However, by the same criteria, the LCM of seven of the ten control cultures from normals showed significant ^{45}Ca release. By comparison, only five of the LCM (without PHA) from eleven patients with a variety of cancers (including three lymphomas, two adenocarcinomas of unknown primary, two head and neck, one chronic lymphocytic leukemia, one thyroid, one liver, and one myxoliposarcoma) were active, causing significant ^{45}Ca release. The averages of the osteolytic activities for the LCM from the normals, cancer patients, and breast cancer patients are given in Table 3. Dose dependency curves of the ^{45}Ca release from the LCM of two breast cancer patients (E/C = 1.98 and 2.05) are given in Fig. 2. The curves are compared to the dose dependency of PTH. Histological sections of the fetal rat bones cultured with the LCM of a breast

TABLE 3. *E/C ^{45}Ca release (mean ± SEM) induced by LCM*[a]

Group	No PHA	With PHA
Normals (10)	1.25 ± 0.13	1.56 ± 0.10
Cancer (11)	1.07 ± 0.08	1.23 ± 0.06[c]
Breast cancer (11)	1.60 ± 0.11[b]	1.61 ± 0.11

[a] Osteolytic activity produced by 10^6 mononuclear cells cultured 72 hr in 1 ml of McCoy's and 10% fetal calf serum—heat inactivated.
[b] Differs significantly from normals ($p < 0.05$); from cancer $p < 0.005$.
[c] Differs significantly from normals and breast cancer patients ($p < 0.005$).

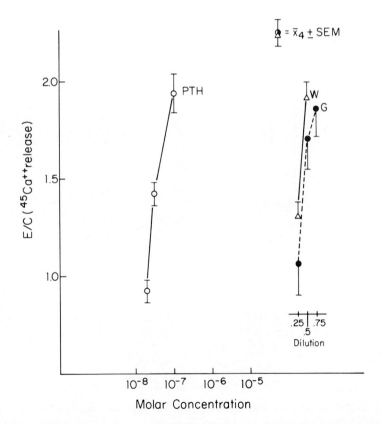

FIG. 2. Dose dependency curves of LCM-derived activity from 2 patients. The dilution and molar scale are to the same scale.

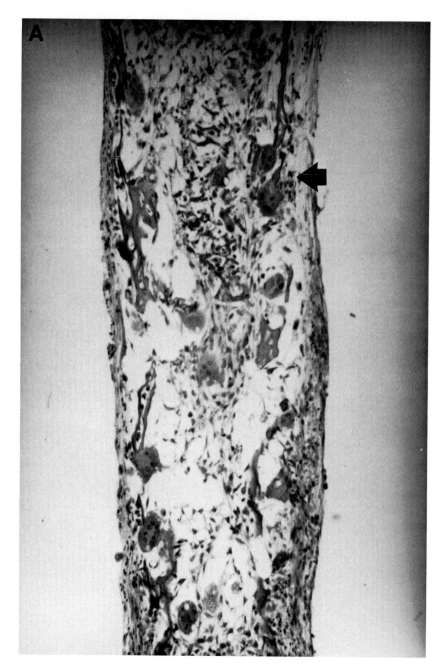

FIG. 3. Explanted fetal rat ulna, shaft portion, that had been exposed for 72 hr to the LCM from a breast cancer patient whose E/C = 2.05. **(A):** Low-power view (×10). **(B):** Same section as **A** at higher power (×25).

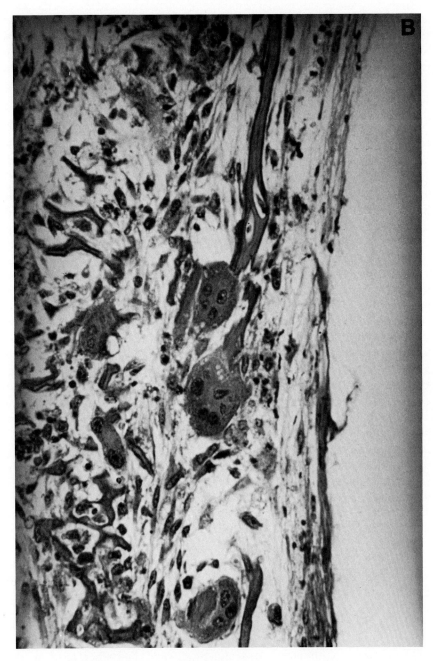

FIG. 3. *(continued)*.

cancer patient whose osteolytic activity was high (E/C = 2.05) are shown in Fig. 3. Marked diminution of bone matrix was evident. Numerous multinucleated and vacuolated osteoclasts were seen, far in excess of those in any PTH- or PGE-treated bones. The majority of the osteoclasts were in contact with the bone matrix, and many osteoclasts were found to be partially engulfing the ends of bone matrix.

CONCLUSION

Circulating Osteolytic Agents

When looked for, elevations of serum immunoreactive parathyroid hormone and PGE could be demonstrated in subpopulations of patients with breast cancer.

iPTH has frequently been demonstrated to be elevated in cancer patients by the carboxyl terminus-specific Mayo assay which was used in this study. It is conceivable in light of the known coincidence of breast cancer and primary hyperparathyroidism (9) that the two patients with elevated iPTH may have had concomitant parathyroid disease, but there were no other supporting clinical findings to indicate this. We plan to reassay the original sera from our patients with another anti-PTH serum and to correlate these data with urinary cyclic AMP levels to ascertain the validity of the assumption that excess (biologically active) PTH is present in these patients. Although it could be suggested that the biologically inactive but immunoreactive carboxyl terminus portion of PTH has a half-life longer than normal in these patients, this possibility seems unlikely. All the patients had normal liver and renal function and presumably normal PTH metabolism.

In our radioimmunoassay serum PGE levels have been found to be significantly elevated in cancer patients compared to normals. The coincident occurrence of hypercalcemia in 15 cancer patients with a variety of solid tumors was not associated with an increased frequency of hyperprostaglandinemia E compared to normocalcemic cancer patients. The nonspecific finding of hyperprostaglandinemia in cancer patients raises questions as to their source. Although breast cancer tissues have been demonstrated to synthesize PGE_2 (3,44), so do adherent mononuclear cells (27; Bockman, *unpublished observations*), which are frequently seen in breast cancer tissues in our experience.

Immune Cells

No evidence of immune cell dysfunction was found when *in vitro* tests were carried out on a similar group of breast cancer patients compared to normals (48). In our study with regard to absolute lymphocyte counts and response to mitogen (PHA) stimulation, no difference compared to normals existed. However, it is clear that total counts of heterogenous populations of cells and response to nonphysiological cell stimulants are crude measures of cell function. Immune cell-derived PGE and lymphokines such as osteoclast-activating factor could have significant biological consequences yet be unmeasured by gross cell counts or cell transformation.

Tumor Tissue

PGE could be measured in the majority of tumor-conditioned media studied. The source of the PGE as previously mentioned cannot necessarily be attributed to the cancer cells since such tissues represent a heterogeneous population of normal tissues (including infiltrating immune cells) and malignant cells. In only one case could significant ($p < 0.05$) osteolytic activity be found in the TCM when assayed in the bone culture system. Interestingly, this same TCM had the highest measurable concentration of PGE, 2.22 ng/2 ml medium (equivalent to 3.15×10^{-9}M), which could have wholly accounted for the amount of bone resorption seen based on the dose dependency curves for PGE_2 in the fetal bone assay. In the two patients whose tumor-bone co-culture demonstrated significant fetal bone resorption, the levels of PGE in the TCM were far too low to account for the osteolytic activity seen. It should be pointed out that the fetal rat bone assay is a delicately balanced *in vitro* system that can probably respond with increased or decreased $^{45}Ca^{++}$ release to a number of physiological and nonphysiological stimuli. Dose dependency and histological evaluation are therefore essential components in the analysis of the bone culture system, but they do not identify nonspecific causes of *in vitro* bone resorption.

Osteoclast-Activating Factor

Since OAF was first described (19), a role for the lymphokine in tumor-induced osteolysis has been sought, and possibly found in the case of multiple myeloma (28). In looking at the unstimulated LCM of the breast cancer patients studied, it was possible to demonstrate significant osteolytic activity in 11 of 11. However, significant osteolysis (E/C > 1.01) could similarly be demonstrated in the unstimulated LCM of 7 of 10 normals. The mean unstimulated LCM activities of breast cancer patients versus normals were 1.60 versus 1.25 and differed significantly ($p < 0.05$) in the two-tailed Student's t-test. No statistically significant difference was noted between normals and 11 patients with a variety of cancer whose disease was associated with a very low incidence of bone metastasis. By contrast, the LCM activity of this latter cancer group was significantly ($p < 0.005$) less than that of the breast cancer group. Dose dependency curves of the LCM osteolysis activity paralleled that previously described for OAF (28).

The chemical nature of the LCM osteolytic activity is unknown at this time. Clearly, the measured osteolytic activity from dose dependency and known PGE levels measured in the LCM cannot be attributed to PGE. Although the dose dependency curves are similar to those of PTH, it is inconceivable that 10^6 lymphocytes (representing 1.0 mg tissue weight) could produce a PTH concentration of 10^{-7}M (equivalent to 1 μg/ml, or 0.1% of the tissue weight), the level of PTH necessary to account for the osteolysis induced in the LCM-treated fetal rat bones. Whatever the substance turns out to be, histological review confirms the appropriateness of the name osteoclast-activating factor for this activity (Fig. 3).

When looked for, a variety of chemical and cellular mediators of osteolysis can be found in the breast cancer population at significant risk to develop bone metastasis. Which if any of these agents correlate with and therefore are suspect in facilitating or promoting tumor metastasis to bone must await the clinical follow-up of these patients. The finding of a probable lymphokine which may cause osteolysis to occur in breast cancer patients at significant risk to develop bone metastases is felt to be relevant to the osteotropism of this cancer. Such data lend support to the concept of tumor recruitment and/or subversion of host defense mechanism to the detriment of the host as evidenced in recent studies (12) in which host macrophages could be shown to carry out osteolysis, creating tumor space and probably facilitating tumor growth in bone. Such data as presented by Galasko and Powles remain consistent with the hypothesis of osteolysis favoring tumor osteotropism, but they do not prove the hypothesis. Further correlative and direct experimental evidence is being sought.

ACKNOWLEDGMENT

The authors would like to express their appreciation to Drs. A. Dimich, D. Bajorunas, R. Ashikari, D. Kinne, and Miss R. Davis for their assistance in accumulating the clinical material; to Mrs. V. Carney, Miss M. Lehr, and Mr. R. Ferguson for their technical assistance; and to Mrs. N. Gavryck for typing the manuscript. This work has been supported in part by National Cancer Institute Grants 08748-10A,B and CA 05826, American Cancer Society Grant PDT-60, and New York State Health Research Council Grant #469.

REFERENCES

1. Abrams, H. L., Spiro, R., and Goldstein, N. (1950): Metastases in carcinoma. *Cancer,* 3:74–85.
2. Arnaud, C. D., Tsao, H. S., and Littledike, T. (1971): Radioimmunoassay of human parathyroid hormone in serum. *J. Clin. Invest.,* 50:21–34.
3. Bennett, A., McDonald, A. M., Simpson, J. S., and Stamford, I. F. (1975): Breast cancer, prostaglandins and bone metastasis. *Lancet,* 1:1218–1220.
4. Benson, R. C., Riggs, B. L., Pickard, B. M., and Arnaud, C. D. (1974): Radioimmunoassay

of parathyroid hormone in hypercalcemic patients with malignant disease. *Am. J. Med.,* 56:821–826.

5. Benson, R. C., Riggs, B. L., Pickard, B. M., and Arnaud, C. D. (1974): Immunoreactive forms of circulating parathyroid hormone in primary and ectopic hyperparathyroidism. *J. Clin. Invest.,* 54:175–181.

5a. Biggers, J. D., Gwatkin, R. B. L., and Heyner, S. (1961): Growth of embryonic avian and mammalian tibiae on a relatively simple chemically defined medium. *Exp. Cell Res.,* 25: 41–58.

6. Böyum, A. (1968): A one-stage procedure for isolation of granulocytes and lymphocytes from human blood. *Scand. J. Clin. Lab. Invest.* [*Suppl. 97*], 21:51–76.

7. Bray, M. A., Gordon, D., and Morley, J. (1974): Proceedings: Role of prostaglandins in reactions of cellular immunity. *Br. J. Pharmacol.,* 52:453P.

8. Currie, G. A. and Basham, C. (1972): Serum mediated inhibition of the immunological reactions of the patients to his own tumor: A possible role for circulating antigen. *Br. J. Cancer,* 26:427.

9. Farr, H. W., Fahey, T. J., Nash, A. G., and Farr, C. M. (1973): Primary hyperparathyroidism and cancer. *Am. J. Surg.,* 126:539.

10. Fell, H. B., and Mellanby, E. (1952): The effect of hypervitaminosis A on embryonic limb-bones cultured *in vitro. J. Physiol.,* 116:320.

11. Fischer, B., Ravdin, R. G., Ausman, R. K., Slack, N. H., Moore, G. E., and Noer, R. G. (1968): Surgical adjuvant chemotherapy in cancer of the breast. *Ann. Surg.,* 168:337.

12. Galasko, C. S. B. (1976): Mechanism of bone destruction in the development of skeletal metastases. *Nature,* 263:507–508.

13. Gerber, F. H., Goodman, J. J., and Kirchner, P. T. (1975): Te-99m-EHDP bone scanning in breast carcinoma. *J. Nucl. Med.,* 16:529.

14. Gordan, G. S., Eisenberg, E., Loken, H. F., Gardner, B., and Hayashida, T. (1962): Clinical endocrinology of parathyroid hormone excess. *Recent Prog. Horm. Res.,* 18: 297–336.

15. Harris, J., and Bagai, R. C. (1972): Immune deficiency states associated with malignant diseases in man. *Med. Clin. North Am.,* 56:501.

16. Hellström, I., and Hellström, K. E. (1969): Studies on cellular immunity and its serum mediated inhibition in Moloney-virus-induced mouse sarcoma. *Int. J. Cancer,* 4:587.

17. Hellström, I., Hellström, K. E., Evans, C. A., Heppner, G. H., Pierce, G. E., and Yang, J. P. S. (1969): Serum mediated protection of neoplastic cells from inhibition by lymphocytes immune to their tumor-specific antigens. *Proc. Natl. Acad. Sci. U.S.A.,* 62:362.

18. Horton, J. E., Oppenheim, J. J., Mergenhager, S. E., and Raisz, L. G. (1974): Macrophage-lymphocyte synergy of the production of osteoclast factor. *J. Immunol.,* 113:1278–1287.

19. Horton, J. E., Raisz, L. G., Simmons, H. A., Oppenheim, J. J., and Mergenhagen, S. E. (1972): Bone resorbing activity on supernatant fluid from cultured human peripheral blood leukocytes. *Science,* 177:793–795.

20. Jessiman, A. G., Emerson, K., Shah, R. C., and Moore, F. D. (1963): Hypercalcemia in carcinoma of the breast. *Ann. Surg.,* 157:377–393.

21. Kersey, J. H., Spector, B. D., and Good, R. A. (1973): Immunodeficiency and cancer. *Adv. Cancer Res.,* 18:211.

22. Kilburn, D. G., Smith, J. B., and Gorczynski, R. M. (1974): Nonspecific suppression of T lymphocyte responses in mice carrying progressively growing tumors. *Eur. J. Immunol.,* 4:784.

23. Kirchner, H., Herberman, R. B., Glaser, M., and Lavrin, S. H. (1974): Suppression of *in vitro* lymphocyte stimulation in mice bearing primary Moloney sarcoma virus induced tumor. *Cell. Immunol.,* 13:32.

24. Lafferty, F. W. (1966): Pseudohyperparathyroidism. *Medicine (Baltimore),* 45:247–260.

25. Luben, R. A., Mundy, G. R., Trummel, C. L., and Raisz, L. G. (1974): Partial purification of osteoclast activating factor from phytohemagglutinin-stimulated human leukocytes. *J. Clin. Invest.,* 53:1473–1480.

26. McCoy, T. A., Maxwell, M., and Kruse, P. F., Jr. (1959): Amino acid requirements of the Novikoff hepatoma *in vitro. Proc. Soc. Exp. Biol. Med.,* 100:115–118.

27. Morley, J. (1974): Prostaglandins and lymphokines in arthritis. *Prostaglandins,* 8:315.

28. Mundy, G. R., Luben, R. A., Raisz, L. G., Oppenheim, J. J., and Buell, C. N. (1974):

Bone-resorbing activity in supernatants from lymphoid cell lines. *N. Engl. J. Med.*, 290: 867–871.

29. Myers, W. P. L. (1973): Hypercalcemia associated with malignant diseases. In: *Endocrine and Nonendocrine Hormone Producing Tumors*, pp. 147–171. Year Book Medical Publishers, Chicago.
30. Pelus, L. M., and Strausser, H. R. (1976): Indomethacin enhancement of spleen-cell responsiveness to mitogen stimulation in tumorous mice. *Int. J. Cancer*, 18:653–660.
31. Plescia, O. J., Smith, A. H., and Grinwich, K. (1975): Subversion of immune system by tumor cells and role of prostaglandins. *Proc. Natl. Acad. Sci. U.S.A.*, 72:1848–1851.
32. Powell, D., Singer, F. R., Murray, T. M., Minkin, C., and Potts, J. T., Jr. (1973): Nonparathyroid humoral hypercalcemia in patients with neoplastic diseases. *N. Engl. J. Med.*, 289:176.
33. Powles, T. J., Clark, S. A., Easty, D., Easty, G. C., and Munro-Neville, A. (1973): The inhibition of aspirin and indomethacin of osteolytic tumour deposits and hypercalcemia in rats with Walker tumour and its possible application to human breast cancer. *Br. J. Cancer*, 28:316–321.
34. Powles, T. J., Dowsett, M., Easty, G. C., Easty, D. M., and Neville, A. M. (1976): Breast-cancer osteolysis, bone metastasis and anti-osteolytic effect of aspirin. *Lancet*, 7960:608–610.
35. Prehn, R. T. (1972): The immune reaction as a stimulator of tumor growth. *Science*, 176: 170–171.
36. Quagliata, F., Lawrence, W. J. M., and Phillips-Quagliata, J. M. (1973): Prostaglandin E 1 as a regulator of lymphocyte function. Selective action on B lymphocytes and synergy with procarbazine in depression of immune responses. *Cell Immunol.*, 6:457.
37. Riggs, B. L., Arnaud, C. D., Reynolds, J. C., and Smith, L. H. (1971): Immunological differentiation of primary hyperparathyroidism from hyperparathyroidism due to nonparathyroid cancer. *J. Clin. Invest.*, 50:2079–2083.
38. Robbins, G. F., Knapper, W. H., Barrie, J., Kripalani, I., and Lawrence, J. (1972): Metastatic bone disease developing in patients with potentially curable breast cancer. *Cancer*, 29:1702.
39. Seyberth, H. W., Segre, G. U., Morgan, J. L., Sweetman, B. J., Potts, J. T., Jr., and Oates, J. A. (1975): Prostaglandins as mediators of hypercalcemia associated with certain types of cancer. *N. Engl. J. Med.*, 293:1278–2183.
40. Sjorgren, H. O., Hellström, I., Bonsal, S. C., and Hellström, H. E. (1971): Suggestive evidence that the "blocking antibodies" of tumor-bearing individuals may be antigen-antibody complexes. *Proc. Natl. Acad. Sci. U.S.A.*, 68:1372.
41. Smith, R. S., Sherman, N. A., and Coffey, R. G. (1974): Effects of pokeweed mitogen, cholera toxin and prostaglandin E 1 on immunoglobin production and cyclic AMP levels in tonsillar lymphocytes. *Int. Arch. Allergy*, 47:586.
42. Strausser, H. R., and Hume, J. L. (1975): Prostaglandin synthesis inhibition: Effect on bone changes and sarcoma tumor induction in BALB/c mice. *Int. J. Cancer*, 15:724.
43. Sykes, J. A. C., and Maddox, I. S. (1972): Prostaglandin production by experimental tumors and effects of anti-inflammatory compounds. *Nature [New Biol.]*, 237:59–61.
44. Tan, W. C., Privett, O. S., and Goldyne, M. E. (1974): Studies of prostaglandins in rat mammary tumors induced by 7,12-dimethylbenz(a)anthracene. *Cancer Res.*, 34:3229–3231.
45. Tashjian, A. H., Voekel, E. F., Goldhaber, P., and Levine, L. (1974): Prostaglandins, calcium metabolism and cancer. *Fed. Proc.*, 33:81–86.
46. Trummel, C. L., Mundy, G. R., and Raisz, L. G. (1975): Release of osteoclast activating factor by normal peripheral blood leukocytes. *J. Lab. Clin. Med.*, 85:1001–1007.
47. Vichayanrat, A., Avramides, A., Gardner, B., Wallach, S., and Carter, A. C. (1976): Primary hyperparathyroidism and breast cancer. *Am. J. Med.*, 61:136–139.
48. Wanebo, H. J., Rosen, P. P., Thaler, T., Urban, J. A., and Oettgen, H. F. (1976): Immunobiology of operable breast cancer. *Ann. Surg.*, 184:258–267.
49. Williams, E. D., Karim, S. M., and Sandler, M. (1968): Prostaglandin secretion by medullary carcinoma of the thyroid. *Lancet*, 1:22–23.

Cancer Invasion and Metastasis: Biologic Mechanisms and Therapy, edited by S. B. Day et al. Raven Press, New York © 1977.

Rationale for Adjuvant Chemotherapy

Frank M. Schabel, Jr.

Southern Research Institute, Birmingham, Alabama 35205

Surgery or radiation therapy fails to cure clinically evident human cancer, in the main, if the disease is systemic (has metastasized) when first recognized, because neither modality can effectively remove or kill distant and/or unrecognized metastases. Starting drug treatment of a tumor when it is first clinically recognized or when it represents, following noncurative surgical or radiological treatment, fails to cure over 90% of cancer in man because the body burden of tumor cells exceeds the tumor cell kill potential of nearly all of the most effective drugs or drug combinations against most tumors. The indicated approach to improving cure rates under these circumstances is to use chemotherapy as an adjuvant to effective (life-prolonging) but noncurative surgical and/or radiological treatment. Surgical adjuvant chemotherapy of carcinoma of the breast and osteogenic sarcoma has already been shown to increase the disease-free interval over that obtained with surgery alone, and the probability of having achieved significant increases in long-term cure rates is high.

Laboratory studies with transplantable metastatic lung, breast, and colon carcinomas and melanotic melanoma, and with a spontaneous breast carcinoma of mice, all of which are uniformly fatal if untreated, have shown that: (a) the incidence of metastatic disease is directly related to tumor mass, (b) surgical cure rates drop as tumor mass at surgery increases, (c) grossly evident primary tumors are generally not curable by drug treatment, and (d) surgical adjuvant chemotherapy increases the long-term cure rates with all of these tumors and significantly increases the life span of treatment failures.

Effective surgical adjuvant chemotherapy is both dose-responsive and related to the body burden of metastatic tumor at time of drug treatment. The effectiveness of surgical adjuvant chemotherapy decreases (a) as the tumor staging is advanced prior to surgery, (b) as the interval from surgery to start of effective chemotherapy is increased, and (c) as the drug doses are reduced. Additionally, and of critical importance to treatment planning, some drugs that are marginally effective or ineffective against the presurgical total body burden of tumor cells are curative in some to all mice with metastatic disease if given shortly after surgical removal of the primary tumor.

451

RATIONALE FOR ADJUVANT CHEMOTHERAPY

Theoretically, cancer arises when one normal cell changes into a malignant neoplastic cell, either by spontaneous mutation or following chemical, viral, or radiation induction. If this mutant neoplastic cell is capable of maintaining uncontrolled cell division, progressive growth leads to clinical presentation. At this point, cure by either surgery or radiation therapy is possible, in the main, only if distant metastatic spread from the primary tumor has not yet occurred. Of the nearly 700,000 people in the United States who currently develop clinically recognized cancer each year, more than 50% will have metastatic disease at the time of diagnosis or will have a high risk of tumor recurrence following the best presently available surgical, radiological, or drug treatment (7). These metastatic tumor foci are the proper target for the chemotherapist and/or the immunotherapist, or, if you choose, the medical oncologist. Anticancer drugs spread throughout the body, with the exception, at least for some drugs, of certain pharmacologic sanctuaries such as the brain, and are able to kill drug-sensitive cancer cells wherever in the body they may be. Drug effectiveness is limited, however, by many factors, chief among which is that drugs kill tumor cells by so-called first-order kinetics. This means that the same percentage, and not the same number, of cancer cells is killed by the highest dose of an effective drug that can be given, essentially irrespective of total body burden (10,18,24,25,26). A variable percentage of human patients with any of 11 tumors may be cured with anticancer drug treatment started when the systemic disease is first clinically recognized, but these tumors represent only about 25% of all cancers and account for only about 8% of all cancer deaths (7). Failure to cure over 90% of clinically recognized systemic cancer with currently available drugs is due, in the main, to a total body burden of tumor cells at the start of drug treatment in excess of the selective cell kill potential for tumor cells over vital normal cells of currently available single drugs or combinations of drugs.

What is the magnitude of the tumor cell kill or tumor cell removal problem? Figure 1 is modified from a recent paper by DeVita, Young, and Canellos (7). That a single cancer cell can establish fatal disease in several mammalian species with a number of histologically different tumor cell types has been repeatedly demonstrated in the laboratory (see refs. 17 and 19 for a review of these data). In addition, immunologic evidence indicates that some myelomas of man and animals originate from one cell, since they produce a single specific immunoglobulin, and monoclonal origin, based on immunologic specificity, appears to be the common process in induction of tumors by chemical carcinogens (3). These observations indicate that total tumor cell removal by surgery, radiation, chemotherapy, or immunotherapy (used alone or as combined modalities) may be required for cure; in the absence of convincing evidence to the contrary, conservative therapeutic

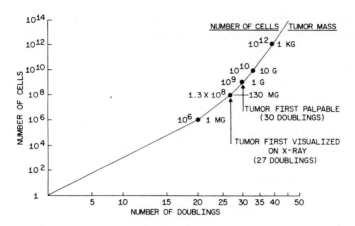

FIG. 1. Theoretical growth curve relating number of tumor doublings to number of tumor cells present and levels of clinical awareness of tumor. (From ref. 7 with permission.)

planning, with cure as the goal, should reach for total tumor cell kill or removal.

In Fig. 1, the number of doublings of one cancer cell and all of its progeny is plotted on the abscissa and the log number of cells on the ordinate. One cancer cell and all of its progeny must go through nearly 30 doublings, to between 10^8 and 10^9 cells, for a single tumor focus to be detectable by X-ray or palpation; therefore, any cancer is far advanced in its natural history from origin to death, when first detected by X-ray or palpation. Each micrometastasis will contain from about 10^8 down to 1 tumor cell, and the total body burden of tumor cells in micrometastases will be the sum of all. In many cases, this total body burden of tumor cells in micrometastases is likely to be large, often in excess of 10^9, and if cure requires reduction of the total body burden to small numbers, perhaps even to less than 1 tumor cell, the job for chemotherapy and immunotherapy is formidable. Clinical experience clearly indicates that most systemic cancers are not curable with drugs (7). As Dr. Joseph Burchenal (2) stated in his James Ewing Lecture in 1975, "You [surgeons] are all painfully aware, as are we [medical oncologists], that the chemotherapy of metastatic solid tumors, with few exceptions, is at best palliative and at worst ineffective and toxic." The selective cell kill potential of our best currently available anticancer drug(s) is below the total body burden of tumor cells in over 90% of patients with clinically evident metastatic tumors.

How do we improve on the cure rates of tumors with unacceptably high metastatic recurrence rates following effective but noncurative surgical and/or radiological treatment of the primary tumor? The obvious and logical answer is to reduce the total body burden of tumor cells by surgical excision and/or radiation cell kill of the grossly apparent and accessible primary tumor and then begin adjuvant drug treatment as soon as possible so that the residual body burden of grossly inapparent metastatic foci is hopefully less than the curative potential of the best or most indicated effective anti-cancer drugs. This concept is being carefully studied in depth, both at home and abroad, in women with breast cancer who have a high risk of metastatic recurrence. The current status of these studies is being regularly reported. The published results are very promising (1,8) and are being updated and reported in this volume. In addition, marked increases in disease-free interval after surgery and probable significantly improved long-term cure rates have also been obtained with surgical adjuvant drug treatment in patients with metastatic osteogenic sarcoma (5,13,25).

INFLUENCE OF TUMOR STAGING ON SURGICAL CURE RATES AND LIKELY TUMOR CELL BURDEN IN METASTATIC FOCI

There is a direct relationship between the size of the primary tumor in carcinoma of the breast in women and both the surgical cure rates and likely metastatic tumor cell body burden; the larger the primary tumor at time of surgery, the lower the long-term cure rate and the shorter the duration of

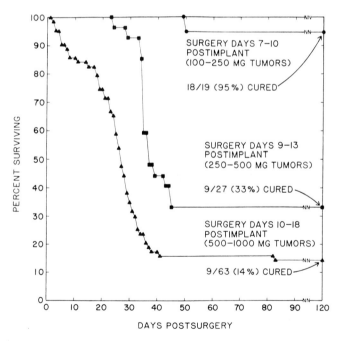

FIG. 2. Cumulative mortality from metastatic C3H mammary carcinoma (line 44) following subcutaneous implant into C3H mice and surgical removal of progressively larger primary tumors. None of the animals plotted showed grossly apparent tumor regrowth at the surgical site at the time of death from demonstrated metastatic lesions. (From ref. 21 with permission.)

life among surgical curative failures (6,22). That the same situation obtains with a metastasizing transplantable breast tumor in C3H mice is illustrated in Fig. 2. Figure 2 is a cumulative mortality plot of C3H mice implanted subcutaneously with a transplantable mammary carcinoma in which progressively larger primary tumors were removed surgically. None of the dying animals showed gross evidence of recurrent tumor at the primary site, and all had extensive metastatic disease at death. Surgical cure rates were inversely related to tumor mass at time of surgery. Additionally, the progressively shorter postsurgical life span in mice dying of metastatic disease as the primary tumor mass at time of surgery increased provides a direct indication of larger metastatic tumor burden with increasing size of the primary tumor (11,21).

Similar relationships have been observed with at least three other metastasizing and uniformly fatal transplantable solid tumors of mice: Lewis lung carcinoma (12,14,16; W. R. Laster, Jr., J. G. Mayo, and F. M. Schabel, Jr., *personal communication*), colon carcinoma (4; T. H. Corbett and D. P. Griswold, Jr., *personal communication*), and B16 melanoma (D. P. Griswold, Jr. and D. J. Dykes, *personal communication*). The above-cited data from both man and animals clearly indicate prompt surgical removal of the smallest primary tumor possible to maximize surgical cure rates and minimize postsurgical metastatic body burden among surgical curative failures.

ACKNOWLEDGMENTS

The experimental work from Southern Research Institute, on which a major part of this chapter is based, was carried out under Contract N01-CM4-3756 from the Division of Cancer Treatment, National Cancer Institute, National Institutes of Health, Department of Health, Education and Welfare; Public Health Service Grant CA-17303 from the National Large Bowel Cancer Project and Division of Cancer Research Resources and Centers, National Cancer Institute, National Institutes of Health, Department of Health, Education and Welfare; and Grant CH-10Q from the American Cancer Society.

The manuscript was submitted at the request of the Editor, Dr. Stacey B. Day. A more complete account from which this report is in part abstracted is in press in *Cancer*, 1977.

REFERENCES

1. Bonadonna, G., Brusamolino, B., Valagussa, V., Rossi, A., Brugnatelli, L., Brambilla, C., De Lena, M., Tancini, G., Bajetta, E., Musumeci, R., and Veronesi, U. (1976): Combination chemotherapy as an adjuvant treatment in operable breast cancer. *N. Engl. J. Med.,* 294:405–410.
2. Burchenal, J. H. (1976): Adjuvant therapy — theory, practice, and potential. The James Ewing Lecture. *Cancer,* 37:46–57.
3. Burnet, F. M. (1971): Immunological surveillance in neoplasia. *Transplant. Rev.,* 7:3–25.
4. Corbett, T. H., Griswold, D. P., Jr., Roberts, B. J., Peckham, J., and Schabel, F. M., Jr.

(1975): A mouse colon-tumor model for experimental therapy. *Cancer Chemother. Rep.*, 5:169–186.

5. Cortes, E. P., Holland, J. F., Wang, J. J., Sinks, L. F., Blom, J., Senn, H., Bank, A., and Glidewell, O. (1974): Amputation and adriamycin in primary osteosarcoma. *N. Engl. J. Med.*, 291:998–1000.

6. Cutler, S. J., and Myers, M. H. (1967): Clinical classification of extent of disease in cancer of the breast. *J. Natl. Cancer Inst.*, 39:193–207.

7. DeVita, V. T., Young, R. C., and Canellos, G. P. (1975): Combination versus single agent chemotherapy: Review of basis for selection of drug treatment of cancer. *Cancer*, 35:98–110.

8. Fisher, B., Carbone, P., Economou, S. G., Frelick, R., Glass, A., Lerner, H., Redmond, C., Zelen, M., Band, P., Katrych, D. L., Wolmark, N., and Fisher, E. R. (1975): L-Phenylalanine mustard (L-PAM) in the management of primary breast cancer. *N. Engl. J. Med.*, 292:117–122.

9. Fugmann, R. A., Martin, D. S., Hayworth, P. E., and Stolfi, R. L. (1970): Enhanced cures of spontaneous murine mammary carcinomas with surgery and five-compound combination chemotherapy, and their immunotherapeutic interrelationship. *Cancer Res.*, 30:1931–1936.

10. Goldin, A., Venditti, J. M., Humphreys, S. R., and Mantel, N. (1956): Influences of the concentration of leukemic inoculum on the effectiveness of treatment. *Science*, 123:840.

11. Griswold, D. P., Jr. (1975): The potential for murine tumor models in surgical adjuvant chemotherapy. *Cancer Chemother. Rep.*, 5:187–204.

12. Humphreys, S. R., and Karrer, K. (1970): Relationship of dose schedules to effectiveness of adjuvant chemotherapy. *Cancer Chemother. Rep.*, 54:379–392.

13. Jaffe, N., Frei, E., III, Traggis, D., and Bishop, Y. (1974): Adjuvant methotrexate and citrovorum-factor treatment of osteogenic sarcoma. *N. Engl. J. Med.*, 291:994–997.

14. Karrer, K., and Humphreys, S. R. (1967): Continuous and limited courses of cyclophosphamide (NSC-26271) in mice with pulmonary metastasis after surgery. *Cancer Chemother. Rep.*, 51:439–449.

15. Martin, D. S., Fugmann, R. A., and Hayworth, P. (1962): Surgery, cancer chemotherapy, host defenses, and tumor size. *J. Natl. Cancer Inst.*, 29:817–834.

16. Mayo, J. G., Laster, W. R., Jr., Andrews, C. M., and Schabel, F. M., Jr. (1972): Success and failure in the treatment of solid tumors. III. "Cure" of metastatic Lewis lung carcinoma with methyl-CCNU (NSC-95441) and surgery-chemotherapy. *Cancer Chemother. Rep.*, 56:183–195.

17. Schabel, F. M., Jr. (1970): Concept and practice of total tumor cell kill. In: *Oncology 1970. Proceedings of the Tenth International Cancer Congress, Vol. 2, Experimental Cancer Therapy*, edited by R. L. Clark, R. W. Cumley, J. E. McCay, and M. M. Copeland, pp. 35–45. Year Book Medical Publishers, Chicago.

18. Schabel, F. M., Jr. (1975): Concepts for systemic treatment of micrometastases. *Cancer*, 35:15–24.

19. Schabel, F. M., Jr. (1976): Concepts for treatment of micrometastases developed in murine systems. *Am. J. Roentgenol.*, 126:500–511.

20. Schabel, F. M., Jr. (1976): Nitrosoureas: A review of experimental antitumor activity. *Cancer Treatment Rep.*, 60:665–698.

21. Schabel, F. M., Jr. (1977): Surgical adjuvant chemotherapy of metastatic murine tumors. *Cancer (submitted for publication)*.

22. Skipper, H. E. (1971): Kinetics of mammary tumor cell growth and implications for therapy. *Cancer*, 28:1479–1499.

23. Skipper, H. E., Schabel, F. M., Jr., Bell, M., Thomson, J. R., and Johnson, S. (1957): On the curability of experimental neoplasms. I. Amethopterin and mouse leukemias. *Cancer Res.*, 17:717–726.

24. Skipper, H. E., Schabel, F. M., Jr., and Wilcox, W. S. (1964): Experimental evaluation of potential anticancer agents. XIII. On the criteria and kinetics associated with curability of experimental leukemia. *Cancer Chemother. Rep.*, 35:1–111.

25. Sutow, W., Gehan, E. A., Vietti, T. J., Frias, A. E., and Dyment, P. G. (1976): Multidrug chemotherapy in primary treatment of osteosarcoma. *J. Bone Joint Surg.*, 58A:629–633.

26. Wilcox, W. S. (1966): The last surviving cancer cell – the chances of killing it. *Cancer Chemother. Rep.*, 50:541–542.

Cancer Invasion and Metastasis: Biologic Mechanisms and Therapy, edited by S. B. Day et al. Raven Press, New York © 1977.

Local Chemotherapy of a Metastasizing Guinea Pig Tumor

Sarkis H. Ohanian, Eliyahu Yarkoni, James T. Hunter, Takao Okuda, Seymour I. Schlager, Herbert J. Rapp, and Tibor Borsos

Laboratory of Immunobiology, National Cancer Institute, National Institutes of Health, Bethesda, Maryland 20014

Malignant tumors would be relatively easy to treat if they were only locally invasive; i.e., cancer death is usually a consequence of metastases. Most animal cancers that are used for studying carcinogenesis, cancer chemotherapy, and immunotherapy are of the nonmetastasizing type. Moreover, most human cancers are carcinomas whereas most of the experimental animal cancers are sarcomas.

We have been studying the immunology and biology of several antigenically distinct chemically induced malignant hepatomas of strain-2 guinea pigs. Cells of line 10, a hepatocellular carcinoma, when injected intradermally (i.d.) into syngeneic guinea pigs, metastasize to the draining lymph nodes (1,2).

The availability of a metastasizing carcinoma permitted us to study the effects of various forms of therapy under conditions where metastases occur "naturally," i.e., the tumor disseminates via the lymphatic system spontaneously after the implantation of the primary tumor. Several years ago it was shown with the line-10 tumor that intratumoral injection of BCG eradicated the primary transplant and microscopically detectable lymph node metastasis, and cured animals resisted subsequent challenge of the same tumor (2). This effect was dependent on dose and time the BCG was administered. Subsequently, we reported that intratumoral injection of certain metabolic inhibitors and chemotherapeutic drugs into line-10 tumors caused regression of local and metastatic lesions. More than 90% of the cured animals were immune to a subsequent challenge with line-10 cells (3,4).

In this chapter the effectiveness of drug treatment started at different times after primary implantation of the tumor is examined and the efficacy of surgery, systemic chemotherapy, and intratumoral chemotherapy are compared.

457

MATERIALS AND METHODS

Animals

Inbred Sewall Wright strain-2 guinea pigs (approximately 250 g) were obtained from the Veterinary Resources Branch, Division of Research Services, National Institutes of Health.

Cells and Reagents

The diethylnitrosamine-induced hepatic line-10 tumor (ascites form) (5) is maintained in strain-2 guinea pigs and is routinely collected as described by Ohanian et al. (6). Each guinea pig received an i.d. injection into the left flank of 10^6 line-10 cells in 0.1 ml of medium 199.

The inhibitors used were: adriamycin (NCI, NSC-123127); 1,3,-bis(2-chloroethyl)-1-nitrosourea (BCNU; NCI, NSC-409962); melphalan (NCI, NSC-8806); 5-fluorouracil (5-FU; Roche Laboratories #771138); and methotrexate (NCI, NSC-740).

Data were evaluated statistically by the Fisher exact test for tumor incidence and by the Mann-Whitney U test for survival.

RESULTS

In the first experiments we have examined the effects of time and dose of administration of drugs on line-10 tumors.

Table 1 shows the results of intralesional therapy carried out 7 days after the i.d. injection of the primary tumors. One intratumoral injection of the chemotherapeutic agents at different dose levels was administered. It can be seen that adriamycin, BCNU, and melphalan were effective in causing tumor regression. Treatment with 5-FU or methotrexate was not effective. Single intratumoral treatment with 5-(3,3-dimethyl-1-triazeno)-imidazole-4-carboxamide (DTIC; 20 mg/kg), higher concentrations of 5-FU or methotrexate, or multiple injections of these drugs were not effective (data not shown). Most of the cured animals when challenged with 10^6 line-10 cells suppressed tumor growth. This effect, however, appeared to be dependent on the dose of drug and is shown most clearly with BCNU.

Table 2 shows the results of intralesional therapy carried out 14 days after the i.d. injection of the primary tumors. It can be seen that drug treatment at this time was not as successful as treatment of the 7-day tumor. In addition, adriamycin and BCNU were toxic for the animals.

In the next experiments we investigated the effect of surgery combined with chemotherapy on 7-day-old line-10 tumors. The primary purpose of these experiments was to determine if removal of the primary tumor site followed by chemotherapy is sufficient to cure animals of their metastasis.

TABLE 1. *Intratumoral chemotherapy of 7-day line-10 tumors*

Treatment	Dose (mg/kg)	Died of toxicity	No. animals alive and at 90 days tumor free/No. treated	Median survival	No. animals resistant to rechallenge/ No. rechallenged[a]
No treatment	—	—	0/9	55	—
Adriamycin	7	2/5	3/5	>94	0/3
	2.4	—	5/5	>94	4/5
	0.8	—	5/5	>94	5/5[b]
BCNU	90	—	4/5	>94	0/4
	30	—	4/5	>94	3/4
	10	—	1/5	89	1/1
5-FU	15	—	1/5	>94	1/1
	5	—	0/5	59	—
	1.7	—	0/5	50	—
Melphalan	2	2/5	3/5	>94	2/3
	0.7	—	3/5	>94	2/3
	0.24	—	2/5	>94	1/2
Methotrexate	90	—	0/5	59	—
	30	—	0/5	55	—
	10	—	0/5	54	—

[a] At 120 days.
[b] One animal developed tumor in the draining lymph node after contralateral rechallenge.

The data in Table 3 summarize the results.

The following are the salient points: (a) Excision of the primary tumor resulted in no recurrence of the tumor at that site; however, nine of ten animals died of their metastases. The lone survivor was not resistant to rechallenge with 10^6 line-10 tumor cells. (b) Intratumoral chemotherapy cured all animals of their tumors and three of four animals were resistant to

TABLE 2. *Intratumoral chemotherapy of 14-day line-10 tumors*

Treatment	Dose (mg/kg)	Died of toxicity	No. animals alive and at 90 days tumor free/No. treated	Median survival	No. animals resistant to rechallenge/ No. rechallenged[a]
No treatment	—	—	0/6	69	—
Adriamycin	5	6/6	—	24	—
	2.5	3/6	0/6	33	—
	0.8	—	2/6	>98	2/2
BCNU	90	4/6	0/6	25.5	—
	30	1/6	1/6	>98	1/1
5-FU	30	6/6	—	15	—
	15	—	0/6	90	—
Melphalan	1.5	—	1/6	>98	1/1
	0.7	—	3/6	>98	3/3
	0.24	—	0/6	>98	—

[a] At 120 days.

TABLE 3. *Intratumoral drug therapy compared with resection of primary tumor*

Group	Treatment at 7 days after tumor inoculation	No. animals alive and at 90 days tumor free/No. treated	No. animals resistant to rechallenge/ No. rechallenged[a]
1	No surgery + 1.4 mg/kg melphalan i.t.	5/5[b]	3/4[c]
2	Excision of primary + 1.4 mg/kg melphalan i.d. ipsilateral	2/10	0/2
3	Excision of primary + 1.4 mg/kg melphalan i.d. contralateral	1/9	0/1
4	Excision of primary + 1.4 mg/kg melphalan i.p.	0/9	
5	No surgery + no drug	0/9	
6	Excision of primary + no drug	1/10	0/1

i.t., intratumoral.
[a] At 120 days.
[b] Difference between groups 1 and 2: $p < 0.025$.
[c] One animal died at 120 days without evidence of tumor.

rechallenge with 10^6 line-10 cells. One animal died at the time of rechallenge without any evidence of tumor. (c) Excision of primary tumor followed by chemotherapy anywhere in the animal, including ipsilateral treatment in such a fashion that the drug drained into the same node where metastatic cells were likely to be, failed to cure most of the animals; none of the three surviving animals was resistant to rechallenge with 10^6 line-10 tumor cells.

The conclusion that may be drawn from this experiment is that surgery followed by adjuvant chemotherapy is unsuccessful in curing animals of their minimal residual metastasis, even when the drug is injected in such a fashion that it drains to the affected lymph node.

DISCUSSION

The experiments reported here are part of an effort to analyze the effectiveness of intratumoral chemotherapy in curing guinea pigs of a metastatic carcinoma. The key point of these experiments is that at the time treatment is started, tumor cells have already spread to the draining lymph node. Three lines of evidence show that by day 7 close to 100% of the animals contain tumor cells in their draining lymph nodes. The first line of evidence comes from histological studies. As illustrated in Fig. 1, tumor cells are present in the peripheral sinuses of draining superdistal axillary lymph node 7 days after implantation of the primary tumor.[1] This observation confirms previous histological studies with this tumor (2).

---

[1] This photomicrograph is from a histological study of the effect of intralesional chemotherapy performed in collaboration with D. Goodman (to be published).

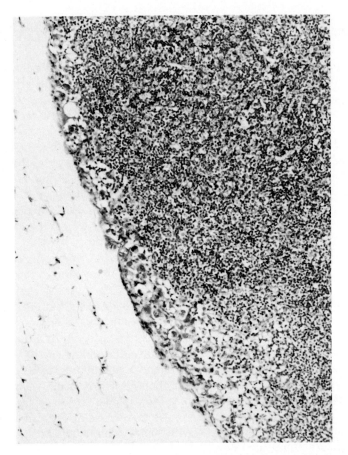

FIG. 1. Line-10 tumor cells in the subcapsular space of the lymph node draining the primary tumor site 7 days after i.d. implantation of 10^6 line-10 cells.

The second line of evidence also confirms previous studies in which implants were removed surgically at day 7; between 80 and 100% of all animals treated this way developed fatal metastatic disease without recurrence of the tumor at the primary site (2). The data shown in Table 3 confirm the ineffectiveness of primary tumor excision in curing the animals. The third line of confirmatory evidence comes from transplantation experiments. In these experiments at day 7 after primary i.d. implantation of line-10 tumor cells, both the primary and the draining lymph node were excised. The draining lymph nodes were then reinjected i.d. into untreated guinea pigs. Several weeks later, line-10 tumors grew at the site of implantation of the draining lymph nodes which led to the death of the animals. The results showed that tumorigenic line-10 cells were present in the draining lymph nodes when surgery was performed (2).

Based on the above evidence we have confirmed with reasonable certainty that at the seventh day after implantation of the primary tumor, the draining lymph node contains microscopically but not clinically detectable viable line-10 tumor cells. Thus local spread of cancer has occurred at the time of treatment. The evidence presented here and elsewhere (3,4) indicates that intralesional chemotherapy with the right drug dosage and time cures guinea pigs of their primary tumor and of draining lymph node metastasis.

It is difficult to understand why one drug works and another does not. For example, adriamycin and DTIC both induce a strong local inflammatory reaction, yet adriamycin is effective although DTIC is not in curing the animals. BCNU, on the other hand, is effective without inducing a strong local inflammatory reaction. In collaboration with D. Goodman, we are doing serial histological studies to elucidate cellular events that occur in the treated primary lesion and the draining lymph node.

The right dose of a drug is the least amount of drug that permanently cures the host of its tumor and the cured host remains immune to the tumor. As seen from Table 2, higher doses of an effective drug may cure a guinea pig of its tumor and its microscopic lymph node metastasis, but the animal fails to reject a challenge with the same tumor. One possibility is that higher doses of the drug are immunosuppressive, possibly interfering with the generation of memory cells. Tests are currently under way to analyze the reasons for successful and for failed immunochemotherapy.

The right time for successful chemotherapy seems to be when the tumor cells in the lymph node are limited to the capsular region of the node, i.e., not later than about 7 days after the implantation of the primary tumor. Treatment started at about 14 days after implantation fails most of the time. These observations are similar to those made with intralesional BCG treatment of line-10 tumors. Why treatment at a later time fails is unclear for at day 14 there seems to be little or no spread of the tumor beyond the draining node. Experiments are under way to analyze various processes including studying local and systemic immune reactions to determine the reasons for the failure of therapy started after 14 days.

REFERENCES

1. Zbar, B., Wepsic, H. T., Rapp, H. J., Whang-Peng, J., and Borsos, T. (1969): Transplantable hepatomas induced in strain-2 guinea pigs by diethylnitrosamine: Characterization by histology, growth, and chromosomes. *J. Natl. Cancer Inst.,* 43:821–831.
2. Zbar, B., Bernstein, I. D., Bartlett, G. L., Hanna, M. G., and Rapp, H. J. (1972): Immunotherapy of cancer: Regression of intradermal tumors and prevention of growth of lymph node metastases after intralesional injection of living *Mycobacterium bovis. J. Natl. Cancer Inst.,* 49:119–130.
3. Bast, R. C., Jr., Segerling, M., Ohanian, S. H., Greene, S. R., Zbar, B., Rapp, H. J., and Borsos, T. (1976): Regression of established tumor and induction of tumor immunity by intratumoral chemotherapy. *J. Natl. Cancer Inst.,* 56:829–832.

4. Borsos, T., Bast, R. C., Jr., Ohanian, S. H., Segerling, M., Zbar, B., and Rapp, H. J. (1976): Induction of tumor immunity by intratumoral chemotherapy. *Ann. N.Y. Acad. Sci.,* 276:565–571.
5. Zbar, B., Bernstein, I. D., and Rapp, H. J. (1971): Suppression of tumor growth at the site of infection with living *Bacillus Calmette-Guerin. J. Natl. Cancer Inst.,* 46:831–839.
6. Ohanian, S. H., Borsos, T., and Rapp, H. J. (1973): Lysis of tumor cells by antibody and complement. I. Lack of correlation between antigen content and lytic susceptibility. *J. Natl. Cancer Inst.,* 50:1313–1320.

Cancer Invasion and Metastasis: Biologic Mechanisms and Therapy, edited by S. B. Day et al. Raven Press, New York © 1977.

Approaches to the Chemotherapy of Lymph Node Metastasis

Shigeru Tsukagoshi and Tomowo Kobayashi

Cancer Chemotherapy Center, Japanese Foundation for Cancer Research, Tokyo, Japan

In order to study the effect of antitumor drugs against metastasis experimentally, one must have an adequate system involving metastasis to specific tissues. Sato et al. reported previously that lymph node metastasis could be induced by inoculation with tumor cells into the mouse tail subcutaneously (s.c.) (1) or into the lymph duct of the rat testis (2), whereas Mizuno et al. (3) studied lung metastasis of Ehrlich ascites cells after repeated inoculation with tumor cells which metastasized to the lung. Koch (4) obtained a strain of Ehrlich tumor which metastasized to the lymph nodes with a high degree of frequency.

It is desirable for the experimental chemotherapy of lymph node metastasis that the control animals die uniformly from tumor growth, accompanied by pronounced metastasis to the tissues, and that there be known antitumor agents effective against the metastasized tumors which may serve as standards. So far, there have not been many animal systems involving lymph node metastasis. In our laboratory, it was found that tumor cells inoculated s.c. at the inner side of the right thigh of experimental animals metastasized primarily to the various lymph nodes and only slightly to the other organs. Since the inoculation method provides an easy means for inducing lymph node metastasis and since there are effective compounds, it was considered that this type of metastatic system could be used in the trials of chemotherapy of lymph node metastasis. In the current study, the influence of therapy was determined against early leukemia L1210 before the occurrence of gross metastasis.

INDUCTION OF LYMPH NODE METASTASIS

About one million L1210 cells maintained as ascites cells in CDF_1 mice were suspended in physiologic saline (0.1 ml) and inoculated s.c. at the inner side of the right thigh. The tumor cells metastasized primarily to the retroperitoneal (mainly lumbar), inguinal, and axillary lymph nodes as shown macroscopically (5). Ascites cells were not formed.

All mice inoculated s.c. with leukemia L1210 died from progressive tumor growth between 8 and 12 days after inoculation, and significant lymph node metastasis was observed. When mice were killed on day 7 for examination of the degree of metastasis, the lymph nodes were observed to be enlarged as shown in Table 1. The histologic examination of various tissues in mice inoculated s.c. with L1210 cells using the present method of inoculation was done on day 7 after inoculation with 10^6 cells, and the results are shown in Table 2. As seen in the table, more tumor cells were found in the various lymph nodes on the right side of the animals, which was where the tumor

TABLE 1. *Size of tumor and lymph nodes in CDF, normal and L1210-bearing mice[a]*

Lymph node or tumor	L1210 mice	Normal mice
Sc	480 ± 92 mm³	—
Re	30 ± 6	6 ± 2 mm³
In	30 ± 3	6 ± 2
Ax	8 ± 2	6 ± 2

[a] Animals were killed 7 days after inoculation (10^6 cells/mouse). Values are the average for 10 mice ($\pm$ SD). Sc, tumor at the inoculation site; Re, right lumbar node; In, right inguinal node; Ax, right axillary node. CDF₁ mice; CDF$_1$ = (BALB/c female $\times$ DBA/2 male) F$_1$.

TABLE 2. *Distribution of L1210 cells in the various tissues on day 7 after s.c. inoculation of 10^6 cells/mouse[a]*

Tissues	Right side		Left side
Lymph nodes			
Lumbar	++		+
Renal	++		+
Inguinal	++		+
Axillary	+		±
Mesenteric		+	
Organs			
Lung	+		+
Liver		++	
Heart		−	
Kidney	−		−
Stomach		−	
Small intestine		−	
Pancreas		−	
Spleen		+	
Uterus and ovary		−	
Adrenal gland	−		±
Salivary gland	−		−

[a] Distribution of tumor cells is indicated as follows: +++, almost 100% of the tissue examined was occupied by the tumor cells; ++, about 50%; +, 1–50%; ±, not clear; −, none.

cells were injected, as compared with the other tissues; however, tumor cells were found to some extent in organs such as the liver, spleen, and lungs in L1210-bearing mice. The retroperitoneal lymph nodes were usually enlarged considerably when assayed on day 7 as can be seen in Table 1, and many more tumor cells were found in the right inguinal and axillary lymph nodes as compared with the left inguinal and axillary lymph nodes.

QUANTITATIVE ASSAY OF LYMPH NODE METASTASIS

So that we could express the chemotherapeutic effect more quantitatively, minced or whole lymph nodes obtained from CDF_1 mice inoculated with 10^6 cells of L1210 were inoculated intraperitoneally into normal CDF_1 mice (six mice per group). The number of L1210 cells in the lymph nodes was calculated using a calibration curve (Fig. 1) which was obtained by plotting average survival days of CDF_1 mice inoculated intraperitoneally with 10^2, 10^3, 10^4, 10^5, 10^6, or 10^7 L1210 cells against the number of inoculated L1210 cells.

Because there was good parallelism between the minced and whole lumbar

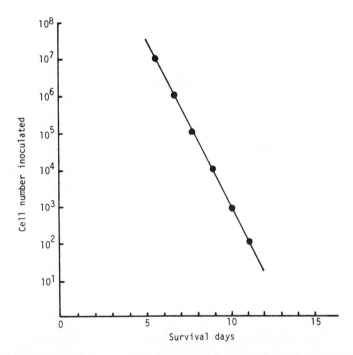

FIG. 1. Relation between number of inoculated tumor cells and mean survival days. A group of 20 CDF_1 mice was inoculated intraperitoneally with 10^2, 10^3, 10^4, 10^5, 10^6, or 10^7 L1210 cells/mouse and the mean survival days were plotted against the number of inoculated cells.

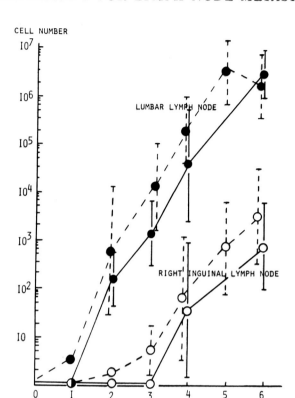

FIG. 2. Number of L1210 cells detected in lumbar or inguinal lymph node. Each right lumbar or inguinal lymph node obtained after s.c. inoculation of 10^6 L1210 cells/mouse (6 mice/group) on the day indicated in this figure was: (a) minced (*dashed lines*) in a 35 × 10 mm plastic dish with scissors aseptically with 0.2 ml Hanks' solution and inoculated intraperitoneally together with two 0.2-ml washings using a capillary or (b) inoculated intraperitoneally without mincing (*solid lines*) using a trocar. Number of L1210 cells proliferating in lymph node was determined using the calibration curve (Fig. 1).

or inguinal lymph node-inoculated groups as shown in Fig. 2, the effect of anticancer agents or those entrapped in liposomes was examined with this assay system, since inoculation of whole lymph node was more convenient than the mincing procedure from various aspects.

QUANTITATIVE ASSAY OF THE EFFECT OF ANTICANCER AGENTS AGAINST LYMPH NODE METASTASIS

The effect of antitumor agents on lymph node metastasis was examined by the quantitative assay system mentioned above.

After subcutaneous inoculation of 10^6 L1210 cells per mouse into CDF_1

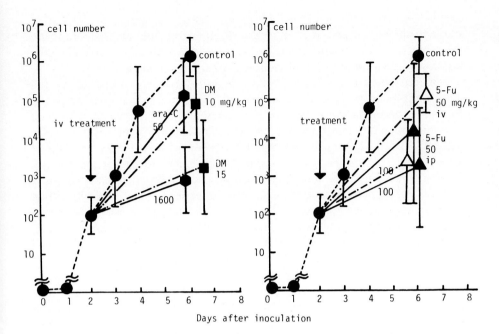

FIG. 3. Comparison of the effect of various anticancer agents on lymph node metastasis. One million L1210 cells/mouse were inoculated s.c. into the right thigh of a group of 6 CDF₁ mice, and cytosine arabinoside (ara-C), daunomycin (DM), or 5-fluorouracil (5-FU) was injected intravenously or intraperitoneally at the doses shown in this figure on day 2. The lumbar lymph node was obtained from each mouse on the day indicated and bioassayed using a calibration curve. △, 5-FU, i.v.; ▲, 5-FU, i.p.

mice, we injected various antitumor agents intraperitoneally or intravenously on day 2 and examined the number of tumor cells in the lumbar lymph node on day 6.

Figure 3 indicates the result of treatment with cytosine arabinoside (ara-C), daunomycin (DM), or 5-fluorouracil (5-FU). As shown in this figure, they could not eradicate the tumor cells in lumbar lymph node even at 1,600 mg/kg of ara-C, 15 mg/kg of DM (close to its LD$_{50}$ value), or 100 mg/kg of 5-FU as far as the effects were determined by day 6 after tumor inoculation.

In order to improve the therapeutic effect of the antitumor drugs against lymph node metastasis, we examined ara-C after entrapping it in liposomes.

THERAPEUTIC TRIALS OF LYMPH NODE METASTASIS WITH ANTICANCER AGENTS ENTRAPPED IN LIPOSOMES

Cytosine arabinoside (1-β-D-arabinofuranosyl cytosine), an important antitumor agent currently used for chemotherapy of human leukemia, is rapidly excreted into urine, mainly as an inactive deaminated metabolite, arabinofuranosyl uracil (6). In order to improve the chemotherapeutic effect of ara-C, it was entrapped into cationic liposomes, and the enhancing antitumor effect on mouse leukemia L1210 was examined.

The liposomes containing cytosine arabinoside were prepared by the slightly modified method of Kinsky et al. (7). The liposomes used in the present experiment were cationic unsonicated ones and were composed of sphingomyelin, cholesterol, and stearylamine hydrochloride in molar ratio of 2:1.5:0.22. Mouse leukemia L1210 cells (1×10^5 cells per mouse) were inoculated intraperitoneally into CDF_1 mice (five mice per group). Twenty-four hours after tumor inoculation, varying doses of aqueous ara-C or ara-C entrapped in the liposomes were injected intraperitoneally. When given as an aqueous solution, a single dose of 50 or 100 mg/kg exerted no significant effect on the survival time of mice bearing leukemia L1210, although increasing doses of the drug had a slight effect. In the case of ara-C entrapped in liposomes, a single dose of 50 mg/kg markedly increased the survival time, giving three long-term survivors out of five mice. Moreover, even with a low dose of 3.1 or 6.3 mg/kg, the effect was comparable to or better than that achieved with 1,600 mg/kg of aqueous ara-C. The admixture of equal doses of aqueous ara-C and the corresponding amount of drug-free liposomes did not affect the life span of mice bearing the tumor (Table 3).

When the effect of ara-C against the lymph node metastasis was assayed quantitatively, ara-C entrapped in liposomes revealed marked effect as shown in Fig. 4. That is, in the analyses of lumbar lymph node on day 6,

TABLE 3. *Effect of cytosine arabinoside entrapped in liposomes on the survival time of mice bearing L1210*

	Dose (mg/kg)	T/C (%)	60-day survivors
Cytosine arabinoside	50	114	0/5
	100	111	0/5
	400	150	0/5
	1,600	189	0/5
Cytosine arabinoside + drug-free liposomes(admixture)	3.1	111	0/5
	12.5	111	0/5
	50	111	0/5
Cytosine arabinoside entrapped in liposomes	3.1	172	0/5
	6.3	208	0/5
	12.5	222	0/5
	25	>358	2/5
	50	>381	3/5
	100	75	0/5

Mean survival time of untreated control was 7.2 days. T/C, mean survival time of the treated group/mean survival time of the control group.

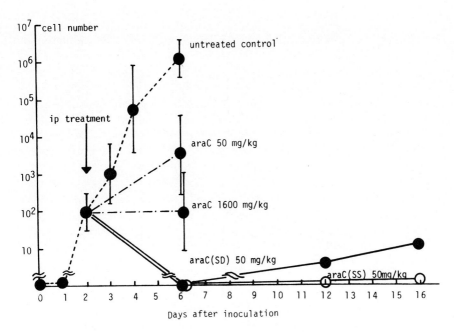

FIG. 4. Comparison of the effect of free and liposome-entrapped cytosine arabinoside (araC) on L1210 cells metastasized to lumbar lymph node.

AraC was injected intraperitoneally into a group of 6 CDF$_1$ mice 2 days after s.c. inoculation of 10^6 L1210 cells/mouse, and the lumbar lymph node was obtained from each mouse on the day indicated in the figure and bioassayed using a calibration curve. AraC (SS) and araC (SD) indicate araC entrapped in liposomes consisting of sphingomyelin, cholesterol, and stearylamine and in those consisting of sphingomyelin, cholesterol, and diacetylphosphate.

ara-C (50 mg/kg) entrapped in liposomes composed of sphingomyelin, cholesterol, and stearylamine was most effective, showing no detectable tumor cells on day 6 and considerably suppressed tumor growth even on day 16. In this case there was a good corelation between the number of tumor cells detected in the lumbar lymph node (Fig. 4) and the life span of the tumor-bearing animals determined in a separate experiment (Fig. 5). Further studies on the effect of anticancer agents entrapped in liposomes against lymph node metastasis are in progress.

DISCUSSION

With the present method of inoculation, when the tumor-bearing mice were killed at various intervals after inoculation, it was found that the tumor cells first metastasized to the retroperitoneal lymph nodes and then to the right inguinal and to the right axillary lymph nodes. At the time of death, however, it was observed that tumor cells had also metastasized to the

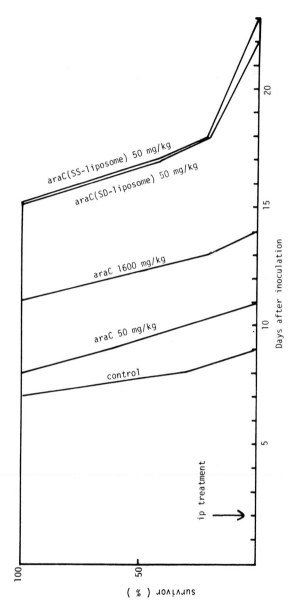

FIG. 5. Effect of free and liposome-entrapped ara-C on the life span of mice with lymph node metastasis. Experimental conditions are the same as indicated in the legend of Fig. 4 except that the number of untreated control mice was 10.

inguinal or axillary lymph nodes on the left side of the animals. In this metastatic system, treatment was started soon after leukemic inoculation, before any extensive metastasis, and inhibition of lymph node metastasis reflected successful therapy of the initial inoculum. Thus, this observed increase of survival time was accompanied by inhibition of lymph node metastasis.

There are many reports (8–12) on the liposomal potentiation of the effect of various antitumor agents, and we found that the antitumor activity of cytosine arabinoside was potentiated by entrapping it in liposomes consisting of sphingomyelin, cholesterol, and stearylamine. That is, schedule dependency of cytosine arabinoside in eliciting the antitumor activity was not observed in the liposome form, which was considerably more effective than free cytosine arabinoside against mouse leukemia L1210 and with a smaller single dose.

In the application of liposomes containing anticancer drugs to this system of lymph node metastasis, cytosine arabinoside entrapped in liposomes was most effective as far as the lumbar lymph node was bioassayed quantitatively. This marked effect of the liposome form of cytosine arabinoside seems to be due to the slow release of cytosine arabinoside and higher degree of distribution of the drug to various lymph nodes *in vivo*. More detailed analyses of these points are currently in progress.

These studies are also currently being extended to other drugs, using both early and advanced metastatic disease. The effectiveness of drugs in such metastatic systems may have implications for clinical tumors having a similar type of metastatic spread.

SUMMARY

When mouse leukemia L1210 cells were inoculated subcutaneously at the inner side of the right thigh of appropriate host animals, metastasis of tumor cells was produced mainly in the retroperitoneal, inguinal, and axillary lymph nodes, with a lesser degree of metastasis to other organs. These experimental metastatic tumor systems were used here to assess the antineoplastic effect of various antitumor agents. Endpoints considered included both animal life span and number of tumor cells in lymph nodes. The number of L1210 cells proliferating in lymph nodes was determined from the calibration curve by bioassay of whole lymph node obtained from CDF_1 mice after subcutaneous inoculation of 10^6 L1210 cells per mouse. Chemotherapy was applied 2 days after inoculation. As the result, the therapeutic effect of various anticancer agents could be expressed quantitatively, but the result was not satisfactory as far as single treatment with cytosine arabinoside, daunomycin, or 5-fluorouracil on day 2 was concerned. However, when cytosine arabinoside entrapped in liposomes consisting of sphingomyelin, cholesterol, and stearylamine was administered intraperitoneally on day 2, no tumor cells were detectable by bioassay of the lumbar lymph node on day 6. The correlation between the increase of survival time and the decrease of tumor cell number in lumbar lymph nodes has been examined using various antitumor agents and those entrapped in liposomes.

ACKNOWLEDGMENTS

This work was supported by Grants-in-Aid for Scientific Research from the Ministry of Education, Science and Culture of Japan, Nos. 1007 and 1064.

REFERENCES

1. Sato, H. (1961): Studies on the role of cancer chemotherapy for prevention of lymph node metastasis. *Cancer Chemother. Rep.*, 13:33–40.
2. Kurokawa, Y., Suzuki, M., and Sato, H. (1968): Experimental studies on lymphatic metastasis using direct inoculation method into lymph vessels. *Proc. Jpn. Cancer Assoc.*, 27:225.
3. Hasegawa, Y., Ishikura, T., and Mizuno, D. (1968): Formation of lung tumor by intravenous transplantation of Ehrlich carcinoma cells and its possible application to the screening for antimetastasizing effects. *Proc. Jpn. Cancer Assoc.*, 27:223.
4. Koch, F. E. (1939): Zur Frage der Metastasenbildung bei Impftumoren. *Z. Krebsforsch.*, 48:495.
5. Tsukagoshi, S., and Sakurai, Y. (1970): Cancer chemotherapy screening with experimental tumors which metastasize to lymph nodes. *Cancer Chemother. Rep.*, 54:311–318.
6. Stewart, C. D., and Burske, P. J. (1971): Cytidine deaminase and the development of resistance to arabinosyl cytosine. *Nature [New Biol.]*, 233:109.
7. Haxby, J. A., Kinsky, C. B., and Kinsky, S. C. (1968): Immune response of a liposomal model membrane. *Proc. Natl. Acad. Sci. U.S.A.*, 61:300.
8. Gregoriadis, G., Swain, C. P., and Wells, E. J. (1974): Drug-carrier potential of liposomes in cancer chemotherapy. *Lancet*, 1:1313–1316.
9. Gregoriadis, G., and Neerunjun, E. D. (1975): Treatment of tumour bearing mice with liposome-entrapped actinomycin D prolongs their survival. *Res. Commun. Chem. Pathol. Pharmacol.*, 10:351–362.
10. Gregoriadis, G., and Neerunjun, E. D. (1975): Homing of liposomes to target cells. *Biochem. Biophys. Res. Commun.*, 65:537–544.
11. Kimelberg, H. K., Tracy, T. F., Jr., Biddlecome, S. M., and Bourke, R. S. (1976): The effect of entrapment in liposomes on the in vivo distribution of ^{3}H-methotrexate in a primate. *Cancer Res.*, 36:2949–2957.
12. Rutman, R. J., Ritter, C. A., Avadhani, N. G., and Hansel, J. (1976): Liposomal potentiation of the antitumor activity of alkylating drugs. *Cancer Treatment Rep.*, 60:617–618.

Cancer Invasion and Metastasis: Biologic Mechanisms and Therapy, edited by S. B. Day et al. Raven Press, New York © 1977.

Adjuvant Chemotherapy

Irwin H. Krakoff

Vermont Regional Cancer Center, University of Vermont, Burlington, Vermont 05401

A large body of experimental evidence in animal systems supports a role for chemotherapy as an adjunct to surgery. Nearly 20 years ago Shapiro and Fugmann (1) reported on the efficacy of chemotherapy as an adjunct to surgery. They made several important observations:

1. ". . . the total number of tumor cells per se . . . [is] responsible for the observed titration of chemotherapeutic response."
2. ". . . the potential value of administering postoperative chemotherapy as an adjunct to surgery is readily apparent." (Fig. 1)
3. ". . . a large tumor mass can protect a small tumor mass against 6-MP therapy in the same animal."

More recently, Schabel (2) has pointed out that "the tumor burden at start of chemotherapy is the major single controlling factor in obtaining drug core." This is substantiated by experience in humans. With relatively few exceptions, large tumors, primary or metastatic, can rarely be eradicated by chemotherapy. Studies by Simpson-Herren et al. (3) have also shown that reducing the tumor burden in the primary site increases the growth fraction of surviving cells in the primary site and in the small tumor cell populations in distant metastases [probably the explanation for the protective effects of large tumors by Shapiro and Fugmann (1)]. Although the growth rate of residual tumor is accelerated, these kinetic differences may make the relatively small tumor cell populations remaining in the primary site or in small metastases vulnerable to destruction by anticancer drugs. Skipper and Schabel (4) have also demonstrated that tumors in mice which could not be cured by surgery alone, or by chemotherapy alone, were curable with surgery and adjuvant chemotherapy. An example is their experiment in the C3H mammary tumor in B6-C3-F1 mice (Fig. 2). They have reported similar results in the Lewis lung carcinoma, a colon tumor in BALB/C mice, the B16 melanoma in BDF1 mice, and others. Figure 2 also demonstrates another point: adjuvant chemotherapy is more effective early (against small tumors) than late (against larger tumors).

The need for better methods for the treatment of breast cancer is obvious. In spite of improvements in surgical techniques and the use of local and

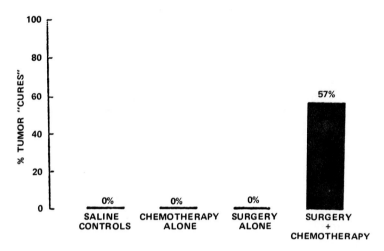

FIG. 1. Effect of surgery (partial surgical excision) plus adjuvant chemotherapy (6-mercaptopurine) on transplanted mammary tumor in mice. (From ref. 1 with permission.)

regional radiotherapy, the overall cure rate for women with breast cancer has not changed in many years. Fisher (5) has noted that for patients with any involvement of axillary nodes by carcinoma, the 5-year recurrence rate is 67%. For patients with four or more positive axillary nodes, the recurrence rate at 5 years is 80%. For patients with axillary nodal involvement and very large primary lesions, the figures are still worse with 5-year recurrence rates as high as 94%. Even with no positive axillary nodes, the recurrence rate is 21% at 5 years and 30% at 10. It is apparent that the long-term survival of patients with localized breast cancer is no better than 70%, and for those with regional nodal metastases it is substantially worse.

Several investigators have studied the possible benefit of postoperative radiotherapy in preventing recurrent disease, and those studies can best be summarized by stating that there is no evidence that postoperative radiotherapy contributes to overall cure rates for patients with breast cancer (6,7). Radiotherapy does appear to influence the site of initial recurrence; as might be expected, those patients who receive radiotherapy have a higher incidence of distant metastases as the initial site of recurrence; those who do not receive radiotherapy appear to develop local recurrences in a slightly higher percentage of cases. Overall, however, radiotherapy provides no benefit in terms of disease-free period or cure rate. In one large review (7) it was suggested that patients with postoperative radiotherapy had a slightly higher recurrence rate overall than did patients who did not receive radiotherapy postoperatively.

The conclusion is inescapable that in a large proportion of cases of breast cancer the disease is disseminated at the time of diagnosis; even though

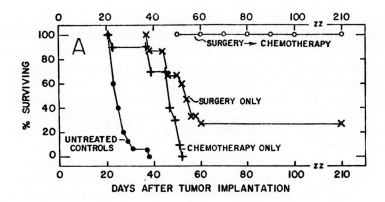

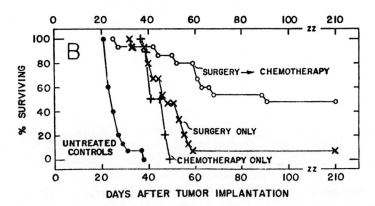

FIG. 2. Effect of surgery plus adjuvant chemotherapy on transplanted mammary tumor in mice. (From ref. 4 with permission.)

metastatic disease cannot be demonstrated, metastases too small to detect must be present. Because of the poor results with local management alone, systemic treatment will be necessary if the disease is to be eliminated.

The role of oöphorectomy done immediately after mastectomy as a systemic adjuvant has been analyzed (8); it appears that oöphorectomy prolongs somewhat the disease-free period (i.e., the period between mastectomy and initial recurrence). However, the period from recurrence to death appears to be shortened and there is no overall advantage to oöphorectomy done in the immediate postmastectomy period, in terms of either greater cure rates or prolongation of survival. Most clinicians prefer to reserve oophorectomy in premenopausal patients until there is evidence of recurrent disease so that they can assess the influence of oöphorectomy on the progress of that disease, using that as a guide for further endocrine therapy.

There has been interest for many years in the possibility that chemotherapy given at and immediately after mastectomy might result in prolonged survival or increased cure rates. Tormey (9) has summarized some of the early clinical trials. In a large study during the 1960s (5) in which patients at risk for recurrence were treated with thio-TEPA it was not possible to demonstrate improvement in survival for the overall group, but the premenopausal patients with more than three positive axillary nodes had a significantly longer median recurrence time and somewhat improved survival at 5 years.

In another study (6) 5-fluorouracil appeared to have a minor effect in decreasing recurrence rates at 3 years post-mastectomy as compared with those of nontreated patients in a group in which there were more than three positive axillary nodes.

In several other studies (10–12), cyclophosphamide was given to patients during the immediate postoperative period with slight improvement in recurrence rates at periods up to 3 years. No data are available yet from those trials concerning survival. A Japanese study (13) in which mitomycin C was given during the immediate postoperative period appeared to indicate a slightly lower recurrence rate in the patients with positive axillary nodes, but insufficient data are available to draw any definitive conclusions.

In some of the studies in which chemotherapy was continued for prolonged periods postoperatively, slightly more encouraging information is available. The study of Long et al. (14) in which thio-TEPA was planned for 1 year post-mastectomy (but actually given for a median of 7.2 months) showed a favorable effect of thio-TEPA in the early postoperative period, but with a longer period of observation no definite benefit was apparent in the treated group. In a similar study (15) using nitrogen mustard intermittently for a mean duration of 9 months there was a lower recurrence rate in the treated group than in the control. The differences were confined to premenopausal patients. There appeared to be minor differences in survival between treated and untreated patients.

Two studies have provided considerable encouragement for the prospect of adjuvant chemotherapy. These deserve somewhat more detailed comment.

The first, that of the National Surgical Adjuvant Breast Project in the United States (16), was published in 1975. The patients included those less than 75 years old who had had a Halsted or modified radical mastectomy for tumors that were T-1, -2, or -3 or -4B with less than 2 cm ulceration. Patients who had one or more positive axillary lymph nodes and no distant metastases were eligible. Patients were randomly allocated to receive either an oral placebo (138 patients) or L-phenylalanine mustard (L-PAM) (148 patients), 0.15 mg/kg/day for 5 days every 6 weeks for 2 years. There were no life-threatening complications. Moderate leukopenia occurred in 60% of the patients who received L-PAM. Nausea and vomiting occurred

in 30% of the patients who received L-PAM and 11% of those who received
the placebo. The data were analyzed by menopausal status and nodal involvement. There were 14 failures (recurrences) in the treated and 29 in
the placebo group (Fig. 3). The difference in failure rate in premenopausal
patients was highly significant (3/42 in the L-PAM group versus 12/43 in
the placebo group). In postmenopausal patients the difference between
treated and untreated patients was not statistically significant. When analyzed by nodal status the difference was significant in those patients with
one to three and those with four or more positive nodes. At the time of the
report, the patients had been followed for 18 months after mastectomy. At
that time it was too early to estimate the effect of treatment on survival, and
that continues to be the case. The beneficial effect of chemotherapy for
patients with breast cancer at high risk for recurrence appears clearly enough
established that present studies of the NSABP are comparing various
chemotherapeutic regimens rather than contrasting a treatment group with
a nontreatment group.

A second important study to be considered is that of Bonadonna et al.
(17). In that study at the National Tumor Institute in Milan, combination
chemotherapy with cyclophosphamide, methotrexate, and 5-fluorouracil
was given because of the demonstrated activity of that combination in
patients with advanced breast cancer (18). The toxicity produced by the

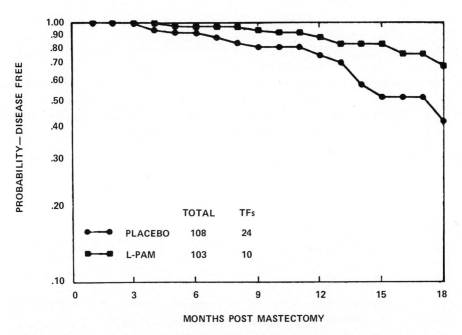

FIG. 3. Effects of surgery plus adjuvant chemotherapy in patients with operable breast
cancer and positive axillary nodes. (From ref. 16 with permission.)

combination was acceptable. Moderate leukopenia occurred in 67% of patients and thrombocytopenia in 57%. Severe myelosuppression was rare. Mucositis, conjunctivitis, and cystitis occurred in 20 to 30% of patients. Partial alopecia was seen in over half the patients and amenorrhea in half of the premenopausal women. Nausea and vomiting occurred to some degree in about 90% of patients. Although the combination of side effects was unpleasant, Bonadonna stated that fewer than 10% of patients experienced a decrease in performance status and that most working women continued to work throughout the period of chemotherapy. On the other hand, there was sufficient resistance to these effects that the original plan to treat the patients for 2 years was altered to 1 year.

After 27 months of study, treatment failure occurred in 24% of 179 control patients and in 5.3% of 207 patients who were treated (Fig. 4). The advantage appeared to be statistically significant in all subgroups of patients. Premenopausal and postmenopausal women achieved similar degrees of benefit, thus refuting the hypothesis that suppression of ovarian function (so-called chemotherapeutic oöphorectomy) was responsible for the delay in recurrence time. Patients with one to three and those with four or more axillary nodes involved were benefited by therapy. No data concerning the effects of therapy on survival are yet available. Follow-up and updating of the Milan data in May 1976 (19) continue to reveal a markedly better re-

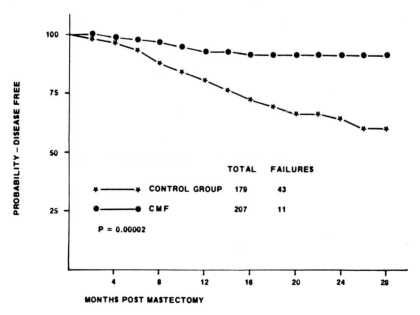

FIG. 4. Effects of surgery plus adjuvant chemotherapy in patients with operable breast cancer and positive axillary nodes. (From ref. 17 with permission.)

currence rate for treated than for untreated patients, although still no survival data are available.

The authors of both of the major adjuvant chemotherapy studies published to date have been circumspect in their interpretations of their data, pointing out that to date only *delay* in recurrence can be claimed. However, it is appropriate to infer that substantial delay, persisting into the post-chemotherapy period, may ultimately be translated into increased *cure* rates.

The short-term toxicity of the various chemotherapeutic regimens studied appears acceptable, from the standpoint of both physician and patient. Concern has been expressed about the possible long-term effects (carcinogenesis, sterility) of protracted treatment with alkylating agents. For patients at high risk (30% or more) for the recurrence of breast cancer, the relative risks of those treatment sequelae appear justified. For patients with less likelihood of recurrence (i.e., those with negative nodes), that question has not yet been answered but studies presently being designed will ask it.

Another systemic modality being studied as a possible adjuvant to surgery is immunotherapy. The demonstration that some patients with neoplastic disease have impaired reactivity to various antigens has led to the attempt to stimulate natural host immunity to cancer by the administration of "immunopotentiators." Among these are *Bacillus Calmette-Guerin* (BCG), a methanol-extractable residue (MER) of BCG, *Corynebacterium parvum*, mixed bacterial vaccines patterned on Coley's toxins, and the antihelmintic levamisole. Each of these agents has been reported to influence favorably the recurrence time or recurrence rate in various tumors; the reports have been generally inconsistent and no clear evidence has yet been presented certifying the benefit to be derived from immunotherapy. One report which requires comment is that of Rojas et al. (20) who administered levamisole to a group of patients with inoperable breast cancer who had been treated with radiotherapy. The recurrence time was distinctly later in the treated group than in a concurrent untreated group, although the ultimate rates were similar. That study and others like it are continuing.

The case for adjuvant chemotherapy can be extended to other kinds of cancer. One of the early demonstrations was in Wilms' tumor. In children not known to have metastases at the time of surgery, nephrectomy alone cures about 15%. Nephrectomy followed by X-ray therapy to the renal bed produces about 50% cures. The addition of actinomycin D to the regimen increases long-term survival to more than 80% (21).

In osteogenic sarcoma it has now been conclusively demonstrated (22) that aggressive chemotherapy started promptly after amputation can result in a high incidence of cures; in patients in whom surgery alone is performed, approximately 85% develop pulmonary metastases within 1 year.

In the modern management of acute lymphoblastic leukemia, the principle is similar, although it has not been referred to as adjuvant chemotherapy. It has been recognized for many years that various drugs could produce "complete remission" in that disease. However, those remissions tended to be brief, and with relapse the development of resistance to further chemotherapy was common. The development of cytokinetic data (23) led to the recognition that complete remission required a reduction in tumor burden of only two logs of leukemic cells, although as many as 10^{13} leukemic cells might be present at the start of therapy. Reduction of that number to 10^{11} did not represent, as was thought 25 years ago, a qualitative change, but merely a relatively minor change in the total number of cells present. When therapeutic programs were changed to require continued "consolidation" and "maintenance" courses of therapy, even in the presence of remission, the cell burden was further reduced and it now appears that a substantial percentage, perhaps a majority, of such patients may actually be cured of disease.

It appears incontrovertible at this time that the appropriate use of chemotherapeutic agents given in the immediate postoperative period and continued for months to years following removal of the primary tumor can result in prolongation of remission and in some diseases increase in cure rates. In breast cancer, prolongation of the disease-free period has clearly been achieved. It is still uncertain whether increases in cure rates will also result. If increased cure rates do not occur with the programs presently in effect, it does not negate the principle of adjuvant chemotherapy, but merely points out that the therapeutic programs used to date are imperfect. However, those programs provide a firm basis for continued study and evaluation of increasingly better therapeutic regimens to achieve better cure rates in a disease which is systemic in the majority of patients when it is detected.

REFERENCES

1. Shapiro, M. D., and Fugmann, R. A. (1957): A role for chemotherapy as an adjunct to surgery. *Cancer Res.,* 17:1098–1101.
2. Schabel, F. M. (1957): Animal models or predictive systems. In: *Cancer Chemotherapy — Fundamental Concepts and Recent Advances.* Year Book Medical Publishers, Chicago.
3. Simpson-Herren, L., Sanford, A. M., and Holmquist, J. P. (1977): Effects of surgery on the cell kinetics of residual tumor. *Cancer Treatm. Rep. (in press).*
4. Skipper, H. F., and Schabel, F. M., Jr. (1977): Quantitative and cytokinetic studies in experimental tumor systems. In: *Cancer Medicine, Ed. 2,* edited by J. F. Holland and E. Frie, III. Lea & Febiger, Philadelphia *(in press).*
5. Fisher, B. (1972): Surgical adjuvant therapy for breast cancer. *Cancer,* 30:1556–1564.
6. Fisher, B., Slack, N. H., Cavanaugh, P. J., Gardner, B., and Ravdin, R. G. (1970): Postoperative radiotherapy in the treatment of breast cancer: Results of the NSABP clinical trial. *Ann. Surg.,* 172:711–728.
7. Stjernsward, J. (1974): Decreased survival related to irradiation postoperatively in early operable breast cancer. *Lancet,* 2:1285–1286.
8. Kennedy, B. J., Mielke, P. W., Jr., and Fortunz, I. E. (1964): Therapeutic castration versus prophylactic castration in breast cancer. *Surg. Gynecol. Obstet.,* 118:524–540.
9. Tormey, D. C. (1975): Combined chemotherapy and surgery in breast cancer: A review. *Cancer,* 36:881–892.
10. Nissen-Meyer, R., Kjellgren, K., and Mansson, B. (1971): A preliminary report from the Scandinavian Adjuvant Chemotherapy Study Group. *Cancer Chemother. Rep.,* 55:561–566.

11. Finney, R. (1971): Adjuvant chemotherapy in the radical treatment of carcinoma of the breast—a clinical trial. *Am. J. Roentgenol.,* 111:137–141.
12. Rieche, K., Berndt, H., and Prahl, B. (1972): Continuous postoperative treatment with cyclophosphamide in breast carcinoma—a randomized clinical study. *Arch. Geschwulstforsch.,* 40:349–354.
13. Yoshida, Y., Miura, S., Murai, H., and Takcuchi, S. (1973): Late results in combined chemotherapy for cure of breast cancer (axillary lymph node metastasis and therapeutic effect). In: *10th Annual Meeting of the Japanese Society for Cancer Therapy,* Abstract 177.
14. Long, R. T. L., Donegan, W. L., and Evans, A. M. (1969): Extended surgical adjuvant chemotherapy for breast carcinoma. *Am. J. Surg.,* 117:701–704.
15. Mrazek, R. G. (1970): Adjuvant chemotherapy with cancer of the breast at one institute. In: *Chemotherapy of Cancer,* edited by W. H. Cole. Lea & Febiger, Philadelphia.
16. Fisher, B., Carbone, P., Economou, S. G., Frelick, R., Glass, A., Lerner, H., Redmond, C., Zelen, M., Band, P., Katrych, D. L., Wolmark, N., and Fisher, E. (and other cooperating investigators) (1975): L-Phenylalanine mustard (L-PAM) in the management of primary breast cancer; a report of early findings. *New Engl. J. Med.,* 292:117–122.
17. Bonadonna, G., Brussolimo, E., Valagussa, R., Rossi, A., Brugnatelli, L., Brambilla, C., DeLena, M., Tancini, G., Bajetta, E., Musemici, R., and Veronesi, U. (1976): Combination chemotherapy as an adjuvant treatment in operable breast cancer. *New Engl. J. Med.,* 294:405–410.
18. Canellos, G. P., De Vita, V. T., Gold, G. L., Chabner, B. A., Schein, P. S. and Young, R. C. (1974): Cyclical combination chemotherapy for advanced breast carcinoma. *Br. Med. J.,* 1:218–220.
19. Rossi, A., Valagussa, P., Bonadonna, G., and Veronesi, U. (1976): Adjuvant treatment with prolonged CMF (Ctx-Mtx-FU) in operable breast cancer with positive axillary nodes. *Proc. A.A.C.R.,* 17:73.
20. Rojas, A. F., Mickiewicz, E., Olivari, E., Carugatti, A., and Lebenstein, M. (1976): Levamisole: A preliminary report on toxicity, clinical action and effect on cellular immunity in cancer patients after 22 months of treatment. *Lancet,* 1:211–215.
21. Burgert, E. O., and Glidewell, O. (1967): Dactinomycin in Wilms' tumor. *J.A.M.A.,* 199: 464.
22. Jaffe, N., Traggis, D., Andonia, S., Chan, D., Sallan, S., Kim, T., and Frei, E., III (1974): "Adjuvant" high dose methotrexate and citrovorum rescue (HDMC) following primary treatment of osteogenic sarcoma. *A.A.C.R. Abstracts,* 15:132.
23. Clarkson, B. D., and Fried, J. (1971): Changing concepts of treatment in acute leukemia. *Med. Clin. North Am.,* 55:561–600.

Note added in proof: More recent data (*personal communication,* November 1976) of the Milan breast cancer study indicate that persistent benefit in this study is restricted to premenopausal patients.

Cancer Invasion and Metastasis: Biologic Mechanisms and Therapy, edited by S. B. Day et al. Raven Press, New York © 1977.

Micrometastasis Therapy: Theoretical Concepts

*Lance A. Liotta, **Gerald Saidel, ***Jerome Kleinerman, and †Charles DeLisi

Laboratory of *Pathology and †Theoretical Biology, National Cancer Institute, National Institutes of Health, Bethesda, Maryland 20014; **Department of Biomedical Engineering, Case Western Reserve University, Cleveland, Ohio 44106; and ***Department of Pathology Research, St. Luke's Hospital, Cleveland, Ohio 44104

The formation of metastases begins with release of tumor cells from the primary tumor. It is generally accepted that most of the circulating tumor cells perish. Only a few survive to form metastases. The question is: how many disseminated tumor cells are needed before the first metastasis is formed? If a tumor is disseminating tumor cells at a continuous rate, when are we certain that micrometastases have been established? The answers to these questions are of great theoretical and practical importance. If we knew more about the factors which determine the timing of micrometastasis formation, a rational basis might exist for planning adjunctive therapy. Furthermore, if we could predict when metastases were initiated, additional information concerning the growth of metastases would lead to estimates of micrometastases size distribution. The success of chemotherapy, radiotherapy, and immunotherapy depends on the number and size of metastases which exist at the time of treatment (1,2).

To develop a theoretical foundation for clarifying concepts in metastasis therapy, we have developed deterministic and stochastic models of metastasis (3,4). Already these models have predicted the course of spontaneous metastasis development in an animal system (4,5). In this chapter we extend the application of these models to the systemic therapy of micrometastases. In particular, we attempt to analyze what factors determine the critical time period when micrometastases are first initiated.

The hematogenous metastatic process from a solid tumor consists of a series of stages:

(a) Vascularization of the neoplasm provides a circulatory entrance route for tumor cells (5,6).

(b) Tumor cells in the tumor mass penetrate the walls of tumor vessels and are dislodged in clumps of various sizes into the tumor venous drainage (7).

(c) Tumor cells are carried by the circulation to the target organ where they arrest in the small blood vessels (8).

(d) A small fraction of the arrested tumor cells survive to traverse the vascular wall and initiate metastases (9,17).

THE MODEL

Basic Concepts

The mathematical model summarized here describes the dynamics of the tumor cell arrival in a target organ with the subsequent initiation and growth of metastatic foci. A detailed derivation of the model using probability concepts can be found elsewhere (4). The main point here is that metastasis formation is inherently a stochastic process; i.e., at any time t there will be some probability of having a given number of metastases. Since only a small fraction of disseminated cells metastasizes, this probability obeys a poisson distribution. Hence if M is the mean number of cells that have metastasized, then by a well-known formula (10),

$$p = exp\ (-M(t)) \qquad [1]$$

is the probability of no metastasis at time t. Thus the problem of determining the probability of no metastasis is reduced to obtaining an expression for the mean number at time t.

An expression for the mean number of metastases at time t is found by solving the differential equations corresponding to the compartment model shown in Fig. 1. Its value is clearly going to depend on:

(a) the rate $\lambda(t)$ at which tumor cells arrest in the target organ;

(b) the probability $\beta_2 m \Delta t$ that an arrested tumor cell will die (or dislodge) in a short time interval, where m is the number of arrested tumor cells;

(c) the probability $\beta_3 m \Delta t$ that an arrested tumor cell will initiate a metastatic focus in a short time interval.

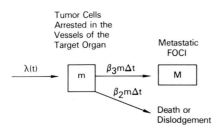

FIG. 1. The formation of metastatic foci can be considered as a stochastic population balance. Tumor cells disseminate from the primary tumor and arrest in the target organ at a rate $\lambda(t)$. The chance of one death in the population of arrested cells $m(t)$ in time Δt is $\beta_2 m \Delta t$. The chance that one metastatic focus will be initiated from the population $m(t)$ in time Δt is $\beta_3 m \Delta t$. The population of metastatic foci is denoted by $M(t)$. See ref. 10 for a comprehensive presentation of stochastic processes and their application to natural sciences.

The death rate β_2 for m tumor cells, which follows first-order kinetics, includes destruction by host defenses, chemotherapy, or radiotherapy. Justification for this form can be found in the studies of Phillips et al. (11) on cellular immune cell killing of tumor cells, of Schabel (1) with regard to chemotherapy, and of Curtis et al. (12) and Schaeffer (13) on radiotherapy. The rate of initiation of metastases by m tumor cells, having the form $\beta_3 m$, can be justified from numerous studies of metastases formation following intravenous injection of graded doses of tumor cells (14,17).

With this background the differential equations for the mean number of tumor cells arrested in the target organ is

$$dm/dt = \lambda(t) - (\beta_2 + \beta_3)m \qquad [2]$$

$$m = 0; \, t = 0 \quad \text{initial conditions.}$$

The rates $-\beta_2 m$ and $-\beta_3 m$ represent the rate at which tumor cells in population m are lost due to death, dislodgment, or metastasis formation. The function $\lambda(t)$ represents the rate at which tumor cells arrest in the vessels of the target organ. This functional form will be determined by the rate at which tumor cells are being released by the primary tumor. Since $-\beta_3 m$ is the rate at which arrested tumor cells initiate metastatic foci, then $+\beta_3 m$ must be the rate at which the number of metastases is increasing. Thus

$$dM/dt = \beta_3 m \qquad [3]$$

$$M = 0; \, t = 0 \quad \text{initial conditions.}$$

Solving these equations yields

$$M(t) = \beta_3/(\beta_2 + \beta_3) \int_0^t \lambda(\tau)\{\exp\left[-(t-\tau)(\beta_2 + \beta_3)\right]\} \, d\tau \qquad [4]$$

Estimates of the parameters β_2 and β_3 can be obtained in experimental systems by the intravenous injection of known numbers of labeled tumor cells. For an intravenous injection all tumor cells with the potential to arrest in the target organ are assumed to do so rapidly (17). Consequently, $\lambda(t)$ is time independent and equal to the number of arrested tumor cells N. Therefore, $\lambda(t) = N$, $t = 0$, and is zero at all other times. With this condition Eq. [4] becomes

$$M(t) = N\beta_3/(\beta_2 + \beta_3) \{1 - \exp\left(-t\,(\beta_2 + \beta_3)\right)\} \qquad [5]$$

AN EMPIRICAL TEST OF THE MODEL

To test this model we applied it to a particular experimental system with a transplantable, poorly immunogenic (T241) murine fibrosarcoma that metastasizes to the lungs (5). Estimates of the parameters β_2 and β_3 can be obtained experimentally following the intravenous injection of tumor cells as described in detail elsewhere (4,15). Briefly, the parameter β_2 for the death rate of tumor cells arrested in the lungs is determined by measuring the initial exponential decay of tumor cells in the lungs following intravenous injection of known numbers of labeled tumor cells. In separate experiments the parameter β_3 is found by counting the total number of metastases formed from an intravenous injection of known numbers of tumor cells. The function $\lambda(t)$ has been experimentally determined by measuring the rate at which tumor cells enter the primary tumor venous drainage (5). Tumor cells entering the venous drainage were tagged with ^{51}Cr and injected intravenously into tumor-bearing mice. Virtually all the cells arrested in the lung within 5 min. Thus it can be assumed in this tumor-host system that the rate at which tumor cells enter the tumor venous drainage is equivalent to their arrest rate in the lungs. Based on experimental data (5), the best functional form is as follows:

$$\lambda(t) = ce^{k(t-\theta)}, \, t > \theta$$
$$= 0; \, t < \theta \qquad [6]$$

where c and k are time-invariant parameters and t is time post-transplant in days. Time delay θ in the above equation represents the number of days after transplantation of the primary tumor that tumor cells first enter the tumor venous drainage; the delay reflects time lag for tumor vascularization (5). Substituting Eq. [6] in Eq. [4], the solution for $t < \theta$ is $M = 0$ and for $t > \theta$:

$$M(t) = \beta_3/(\beta_2 + \beta_3) \, \{c[1/k \, (e^{k(t-\theta)} - 1) + 1/(k + \beta_2)$$
$$(e^{k(t-\theta)} - e^{-\beta_2(t-\theta)})]\} \qquad [7]$$

When $t \gg \theta$, the solution is approximately

$$M(t) = \beta_3/(\beta_2 + \beta_3) \, \{ce^{kt}[1/k + 1/(k + \beta_2)]\}$$

In Fig. 2 the predicted probability of surgical cure is compared with experimental data. The experimentally determined parameter values are: $\beta_2 = 4.2$ days^{-1}; $\beta_3/\beta_2 = 1 \times 10^{-4}$; $k = 0.48$ days^{-1}; $c = 1,440$ cells/day; and $\theta = 4.0$ (days). The model shows a good fit with the data.

In this system the presence of micrometastases is determined early in the course of tumor growth. There exists a critical time period during which the probability that no metastases exist rapidly falls to zero. This critical time period exists in other experimental tumors which metastasize such as the Lewis lung carcinoma (6). An understanding of the factors which determine the onset and duration of this critical period may provide insights into the timing of therapy.

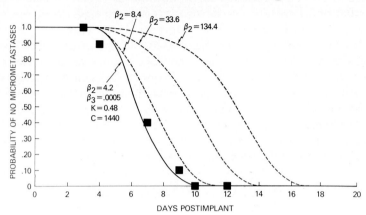

a. EFFECT OF INCREASING DEATH RATE (β_2)

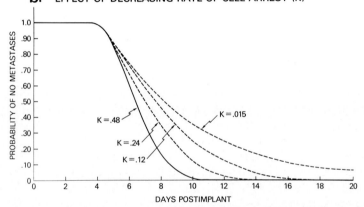

b. EFFECT OF DECREASING RATE OF CELL ARREST (K)

FIG. 2. Comparison of model prediction with experimental data for the probability of no micrometastases existing (equal to the probability of surgical cure) at the time of tumor excision at a sequence of times following transplantation. The tumor was excised by amputating the tumor-bearing limb. Fourteen days after amputation, mice were sacrificed for pulmonary metastasis assay. This waiting period allowed microscopic metastases existing at the time of amputation to grow to sufficient size for recognition. The lungs of sacrificed mice were inflated with neutral buffered formalin and fixed for 7 days. Metastases were identified both macroscopically in individual lung lobes and microscopically in lobe serial sections. The data (■) in **(a)** are the proportions of 10 mice with no metastases. The solid curves are the solutions of Eq. 1 for *M* given by Eq. 7 for the parameter values listed. The parameter values were determined experimentally. Dashed curves are solutions of Eq. 3 when a specified parameter is varied.

The solution of the equation for p for various parameter values demonstrates that an increase in the death rate (β_2) of metastasizing tumor cells causes a delay in the critical time period with little effect on the slope or duration of the period (Fig. 2a). Decreasing the rate of tumor cell arrest in the target organ (k) serves to change the slope of the critical time period and lengthen its duration (Fig. 2b). Because of their rapid death rate in this experimental system, residual tumor cells arrested in the vessels of the target organ at the time of tumor excision make little contribution to the overall probability of having no established micrometastases. This can be seen from inspection of the second negative exponential term in Eq. [7], which decays rapidly when $\lambda(t)$ is set to zero.

MICROMETASTASES THERAPY

The probability model of metastases formation can be extended to include the therapy of established, growing micrometastases if certain presuppositions are made about metastasis growth and susceptibility to therapy. Recognizing that larger micrometastases are less responsive to therapy (1,16), we may choose a micrometastasis of size s which is too large to be completely eradicated by therapy at a given systemic dose d. We are interested in the probability that at time t no metastases have exceeded size s. This can be obtained as follows: if a newly initiated metastasis requires a time $l(s)$ to reach a size s, then any metastasis that has not been established by time $t - l(s)$ cannot reach the critical size. Hence, we are interested in the probability that no micrometastases have been initiated by time $t - l(s)$. This is just given by Eq. [1] with t replaced by $t - l(s)$. Based on this simplified approach, the time-dependent curves for the probability of overall cure by adjuvant therapy at a dose d would be the same as those shown in Fig. 2 but would be shifted to the right by an amount $l(s)$. The curves would retain the qualitative character of a rapid decay phase beyond which eradication of all micrometastases would be very unlikely for a given adjuvant dosage. The dose of adjuvant therapy necessary to cure the patient is therefore dependent on the time of surgical intervention as well as the growth rate of micrometastases.

In summary, the major conclusions generated by a theoretical analysis of micrometastases formation are as follows:

1. The initiation of micrometastatic foci can be modeled as a poisson process.

2. During the growth of a transplanted tumor there exists a critical time period when the probability that no micrometastases exist (one minus this value is the probability that at least one or more metastases have been established) rapidly decays to zero. The timing and slope of this critical period are determined by the rate at which tumor cells are released from the tumor and arrest in the target organ and by survival parameters for arrested tumor cells.

3. The small number of residual circulating tumor cells or tumor cells arrested in target organ vessels at the time of surgical primary tumor removal make little contribution to overall survival. This is based on the low probability that a residual arrested cell metastasizes. Therapy of these residual cells would not affect overall survival. Therapy should instead be focused on established micrometastases.

4. The success of systemic adjuvant therapy in which each micrometastatic focus can be assumed to be exposed to the same local dosage is dependent on micrometastasis size, not number.

We acknowledge that metastasis formation is a complex phenomenon. However, factors that influence this process can be grouped into the three rates depicted in Fig. 1. Thus we can establish a framework for analyzing metastasis formation. Although the conclusions stated above may be applicable only to experimental systems, they can serve to pinpoint future research directions.

REFERENCES

1. Schabel, F. M., Jr. (1975): Concepts for systemic treatment of micrometastases. *Cancer*, 35:15–24.
2. Hoover, H. C., Jr., and Ketcham, A. S. (1975): Techniques for inhibiting tumor metastases. *Cancer*, 35:14.
3. Saidel, G. M., Liotta, L. A., and Kleinerman, J. (1976): System dynamics of a metastatic process from an implanted tumor. *J. Theor. Biol.*, 56:417–434.
4. Liotta, L. A., Saidel, G. M., and Kleinerman, J. (1976): Stochastic model of metastases formation. *Biometrics*, 32:535–550.
5. Liotta, L. A., Kleinerman, J., and Saidel, G. M. (1974): Quantitative relationships of intravascular tumor cells, tumor vessels, and pulmonary metastases following tumor implantation. *Cancer Res.*, 34:997–1004.
6. James, S. E. and Salsbury, A. J. (1974): Effect of (+)-1,2-bis(3,5-dioxopiperazin-1-yl) propane on tumor blood vessels and its relationship to the antimetastatic effect in the Lewis lung carcinoma. *Cancer Res.*, 34:839–842.
7. Liotta, L. A., Kleinerman, J., and Saidel, G. M. (1976): The significance of hematogenous tumor cell clumps in the metastatic process. *Cancer Res.*, 36:889–894.
8. Coman, D. R. (1953): Mechanisms responsible for the origin and distribution of bloodborne tumor metastases: A review. *Cancer Res.*, 13:397–404.
9. Fidler, I. J. (1970): Metastases: Quantitative analysis of distribution and fate of tumor emboli labeled with 125 I-5-iodo-2' deoxyuridine, *J. Natl. Cancer Inst.*, 45:775–782.
10. Bailey, T. J. (1964): *The Elements of Stochastic Processes with Applications to the Natural Sciences.* John Wiley and Sons, New York.
11. Phillips, R. A., Clark, D. A., Schilling, R. M., and Miller, R. G. (1974): Quantitation and characterization of effector cells and their progenitors. In: *Cell Biology and Tumor Immunology, Vol. 1, Proceedings of the XI International Cancer Congress*, edited by P. Bucalossi, U. Veronesi, and N. Cascinelli, pp. 264–336. American Elsevier, New York.
12. Curtis, S. B., Barendsen, G. W., and Hermens, A. F. (1973): Cell kinetic model of tumour growth and regression for a rhabdomyosarcoma in the rat: Undisturbed growth and radiation response to large single doses. *Eur. J. Cancer*, 9:81–87.
13. Schaeffer, J., El-Mahdi, A. M., and Constable, W. C. (1973): Radiation control of microscopic pulmonary metastases in C3H mice. *Cancer*, 32:346–351.
14. Fisher, B., and Fisher, R. (1967): Metastases of cancer cells. In: *Methods in Cancer Research, Vol. 1*, edited by H. Busch, pp. 243–286. Academic Press, New York.
15. Liotta, L. A., and DeLisi, C. (1977): A mathematical method for differentiating tumor cell

removal rate from invasion rate in experimental metastases. *Cancer Res. (submitted for publication).*

16. Holland, J. F. (1976): Breast cancer and chemotherapy. *Science,* 192:1062–1063.
17. Fidler, I. J. (1976): Patterns of Tumor Cell Arrest and Development. In: *Fundamental Aspects of Metastasis,* edited by L. Weiss, pp. 275–289. North Holland Publishing Co., Amsterdam.

Cancer Invasion and Metastasis: Biologic Mechanisms and Therapy, edited by S. B. Day et al. Raven Press, New York © 1977.

Comments Regarding the Distribution and Fate of Circulating Tumor Cells

J. W. Proctor

Division of Radiation Oncology, Clinical Radiation Therapy Research Center, Allegheny General Hospital, Pittsburgh, Pennsylvania 15212

Radiolabeled cells from solid nonlymphoid tumors, when injected into the venous system of animals that have not previously encountered a tumor, tend to hold up in the first capillary bed they encounter regardless of the model, e.g., lung and liver following peripheral and portal injections, respectively. Some of them such as the B_{16} mouse melanoma reported on by Fidler (1) pass through to other organs via the systemic circulation after a short-lived stopover in the lungs, whereas others such as our rat sarcomas apparently never leave the lung in significant numbers (2). These differences, which in rabbits according to Zeidman (3) are not due to differences in cell size, reflect the differing biological patterns of spontaneous metastatic spread of the various tumor models from solid extravascular implants. Thus the peripherally placed locally growing sarcomas almost never spread to any organ other than the lung (2,4), whereas the B_{16} not infrequently spreads to heart, brain, kidneys, and adrenals (1). In most such models, an exception being the allogeneic intraperitoneal BP8 tumor model used by Porteous and Munro (5), the radiolabel disappears rapidly from the animal. This rapid loss of radiolabel reflects the rate of cell death and thus the large number of cells required to produce tumor growth in most models. In other systems, possibly including the BP8 model, tumors are reputed to grow from only a single cell, and it is possible that in these the initial loss of radiolabel will not occur.

Studies such as those mentioned by Peters (*this volume*) and our own indicate that radiolabel loss is due to the death of the tumor cells and probably also that this occurs in the target organ itself. The question as to whether the loss of tumor cells is due to passive deterioration as claimed by Peters or to active destruction as claimed by Alexander has not been answered satisfactorily. However, the fact that increasing the numbers of injected cells leads to a smaller percentage loss as does pretreatment with cyclophosphamide (Peters) would, as claimed by Alexander although refuted by Peters (*this volume*), weigh in favor of an active destructive mechanism. It is apparent that the loss of cells is low in 1-week-old rats (Peters and ourselves) compared to that in older rats indicating a defective destruction mechanism (our contention) or an inherent unspecified difference in the microenvironment of the lungs of 1-week-old and adult rats which allows for "passive" survival in the former (Peters' contention).

It has been suggested by Woodruff and Dunbar (6), by us (2), and again by Alexander (*this volume*) that the destruction of tumor cells in previously unsensitized animals might be macrophage mediated. The data presented by Peters (*this volume*), like those reported by Bomford and Olivotto (7), do not support such a contention, but there again none of these findings rules out a mechanism in which monocytes are rapidly recruited *de novo* from the bone marrow.

Nonimmune factors that determine patterns of organ distribution were discussed also. The data of Nicolson and co-workers (8,9) demonstrate clearly that tumor cells can display organotropism. The question raised by such findings relates to their significance in the biology of blood-borne tumor spread. Were these cells selected from the wild tumor as a subpopulation with a special affinity for the lung or were they a population which adapted to a new environment and acquired special characteristics over several cycles through a foreign tissue? The comments of Nicolson tended to suggest that the cell lines would revert to less organotropic populations if the selective pressure was released indicating that "modulation or adaptation" rather than "selection" was the likely mechanism involved. These findings raise the further questions of (a) the importance of tertiary spread (10), which despite the lack of definitive experimental evidence is still a generally accepted phenomenon, and (b) Paget's "soil seed" (11) and Ewing's "mechanical" factors (12). Modulation or adaptation need not be of great significance in secondary spread and possibly not even in tertiary spread since it appears to require several cycles for processes such as those described by Nicolson to become manifest.

Data from our rat sarcoma model support the concept of Ewing almost absolutely in that tumor cells injected intravenously hold up and grow almost exclusively in the first target organ they reach. However, similar cells injected into the systemic circulation show a marked predilection for the adrenal gland and ovaries in particular (4). Thus about 2,000 tumor cells 10 min after injection give rise to approximately the same amount of tumor in the adrenal glands (2.0 g) 4 weeks later, as do more than 100,000 cells in the lungs of the same animal (Fig. 1). In this experiment approximately 500 cells in the ovaries produced more than 4 g of tumor.

Our conclusion was that the organ pattern of secondary spread from this particular tumor was determined by "mechanical" factors, whereas tertiary spread was influenced largely by "soil seed" considerations as suggested by Paget before the turn of the century. As Fisher remarked (*this volume*), the actual significance of tertiary spread in the clinic is unknown.

The question of influence of specific immunity on the fate of circulating

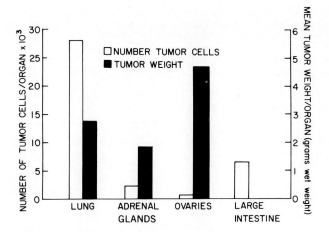

FIG. 1. Approximately 2×10^5 MCI ^{125}IUdR-labeled cells registering approximately 1 cpm/8 cells and with a labeling index of >7% were injected under ether anesthesia into the aortas of 8-week-old female syngeneic rats from the strain of origin. The number of cells/organ was based on cpm/organ 10 min after injection and the weight of tumor/organ established 4 weeks later.

cells was raised by data presented separately in this volume by Glaves and co-workers (13) and Fidler, demonstrating a redistribution of tumor cells to different organs in two different animal models. This phenomenon has not been observed by us in rat sarcoma model (2), underlining the heterogeneity of animal tumor models, a property which, as emphasized by Fisher, is shared by human cancers.

In summary with regard to therapy, the distribution and growth patterns of metastases are likely to become important because the effect of chemotherapy at one site may differ from that at another (14), as quite possibly might the effect of immunotherapy, although the lack of success of this latter modality at present precludes a definitive comment. The likelihood is that the relative importance of the significant factors will vary from one cancer to another as it does from one animal model to another, and that only by carefully defining the factors significant for each form of cancer will it be possible to exploit these properties.

REFERENCES

1. Fidler, I. J. (1970): Metastasis: Quantitative analysis of distribution and fate of tumor emboli labelled ^{125}I-5-iodo-2' deoxyuridine. *J. Natl. Cancer Inst.,* 45:773–782.
2. Proctor, J. W., Auclair, B. G., and Rudenstam, C. M. (1976): The distribution and fate of blood borne ^{125}IUdR labelled tumor cells in immune syngeneic rats. *Int. J. Cancer,* 18: 255–262.
3. Zeidman, I. (1961): The fate of circulating tumor cells. I. Passage of cells through capillaries. *Cancer Res.,* 21:38–39.
4. Proctor, J. W. (1977): Support for the "soil seed" hypothesis and the "mechanical" theory derived from a rat sarcoma model. *Br. J. Cancer (in press).*

5. Porteous, D. D., and Munro, T. R. (1972): The kinetics of the killing of mouse tumor cells "in vivo" by immune responses. *Int. J. Cancer,* 10:112–117.
6. Woodruff, M. F. A., and Dunbar, B. (1974): The effect of cell dose and distribution on the development of a transplanted tumor. *Eur. J. Cancer,* 10:533–547.
7. Bomford, R., and Olivotto, M. (1971): The mechanism of inhibition by *Corynebacterium parvum* of the growth of lung nodules from intravenously injected tumor cells. *Int. J. Cancer,* 14:226–235.
8. Nicolson, G. L., and Winkelhake, J. L. (1975): Organ specificity of blood borne metastases determined by cell adhesion. *Nature,* 255:230–232.
9. Fidler, I., and Nicolson, G. L. (1976): Organ selectivity for implantation survival and growth of B16 melanoma variant tumor lines. *J. Natl. Cancer Inst.,* 57:1199–1202.
10. Sugarbaker, E. V., Cohen, A. M., and Ketcham, A. S. (1971): Do metastases metastasize? *Ann. Surg.,* 174:161–166.
11. Paget, S. (1889): The distribution of secondary growths in cancer of the breast. *Lancet,* 1:571–573.
12. Ewing, J. (1928): In: *Neoplastic Diseases, Ed. 3,* pp. 86–87. W. B. Saunders Co., Philadelphia.
13. Weiss, L., Glaves, D., and Waite, D. A. (1974): The influence of host immunity on the arrest of circulating cancer cells and its modification by neuraminidase. *Int. J. Cancer,* 13:850–862.
14. Pugh, R. P., Jacobs, E. M., Bateman, J. R., and Bull, F. E. (1975): CCNU vs CCNU + Vincristine in disseminated melanoma. A.S.C.O. Abstracts, No. 1103, p. 246.

Cancer Invasion and Metastasis: Biologic Mechanisms and Therapy, edited by S. B. Day et al. Raven Press, New York © 1977.

Some Observations on the Biology of Metastasis

J. Norris Childs

Chester Beatty Research Institute, Royal Cancer Hospital, Belmont, Sutton, Surrey, England

The need for understanding the biology of metastases is underlined by the presence of metastases, either apparent or soon to be apparent, in many cancer patients at the time of diagnosis. In transplanted tumors in animals, there is good evidence from cytology and bioassay studies that tumor cells are shed from the primary and appear in the blood and distant organs by days 4 to 9 of tumor growth (4,5,7). The kinetics of growth of the primary and its concurrent metastases and the increase in numbers of cells shed into the blood over time have all been described in elegant mathematical form (1,6,8), leaving, however, an unknown blank in the period after the removal of the primary.

Experimental treatment of metastases in animals and man has been approached from several angles: treating the animal soon after tumor transplantation and thereby preventing metastases; treating animals late in tumor bearing with X-rays, cytotoxic drugs, anticoagulants, and either decreasing the number of metastatic nodules in a lung or reducing their size, but rarely achieving a cure; treating patients usually in combination with surgical removal of the primary and changing 5-year survival. This latter approach is the only system seemingly relevant to humans, but it is not much different from fiddling with number or size of metastases, since the end result is usually death from metastases later. Any cures these approaches achieve seem at present fortuitous rather than consistent, and really provide no new information about the early growth and development of metastases.

I have been studying metastases of chemically induced transplantable sarcomata in syngeneic rats. These solid tumors, when grown in the leg and excised at day 14 (a time when autopsied animals would have no gross or microscopic metastases), have a finite rate of metastases to lymph nodes or lungs if the animals are allowed to live out their life. It is puzzling why in these syngeneic animals with similar tumor innocula to start, same duration of tumor growth, and same size of tumor at the time of surgery, only 20% of the animals develop lung metastases.

I feel the way to approach this question is by studying the period immediately after removal of the primary tumor, an approach that has been neglected up to the present. To study these inapparent future metastases, one must be able to detect them. Histology, immunochemistry, and cytology all fall short of the mark and say nothing about viability; a bioassay seems to be the only possible approach. Many are described in the literature, from the all-or-none "organ brei" assay of Goldie et al. (3) to the extraordinarily tedious "quantitative" volume growth rate assay of DeWys (2). A quantitative bioassay is necessary for the study of small numbers of cells, and the assay which holds promise of being that involves exsanguinating the animal to be studied, removing the lungs, washing them four times in normal saline, cutting them up finely with scissors, trypsinization for 2 to 4 hr, washing once with medium 199, then injecting various dilutions i.p. in a volume of 5 ml into preirradiated weanling rats. To date this bioassay has been used to study residual tumor cells in the lungs after surgical removal of the primary. The following are some early results that have been obtained.

One tumor studied (HSBPA) will grow from 10^4 cells when injected i.m. and 10^3 cells if injected i.v. or i.p. (when injected alone or mixed with trypsinized normal lung). If a leg primary approximately $2\frac{1}{2}$ cm in diameter is excised at day 14, 0 to 10% of the animals develop lung metastases. In one series of experiments, 1/22 animals developed postsurgical metastases. Of another 29 animals killed 7 days post-excision, none had gross lung metastases, but 6 of these 29 were bioassay positive for tumor cells in the lung, suggesting that as late as 7 days after surgery there may be more than 1,000 cells in the lungs of animals that would not develop metastases, and that these cells may be lying dormant. Animals that had borne the HSBPA tumor for 14 days were then treated 7 days after tumor excision with BCNU, cyclophosphamide, or whole body irradiation, and either bioassayed 3 days later or kept as spontaneous metastasis controls. With BCNU 15 mg/kg i.p., 1/8 developed postamputation node metastasis, and 3/8 had bioassay-positive lungs. With cyclophosphamide 180 mg/kg i.p., 0/8 developed postamputation metastases, and 0/8 were bioassay positive. With 500 rads whole body irradiation, 2/8 developed postsurgical metastases, whereas 5/8 were bioassay positive. These data support the idea that the number of residual tumor cells in the lung is affected by postsurgical adjuvant therapy, and that this effect can be analyzed in the bioassay system.

In order to study what happens to numbers of tumor cells in the lungs after surgery when the supply of new tumor cells via the blood ceases, the quantitative, dilutional bioassay that will detect smaller numbers of cells is needed. A different tumor (MC3) which will grow from 10 cells i.p. is better suited to these studies. In a preliminary experiment with this tumor, 0/7 rats that had borne the primary for 14 days developed postexcisional metastases; 0/8 had gross metastases at autopsy 7 days post-excision, but 4 of these 8 had bioassay-positive lungs. With this tumor, the percentage of animals with metastases increases as the primary is left to grow longer before surgery, and hence the route is open to relating the occurrence of metastases to the number of cells left in the lungs.

While the primary tumor is present, the number of tumor cells in the lung is a function of their rate of release from the primary, their rate of death in the lung, and their rate of growth in the lung. For these rat tumors and human tumors, clinically negative for metastases at the time of surgery, three factors must be in near equilibrium. After the primary is removed, the influx of new cells ceases and cell death continues as do division and growth of some of the cells that are there. The total number of cells should thus decrease to a nadir after which growth outstrips death if metastases are to occur. This suggests that in tumors with a finite rate of metastatic occurrence, the ultimate growth or lack of growth of metastases depends on how low the number of tumor cells falls, and that success in treatment of micro-metastases will be related to reducing the number of tumor cells below a threshold under which they cannot grow. Studying the biology, numbers, and time-related growth characteristics of tumor cells in the period immediately following removal of the primary will hopefully suggest timings and modes of adjuvant chemo- and radiotherapies which will be of use in the control of metastatic growth.

ACKNOWLEDGMENT

This work was supported by NCI fellowship number 5 F32 CA 05100–02.

REFERENCES

1. Butler, T. P., and Gullino, P. M. (1975): Quantitation of cell shedding into efferent blood of mammary adenocarcinoma. *Cancer Res.,* 35:512.
2. DeWys, W. D. (1972): A quantitative model for the study of the growth and treatment of a tumor and its metastases with correlation between proliferative state and sensitivity to cyclophosphamide. *Cancer Res.,* 32:367.
3. Goldie, H., Jeffries, B. R., Jones, A. M., and Walker, M. (1953): Detection of metastatic tumor cells by intraperitoneal inoculation of organ brei from tumor bearing mice. *Cancer Res.,* 13:566.
4. Greene, H. S. N., and Harvey, E. K. (1964): The relationship between the dissemination of tumor cells and the distribution of metastases. *Cancer Res.,* 24:799.
5. Julian, L. (1958): The metastatic process of a transplantable lymphocytic tumor of chickens (RPL 16). I. The time of metastasis. *Cancer Res.,* 18:247.
6. Liotta, L. A., Kleinerman, J., and Saidel, G. M. (1974): Quantitative relationships of intra-vascular tumor cells, tumor vessels, and pulmonary metastases following tumor implantation. *Cancer Res.,* 34:997.
7. Romsdahl, M. D., Chu, E. W., Hume, R., and Smith, R. R. (1961): The time of metastasis and release of circulating tumor cells as determined in an experimental system. *Cancer,* 14:883.
8. Simpson-Herren, L., and Lloyd, H. H. (1970): Kinetic parameters and growth curves for experimental tumor systems. *Cancer Chemother. Rep.,* 54:143.

Cancer Invasion and Metastasis: Biologic Mechanisms and Therapy, edited by S. B. Day et al. Raven Press, New York © 1977.

Concluding Remarks on Cancer Dissemination and Metastases

Silvio Garattini

Istituto di Ricerche Farmacologiche "Mario Negri," Milan, Italy

It is always difficult to sum up a volume. Since the volume consists of 43 chapters and discussions, I will try to make a few pertinent remarks rather than attempt a complete summary. But my remarks will labor under a major handicap: they will be biased by my pharmacological origins.

One point I would like to comment on is what has been called the *metastatic potential* of cancer cells, stressing the difficulty of predicting whether cancer cells of a given experimental tumor will or will not disseminate and/or metastasize. How do we test this potential? Only by using a host organism. Therefore we immediately have another factor to consider, and, as has repeatedly been pointed out, we cannot discuss metastases without considering the two facets of the question: properties of cancer cells and conditions of the host organism.

The site of implantation is of key importance: after all, not all human tumors are located s.c. or i.m.. We know that the pattern of dissemination and metastasis may change depending on the site of implantation. Certain tumors induce metastases in lymph nodes when they are implanted in a bone cavity but have little capacity to metastasize when they are implanted i.m. (1). Implantation in the intestinal wall may facilitate the formation of liver metastasis; tumors that normally metastasize widely, such as the Lewis lung carcinoma (3LL), become nonmetastatic when implanted in the peritoneal cavity. If we push these observations to the extreme we may find that metastatic potential is only a relative term because cancer cells with metastasizing capacities may not metastasize when implanted in "unfavorable sites" or in hosts with effective defenses. The opposite may be true when cancer cells with low metastasizing capacity are implanted in sites favorable for dissemination (e.g., the brain) or in animals with weak defenses (2).

Our concept of defenses is probably changing because a great complexity of factors may play a role in metastasis, including immunological mechanisms (first or second line of defense), hemostatic mechanisms, endothelial properties, and a number of local factors that may facilitate or inhibit leakage of cancer cells from the primary tumor or the take of disseminated cancer cells into normal tissue. These factors combine in a very delicate balance on which hangs the possibility of cells migrating, surviving in the hematogenous or lymphatic circulation, arresting in given tissues, and establishing themselves there. I am sure that the future will see a large number of studies to evaluate which of these many factors have biological significance for the question of metastases.

Connected with the problem of metastatic potential is the difficulty of finding what characteristics distinguish tumors that metastasize from those that do not. Several aspects have been discussed in this volume, such as adhesion, aggregability, release of cells as clumps, loss of anchorage dependence, release of tumor angiogenic factors (TAF), production of plasminogen activators or other proteases, and production of prostaglandins or other osteolytic factors.

Even more important for therapeutic implications is the question of establishing whether, within a given tumor which metastasizes, all the cancer cells or only a fraction of them have the same properties. In other words, can we predict which cells are going to disseminate and, among them, which ones are going to "take" and give rise to a metastatic nodule?

We know that many cells disseminate but only few metastases are formed. Is this a random effect or are certain cells "committed" to make metastases?

I believe that some facts emerged in this respect in this volume, suggesting that some cancer cell subpopulations may have special properties, such as the presence of epiglycanin or other glycoprotein (GP-1), receptors for *Vicia graminea,* or capacity to solubilize collagen, which put them in more favorable conditions to disseminate. The fact that B16 melanoma yields lines capable of metastasizing selectively in different organs is a good indication of the presence of different kinds of cells in this tumor. The same applies for cells that become resistant to attack by specifically immunized lymphocytes.

However, when the cells disseminate and arrest in given tissues, metastases do not always grow. We come therefore to the problem of cancer cell dormancy. Can cancer cells sleep for many years and then wake up? What factors are involved? Is it the cells which do not proliferate, or the host which inhibits proliferation? Or is a steady-state condition achieved in which the cancer cells do proliferate but not beyond the rate of cell destruction? This may seem merely an academic problem, but here we have learned that models may be available to study dormancy. Depending on which model is used, the factors operative for dormancy may be antibodies, cell-mediated immunity, or macrophages.

Much discussion and many presentations have dealt with selecting proper models. It is true that any model may be suitable if properly understood, but it is clear that certain experimental models may be closer to clinical situations. For therapeutic purposes it may be highly desirable to have in the same animals the growth of a primary tumor, a process of dissemination, and the appearance of metastatic nodules before the animals die. This pattern must be reproducible in order to permit quantitative evaluation of the various treatments (surgery, irradiation, chemotherapy, or immunotherapy). In these models it should be possible to establish the precise reason for the death of tumor-bearing animals as the burden of the primary tumor, the presence of metastases in vital organs, or other unrelated factors such as thrombosis or infections. This may obviously influence the interpretation of all findings.

For example, one agent may provide good antimetastatic treatment, but it may not be effective in prolonging the survival of the animals, for the simple reason that the host is not killed by the metastases. Concerning models, it became apparent in this volume that there is a difference between so-called spontaneous metastases deriving from a primary tumor and artificial metastases obtained, for instance, by intravenous injection of cells.

The number of circulating cancer cells is different in the two models with at least 20 times more in artificial than in spontaneous metastases. The presence of the primary tumor may affect the arrest of cancer cells and their subsequent evolution.

The burden of antigens is different, and this has been suggested as an explanation of why T lymphocytes are active in the artificial model, but B lymphocytes decrease metastases in the spontaneous model. Hemostatic parameters are different as well. At an early stage but not at a late stage in the 3LL model a decrease in platelets is noted in the artificial model whereas the opposite occurs in the spontaneous model. The spontaneous model shows anemia and an increased fibrinogen level but this does not occur in the artificial system. The thymidine index indicating the rate of cell proliferation is lower in the spontaneous than in the artificial system. Drugs are usually more effective in the artificial model, because only in the spontaneous system is there a continuous leakage of cancer cells from the primary tumor into blood and/or lymphatic vessels. Then, too, certain treatments such as cyclophosphamide may increase metastases in the artificial system although they block them in the spontaneous model. Discussing the therapeutic problem of metastases, it is equally important to know which agents increase metastases and which decrease them. We have heard that X-irradiation, glucocorticoids, general anesthetics, and probably many other drugs may increase metastases, and this should be carefully considered particularly at the clinical level where polytherapy is the current practice. On the other hand, it seems to me that the concept of antimetastatic therapy may represent a useful additional concept for achieving a therapeutic strategy.

Even considering classic chemotherapy for metastases, new aspects may emerge. We have been exposed to the idea that micrometastases may be more sensitive than the primary tumor to antiproliferating agents for several reasons, including their higher proliferative rate and greater vascularity. In addition, it may be shown that the concentration of a drug, such as adriamycin, in a tumor is within certain limits inversely proportional to the weight of the vegetating part of the tumor. Accordingly, still for adriamycin, but for other drugs too, it can be shown that the total exposure of metastases to the drug is much higher than for the primary tumor when data are expressed per unit of tissue weight (Table 1). This may help explain why adriamycin shows more activity on metastases than on primary tumor in these experimental models (3). Perhaps even more important is the concept of *antimetastatic therapy* in order to find cell kill mechanisms other than antiproliferation. The effect on proliferation has been the basis of cancer chemotherapy but is also its limit because of the poor specificity of cancer cells compared to normal tissues.

Dealing with the processes of dissemination and metastasis formation at stages independent from proliferation, it may be possible to become more selective and less toxic for the host. A very incomplete and purely theoretical list of possible points of attack for antimetastatic chemotherapy includes effects on surface glycoproteins, plasminogen activators, collagenase, physical properties of the surface (adhesion, charge, aggregability, and motility), contractile proteins of the membrane, vascularization, angiogenic factors, endothelial organ determinants, size of capillaries, local factors such as chalones, osteolytic factors, platelets, fibrinogen, coagulation factors, and stimulation of cell subpopulations with immunological effects.

TABLE 1. *Higher accumulation of adriamycin in metastases than in primary tumors*

Experimental tumor	Weight ($\pm$ SE)	Adriamycin exposure area under the curve (μg/g $\times$ min $\pm$ SE)
1. Lewis Lung carcinoma i.m. (C_{57}B1/6J mice)		
Primary tumor (whole)	7.2 $\pm$ 1.1 g	1,813 $\pm$ 143
(vegetating part)		2,809 $\pm$ 377
Lung metastases	169 $\pm$ 36 mg	11,576 $\pm$ 1,411
2. S 180 intratibial (CD$_1$ mice)		
Primary tumor	7.5 $\pm$ 0.3 g	<1
Renal lymph nodal metastases	195 $\pm$ 30 mg	2,435 $\pm$ 339
Iliac lymph nodal metastases	370 $\pm$ 42 mg	3,619 $\pm$ 537
3. Walker carcinoma i.m. (CD rats)		
Primary tumor	31.2 $\pm$ 7 g	4,748 $\pm$ 980
Lymph nodal metastases	4.0 $\pm$ 1.2 g	10,945 $\pm$ 2,111

Adriamycin was injected i.v. at the dose of 15 mg/kg (experiments 1 and 2) or 10 mg/kg (experiment 3). The area under the curve was calculated 24 hr after administration, and in all cases adriamycin was determined according to the method of Schwartz (4) at 8 different times.

The availability of drugs with the above-mentioned mechanisms need not be seen as a type of single therapy but more as a new approach which can be added to the existing armamentarium and used with other treatment methods.

There is therefore no lack of opportunity to design anticancer agents more rationally. The antimetastatic drugs discussed in this volume including immunostimulants, ICRF 159, warfarin, polymers, nonionic detergents, polysaccharides, aspirin, and indomethacin, should be regarded simply as prototypes of many other drugs which we hope will be available in the not too distant future.

REFERENCES

1. Franchi, G., Reyers-degli Innocenti, I., Rosso, R., and Garattini, S. (1968): Lymph-node metastases after intratibial transplantation of tumors. *Int. J. Cancer,* 3:765–770.
2. Rosso, R., Donelli, M. G., and Garattini, S. (1967): Studies on cancer dissemination. *Cancer Res.,* 27:1225–1231.
3. Donelli, M. G., and Garattini, S. (1977): Differential accumulation of anticancer agents in metastases as compared with primary tumors in experimental models. In: *Recent Advances in Cancer Treatment* (A Monograph of the European Organization for Research on Treatment of Cancer), edited by H. J. Tagnon and M. J. Staquet. Raven Press, New York (*in press*).
4. Schwartz, H. S. (1973): Mechanisms and selectivity of anthracycline aminoglycosides and other intercalating agents. *Biochem. Med.,* 7:396–404.

Subject Index

A

Abdominal lesions, 334
Ablation, irradiation, metastasis
    after, 229-234
ABO hemolytic disease, 69
Abortions in genotype *pp* families,
    76-77f
ACR, *see* Adenomatosis of the colon
    and rectum, hereditary
Actin
    cables, distribution of, 387t
    matrices
        deformed, 383
        intracellular, 384, 386
Actinomycin D, 411, 481
ADCC, *see* Antibody-dependent
    cellular cytotoxicity
Adenocarcinoma
    Blood group antigens in, 69-73
    immunotherapy for, with anti-A
        and anti-P_1, 75-78
    pancreatic duct, metastasis in,
        81-93
    transplantable, 357
Adenomatosis of the colon and
    rectum (ACR), hereditary,
    382-392, 395
    cells, transformation of, 389-391
Adherence, tumor cell, 248-249
Adhesive properties of tumor cells,
    170-171
Adriamycin, 221-223, 458, 459t, 462
    504
Agar sulfate (Aga-S), 368-370
Agglutinogen p, 75
Alginic acid, sulfated (Alg-S), 368-370
Allogeneic mice, 286-288, 291-292
ϵ-Aminocaproic acid (EACA), 368
Anchorage
    independence, 389
    loss of, 383
Anemia, microangiopathic hemolytic,
    155
Anesthesia
    role of, 415-416
    tribromoethanol, 418

Angiogenesis, 391; *see also*
    Vascularization
    cell shedding and, 100-101
    dormancy and, 101
    invasiveness and, 102
    tumor, 95-102
Angiogenic factor, 391
Angiotensin-induced hypertension,
    146-148
Anti-A antibody, 78
Anti-Fc antibody, 254
Anti-P_1 antibody, 77-78
Antibody
    anti-A, 78
    anti-Fc, 254
    anti-P_1, 77-78
    anticytoplasmic, 253-254
    antigen versus, 317-318
    antimembrane, 249-250, 253
    antitumor, 246, 247-250
    "arming" of lymphocytes by, 316
    auto-anti-idiotypic, 253-255
    circulating, 246
    complement-dependent cytotoxic,
        247
    -dependent cellular cytotoxicity
        (ADCC), 222-223
Anticancer agents against lymph
    node metastasis, 468-469
Anticoagulative therapy, 416
Anticytoplasmic antibody, 253-254
Antidisseminative, selective, 214
Antifibrinogen, 368
Antigen
    antibody versus, 317-318
    balance of, 355
    blood group, in adenocarcinoma,
        69-73
    membrane, tumor-associated, 112
    p, 78
    serum carcinoembryonic (CEA),
        208-209
    T, 69, 78
    tumor, free, 311-315
Antigenic modulation, 38, 112
Antimembrane antibody, 249-250,
    253